Nano Drug Delivery Systems for Cancer Therapy

This book explores cutting-edge research and applications in the field of nanomedicines for cancer imaging, diagnosis, and therapy. It begins by highlighting the pivotal role of engineered silica-based nanoparticles in the precise delivery of anticancer drugs. The book further delves into the versatile utilization of metallic nanoparticles for hyperthermia and chemotherapy, showcasing their efficacy in combating cancer and reducing treatment-related discomfort. Additionally, it examines the applications of functionalized nanomaterials in the emerging field of cancer stem cell therapy and the use of radioactive nanoparticles for precise cancer diagnosis and therapy. The book also provides a thorough review of the potential of functionalized lipid-based nanoparticles for precision and targeted treatment. It discusses the roles of dendrimer-based nanomaterials, carbon-based nanomedicines, inorganic nanostructured materials, and polymeric nanomaterials in the realms of cancer diagnosis and personalized, targeted cancer therapies. Finally, the book delves into the commercial aspects of nanomedicines, addressing the challenges and future prospects of introducing these groundbreaking technologies to the forefront of cancer care.

Key Features:

- Provides a comprehensive overview of the latest advancements in nanomedicines for cancer diagnosis and therapy
- Emphasizes the pivotal role of engineered silica-based nanoparticles for precise anticancer drug delivery
- Explores the use of metallic nanoparticles for hyperthermia and chemotherapy
- Discusses radioactive nanoparticles for precise diagnosis and functionalized lipid-based nanoparticles for targeted treatment
- Addresses the commercial aspects of nanomedicines, offering insights into the challenges and future prospects of these innovative technologies in the field of cancer care

This book is an invaluable resource for researchers and scientists in the fields of nanomedicine, oncology, and drug delivery systems.

Nano Drug Delivery Systems for Cancer Therapy

Edited by
Sanjukta Patra and Manashjit Gogoi

CRC Press
Taylor & Francis Group
Boca Raton London New York

CRC Press is an imprint of the
Taylor & Francis Group, an **informa** business

First edition published 2027
by CRC Press
2385 NW Executive Center Drive, Suite 320, Boca Raton FL 33431

and by CRC Press
4 Park Square, Milton Park, Abingdon, Oxon, OX14 4RN

CRC Press is an imprint of Taylor & Francis Group, LLC

ISBN: 978-1-041-36262-3 (hbk)
ISBN: 978-1-041-35794-0 (pbk)
ISBN: 978-1-003-79935-1 (ebk)

DOI: 10.1201/9781003799351

Typeset in Times
by Apex CoVantage, LLC

Contents

Preface

Cancer management continues to be one of the most formidable challenges in modern medicine, demanding innovative therapeutic strategies that go beyond the purview of conventional approaches. Despite significant advances in diagnosis and treatment, limitations such as non-specific drug distribution, systemic toxicity, multidrug resistance, and suboptimal therapeutic efficacy persist. Nanotechnology has emerged as an instrumental and transformative tool, offering unprecedented opportunities to enhance the precision, efficacy, and safety of cancer therapy.

This book, *Nano Drug Delivery Systems for Cancer Therapy*, is a comprehensive resource that brings together contemporary research and developments in the field of nanomedicines for cancer therapy. The chapters reflect a multidisciplinary convergence of biomedical engineering, materials science, computational biology, and pharmaceutical sciences, highlighting both fundamental principles and translational perspectives.

This book covers a wide spectrum of topics, beginning with an overview of nanomedicines for cancer therapy, followed by insights into computational modeling approaches that aid in the design and optimization of nano drug delivery systems. Subsequent chapters explore various nanocarriers, including lipid-based nanoparticles, polymeric nanoparticles, silica-based systems, and inorganic nanostructures, each offering unique advantages in targeted drug delivery. Special emphasis has been placed on emerging areas, such as functionalized nanomaterials for cancer stem cell therapy, magnetic nanomaterials for hyperthermia and drug delivery, and advanced platforms, such as graphene-based nanostructures for photothermal therapy. Additionally, the integration of nanotechnology in cancer imaging and diagnosis is addressed, underscoring the growing importance of theranostics in personalized medicine.

The contributions in this volume are authored by researchers and academicians from reputed institutions, reflecting diverse expertise and perspectives. Their collective efforts provide valuable insights into current challenges, technological advancements, and future directions in nano-enabled cancer therapeutics.

This book is intended for researchers, clinicians, postgraduate students, and professionals engaged in cancer research, nanotechnology, and drug delivery. It aims to serve as both a reference text and a knowledge source for further innovation in the field.

We express our sincere gratitude to all the contributors for their scholarly work and commitment. We also acknowledge the support of their respective institutions in facilitating this collaborative effort. This book will meaningfully contribute to the advancement of nanomedicine, leading to improved outcomes in cancer therapy.

Acknowledgments

The editors would like to thank almighty God for the opportunity, motivation, and strength to complete the endeavor of editing this book.

They sincerely thank Dr. Bhavik Sawhney, Senior Editor (Life Sciences), CRC Press, Taylor & Francis, and all the editorial board members for their approval and for granting us this opportunity to edit this book. They would like to express their sincere gratitude to the editorial team of Taylor & Francis for constantly following up on the editing process and helping complete this assignment.

The editors gratefully acknowledge all the contributors for their valuable chapters and insights, as well as for their patience throughout the process of completing this edited book. Their commitment and cooperation have been vital in bringing this volume to fruition.

Dr. Sanjukta Patra expresses heartfelt thankfulness to little Paridhi and her husband, Rajesh Kumar. It is their shared time that has brought this book in black and white. She is thankful to all her family members for their constant support and blessings.

Dr. Manashjit Gogoi expresses his thankfulness to his beloved sons, Adityavardhan and Atanu, and wife, Mayuri, who sacrificed a lot and kept him inspired to finish this task. He is also thankful to his sister-in-law, Hewali, and his parents, brothers, and in-laws for their constant support, unconditional love, and blessings.

About the Editors

Sanjukta Patra is a faculty member in the Department of Medical Sciences and Technology at the Indian Institute of Technology Madras. Prior to this, she was at the Department of Biosciences and Bioengineering at the Indian Institute of Technology Guwahati. She has nearly two decades of academic and research experience. Her research interests include diagnostics and therapeutics, enzyme and microbial technologies, and recombinant biomolecule production for healthcare applications. Dr. Sanjukta has led and contributed to several externally funded projects supported by DBT, ICMR, MEITY, CSIR, SERB, and ANRF. She also has consultancy projects to her credit. She has contributed and collaborated on several research and development projects, including biosensor development for tuberculosis, candida, and malaria and whole cell biosensors for small molecules on various platforms. She has been granted patents on technology development and has published in international peer-reviewed journals, as well as contributed to edited books and conference proceedings.

Manashjit Gogoi is a faculty member in the Department of Biomedical Engineering at North-Eastern Hill University (NEHU), Shillong, India. He holds a PhD in biomedical engineering from IIT Bombay, an MTech in bioelectronics from Tezpur University, and a BE in chemical engineering from Gauhati University. His research focuses on nanomedicine, biosensors, microfluidics, point-of-care diagnostics, cancer drug delivery, and magnetic nanoparticle-based therapeutics. He has over a decade of academic and research experience. Dr. Gogoi has led and contributed to several externally funded projects supported by DBT, SERB, and ANRF. He has supervised multiple PhD and postgraduate students and has published widely in reputed international journals, along with contributions to edited books and book chapters. He is a chartered engineer and a member of several professional societies and editorial boards. His work has been recognized through national awards, including MeitY TIDE 2.0 and ABLE-BEST.

1 Nanomedicines for Cancer Therapy

Angelina Gogoi,[1] Anjan Boro,[1] Kaushiki Bora,[1]
Luish Pritam Das,[1] and Manashjit Gogoi
[1]Department of Biomedical Engineering, North-Eastern Hill University, Shillong, Meghalaya, India

1.1 INTRODUCTION

Cancer is a group of diseases that causes rapid proliferation of abnormal cells due to multiple genetic mutations that lead to the formation of a tumor mass consisting of a large group of abnormal cells. Globally, approximately 10 million deaths were confirmed due to cancer in the year 2020 (Ferlay et al. 2019). According to the World Health Organization (WHO) statistics for 2019, cancer is the primary or second major cause of mortality before the age of 70 in 112 of 183 countries and ranks third or fourth in another 23 countries.

Conventional methods of treatment for cancer are chemotherapy, radiotherapy, surgery, hormonal therapy, immunotherapy, consisting of immune checkpoint inhibitor therapy, monoclonal antibody therapy, and non-specific immunotherapy. Therapies are given according to the stage of the cancer patient grade of the tumor and the condition of the patient. Therapies are mostly given with a combination of various therapies, but still, the efficacy of the therapies remains obscure. The therapies are cytotoxic (especially chemotherapy and radiation therapy), lacking specificity, and multidrug resistance is creating a significant challenge for cancer treatment (Gavas et al. 2021). Multidrug resistance is mostly seen in the treatment procedures due to the refluxing of drugs out of the cells, change in drug metabolism, reduced amount of absorption of drugs, apoptosis pathway blocking, change of chemotherapeutic agent target, epigenetic altering, etc.

In the last few decades, a large number of nanoparticles (NPs) have been investigated for efficient drug delivery, diagnosis, medical imaging, and nanomedical equipment. Nanotechnology has the potential to revolutionize the treatment of cancer, as the NPs used have advantages, such as being biocompatible, having reduced toxicity, targeted payload delivery, and excellent stability (Gavas et al. 2021). NPs are particles in the size range of 1–100 nm, which can be found in 0-dimension, 1-dimension, 2-dimension, and 3-dimension (Tiwari et al. 2012) (Laurent et al. 2008). After the introduction of drug-loaded NPs in the bloodstream of the patient, the NPs continue to circulate in the bloodstream and eventually reach the target site via ligands or internal or external stimuli. They have a greater surface area, as their sizes are minute, which helps them to encapsulate or attach a higher number of therapeutic payloads, further enabling them to enter into cells easily. Nanocarriers can enhance the half-life of drugs, which helps in their aggregation into tumors (Shin et al. 2016) (Bertrand et al. 2014). So, we see that nanomedicine has many advantages over conventional ways.

Nanotechnology has opened a new pathway for treating cancer with NPs in recent years. This review focuses on conventional therapies for cancer and their drawbacks, types of nanomedicine, active and passive targeting, triggered release, and challenges of nanomedicine.

DOI: 10.1201/9781003799351-1

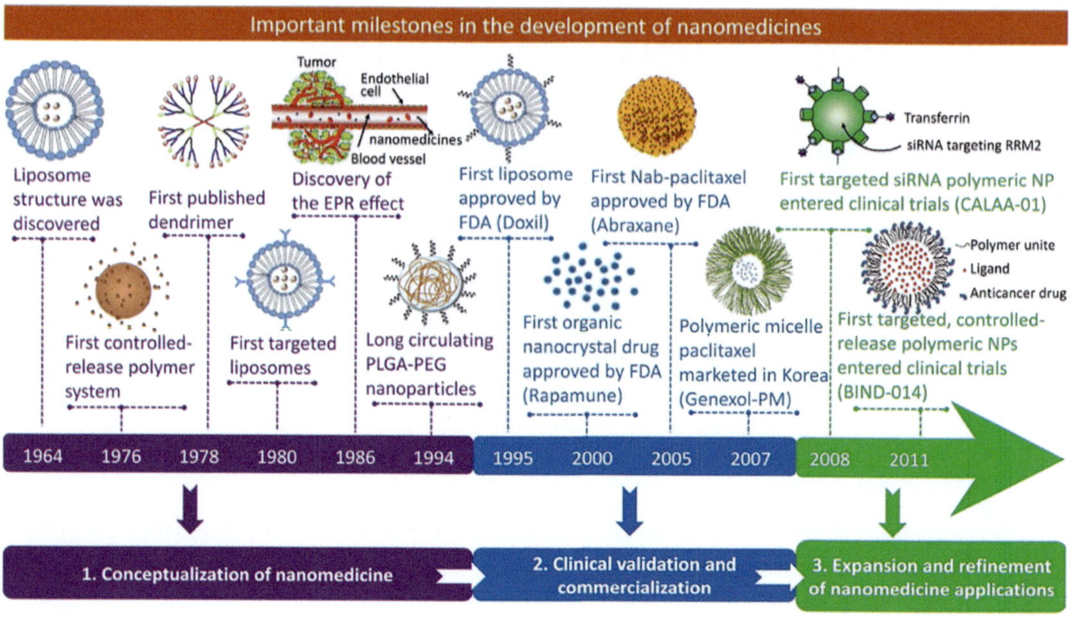

FIGURE 1.1 Important milestones achieved in nanomedicine research and development. As discussed above, liposome was the first nanomedicine discovered in 1964. After that, a series of other types of nanomedicines were discovered. The first liposome nanomedicine was approved by the Food and Drug Administration (FDA) in 1995. In 2011, polymeric NPs were the first NPs to have been targeted with controlled release, which entered for the clinical trials.

Source: Zhang et al. 2020.

1.2 CONVENTIONAL THERAPIES AND THEIR DRAWBACKS

There are a notable number of conventional treatments that have been adapted to treat cancer. These are discussed in the following sections. These therapeutic modalities are used either alone or in combination. However, the therapeutic outcome is far from satisfactory.

1.2.1 Chemotherapy

In chemotherapy, highly toxic or life-threatening anticancer drugs inhibit advancement of tumor cells. These drugs are delivered orally, by injecting directly into a vein, as a shot, the body cavity, or the tumor (Nakamura and Maeda 2023), or in the form of creams, which can be applied directly on the skin. They harm both malignant and normal cells; as a result, this treatment method causes side effects during therapy, such as headache, burning sensation in the applied areas of the body, pain, fatigue, anorexia, vomiting, severe weight loss problems, skin problems, frequent changes in mood, hair loss, sleep problems, change in appetite, constipation, and diarrhea in patients (source: https://www.cancer.net/navigating-cancer-care/how-cancer treated/chemotherapy/side-effects-chemotherapy).

1.2.2 Surgical Method

In the surgical method, the surgeon removes the tumor mass directly with the best possible minimally invasive surgery. However, this method has its drawbacks, such as pain in the body, potential internal and external bleeding and blood clotting infection at the surgical site, and damage to the neighboring healthy tissue around the surgical incision (Tohme et al. 2017).

1.2.3 Radiation Therapy

Radiation therapy for cancer treatment uses high-energy ionizing radiation either internally or externally (Baskar et al. 2012) to kill the cancer cells by targeting the genes, resulting in the inability of the cells to reproduce and grow further. There are two ways to irradiate cancer cells. The first is by using photon beams, such as X-rays and gamma rays, to target tumors present deep inside the body (Baskar et al. 2012). The second is by the use of particle radiation, such as electrons and proton, to target cancer cells present close to the body surface (Thomas et al. 2010). Despite its successful use in cancer treatment, radiation therapy possesses side effects, such as loss of energy after therapy, various skin problems, hair loss, inflammation inside the mouth, taste loss, memory loss, unsteady walking, poor vision, and complications in fertility.

1.2.4 Hormone Therapy

Endocrine treatment or secretory medicine or hormone therapy is a type of cancer treatment that employs hormones to reduce or stop the growth of cancer. This type of therapy works by blocking the body's ability to produce hormones and interferes with how hormones function and react within the body (source: https://www.cancer.gov/about-cancer/treatment/types/hormone-therapy). It is widely acknowledged that the changed endocrine environment brought on by hormone therapy causes vasomotor, atrophic, and metabolic alterations (Dennerstein et al. 1979). Other side effects include tiredness, digestive system problems, impotence, hot flushes and sweating, risk of heart problems etc.

1.2.5 Immunotherapy

In cancer immunotherapy, also known as immuno-oncology, the lymphatic system consisting of white blood cells, organs, and tissues is used to prevent, run and eliminate cancer through the use of the body's own defenses (source: https://www.cancer.gov/about-cancer/treatment/types/immunotherapy%20(accessed%20Apr.%2004,%202023). Eleven monoclonal antibodies, including unmodified antibodies and antibodies laced with toxins or radionuclides, have received approval for treatment of cancer and another potential strategy in cancer immunotherapy is the elimination of distributed tumor cells that are present in the blood circulation and micro-metastases in distant organs (source: https://www.cancer.gov/about-cancer/treatment/types/immunotherapy%20(accessed%20Apr.%2004,%202023)). Side effects of this therapy varies from person to person as it is not specific, immune response of the person can vary, and due to concentrated or diluted concentration of the therapy. Some of the effects include swelling, weight gain from retaining fluid, rash, heart palpitations, itchiness, sinus congestion, organ inflammation etc.

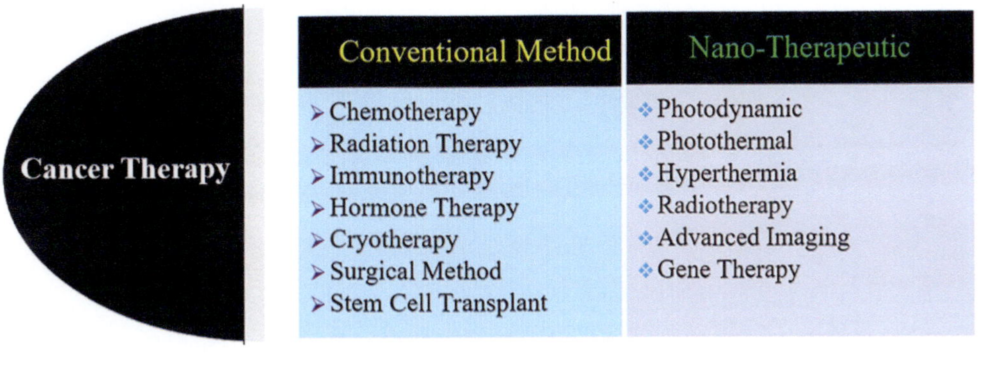

FIGURE 1.2 Conventional methods and the diverse use of nanomedicine for cancer therapy.

1.3 NANOMEDICINE-BASED STRATEGIES FOR CANCER THERAPY

Nanomedicine has been recently introduced and studied broadly for their use in cancer treatment. The application and development of NPs have paved a way in introducing targeted drug delivery system, which have better possibilities than the conventional method of therapies.

1.3.1 Targeted Drug Delivery

Targeted drug delivery delivers medication by specifically targeting the cancer site. This increases the concentration of drug in that specific area, thus overcoming the drawback of the conventional methods discussed above, which lack delivery of drugs in the targeted site and as a result damage the normal cells as well. Henceforth, targeted drug delivery aids in overcoming the shortcoming of conventional therapy methods. It is designed to hold the drugs in place until the target site is reached and released. It improves the pharmaceutical activity, reducing side effects in addition to reduction in the dose administered. Targeted drug delivery is feasible either as active targeting or passive targeting.

1.3.1.1 Active Targeting

In active targeting, drug-loaded NPs are conjugated with ligands, such as proteins, carbohydrates, peptides, and antibodies, specific to the disease-infected cells or tissues. These ligands guide the nanocarriers to reach the target site. Thus, active targeting targets cancerous sites by direct interaction between ligand and receptor. This targeting method to deliver drugs is used in cancer therapy, enhancing the selectivity of medications to tumor sites, significant accumulation of drugs, and enhancing anticancer effects in tumor cells (Muhamad et al. 2018). This minimizes harm to normal cells. However, this approach of targeting is most useful when the nanocarrier successfully reaches the targeted site.

Transferrin-conjugated NPs (Yao et al. 2020) are used to deliver drugs in cancer therapy. The function of transferrin is to transport iron into cells in the body. In tumor cells, they are expressed more than in normal cells. In another instance, human EGF receptor-2 (HER2) is expressed more

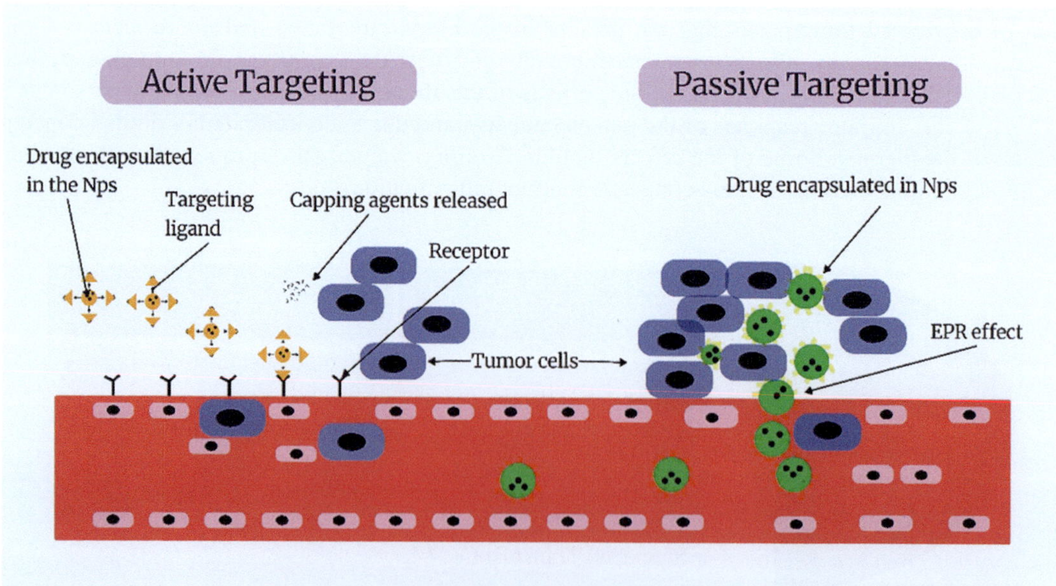

FIGURE 1.3 Illustration of how active and passive targeting strategies are used by nanomedicine in the field of drug delivery to target tumor cells.

in tumor cells of breast cancer. It is targeted using herceptin. In order to reduce cell toxicity, HER2-targeted PEGylated liposomal doxorubicin was developed (Gavas et al. 2021).

1.3.1.2 Passive Targeting

For passive targeting, a phenomenon was observed where the blood arteries around a tumor are leakier and more tangled together than they are in healthy tissues, which increases the accumulation and retention of macromolecules, including NPs, in the neoplastic tissue, it is stated as enhanced permeability and retention effect (Iyer et al. 2006) (Wang et al. 2023). It is observed when blood-borne nanocarriers target the interstitial spaces of tumor tissues and collect there as a result of compromised lymphatic outflow (BAZAK et al. 2014). Some chemotherapeutic medications diffuse poorly into cells, which makes it difficult to control tumor cells. Multiple-drug resistance may result from this lack of control, which lowers the efficiency of conventional therapy for cancer cell treatment. Cancer cells' uncontrolled behavior has the potential to alter membrane transport proteins, which would otherwise block the effects of a common medicine (Sriraman et al., 2014). Small compounds can achieve improved pharmacokinetics, tumor selectivity, and fewer adverse effects by being enclosed in nanosized therapeutic carriers. In contrast to conventional ones, passive tumor targeting relies on carrier features such as size and circulation duration rather than the ligands for targeted tissue and organ binding. In addition to the EPR effect, nanomedicines are also passively administered through the tumor microenvironment. There are some shortcomings to passive targeting, such as heterogeneous drug distribution, restricted EPR effects, and varying blood artery permeability depending on the kind of tumor (Ediriwickrema and Saltzman 2015). Sclareol compound found in Salvia sclarea plants was loaded in solid lipid nanoparticles (SLNs) was released to human lung epithelial cancer cell had inhibited the growth and proliferation of cancer cells rather than free drug (Ali et al. 2021) (Cerri et al. 2019).

1.3.2 Stimuli Response of Nanomedicines

After the scientific breakthrough of the enhanced permeability and retention (EPR) effect and the active targeting strategies NPs have been recognized as potential drug delivery platforms for tumors (Zhang et al. 2017a) (Gao et al. 2016) (van der Meel et al. 2019) (Zhang and Khademhosseini 2017). Nanocarriers optimize pharmacotherapeutic outcomes by loading payloads such as antibodies, anticancer drugs, imaging agents, nucleic acids, etc. (Chen et al. 2018) (Yi et al. 2018). Nevertheless, it encounters several obstacles throughout circulation or in malignancies (Maeda et al. 2000), namely degeneration, leakage of bioactive compounds, and detection and removal by the reticuloendothelial system (RES). After overcoming all these problems, once the nanocarriers reach the target site(s), stimuli-response nanocarriers release and activate bioactive compounds in the specific sites in response to internal or external triggered responses. The types of endogenous and exogenous responsive responses are discussed in the following section.

1.3.2.1 Endogenous/Internal-Stimuli Response

Certain environments prevailing inside the cancer cells such as low pH, hypoxia, and redox potential among others may act as desirable conditions for triggered response to achieve tumor imaging and treatment, pharmaceutical release, prodrug activation, and endosome or lysosome rejection (Peer et al. 2007).

1.3.2.1.1 pH Response

Tumor microenvironments are highly acidic due to the generation of lactic acid in the tumors and protons that are hydrolyzed during ATP (Mi et al. 2017). Therefore, they have a low pH value in contrast to normal healthy tissues. So, NPs are synthesized to achieve triggered release at low pH by accumulating disulfide linkers and hydrazone bonds, which are sensitive to pH change. Until now, certain types of nanomedicines have been developed that react to pH, such as $CaCO_3$ NPs (Dong et al. 2016) (Wang et al. 2018), liposomes (Vila-Caballer et al. 2016), dendrimers (Wang et al. 2015), and nanogels (Zhan et al. 2011) (Madhusudana Rao et al. 2015) (Huang et al. 2019b).

1.3.2.1.2 Reactive Oxygen Species Response

Cancers tend to create a high amount of intracellular reactive oxygen species (ROS), and hence, ROS-triggered nanomedicines could be created to achieve drug delivery (Li et al. 2021). The tumor cells create H_2O_2 abundantly and so nanomedicines are created that react as H_2O_2 catalysts for producing O_2 and eliminate the anaerobic tumor microenvironment. These nanomedicines as they get into contact with the tumor cells undergo physical and chemical changes (Juan et al. 2021). Manganese oxide composition NPs along with doxorubicin helps in reducing the hypoxic environment of cancer cells by generating molecular oxygen leading to production of ROS and effective application of doxorubicin (Yang et al. 2017).

1.3.2.1.3 Enzyme Response

Particular enzyme's uncontrolled activity in neoplastic circumstances might serve as a cause for enzyme-responsive delivery of the drug. Multiple enzyme-responsive nanocarriers have been designed to carry targeted payload release to tumor sites in patients, prodrug/ligand activation, and morphological alteration (Li et al. 2020) which includes mesoporous silica NPs (Naz et al. 2019), magnetic NPs (Alromi et al. 2021), dendrimers (Bober et al. 2022), liposomes (Fouladi et al. 2017), etc. Furthermore, the prodrug method is commonly used to safeguard the potency of the nanocarriers along with the ligands and the drugs while they circulate in the bloodstream of the patient to maximize the therapeutic applicability so the prodrugs will get activated by the enzymes (Dong et al. 2022).

1.3.2.1.4 Hypoxic Response

Hypoxia is prone to arise inside tumor cells due to inadequate vascularization, which plays a significant factor in tumor growth, such as loco-regional expansion and malignant transformation (Blanco et al. 2015). Hypoxia promotes tumor formation, which has a detrimental influence on diagnosis and treatment and results in susceptibility to conventional treatment. So, several nanocarriers have been developed that are activated by hypoxia- and they treat tumors by increasing the oxygen level (Naz et al. 2019) (Mi 2020). Till now, several NPs have been developed to target the tumor microenvironments suffering from hypoxia such as liposomes (Liu et al. 2017a), silica (Im et al. 2019), polymeric micelles (Yang et al. 2019), albumin NPs (Yang et al. 2019) etc which could be conjugated with contrast agents, ligands, anticancer drugs etc (Liu et al. 2014).

1.3.2.1.5 Multimodal Response

Several nanocarriers have been developed to respond to multiple stimuli response to gain high specificity and efficacy. Nanocarriers such as platinum NPs have been designed to respond to pH as well as Glutathione (GSH) (Jia et al. 2021a). Multiple stimuli-responsive nanocarriers have a strong capability for prolonged circulation, tumor accumulation, increased penetration in cancerous tissue, absorption into cancer cells, and endosome escape (Li et al. 2016) (Mi 2020).

1.3.2.2 EXO/External-Triggered Release

The intervention of external stimuli, which include light, temperatures or magnetic fields, to trigger the release of drug via the nanocarrier that is precisely at the targeted site within the body is known as external stimulus-triggered drug delivery. By doing this, the risk of injury to healthy cells is diminished because the medicine can only be delivered when it is required. The medicine's therapeutic effectiveness is further increased by its targeted release, that means that lesser of the drug is required to attain the intended result, lowering the risk of negative side effects (Wang and Kohane 2017). Substances used to formulate such drug conveyance mechanisms are responsive to an array of external stimulation which are discussed below:

1.3.2.2.1 Temperature-Triggered Release

Heat-sensitive polymerization inside Magnetically Controlled Nanocarriers (MCNC) breaks fragile bonding to unleash the subatomic particle. Super magnetic force of Fe2O3 NPs in the aquaphobic cavity of MCNC unleash heating in reaction with AMF (alternating magnetic field) (Jia et al. 2021b). A PEG-PLA capping is applied with the solid lipid NPs to increase their hydrophobic nature and emulsion cohesion (Mishra et al. 2010). A quick method for producing nanocomposites known as fast nanoprecipitation which is extensible and offers shape as well as thickness customization, is used to form synthetic Magnetically Controlled Nanocarriers. Selective magnetic force contours are able to precisely regulate the level of discharge, which is controllable by alternating magnetic field density (Wang and Kohane 2017).

1.3.2.2.2 Ultrasound

The area to be applied for ultrasound triggered release is targeted on and localized using ultrasonic wave. Whenever stimuli-responsive hydrogels are subjected to ultrasonic transducers, the process involved in conveying energy to cause a reaction is applied through sound wave pathways. A sensitive hydrogel uses the ultrasound waves for energizing transference via either thermally and non-thermally (Yeingst et al. 2022).

1.3.2.2.3 Light-Triggered Release

The production of oxidants from O_2 in photothermal therapeutic intervention, results in the combustion of beam at various spectra waves, or conversion of energy into various forms which causes formation of soaked up light causing biochemical interactions in delivered or intracellular biomolecules. As well as diagnostics such as light microscopy and curative purposes are emerged from such procedures. They are used for therapeutics that is stimulated by light (Sharma et al. 2018).

These triggering pathways have the efficiency to penetrate epithelium and epidermis penetration to such an extent that results in antitumor efficacy. Considering characteristics that vary depending upon specific application field, like encapsulate of biomolecules, preservation of its pharmacological or therapeutic action throughout encapsulating and retention, regulated and maintained discharge at chosen specific regions, this seems to be an extremely difficult operation. ThermoDox is brand-new thermal—responsive liposome that requires active target and it depends upon external stimulation to discharge Dox once it having accumulated inside the tumor (Thorat and Bauer 2020).

Since those elements are able to respond quickly, the doctor or the patient can remotely and so forth stimulate that delivery of the medicines. Existence of NPs inside the target location can be confirmed, and their intensity can be measured using common screening techniques such as spectroscopy, MRI, ultrasound etc. along with anticipation of possible nanoparticles (Naz et al. 2019). This enables detailed, image-guided intervention. However, it's allowed to anticipate traits that are distinctive for every patient or customize individualized therapy throughout timely manner (Busatto et al. 2019a). Meticulous anticancer drug dosages could be delivered and then tracked utilizing visual information that is easily accessible at the moment of molecular targeted delivery. Over the temporal aspect, external stimulation enables far more discretion. External triggered release system allows the doctor to "switch treatments on and shut down" at will, that is not possible with normal approaches. This allows for exact modulation about the scheduling and length of intervention (Wang and Kohane 2017).

1.3.3 Interaction of Nanomedicines with Cells

Nanoparticles have shown great potential in delivering drugs due to their minute size. As the volume decreases, surface area increases, and hence a good number of drugs could be incorporated into the nanocarriers which are internalized in the human body by cell endocytic mechanism. When the NPs interact with the cell surface, for their binding with the cell membrane and possible linking with the receptors, specific ligands are used. Transferrin and folate target the tumor cells which constitutively activates correlating receptors (Sudimack and Lee 2000) (Daniels et al. 2012) or hyaluronic acid which guides the nanocarriers to target the CD44-overexpressing tumor cells (Mattheolabakis et al. 2015). Another difficulty is when nanocarriers make contact with the body's interior environment they form corona, which could be avoided by conjugating polyethylene glycol (PEG) or making acquaintance with zwitterion on the surface of the nanocarriers (Milton Harris et al. 2001) (Howard et al. 2008) (García et al. 2014) (Safavi-Sohi et al. 2016).

After interacting with the cell surface, they are internalized by the cells via endocytosis. The most common mechanism analyzed is clathrin-mediated endocytosis (CME) (Kou et al. 2013; Manzanares and Ceña 2020) where several biomolecules including low-density lipoprotein for cholesterol uptake and transferrin for iron uptake could be done (Dambournet et al. 2018) (Loebrich 2014) (Qin et al. 2019). Macropinocytosis is another mechanism where extracellular fluids are absorbed by the protusions present in the membrane (Bridgewater et al. 2012; Chen et al. 2017; Fekri et al. 2019; Grimmer et al. 2002; Lee et al. 2014). Caveolae-mediated endocytosis makes use of both receptor dependent and independent mechanism (Corrotte et al. 2021; Jung et al. 2018b; Muro 2018a), where caveolae are invaginations of 50–80nms (Chaudhary et al. 2014; Muro 2018b), but the topic is still being discussed. Besides all these mechanisms phagocytosis is another one, which can internalize large particles of above 0.5μm (Gordon 2016). The nanomedicines are then finally internalized based on their morphology such as size, shape, charge, hydrophobicity, rigidity, roughness, and surface functionalization.

1.4 NANOMEDICINES FOR CANCER THERAPY

Nanomedicine is the branch of science that deals with medicine for the betterment of human health using nanotechnology. Nanomedicine has generated a new pathway for the delivery of drugs and medical imaging for cancer treatment. Some of the most common nanoparticles conjugated with ligands and drugs for cancer therapy are liposomes, magnetic nanostructures, polymers, and micelles. Liposomal doxorubicin was the first clinically approved nanomedicine used to treat cancer (Barenholz 2012).

Some of the nanomedicines used to treat cancer are discussed below:

1.4.1 Liposome

Liposomes are spherical vesicles made of phospholipids. These self-assembled vesicles have a hydrophilic head and hydrophobic tail. In the aqueous core of liposome, hydrophilic drug is encapsulated while the membrane encapsulates a hydrophobic drug. Liposome shows excellent biocompatibility, biodegradable and low toxicity nature (Daraee et al. 2016). Also, their surface can be modified to alter biodistribution, increase blood circulation time, alter drug distribution as per size and can be used for triggered drug release. Comparable efficacy in breast cancer (Gabizon 2006) and Kaposi curcuma in HIV patients were treated using polyethylene glycol (PEG) liposomes loaded with Doxorubicin (DOX) (Geisberg and Sawyer 2010). Curcumin conjugated liposomes are used in the treatment of several cancers such as breast cancer, liver carcinoma, prostate cancer. Paclitaxel loaded magnetic liposomes have been successfully used to treat cancer cells (Mahato et al. 2021). Skin mucosal sarcoma using long circulating liposome modified with doxorubicin is used to passively target tumor cells (Rommasi and Esfandiari 2021). In another instance, folic acid is used as a targeting ligand with liposome to target specific sites of ovarian, breast, lung, colon, kidney and brain tumors where folate receptors are expressed in a greater amount (Deshpande et al. 2013). High cost of production of liposome, short half-life, low stability is some of the shortcoming of liposomes.

1.4.2 Solid-Lipid Nanoparticles

Although pharmaceutical agility inside the solid-lipid nanoparticles (SLN) ought to be significantly lesser than aqueous oil. SLNs are prepared to address the drawbacks of particulate transporters, like emulsions or polymeric nanocomposites, due to their benefits including the potential for regulated

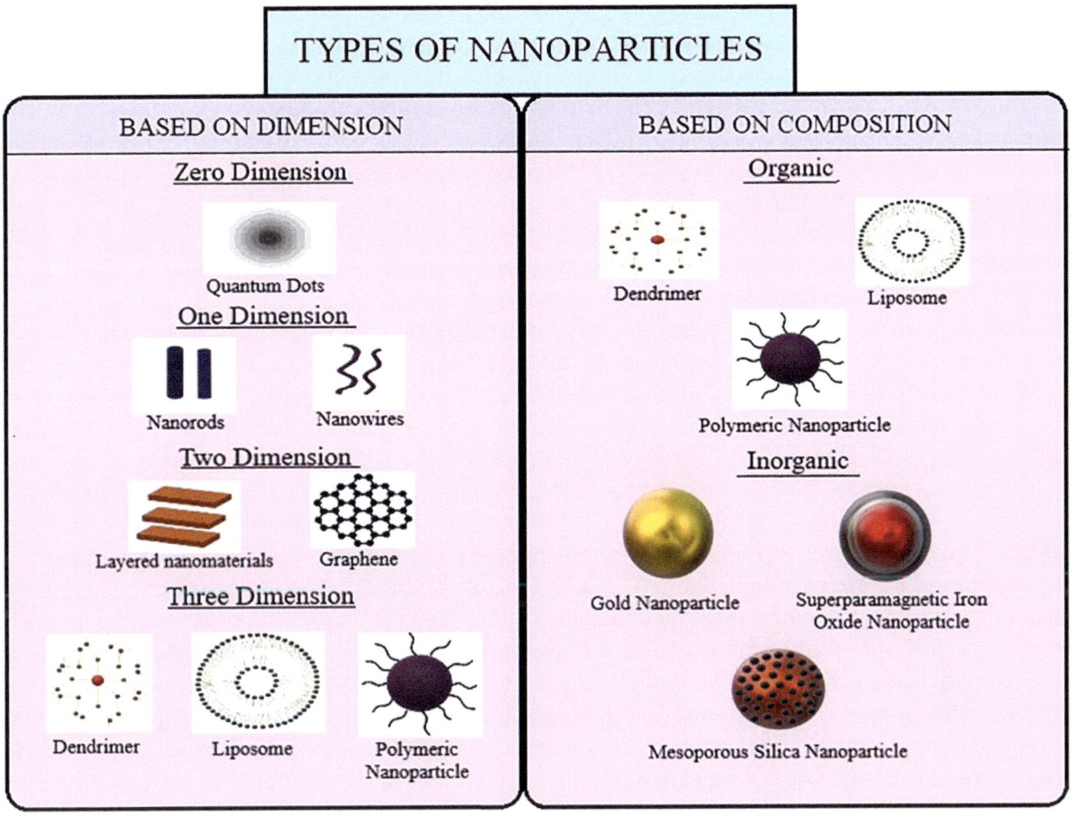

FIGURE 1.4 Different types of nanoparticles classified based on their dimension and composition. The composition and size of nanoparticles can alter their physiochemical attributes, including solubility, stability and reaction time which may impact their possible uses.

delivery of drugs as well as drug targeted specific (Mehnert and Mäder 2012). They enhanced drug cohesion, and capability to incorporate both lipid soluble and water—soluble drugs and also lack biotoxicity, do not require the usage of natural cleaning agents, and pose no issues with mass manufacturing including sterilization (Siram et al. 2019). Nanoparticles are analyzed using various electron microscopy (SEM, AFM, TEM etc.) and range in size from 40 to 1000 nm. Roughly about 0.1 to 30 (% w/w) percent unsaturated fats that is disseminated in a liquid media makes up solid lipid nanoparticles. To improve endurance, stabilizers are utilized in quantities ranging from 0.5 to 5% (Naseri et al. 2015). In thermoregulation, their lipids elements remain rigid. Lipids employed inside the creation of SLNs encompass hydrocarbons, monoacylglycerols, diacylglycerols, and cholesterol as well as unsaturated fats, and growth hormones (Haider et al. 2020) (Mehnert and Mäder 2012).

1.4.3 Extracellular Vesicles Nanoparticles

Extracellular vesicles (EVs) are a wide array of tiny, lipid-bound nanocomposites that perform the pivotal role across several physio/pathological phenomena. Segments containing EVs that coincide on dimension and have different compositions and bioactivities are released by cells (Witwer and Wolfram 2021). Utilizing the inherent epithelial characteristics, nanoparticles are being additionally investigated again for the transport of anticancer drug cargoes to the targeted site or cells (Busatto et al. 2019b). EVs and liposomes are composed of phospholipids, so both are equivalent from the standpoint of therapeutic agents. It is possible that numerous EVs have therapeutic uses, including (i) fluid biopsy, enabling tracking of tumor growth, including malignancy. Such malignancies can be monitored by isolating receptacles through liquids and obtaining a portrait about the creator tissue at the time of membrane synthesis. (ii) The second use is engagement during therapy, which enables routing receptacles toward disease cells. It also enables the concentration of the pharmacological response of the EVs on the diseased cells or decreases pathological indications on them. (iii) The third use is the transportation of drugs, which helps deliver curative RNAs employing the EV supply chain —for example, localizing drugs toward targeted cells or regions (Witwer and Wolfram 2021) (Phillips et al. 2021; Willms et al. 2018).

1.4.4 Micelles

Micelles are an assemblage of molecules in a colloidal solution with a hydrophobic tail and a hydrophilic head. They are round or spherical in shape with a hydrophobic center. Nanomicelles are being used for delivering drugs owing to their small structure, simple preparation methods, low cost, impressive biocompatibility, and successful entrapping of lipophilic drugs in their core. Micelles enhance drug solubility, tissue penetration, targeting of specific sites, and circulation time and reduce toxicity; hence, they are used extensively and considered suitable for various biological uses in addition to drug delivery (Hanafy et al. 2018). Doxorubicin is encapsulated in the core of micelle, which is used for active targeting in the treatment of human Kaposi's sarcoma, greatly enhancing internalization in tumor endothelial cells (Oerlemans et al. 2010). Quercetin-loaded micelles are used in the treatment of lung cancer; nanomicelles made from the diblock copolymer and polyethylene glycol (PEG)-derivatized phos-phatidylethanolamine (PE) played a critical role in the enhancement of anticancer activity and the reduction of toxicity to the intestinal epithelium (Mahato et al. 2021). Cisplatin-loaded micelles are used in targeting solid tumors, and paclitaxel-loaded micelles are used in the treatment of breast cancer, pancreatic cancer, lung cancer. In lung cancer treatment they are used in combination with carboplatin; pancreatic cancer, in combination with gemcitabine; and ovarian cancer, in combination with carboplatin (Wang et al. 2007). Paclitaxel was used to actively target follicle receptor and improve the cytotoxicity of tumor cells (Wang et al. 2007).

1.4.5 Nanoemulsion

A nanoemulsion is a micron-sized organic nanoparticle carrier system that acts as a colloidal particulate system (Gavas et al. 2021). There is a wide range of sizes between 10 and 1,000 nm. Essentially, it is an aqueous heterogeneous mixture of oil droplets ranging in size from 10–1000 nm (Ma et al. 2009). It consists primarily of oil, emulsifying agents, and aqueous phases (Jaiswal et al. 2015). A crude temporary emulsion may be created by mixing oil with water. After standing, the dispersed globules will coalesce into two distinct phases. The characteristics of nanoemulsions are different from those of liposomes, such as optical quality, stability, and biodegradability (Dianzani et al. 2020). Nanoemulsions containing paclitaxel and spirulina have improved anti-neoplastic effects through altering immunity via TLR4/NF-kB signaling pathways (Hung et al. 2021). Applied topically on the skin, cetostearyl alcohol, a non-ionic surfactant, stagnates the hydrocortisone butyrate in the emulsion (Piérard et al. 1996). These nanoemulsions are not toxic and do not irritate when injected. However, due to the high temperature and pressure needed, as well as the expensive cost of equipment, such as homogenizers and microfluidizers, therapeutic uses of nanoemulsions are troublesome. However, their physical stability was found to be enhanced. Nanoemulsions have a significantly higher absorption rate because they are composed of minute droplets with a substantial surface area.

1.4.6 Polymeric Nanoparticles

Polymeric nanoparticles (PNPs) are colloidal nanoparticles made of polymer in the size range of 1–1000nm. Polymeric NPs are further classified into two types based on structure:

Nanosphere—Drugs adhere to the surface of the NP.
Nanocapsule—Drugs are encapsulated in the NP.

Polymethyl methacrylate (PMMA), polystyrene, polyacrylates, etc. were used previously (Han et al. 2020; Vijayan et al. 2013), which were not biocompatible due to their toxicity as they were difficult to degrade or excrete. To avoid toxicity, biodegradable polymeric NPs are introduced such as poly-lactic acid (PLA), poly (lactic-co-glycolic acid) (PLGA), poly(ε-caprolactone) (PCL), and natural polymers including chitosan, alginate, gelatin, and albumin. PNPs are low-cost, biocompatible, and biodegradable. Because of their characteristics and morphologies, these enhanced polymeric NPs aid in the stabilization of unstable therapeutic drugs and have greater loading ability. Further, PNPs offer various drug delivery modalities such as oral and intravenous (IV). PNPs protect the tissues from toxicity due to the unwanted degradation of drugs. PNPs containing cisplatin, such as dexamethasone or -tocopheryl succinate, have been used in chemotherapy to avoid cisplatin-induced ototoxicity (VP 2003).

1.4.7 Hydrogel

Hydrogels are three-dimensional network polymeric materials with the ability to contain large number of fluids because of their hydrophobic construction (Gao et al. 2016) (Zhang et al. 2017b). Hydrogels exhibit distinctive characteristics such as less toxicity, amplifying the benefits of the anticancer drug, possessing impressive controlled drug release attributes, and providing protection to the drugs. PAA, chitosan and alginate, and PVA are used in hydrogel-based phototherapy for treating cancer (Zhang et al. 2017b). Although research in the application of hydrogels is persistent, there have been challenges. For example, swelling (Zhang and Khademhosseini 2017) is a common disadvantage, as the longer duration in aqueous surroundings weakens the network of hydrogels. Glycol chitosan hydrogel and doxorubicin hydrochloride-formed GC10/dox is used in the treatment of thyroid cancer (Yoo et al. 2018). Controlled drug delivery using STINGels (Leach et al. 2018) showed improvement in neck and head cancer. Two percent poloxamer is used to deliver carboplatin drug for cervical cancer recurrence (Narayanaswamy and Torchilin 2019).

1.4.8 Carbon-Based Nanoparticles

Carbon-based nanoparticles (CNPs) particles were assumed to be carbon-based nanoparticles if they are 10 nm in size or less. Molecular fluorophores are responsible for the luminescent properties of carbon nanoparticles, which have been modified (Xiong et al. 2018). Because of their natural optical properties, CNPs can serve as good mediators in phototherapy, as well as drug delivery vehicles for a variety of anticancer cancer drugs (Tang et al. 2021). Carbon nanotubes, graphene, fullerene, quantum dots, and other materials are some examples of CNPs (Klochkov et al. 2021).

1.4.9 Graphene

The graphene molecule is a two-dimensional structure composed of a honeycomb lattice formed by sp2-hybridized carbon atoms. Because of its magnetic, optic, heat, physical, and electronic capabilities, graphene may be employed in practically every scientific discipline (Sanchez et al. 2012a), and it has the ability to transport drugs and monitor cells in real time. According to the study, materials based on graphene have a higher permeability, which makes them potential candidates for the creation of triggered release and biocompatible for next-generation delivery systems (Hoseini-Ghahfarokhi et al. 2020; Sattari et al. 2021). Highly diffused in PBS solution, graphene oxide nanoparticles enhanced with polyethylene glycol (PEG) and encapsulated with polymethylmethacrylic acid (PMMA) served as an effective drug delivery system (Zhao et al. 2015).

1.4.10 Fullerene

Fullerene (C60) is a carbon allotrope that looks like a closed cage. There are many potential medical applications for the fullerene family, particularly C60, which has attractive physical and electrochemical properties (Sanchez et al. 2012b). It has been demonstrated that fullerene substrates can enter the hydrophobic region of HIV proteases, preventing substrates from reaching the enzyme's catalytic site. A wide range of applications have been made possible by fullerenes and their derivatives in the medical field. They can be used as sensitizers for photodynamic therapy and as targeting vectors for mineralized bone (Chen et al. 2012). Upon injection into the blood vessel, fullerene and its variants are rapidly absorbed by all tissues and are hypo toxic. Employing fullerene derivatives as carriers offers a novel method for creating tissue-targeted medications (Qingnuan et al. 2002a).

1.4.11 Carbon Nanotubes

A carbon nanotube (CNT) is a cylindrical nanostructure made up of large number of carbon molecules and is employed for drug administration due to its distinct medical, mechanical, and chemical properties. In addition to doxorubicin, paclitaxel, and methotrexate siRNA, they have been used as therapeutic payloads for cancer treatment (Madani et al. 2011). The two types of CNTs are single-walled and multi-walled, respectively. By interacting with immune cells, carbon-based compounds can elicit an immune response, thereby suppressing tumor growth. One example would be the use of fluorescent single-walled CNTs implanted with mAb that encapsulates doxorubicin to target colon cancer cells (Dadwal et al. 2018) (Qingnuan et al. 2002b). The cancer cells take up this complex of CNTs, while it remains in the cytoplasm, which induces the intracellular release of doxorubicin. Nanotubes possess multiple covalent functionalization on the sidewalls or tips that make it possible to carry multiple molecules simultaneously, which has proven to be valuable in treating cancer (Wang et al. 2008).

1.4.12 Dendrimers

Dendrimers are symmetrical macromolecules with hyperbranched dendrons and in the size range of 1–10 nm. The dendrimer is divided into three parts: core, branches, and terminal functional groups. Dendrimers have improved solubility, adaptable modifiable branching, specified molecular weight, high drug loading capacity, the bioavailability of hydrophobic therapeutics, and a polydispersity index (Majoros et al. 2005). In dendrimers, anti-neoplastic drug is either covalently conjugated to the dendrimer's peripheral groups or loaded within the empty spaces. Dendrimers for cancer therapeutics are polyamidoamine (PAMAM), polyethylene glycol (PEG), 2,2-bishydroxymethylpropionic acid (Bis-MPA), triethanolamine (TEA), polypropylene imine (PPI) and poly-l-lysine (PLL) (Martín-Saldaña et al. 2017) (Majoros et al. 2005). Dendrimers with cationic charges like PMMA, PPI, and PLL can deliver nucleic acids. When doxorubicin (DOX) and tumor necrosis factor-related apoptosis-inducing ligand (TRAIL) plasmids were encapsulated in dendrimer, they had better anticancer effects than carriers containing DOX and TRAIL plasmids alone. Dendrimers have good potential to work as cancer nanotherapeutics if they are used as a hybrid therapy and modified (Ali et al. 2021).

1.4.13 Cyclo-Dextrin Nanoparticles

The use of cyclodextrins (CDs) can improve overall solubility for medications that dissolve inadequately in liquid. CDs provide a notable capacity to induce biomolecules' potential host interplay due to the resonator frame as well as non-polar layout morphology. CDs induce interference throughout related to NPs, which boost drug concentration, increase solubility, reconfigure drug metabolic rate, and lower cytotoxic effects (Soe et al. 2022). In catalytic breakdown of starches from corn, potatoes, and different grains, amphiphilic cyclic oligosaccharides that have at least six D-(+)

glucopyranose units and -(1, 4) glycosidic linkages are produced. When water-insoluble medicinal particles are delivered across the liquid exterior of lipid-soluble cellular membranes obstacles, cyclodextrins function like genuine transporters. Furthermore, CDs have such potentiality toward innovative drug delivery mechanisms because they have self-assembly characteristics onto nano-level complexes in dilute solutions (Li et al. 2023; Salústio et al. 2011).

Either nanospheres or nanocapsules will form depending on the preparation method. Encapsulation may be performed straight throughout production by employing drug: CD aggregates that have already been generated or by combining both pre and high loading. Whereas the polymeric nanocomposites outside coatings are made with β—cd, their interiors are made with biopolymers. Pharmaceuticals may therefore be added to polymeric Np' center or may be coupled to β—cd in the outermost cavity. Diffusion of premade polymeric materials or polymerization are two methods of creating nanomaterial structures (Gadade and Pekamwar 2020; Krauland and Alonso 2007).

1.4.14 Magnetic Nanostructures

Magnetic NSs are widely used in the field of medical imaging, such as magnetic resonance imaging (MRI) and drug delivery, which is done by containing metal and metal oxides. They are often coated with organic compounds such as polymers and fatty acids (Schroeder et al. 2011) to improve stability and lower cytotoxicity. The magnetic NSs conjugated with drugs are introduced into the patient's body, which is guided by an external magnetic field and targets the cancer cells; as a result, the adverse effects of traditional therapies are reduced. Because of their biocompatibility and simplicity of synthesis, iron-oxide-based NSs like magnetite and maghemite are widely used for MRI, cancer hyperthermia, MDT, and drug delivery applications (Jaiswal et al. 2014). For the use of MSs, their magnetic moment is the most important criterion (Gogoi 2021). LHRH-conjugated superparamagnetic iron oxide nanoparticles are effective in the targeting and medical imaging of tumors of breast cancer (Castaneda et al. 2011). Magnetic NSs are also used to treat cancer patients by giving hypothermia to destroy tumor cells by thermal ablation (Basoglu et al. 2018; Meng et al. 2009). Feridex® and Resovist® are magnetic NSs currently undergoing clinical trials and possibly might be administered to patients for liver metastasis and colon cancer (D.V.M. et al. 2017).

1.4.15 Silica Nanoparticles

Silica NPs are silica in the size range of 10–500 nm. Silica NPs are conjugated with amino-silicanes on the surface and deliver genes (Meng et al. 2009). Mesoporous silica nanoparticles (MSNs) have recently gained attraction for intracellular siRNA delivery and are identified to be one of the efficient drug carriers due to their superior pharmacokinetic qualities and are thus used for immunotherapy. Colorectal cancer cells efficiently absorbed camptothecin-loaded mesoporous silica NPs (D.V.M. et al. 2017). Mesoporous silica NPs are recommended as an effective method for fluorescent cell tracking. Lipid-coated MSNPs are suggested as a beneficial method of treating cancer by delivering and sustaining therapeutic medication concentrations at the tumor site without causing systemic negative effects (Legge et al. 2019).

1.4.16 Metallic Nanostructure

Metallic NSs that are frequently used as nanomedicine are iron-based, gold, silver, and copper. Since these metallic NSs have good optical, magnetic, and photothermal capabilities, they are used as biological imaging and drug delivery systems. Metallic NSs are often conjugated with liposomes, dendrimers, etc. for drug delivery. As the gold NSs' size and surface could be effectively controlled (Lo et al. 2013) and are easily detectable inside the patient body, they are usually favored for intracellular targeting. "Anti-HER2 functionalized gold-on-silica nanoshells" have been shown to attack HER2-positive breast cancer cells (Bagalkot et al. 2007). Feraheme®, an iron oxide NS formulation including ferumoxytol, was authorized by the FDA in June 2009 to treat nodal metastases in prostate and testicular cancer (Mousa and Bharali 2011; Xu et al. 2006).

1.4.17 Calcium Phosphate Nanoparticles

Calcium phosphate (CaP) is an inorganic mineral, and it chemically resembles human hard tissues. They are highly biocompatible, biodegradable, and nontoxic. They are prominently used as carriers to deliver drugs and biomolecules, which otherwise would not have been able to enter cells alone. The chief quality that makes them an excellent delivery vehicle includes their ability to contain drugs both on the surface and inside in addition to holding them till they reach the target site (Sokolova and Epple 2021). Calcium phosphate nanoparticles are also utilized in delivering and releasing siRNA inside a cell. The new generation of controlled drug delivery carriers in cancer therapy identifies the use of calcium phosphate nanocomposites (Dan Son and Kim 2017). Furthermore, a greater application of calcium phosphate nanoparticles could be seen in cancer therapy because of their non-toxic nature and drug release in specific target sites in addition to their size similar to cell ligands, channels that elevate the biocompatible nature of the particle. However, they show complications in drug load beyond a limit, initial burst release, and short-term release of drug (Dan Son and Kim 2017) (Khalifehzadeh and Arami 2020). Lipid-coated CaP is used to target folic acid for delivering siRNA to breast cancer, polyethylene glycol-arginyl glycyl aspartic acid-coated CaP is used in the delivery of drug resistance inhibitors and chemotherapeutic agents to hepatocellular carcinoma, lipid-coated CaP is used to deliver siRNA to hepatocellular carcinoma, poly acrylic acid/polyethylene glycol/gold nanorod-coated CaP is used for DOX delivery and photothermal therapy of liver cancer. These are some of the applications of calcium phosphate nanoparticle application in targeting cancer (Ding et al. 2017; Huang et al. 2019a).

1.4.17.1 Nanomedicines with Multiple Functionalities

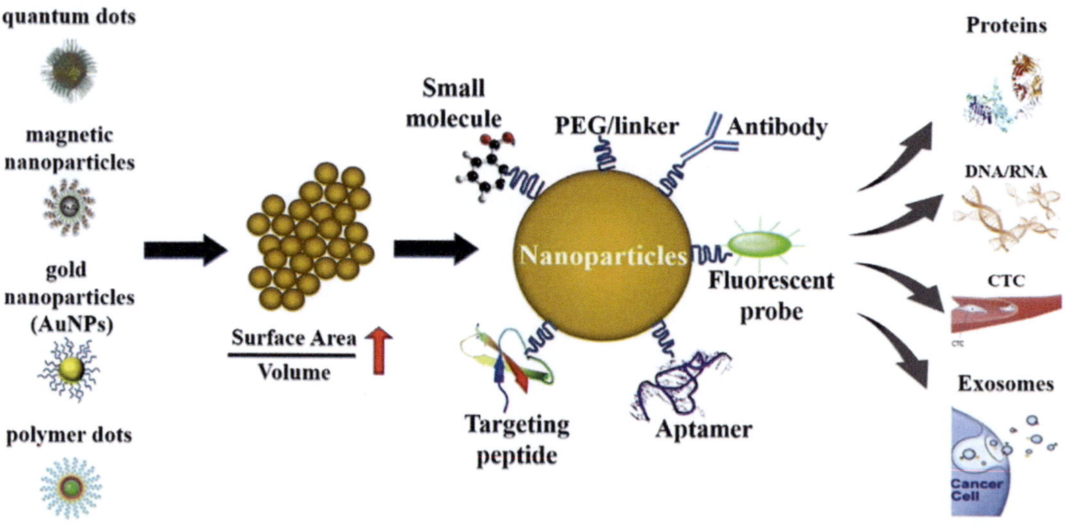

FIGURE 1.5 Illustration of how different kinds of NPs are conjugated with antibody, aptamer, ligands, contrasting agents, linkers, etc. to treat or diagnose a specific disease. As the volume of the NPs decreases, surface area increases, resulting in more conjugation of the linkers, antibodies etc. The interaction phenomenon will subsequently be turned into a quantitative signal that can be monitored.

Source: Zhang et al. 2019.

1.4.17.1.1 Nanomedicine for Drug Delivery and Hyperthermia

Hyperthermia is application of heat at the targeted tumor site. It is done by gradually raising the temperature in the tumor microenvironment until the cells die by apoptosis or necrosis. The treatment is categorized based on how much the temperature rises and the application of hyperthermia in the local, regional or whole body. In terms of temperature, there is thermal ablation, where the temperature is more than 46°C and reaches up to 56°C, leading to cell necrosis, moderate hyperthermia, where the temperature is between 41 and 46°C, leading to protein denaturation, and diathermia, where there is the usage of low temperature—that is, below 41°C. The heat is generated by superparamagnetic NPs with the help of an alternating magnetic field (AMF) using Néel relaxation and Brownian relaxation or by multi-domain magnetic NPs (MNPs) using hysteresis loss (Gogoi 2021) (Ahmed et al. 2020).

The MNPs used for drug delivery in hyperthermia is based on two types of mechanism—the MNP is conjugated with drugs using a linker and with the help of AMF, the drug is released because of the heating of the linker (Derfus et al. 2007). The second approach is the release of drugs from a polymeric matrix encapsulated with MNPs with the help of AMF or EMF (electromagnetic field) (Martín-Saldaña et al. 2018). A good number of iron oxide-based, as well as the oxides of the nanostructures such as Fe, Co, Ni, Zn, Mn, Gd, and Mg, are used as hyperthermia agents. The most common is the magnetite (Fe3O4) NPs that are equilibrated using ligands such as cationic liposomes, dextran, hydro-gel, polyvinyl alcohol, etc., and the maghemite (γ-Fe2O3) NPs equilibrated using dextran as ligand. There is also seen the use of ferrite-based NPs such as cobalt ferrite, nickel ferrite, manganese ferrite among others, and ferromagnetic NPs. The main principle governing the heating of the MNPs is magnetic energy dissipation, which is based on the size of the MNPs, the viscosity of the carrier—that is, the solvent used for the MNPs, increase in anisotropy of the MNPs, and stability of the ligands.

Several clinical trials had undergone using MNPs as agents for drug delivery in hyperthermia. Dextran magnetite-loaded magnetic liposomes were effective in treating AH60C tumors in rats (Shinkai et al. 1996). Magnetic cationic liposomes were effective in treating solid tumors in various types of animals with repeated hyperthermia (Lu et al. 2005) (Masuko et al. 2008) (Ito et al. 2003). The European Union has approved the use of aminosilane-coated superparamagnetic iron oxide NP (SPION) known as Nanotherm® for hyperthermia accompanied by radiation therapy for periodic glioblastoma patients in 2010 and again it was also approved by FDA in the USA for clinical trials on prostate cancer patients (Kok et al. 2020).

1.4.17.1.2 Nanomedicine for Drug Delivery and Photothermal Therapy

The transport action of nanaparticles is done by anchoring drugs which is designed accordingly to target the malignant tissue. These medications are then released into the cancerous sites to initiate the process of elimination. The presence of genomic antioxidants and conventional chemotherapeutic drugs within the nano-carriers strongly suggests that these NPs are suitable for use in respective cytotoxicity and genomic therapeutics (Yao et al. 2020).

In photothermal therapy, elements that accumulate EM energy are utilized and transformed into heat energy which induces apoptosis of melanoma cells, releasing malignant cells with a specific immunizing agent that can be absorbed and introduced by antigen-presenting cells, activating immune organelles, as well as inducing an anticancer inflammatory system reaction. Photothermal therapy and immunoadjuvant combined may result in the production of an in situ autologous cancer vaccine (InCVAX). With this approach, the significant autoimmune symptoms that are typically present during surgical treatment are avoided, as well as the adverse symptoms of chemotherapeutic medications (Liu et al. 2017b) (Shang et al. 2020). Both inorganic and organic photothermal agents (PTA) have been utilized to maximize the efficiency of cancer therapy. These substances possess a significant near infrared region to increase the thermal rate of exchange (Shang et al. 2020).

Polythermal agents are made of inorganic materials, such as Au NPs, Carbon NPs, black phosphorus quantum dots loaded by PLGA, FeS NPs, palladium nanosheets, and Cu-based nanoparticles (Shi et al. 2017). The typical biocompatibility of inorganic compounds is weak, resulting in rapid elimination as well as cytotoxicity in vivo. Protein-based PTAs, synthesized polymers, liposome/micelle-encapsulated near-infrared markers, and other organic-based photothermal agents generally work by excreting light generated by near-infrared radiation. Organic-based PTAs are more biocompatible, biodegradable, can also be reliably reconfigured to accomplish versatility like the capability to locate and target the tumors as well as to perform theragnostic (Shi et al. 2017) (Jung et al. 2018a).

1.4.17.1.3 Nanoparticles for Drug Delivery and Photodynamic Therapy

In photodynamic theory, light absorbing molecules called photosensitizers are administered into the body and they generate reactive oxygen species that damage the cancerous tumor at specific wavelength of light. Synthesizing ultra-low size organically modified silica nanoparticles (SiNPs) covalently linked with iodobenzylpyropheophorbide by the alkaline hydrolysis and polycondensation of the organotrialkoxysilane precursors within the nonpolar core of Tween-80/water microemulsion showed that the prepared SiNPs had a great affinity for cancer cells demonstrating that they possess potential for cancer treatment and diagnosis by photodynamic therapy (Bechet et al. 2008; Ohulchanskyy et al. 2007). Aluminum phthalocyanine tetrasulfonate (AlPcS4)-loaded liposomes acts as an effective and safe strategy for PDT of superficial bladder cancer (Derycke et al. 2004). Nanoparticle hydrogels loaded with the PS temoporfin (mTHPP) were rendered suitable as carriers for Photodynamic therapy (PDT) (Kamuhabwa et al. 2004). Rose Bengal (RB)-loaded polyamidoamine dendrimers acted acts as a suitable drug delivery system releasing above 80% of RB in 72 h. RB-loaded dendrimer exhibited minimized dark toxicity and enhanced phototoxicity to Dalton's Lymphoma As cite cancer (DLA) cells thus demonstrating as a promising drug delivery system for PDT (Rak et al. 2023) (Reza Saboktakin et al. 2011). Nanoassemblies based on heptakis (2-oligo(ethyleneoxide)-6-hexadecylthio-)-β-CD (SC16OH) and zinc-phthalocyanine (ZnPc) demonstrated potential photodynamic anticancer effects in HeLa cancer cells, suggesting a promising Zn-Pc delivery system (Conte et al. 2014; Karthikeyan et al. 2011). PDT is high selectivity in targeting only cancer cells, enhancing its permeability and retention effect, increasing its retention time in malignant tissue, reduces targeting normal tissues and hence possessing less threat to them.

1.4.17.1.4 Nanomedicine for Drug Delivery and Radiotherapy

Nanomaterials can be employed as exposure levels adjuvants (synthetic NPs), radioactive sensitizers, and contrasting reagents in X-Ray, CT, MRI, and PET for improved imaging. Radiotherapy has abstracted almost exclusively on the malignancy cell themselves, omitting the complicated biological synergy intervening tumors and the epithelium in which they develop, it is determined as tumor microenvironment (TME) (Chatterjee et al. 2013). Radiation-responsive malignant endothelial cells cause the pathway of inflammation to begin when they die. External beam radiotherapy (EBRT) and internal radio isotope therapy (RIT) are the two primary categories of radiotherapy. Regarding EBRT, exogenous high radiation could cause the extinction of malignant organelles despite being constrained by deep penetration. As a result, it is frequently employed to treat a variety of distant solid tumors (such as ductal and lobular carcinoma, prostate tumors, malignant lung tumor, colorectal, hepatocellular carcinoma, and esophageal) (Barker et al. 2015; Hill 2017). For internal RIT, therapeutic radioactive isotopes are often injected into the tumor using minimally invasive techniques. For instance, it is viable to intravenously introduce lipid NPs, antibodies, or NPs with malignant cells targeting receptors as ideal tumor-homing agents as well as to effectively insert radioactive isotopes into the tumors. RIT can use therefore treatment of both metastatic and local solid cancers (Rocca et al. 2015).

The combination of chemotherapeutics with radiation dose-enhancing nanoparticles for superior tumor control nanoparticles which release their payload upon exposure to a reducing agent, such as RT delivers both chemotherapeutics and radiopharmaceuticals (Good and Harrington

2013). Numerous chemotherapeutic agents, such as camptothecin, docetaxel, paclitaxel, doxorubicin, cisplatin, and ATM-kinase inhibitors, have been researched for nanoparticle augmented CRT with optimistic outcomes suggesting higher benefit over chemotherapeutic or radiotherapy alone (Hagan et al. 2018; Harrington et al. 2007). The immunosuppressive microenvironment induced by melanoma can be addressed by radiotherapy by unleashing tumor-associated antigens (TAA). Furthermore, Infrared alters the tumor microenvironment and stimulates cascades involved in attracting inflammatory responses, which might also improve the penetration of given immunotherapeutic (DuRoss et al. 2019; Shams et al. 2022). Gold NPs are used as a radiosensitizer in radiation therapy—for example, AuNps-PEG-Cetuximab, which is combined of gold NPs with the drug Cetuximab (Chen et al. 2020). Iron-oxide NPs were used in radiation therapy to enhance the delivery of radiation to the tumor site—for example, Ferumoxytol, which is an iron oxide NPs used as a contrast agent in MRI scans (Canese et al. 2021).

1.4.17.1.5 Nanomedicine for Drug Delivery and Imaging

There is ongoing research and development for the use of nanomedicine in drug delivery and imaging, which possess the potential to significantly increase the efficacy and security of medical therapies. Clinicians may visualize specific bodily regions and monitor the absorption and effectiveness of drugs by using nanoparticles in imaging. This may be done using methods including fluorescence microscopy, ultrasonography, single photon emission computed tomography (SPECT), positron emission tomography (PET), computed tomography (CT) scans, and magnetic resonance imaging (MRI) (Koo et al. 2005). Several different forms of nanoparticles, including liposomes, dye-molecule-doped silica nanoparticles, Quantum dots, gold nanoparticles, immunotarget nanoshells, perfluorocarbon nanoparticles, nanoshells, and magnetic nanocrystals, are now utilized in molecular imaging to identify cancer (Liu et al. 2007).As we evaluate liposomes for in vivo imaging, investigations revealed that breast cancer cells accumulated considerably more sterically stabilized liposomes encapsulating 99 mTc-HMPAO with and without covalently coupled Vasoactive intestinal peptide binders than normal breast tissues (Dagar et al. 2003). Superparamagnetic iron oxide nanoparticles are used in MRI for the passive identification of prostate cancer lymph node metastases because they are made of biodegradable iron that is biocompatible and can therefore be reused by cells using regular biochemical pathways for iron metabolism. MRI with this superparamagnetic nanoparticle successfully identified all patients with translational metastases and a node-by-node assessment had a substantially higher sensitivity than conventional MRI (Bulte and Kraitchman 2004; Harisinghani et al. 2003). Advances in biological research and clinical diagnostics have made great use of fluorescence labelling methods. For example, to achieve sensitive detection, there is a rising demand for fluorescent labelling probes which are more intense, stable, and sensitive. By doping a fluorescent dye (Rubpy) into silica nanoparticles, researchers have created a novel type of highly luminous and photostable nanoparticle (Zhao et al. 2004). Overall, the small size for easy detection, specific imaging properties like magnetic, metallic fluorescent or bioluminescent, and target specific delivery of nanoparticles to the tissue makes them particularly useful for imaging applications in medicine.

1.5 CHALLENGES OF NANOMEDICINES

Although the field of nanomedicine is growing challenges still persist for overall application of nanomedicine in cancer therapy. Nanomedicine has to be effectively circulated so that medication is distributed in the required site. The ability of nanomedicine to penetrate tumor cells greatly depends on the size of the pore of tumor (Fisher et al. 2013). Although there has been impressive progress in this field, research is still sparse due to technological factors, lack of knowledge in this area, and lack of proper lab space. In heterogeneous tumors, a minor subgroup of tumor cells can greatly vary the composition of the tumor cells and their heterogeneous growth. This factor influences the survival rate of the tumor as various subgroups occupy different space inside the tumor, and the endurance of such a model surpasses individual subpopulation (Rasool et al. 2022). There is hindrance in areas of biological, technological, and design of nanomedicine. New developments in nanomedicines need to take care of challenges such as their successful biodistribution, effective synthesis of nanoparticles, minimizing toxicity, overcoming biological barriers, suitable administration route, overall productivity of nanomedicine and its size for their effective working (Gavas et al. 2021).Scientific reasons such as insufficient understanding of the interacting mechanisms of magnetic nanoparticles, different behavior in in vitro and in vivo experiments, clinical reasons such as high cost of clinical trials, incorect chosen target, errors in the dosage and duration of treatment, and various other marketing reasons obstruct the widespread practical use of magnetic nanoparticles (Koksharov et al. 2022). Despite the popularity of nanomedicine, the number passing through clinical trials is less. Also, most of it cannot pass beyond in vivo and in vitro trials.

Nano formulations that reach the market today are low in number, although the amount of nanomedicine developed for treatment of different type of cancers is huge. This is because a nanocarrier formulation has to go through a series of evaluation procedures before it is suitable for the market (Metselaar and Lammers 2020). Development of devices with accurate sensitiveness, cost effective and effortless in use is required. A significant number of devices are made for

TABLE 1.1
Nanomedicines Approved by One or More Regulatory Bodies

Product	Nanoplatform/agent	Indication	Status	Company
Doxil	PEGylated liposome/ doxorubicin hydrochloride	Ovarian cancer	Approved 11/17/1995 FDA50718	Ortho Biotech (acquired by JNJ)
Myocet	Non-PEGylated liposomal doxorubicin nanomedicine	Metastatic breast cancer	Approved in Europe and Canada, in combination with cyclophosphamide	Sopherion Therapeutics, LLC in North America and Cephalon, Inc. in Europe
DaunoXome	Lipid encapsulation of daunorubicin	First-line treatment for patients with advanced HIV-associated Kaposi's sarcoma	Approved in the USA	Galen Ltd.
ThermoDox	Heat-activated liposomal encapsulation of doxorubicin	Breast cancer, primary liver cancer	Received Fast Track Designation, approval expected by 2013	Celsion
Abraxane	Nanoparticulate albumin/ paclitaxel	Various cancers	Approved 1/7/2005 FDA21660	Celgene
Rexin-G	Targeting protein tagged phospholipid/microRNA-122	Sarcoma, osteosarcoma, pancreatic cancer, and other solid tumor	Fully approved in Philippine Phase II/III in USA	Epeius Biotechnologies Corp.
Oncaspar	PEGylated asparaginase	Acute lymphoblastic leukemia	Approved 24/06/2006	Enzon Pharmaceuticals, Inc.
Resovist	Iron oxide nanoparticles coated with carboxydextran	Liver/spleen lesion imaging	In 2001, approved for the European market	Bayer Schering Pharma AG
Feridex	Iron oxide nanoparticles coated with dextran	Liver/spleen lesion imaging	Approved by US-FDA in 1996	Berlex Laboratories
Endorem	Iron oxide nanoparticles coated with dextran	Liver/spleen lesion imaging	Approved in Europe	Guerbet

Source: Zhang et al. 2020.

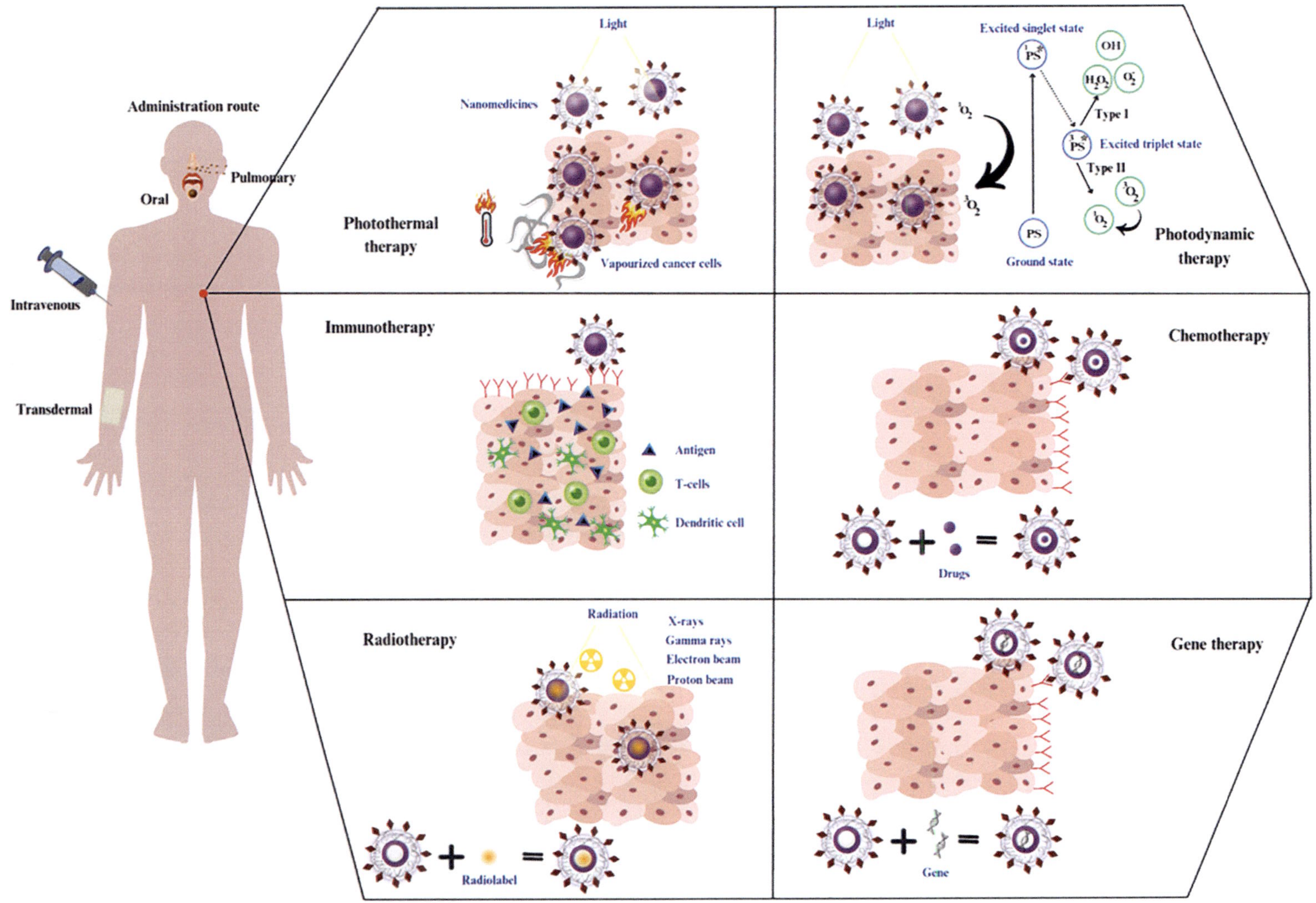

FIGURE 1.6 This image depicts various nanomedicine-based cancer therapy approaches and administration routes, including oral, pulmonary, intravenous, and transdermal methods. Therapies illustrated include photothermal therapy, photodynamic therapy, immunotherapy, chemotherapy, radiotherapy, and gene therapy, showcasing their mechanisms such as light activation, immune response, radiation, and genetic modification, all targeting cancer cells with precision for enhanced therapeutic outcomes.

simple laboratory uses and are unfit for use in large trials. Thus, there remains a challenge to overcome this issue and develop more compatible devices. Other challenges arise due to the toxicity of nanoparticles which could lead to overexposure of drugs, irregular changes in biodistribution of drugs, unexpected immunological responses, which are difficult to predict based on studies in small laboratory animals (Mahato et al. 2021).

1.6 CONCLUSION AND FUTURE PROSPECTS

Cancer is a leading cause of death around the globe. It is grouped into six chief groups based on cell genesis, caused due to various intrinsic and extrinsic factors. The statistical review presented in this review paper shows global cancer deaths from 2008–2019, global cancer data in 2019 in Asia, Europe, America, Africa and Oceania in addition to specifically showing the cancer cases in Asian continent in 2020 and types of cancers in Asian continent in 2020. There have been various conventional therapies practiced to treat cancer like radiation therapy, chemotherapy, surgery, hormone therapy, immune therapy. Despite their popular use, drawbacks persist. Therefore, introduction of nanomedicine helped to overcome these disadvantages in cancer therapy. Following it, various organic (polymeric, dendrimers, monoclonal antibodies, EVs, liposomes, solid lipid nanoparticle, micelles, nanoemulsions, cyclo-dextrin nanosponges carbon), inorganic (quantum dots, metallic, magnetic, silica, calcium phosphate) and hybrid nanoparticles (lipid-polymer, liposome-silica, hydrogels, chitosan-carbon nanotubes, cell membrane-coated nanoparticles) are discussed. Drug delivery is done by two types of triggered release namely, internal and external. Furthermore, drugs can be delivered to the target site by active or passive targeting. Despite the efficient use of nanoparticles in drug delivery and therapy it has certain challenges which are discussed in this review paper.

To enhance nanomedicine translation and performance a specific drug decision-making framework such as AstraZeneca's 5R principle: right target/efficacy, right tissue/exposure, right safety, right patient, and right commercial potential needs to be adopted. To achieve the goals, an improved understanding of the heterogeneity of cancer and biological factors influencing the behavior of nanomedicine in tumors is essential; a transition from formulation-driven research to disease-driven development needs to be worked upon; the implementation of more relevant animal models and testing protocols for effective application in human tumor; and the pre-selection of the patients most likely

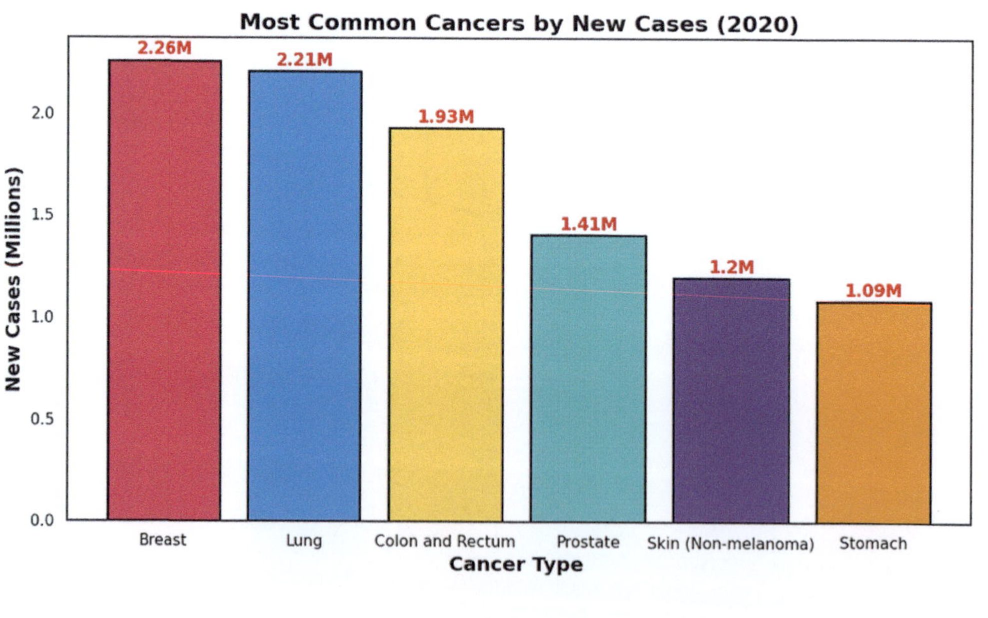

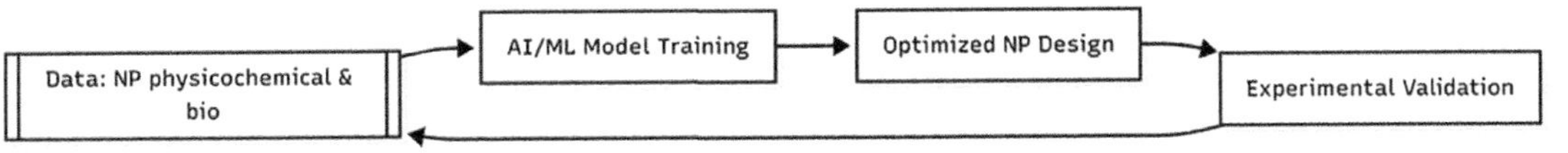

to respond to nanomedicine therapies are some of the ways which are required to be adopted in order for a successful cancer therapy. Overcoming these challenges to improve the development of nanomedicine and their clinical translation are the key to establish superior therapies. Nanoparticles play a prominent role in developing target specific drug delivery systems. In recent days, mathematical modeling and simulation plays an important role in optimization of various parameters like nanoparticle-based drug dose, dissolution of drug particles, and adverse reaction from the nanoparticles. With the help of modeling and simulation, determining or optimizing the type, shape, and size of the nanoparticles and its influence on the targeted cells/tissues can be achieved.

REFERENCES

Ahmed S, Rajak BL, Gogoi M, Sarma HD. Magnetic nanoparticles mediated cancer hyperthermia. Smart Healthcare for Disease Diagnosis and Prevention. Academic Press; 2020 Jan 1;153–73.

Ali ES, Sharker SM, Islam MT, Khan IN, Shaw S, Rahman MA, et al. Targeting cancer cells with nanotherapeutics and nanodiagnostics: Current status and future perspectives. Semin Cancer Biol. Academic Press; 2021 Feb 1;69:52–68.

Alromi DA, Madani SY, Seifalian A. Emerging application of magnetic nanoparticles for diagnosis and treatment of cancer. Polymers [Internet]. Multidisciplinary Digital Publishing Institute; 2021 Nov 27 [cited 2023 Apr 4];13(23):4146. Available from: https://www.mdpi.com/2073-4360/13/23/4146/htm

Bagalkot V, Zhang L, Levy-Nissenbaum E, Jon S, Kantoff PW, Langery R, et al. Quantum dot-aptamer conjugates for synchronous cancer imaging, therapy, and sensing of drug delivery based on bi-fluorescence resonance energy transfer. Nano Lett [Internet]. Nano Lett; 2007 Oct [cited 2023 Apr 5];7(10):3065–70. Available from: https://pubmed.ncbi.nlm.nih.gov/17854227/

Barenholz Y. Doxil®—the first FDA-approved nano-drug: Lessons learned. J Control Release [Internet]. J Control Release; 2012 Jun 10 [cited 2023 Apr 4];160(2):117–34. Available from: https://pubmed.ncbi.nlm.nih.gov/22484195/

Barker HE, Paget JTE, Khan AA, Harrington KJ. The tumour microenvironment after radiotherapy: Mechanisms of resistance and recurrence. Nat Rev Cancer [Internet]. Nat Rev Cancer; 2015 Jul 26 [cited 2023 Apr 5];15(7):409–25. Available from: https://pubmed.ncbi.nlm.nih.gov/26105538/

Baskar R, Lee KA, Yeo R, Yeoh KW. Cancer and radiation therapy: Current advances and future directions. Int J Med Sci [Internet]. Int J Med Sci; 2012 Feb 27 [cited 2023 Apr 4];9(3):193–9. Available from: https://pubmed.ncbi.nlm.nih.gov/22408567/

Basoglu H, Goncu B, Akbas F. Magnetic nanoparticle-mediated gene therapy to induce Fas apoptosis pathway in breast cancer. Cancer Gene Ther [Internet]. Cancer Gene Ther; 2018 Jun 1 [cited 2023 Apr 5];25(5–6):141–7. Available from: https://pubmed.ncbi.nlm.nih.gov/29593359/

Bazak R, Houri M, Achy SEL, Hussein W, Refaat T. Passive targeting of nanoparticles to cancer: A comprehensive review of the literature. Mol Clin Oncol [Internet]. Mol Clin Oncol; 2014 Nov [cited 2023 Apr 4];2(6):904–8. Available from: https://pubmed.ncbi.nlm.nih.gov/25279172/

Bechet D, Couleaud P, Frochot C, Viriot ML, Guillemin F, Barberi-Heyob M. Nanoparticles as vehicles for delivery of photodynamic therapy agents. Trends Biotechnol. 2008 Nov;26(11):612–21.

Bertrand N, Wu J, Xu X, Kamaly N, Farokhzad OC. Cancer nanotechnology: The impact of passive and active targeting in the era of modern cancer biology. Adv Drug Deliv Rev [Internet]. NIH Public Access; 2014 [cited 2023 Apr 3];66:2. Available from: /pmc/articles/PMC4219254/

Blanco E, Shen H, Ferrari M. Principles of nanoparticle design for overcoming biological barriers to drug delivery. Nat Biotechnol [Internet]. Nat Biotechnol; 2015 Sep 8 [cited 2023 Apr 4];33(9):941–51. Available from: https://pubmed.ncbi.nlm.nih.gov/26348965/

Bober Z, Bartusik-Aebisher D, Aebisher D. Application of dendrimers in anticancer diagnostics and therapy. Molecules [Internet]. Multidisciplinary Digital Publishing Institute (MDPI); 2022 May 1 [cited 2023 Apr 4];27(10). Available from: /pmc/articles/PMC9144149/

Bridgewater RE, Norman JC, Caswell PT. Integrin trafficking at a glance. J Cell Sci [Internet]. Company of Biologists; 2012 Aug 15 [cited 2023 May 1];125(16):3695–701. Available from: /pmc/articles/PMC3462077/

Bulte JWM, Kraitchman DL. Iron oxide MR contrast agents for molecular and cellular imaging. NMR Biomed [Internet]. NMR Biomed; 2004 Nov [cited 2023 Apr 5];17(7):484–99. Available from: https://pubmed.ncbi.nlm.nih.gov/15526347/

Busatto S, Pham A, Suh A, Shapiro S, Wolfram J. Organotropic drug delivery: Synthetic nanoparticles and extracellular vesicles. Biomed Microdevices [Internet]. Biomed Microdevices; 2019a Jun 1 [cited 2023 Apr 4];21(2). Available from: https://pubmed.ncbi.nlm.nih.gov/30989386/

Busatto S, Pham A, Suh A, Shapiro S, Wolfram J. Organotropic drug delivery: Synthetic nanoparticles and extracellular vesicles. Biomedical Microdevices [Internet]. Springer; 2019b Apr 15 [cited 2023 Apr 5];21(2):1–17. Available from: https://link.springer.com/article/10.1007/s10544-019-0396-7

Canese R, Vurro F, Marzola P. Iron oxide nanoparticles as theranostic agents in cancer immunotherapy. Nanomaterials [Internet]. Multidisciplinary Digital Publishing Institute (MDPI); 2021 Aug 1 [cited 2023 Apr 4];11(8). Available from: /pmc/articles/PMC8399455/

Castaneda RT, Khurana A, Khan R, Daldrup-Link HE. Labeling stem cells with ferumoxytol, an FDA-approved iron oxide nanoparticle. J Vis Exp [Internet]. J Vis Exp; 2011 [cited 2023 Apr 5]; (57). Available from: https://pubmed.ncbi.nlm.nih.gov/22083287/

Cerri GC, Lima LCF, Lelis D de F, Barcelos L da S, Feltenberger JD, Mussi SV, et al. Sclareol-loaded lipid nanoparticles improved metabolic profile in obese mice. Life Sci. Pergamon; 2019 Feb 1;218:292–9.

Chatterjee DK, Wolfe T, Lee J, Brown AP, Singh PK, Bhattarai SR, et al. Convergence of nanotechnology with radiation therapy—insights and implications for clinical translation. Transl Cancer Res [Internet]. NIH Public Access; 2013 Aug 8 [cited 2023 Apr 5];2(4):256. Available from: /pmc/articles/PMC4179207/

Chaudhary N, Gomez GA, Howes MT, Lo HP, McMahon KA, Rae JA, et al. Endocytic crosstalk: Cavins, caveolins, and caveolae regulate clathrin-independent endocytosis. PLoS Biol [Internet]. PLoS Biol; 2014 [cited 2023 May 1];12(4). Available from: https://pubmed.ncbi.nlm.nih.gov/24714042/

Chen H, Gu Z, An H, Chen C, Chen J, Cui R, et al. Precise nanomedicine for intelligent therapy of cancer. Sci China Chem [Internet]. Science China Press; 2018 Dec 1 [cited 2023 Apr 4];61(12):1503–52. Available from: /doi/10.1007/s11426-018-9397-5

Chen PH, Yao H, Huang LJS. Cytokine receptor endocytosis: New kinase activity-dependent and -independent roles of PI3K. Front Endocrinol (Lausanne) [Internet]. Frontiers Media SA; 2017 May 1 [cited 2023 May 1];8(MAY). Available from: /pmc/articles/PMC5410625/

Chen Y, Yang J, Fu S, Wu J. Gold nanoparticles as radiosensitizers in cancer radiotherapy. Int J Nanomedicine [Internet]. Dove Press; 2020 [cited 2023 Apr 4];15:9407. Available from: /pmc/articles/PMC7699443/

Chen Z, Mao R, Liu Y. Fullerenes for cancer diagnosis and therapy: Preparation, biological and clinical perspectives. Curr Drug Metab. Bentham Science Publishers; 2012 Sep 16;13(8):1035–45.

Chen Y, Yang J, Fu S, Wu J, Gold Nanoparticles as Radiosensitizers in Cancer Radiotherapy. International Journal of Nanomedicine, 2020; 15, 9407–9430. https://doi.org/10.2147/IJN.S272902

Conte C, Scala A, Siracusano G, Leone N, Patanè S, Ungaro F, et al. Nanoassembly of an amphiphilic cyclodextrin and Zn(II)-phthalocyanine with the potential for photodynamic therapy of cancer. RSC Adv [Internet]. R Soc Chem; 2014 Sep 16 [cited 2023 Apr 5];4(83):43903–11. Available from: https://pubs.rsc.org/en/content/articlehtml/2014/ra/c4ra07847k

Corrotte M, Cerasoli M, Maeda FY, Andrews NW. Endophilin-A2-dependent tubular endocytosis promotes plasma membrane repair and parasite invasion. J Cell Sci [Internet]. Company of Biologists; 2021 Mar 3 [cited 2023 May 1];134(5). Available from: /pmc/articles/PMC7725609/

Dadwal A, Baldi A, Kumar Narang R. Nanoparticles as carriers for drug delivery in cancer. https://doi.org/10.1080/21691401.2018.1457039 [Internet]. Taylor & Francis; 2018 Nov 5 [cited 2023 Apr 5];46(sup2):295–305. Available from: https://www.tandfonline.com/doi/abs/10.1080/21691401.2018.1457039

Dagar S, Krishnadas A, Rubinstein I, Blend MJ, Önyüksel H. VIP grafted sterically stabilized liposomes for targeted imaging of breast cancer: In vivo studies. J Controlled Release [Internet]. Elsevier; 2003 Aug 28 [cited 2023 Apr 5];91(1–2):123–33. Available from: https://pubmed.ncbi.nlm.nih.gov/12932644/

Dambournet D, Sochacki KA, Cheng AT, Akamatsu M, Taraska JW, Hockemeyer D, et al. Genome-edited human stem cells expressing fluorescently labeled endocytic markers allow quantitative analysis of clathrin-mediated endocytosis during differentiation. J Cell Biol [Internet]. The Rockefeller University Press; 2018 Sep 9 [cited 2023 May 1];217(9):3301. Available from: /pmc/articles/PMC6123002/

Dan Son K, Kim YJ. Anticancer activity of drug-loaded calcium phosphate nanocomposites against human osteosarcoma. Biomater Res [Internet]. BioMed Central Ltd.; 2017 Jun 24 [cited 2023 Apr 5];21(1):1–8. Available from: https://biomaterialsres.biomedcentral.com/articles/10.1186/s40824-017-0099-1

Daniels TR, Bernabeu E, Rodríguez JA, Patel S, Kozman M, Chiappetta DA, et al. The transferrin receptor and the targeted delivery of therapeutic agents against cancer. Biochimica et Biophysica Acta (BBA)—General Subjects. Elsevier; 2012 Mar 1;1820(3):291–317.

Daraee H, Etemadi A, Kouhi M, Alimirzalu S, Akbarzadeh A. Application of liposomes in medicine and drug delivery. Artif Cells Nanomed Biotechnol [Internet]. Artif Cells Nanomed Biotechnol; 2016 Jan 1 [cited 2023 Apr 4];44(1):381–91. Available from: https://pubmed.ncbi.nlm.nih.gov/25222036/

Dennerstein L, Burrows GD, Hyman GJ, Sharpe K. Hormone therapy and affect. Maturitas. Elsevier; 1979 Jun 1;1(4):247–59.

Derfus AM, Von Maltzahn G, Harris TJ, Duza T, Vecchio KS, Ruoslahti E, et al. Remotely triggered release from magnetic nanoparticles. Advanced Materials [Internet]. John Wiley & Sons, Ltd; 2007 Nov 19 [cited 2023 Apr 5];19(22):3932–6. Available from: https://onlinelibrary.wiley.com/doi/full/10.1002/adma.200700091

Derycke ASL, Kamuhabwa A, Gijsens A, Roskams T, De Vos D, Kasran A, et al. Transferrin-conjugated liposome targeting of photosensitizer AlPcS4 to rat bladder carcinoma cells. J Natl Cancer Inst [Internet]. J Natl Cancer Inst; 2004 Nov 3 [cited 2023 Apr 5];96(21):1620–30. Available from: https://pubmed.ncbi.nlm.nih.gov/15523091/

Deshpande PP, Biswas S, Torchilin VP. Current trends in the use of liposomes for tumor targeting. Nanomedicine (Lond) [Internet]. Nanomedicine (Lond); 2013 [cited 2023 Apr 4];8(9):1509–28. Available from: https://pubmed.ncbi.nlm.nih.gov/23914966/

Dianzani C, Monge C, Miglio G, Serpe L, Martina K, Cangemi L, et al. Nanoemulsions as delivery systems for poly-chemotherapy aiming at melanoma treatment. Cancers [Internet]. Multidisciplinary Digital Publishing Institute; 2020 May 9 [cited 2023 Apr 5];12(5):1198. Available from: https://www.mdpi.com/2072-6694/12/5/1198/htm

Ding Y, Zhai K, Pei P, Lin Y, Ma Y, Zhu H, et al. Encapsulation of cisplatin in a pegylated calcium phosphate nanoparticle (CPNP) for enhanced cytotoxicity to cancerous cells. J Colloid Interface Sci. Academic Press Inc.; 2017 May 1;493:181–9.

Dong X, Brahma RK, Fang C, Yao SQ. Stimulus-responsive self-assembled prodrugs in cancer therapy. Chem Sci [Internet]. Royal Society of Chemistry; 2022 Apr 4 [cited 2023 Apr 4];13(15):4239. Available from: /pmc/articles/PMC9006903/

Dong Z, Feng L, Zhu W, Sun X, Gao M, Zhao H, et al. CaCO3 nanoparticles as an ultra-sensitive tumor-pH-responsive nanoplatform enabling real-time drug release monitoring and cancer combination therapy. Biomaterials [Internet]. Biomaterials; 2016 Dec 1 [cited 2023 May 1];110:60–70. Available from: https://pubmed.ncbi.nlm.nih.gov/27710833/

DuRoss AN, Neufeld MJ, Rana S, Thomas CR, Sun C. Integrating nanomedicine into clinical radiotherapy regimens. Adv Drug Deliv Rev [Internet]. NIH Public Access; 2019 Apr 1 [cited 2023 Apr 5];144:35. Available from: /pmc/articles/PMC6745263/

D.V.M. PJH, D.V.M. KLM, Petryk AA, Petryk JD, Sechrist S, Gladstone DJ, et al. Hypo-fractionated radiation, magnetic nanoparticle hyperthermia and a viral immunotherapy treatment of spontaneous canine cancer. https://doi.org/10.1117/12.2256213 [Internet]. SPIE; 2017 Feb 22 [cited 2023 Apr 5];10066:24–32. Available from: https://www.spiedigitallibrary.org/conference-proceedings-of-spie/10066/1006605/Hypo-fractionated-radiation-magnetic-nanoparticle-hyperthermia-and-a-viral-immunotherapy/10.1117/12.2256213.full

Ediriwickrema A, Saltzman WM. Nanotherapy for cancer: Targeting and multifunctionality in the future of cancer therapies. ACS Biomater Sci Eng [Internet]. Am Chem Soc; 2015 Feb 9 [cited 2023 Apr 4];1(2):64–78. Available from: https://pubs.acs.org/doi/full/10.1021/ab500084g

Fekri F, Abousawan J, Bautista S, Orofiamma L, Dayam RM, Antonescu CN, et al. Targeted enhancement of flotillin-dependent endocytosis augments cellular uptake and impact of cytotoxic drugs. Sci Rep [Internet]. Nature Publishing Group; 2019 Dec 1 [cited 2023 May 1];9(1). Available from: /pmc/articles/PMC6882852/

Ferlay J, Colombet M, Soerjomataram I, Mathers C, Parkin DM, Piñeros M, et al. Estimating the global cancer incidence and mortality in 2018: GLOBOCAN sources and methods. Int J Cancer [Internet]. Int J Cancer; 2019 Apr 15 [cited 2023 May 2];144(8):1941–53. Available from: https://pubmed.ncbi.nlm.nih.gov/30350310/

Fisher R, Pusztai L, Swanton C. Cancer heterogeneity: Implications for targeted therapeutics. Br J Cancer [Internet]. Br J Cancer; 2013 Feb 19 [cited 2023 Apr 5];108(3):479–85. Available from: https://pubmed.ncbi.nlm.nih.gov/23299535/

Fouladi F, Steffen KJ, Mallik S. Enzyme-responsive liposomes for the delivery of anticancer drugs. Bioconjug Chem [Internet]. Bioconjug Chem; 2017 Apr 19 [cited 2023 Apr 4];28(4):857–68. Available from: https://pubmed.ncbi.nlm.nih.gov/28201868/

Gabizon AA. Applications of liposomal drug delivery systems to cancer therapy. Nanotechnology for Cancer Therapy [Internet]. CRC Press; 2006 Dec 19 [cited 2023 Apr 4];595–611. Available from: https://www.taylorfrancis.com/chapters/edit/10.1201/9781420006636-29/applications-liposomal-drug-delivery-systems-cancer-therapy-alberto-gabizon

Gadade DD, Pekamwar SS. Cyclodextrin based nanoparticles for drug delivery and theranostics. Adv Pharm Bull [Internet]. Adv Pharm Bull; 2020 [cited 2023 Apr 5];10(2):166–83. Available from: https://doi.org/10.34172/apb.2020.022

Gao W, Zhang Y, Zhang Q, Zhang L. Nanoparticle-hydrogel: A hybrid biomaterial system for localized drug delivery. Ann Biomed Eng [Internet]. Ann Biomed Eng; 2016 Jun 1 [cited 2023 Apr 4];44(6):2049–61. Available from: https://pubmed.ncbi.nlm.nih.gov/26951462/

García KP, Zarschler K, Barbaro L, Barreto JA, O'Malley W, Spiccia L, et al. Zwitterionic-coated "stealth" nanoparticles for biomedical applications: Recent advances in countering biomolecular corona formation and uptake by the mononuclear phagocyte system. Small [Internet]. John Wiley & Sons, Ltd; 2014 Jul 1 [cited 2023 Apr 4];10(13):2516–29. Available from: https://onlinelibrary.wiley.com/doi/full/10.1002/smll.201303540

Gavas S, Quazi S, Karpiński TM. Nanoparticles for cancer therapy: Current progress and challenges. Nanoscale Res Lett [Internet]. Springer; 2021 [cited 2023 Apr 3];16(1). Available from: /pmc/articles/PMC8645667/

Geisberg CA, Sawyer DB. Mechanisms of anthracycline cardiotoxicity and strategies to decrease cardiac damage. Curr Hypertens Rep [Internet]. Springer; 2010 Dec 15 [cited 2023 Apr 4];12(6):404–10. Available from: https://link.springer.com/article/10.1007/s11906-010-0146-y

Gogoi M. Magnetic nanostructures for cancer theranostic applications. Curr Pathobiol Rep [Internet]. Springer; 2021 Sep 1 [cited 2023 Apr 5];9(3):71–8. Available from: https://link.springer.com/article/10.1007/s40139-021-00224-2

Good JS, Harrington KJ. The hallmarks of cancer and the radiation oncologist: Updating the 5Rs of radiobiology. Clin Oncol (R Coll Radiol) [Internet]. Clin Oncol (R Coll Radiol); 2013 Oct [cited 2023 Apr 5];25(10):569–77. Available from: https://pubmed.ncbi.nlm.nih.gov/23850153/

Gordon S. Phagocytosis: An immunobiologic process. Immunity. Cell Press; 2016 Mar 15;44(3):463–75.

Grimmer S, van Deurs B, Sandvig K. Membrane ruffling and macropinocytosis in A431 cells require cholesterol. J Cell Sci [Internet]. J Cell Sci; 2002 Jul 15 [cited 2023 May 1];115(Pt 14):2953–62. Available from: https://pubmed.ncbi.nlm.nih.gov/12082155/

Hagan CT, Medik YB, Wang AZ. Nanotechnology approaches to improving cancer immunotherapy. Adv Cancer Res [Internet]. Adv Cancer Res; 2018 Jan 1 [cited 2023 Apr 5];139:35–56. Available from: https://pubmed.ncbi.nlm.nih.gov/29941106/

Haider M, Abdin SM, Kamal L, Orive G. Nanostructured lipid carriers for delivery of chemotherapeutics: A review. Pharmaceutics [Internet]. Multidisciplinary Digital Publishing Institute; 2020 Mar 23 [cited 2023 Apr 5];12(3):288. Available from: https://www.mdpi.com/1999-4923/12/3/288/htm

Han B, Yang Y, Chen J, Tang H, Sun Y, Zhang Z, et al. Preparation, characterization, and pharmacokinetic study of a novel long-acting targeted paclitaxel liposome with antitumor activity. Int J Nanomedicine [Internet]. Dove Press; 2020 [cited 2023 Apr 5];15:553. Available from: /pmc/articles/PMC6986409/

Han X, Xu K, Taratula O, Farsad K. Applications of nanoparticles in biomedical imaging. Nanoscale [Internet]. NIH Public Access; 2019 Jan 1 [cited 2023 Apr 4];11(3):799. Available from: /pmc/articles/PMC8112886/

Hanafy NAN, El-Kemary M, Leporatti S. Micelles structure development as a strategy to improve smart cancer therapy. Cancers (Basel) [Internet]. Multidisciplinary Digital Publishing Institute (MDPI); 2018 Jul 20 [cited 2023 Apr 5];10(7). Available from: /pmc/articles/PMC6071246/

Harisinghani MG, Barentsz J, Hahn PF, Deserno WM, Tabatabaei S, van de Kaa CH, et al. Noninvasive detection of clinically occult lymph-node metastases in prostate cancer. N Engl J Med [Internet]. N Engl J Med; 2003 Jun 19 [cited 2023 Apr 5];348(25):2491–9. Available from: https://pubmed.ncbi.nlm.nih.gov/12815134/

Harrington K, Jankowska P, Hingorani M. Molecular biology for the radiation oncologist: The 5Rs of radiobiology meet the hallmarks of cancer. Clin Oncol. 2007 Oct;19(8):561–71.

Hill RP. The changing paradigm of tumour response to irradiation. British Journal of Radiology. British Institute of Radiology; 2017;90(1069).

Hoseini-Ghahfarokhi M, Mirkiani S, Mozaffari N, Abdolahi Sadatlu MA, Ghasemi A, Abbaspour S, et al. Applications of graphene and graphene oxide in smart drug/gene delivery: Is the world still flat? Int J Nanomedicine [Internet]. Dove Press; 2020 Nov 27 [cited 2023 Apr 5];15:9469–96. Available from: https://www.dovepress.com/applications-of-graphene-and-graphene-oxide-in-smart-druggene-delivery-peer-reviewed-fulltext-article-IJN

Howard MD, Jay M, Dziubla TD, Lu X. PEGylation of nanocarrier drug delivery systems: State of the art. J Biomed Nanotechnol. American Scientific Publishers; 2008 Jun;4(2):133–48.

Huang D, He B, Mi P. Calcium phosphate nanocarriers for drug delivery to tumors: Imaging, therapy and theranostics. Biomater Sci. Royal Society of Chemistry; 2019a Oct 1;7(10):3942–60.

Huang K, He Y, Zhu Z, Guo J, Wang G, Deng C, et al. Small, traceable, endosome-disrupting, and bioresponsive click nanogels fabricated via microfluidics for CD44-targeted cytoplasmic delivery of therapeutic proteins. ACS Appl Mater Interfaces [Internet]. ACS Appl Mater Interfaces; 2019b Jun 26 [cited 2023 May 1];11(25):22171–80. Available from: https://pubmed.ncbi.nlm.nih.gov/31190543/

Hung W-H, Chen P-K, Fang C-W, Lin Y-C, Wu P-C, Chen-H, et al. Preparation and evaluation of azelaic acid topical microemulsion formulation: In vitro and in vivo study. Pharmaceutics [Internet]. Multidisciplinary Digital Publishing Institute; 2021 Mar 19 [cited 2023 Apr 5];13(3):410. Available from: https://www.mdpi.com/1999-4923/13/3/410/htm

Im S, Lee J, Park D, Park A, Kim YM, Kim WJ. Hypoxia-triggered transforming immunomodulator for cancer immunotherapy via photodynamically enhanced antigen presentation of dendritic cell. ACS Nano [Internet]. ACS Nano; 2019 Jan 22 [cited 2023 May 1];13(1):476–88. Available from: https://pubmed.ncbi.nlm.nih.gov/30563320/

Ito A, Tanaka K, Honda H, Abe S, Yamaguchi H, Kobayashi T. Complete regression of mouse mammary carcinoma with a size greater than 15 mm by frequent repeated hyperthermia using magnetite nanoparticles. J Biosci Bioeng [Internet]. J Biosci Bioeng; 2003 [cited 2023 Apr 5];96(4):364–9. Available from: https://pubmed.ncbi.nlm.nih.gov/16233538/

Iyer AK, Khaled G, Fang J, Maeda H. Exploiting the enhanced permeability and retention effect for tumor targeting. Drug Discov Today. Elsevier Current Trends; 2006 Sep 1;11(17–18):812–8.

Jain RK. Barriers to drug delivery in solid tumors. Sci Am [Internet]. Sci Am; 1994 [cited 2023 Apr 4]; 271(1):58–65. Available from: https://pubmed.ncbi.nlm.nih.gov/8066425/

Jaiswal M, Dudhe R, Sharma PK. Nanoemulsion: An advanced mode of drug delivery system. 3 Biotech [Internet]. 3 Biotech; 2015 Apr 1 [cited 2023 Apr 5];5(2):123–7. Available from: https://pubmed.ncbi.nlm.nih.gov/28324579/

Jaiswal MK, Gogoi M, Dev Sarma H, Banerjee R, Bahadur D. Biocompatibility, biodistribution and efficacy of magnetic nanohydrogels in inhibiting growth of tumors in experimental mice models. Biomater Sci [Internet]. Biomater Sci; 2014 Mar [cited 2023 Apr 5];2(3):370–80. Available from: https://pubmed.ncbi.nlm.nih.gov/32481863/

Jia R, Teng L, Gao L, Su T, Fu L, Qiu Z, et al. Advances in multiple stimuli-responsive drug-delivery systems for cancer therapy. Int J Nanomedicine [Internet]. Dove Press; 2021a [cited 2023 Apr 4];16:1525. Available from: /pmc/articles/PMC7920594/

Jia R, Teng L, Gao L, Su T, Fu L, Qiu Z, et al. Advances in multiple stimuli-responsive drug-delivery systems for cancer therapy. Int J Nanomedicine [Internet]. Dove Press; 2021b [cited 2023 May 2];16:1525. Available from: /pmc/articles/PMC7920594/

Juan CA, de la Lastra JMP, Plou FJ, Pérez-Lebeña E. The chemistry of Reactive Oxygen Species (ROS) revisited: Outlining their role in biological macromolecules (DNA, lipids and proteins) and induced pathologies. International Journal of Molecular Sciences [Internet]. Multidisciplinary Digital Publishing Institute; 2021 Apr 28 [cited 2023 Apr 4];22(9):4642. Available from: https://www.mdpi.com/1422-0067/22/9/4642/htm

Jung HS, Verwilst P, Sharma A, Shin J, Sessler JL, Kim JS. Organic molecule-based photothermal agents: an expanding photothermal therapy universe. Chem Soc Rev [Internet]. R Soc Chem; 2018a Apr 3 [cited 2023 Apr 5];47(7):2280–97. Available from: https://pubs.rsc.org/en/content/articlehtml/2018/cs/c7cs00522a

Jung WR, Sierecki E, Bastiani M, O'Carroll A, Alexandrov K, Rae J, et al. Cell-free formation and interactome analysis of caveolae. J Cell Biol [Internet]. The Rockefeller University Press; 2018b Jun 6 [cited 2023 May 1];217(6):2141. Available from: /pmc/articles/PMC5987714/

Kamuhabwa A, Agostinis P, Ahmed B, Landuyt W, Van Cleynenbreugel B, Van Poppel H, et al. Hypericin as a potential phototherapeutic agent in superficial transitional cell carcinoma of the bladder. Photochemical and Photobiological Sciences. 2004 Aug 4;3(8):772–80.

Karthikeyan K, Babu A, Kim SJ, Murugesan R, Jeyasubramanian K. Enhanced photodynamic efficacy and efficient delivery of Rose Bengal using nanostructured poly(amidoamine) dendrimers: Potential application in photodynamic therapy of cancer. Cancer Nanotechnol [Internet]. BioMed Central; 2011 Dec 13 [cited 2023 Apr 5];2(1–6):95–103. Available from: https://cancer-nano.biomedcentral.com/articles/10.1007/s12645-011-0019-3

Khalifehzadeh R, Arami H. Biodegradable calcium phosphate nanoparticles for cancer therapy. Adv Colloid Interface Sci [Internet]. Adv Colloid Interface Sci; 2020 May 1 [cited 2023 Apr 5];279. Available from: https://pubmed.ncbi.nlm.nih.gov/32330734/

Klochkov SG, Neganova ME, Nikolenko VN, Chen K, Somasundaram SG, Kirkland CE, et al. Implications of nanotechnology for the treatment of cancer: Recent advances. Semin Cancer Biol. Academic Press; 2021 Feb 1;69:190–9.

Kok HP, Cressman ENK, Ceelen W, Brace CL, Ivkov R, Grüll H, et al. Heating technology for malignant tumors: A review. Int J Hyperthermia [Internet]. Int J Hyperthermia; 2020 Jan 1 [cited 2023 Apr 5];37(1):711–41. Available from: https://pubmed.ncbi.nlm.nih.gov/32579419/

Koksharov YA, Gubin SP, Taranov I V., Khomutov GB, Gulyaev Y V. Magnetic nanoparticles in medicine: Progress, problems, and advances. Journal of Communications Technology and Electronics [Internet]. Nature Publishing Group; 2022 Feb 1 [cited 2023 Apr 5];67(2):101. Available from: /pmc/articles/PMC8988108/

Koo OM, Rubinstein I, Onyuksel H. Role of nanotechnology in targeted drug delivery and imaging: A concise review. Nanomedicine [Internet]. Nanomedicine; 2005 Sep [cited 2023 Apr 5];1(3):193–212. Available from: https://pubmed.ncbi.nlm.nih.gov/17292079/

Kou L, Sun J, Zhai Y, He Z. The endocytosis and intracellular fate of nanomedicines: Implication for rational design. Asian J Pharm Sci [Internet]. Shenyang Pharmaceutical University; 2013 [cited 2023 Apr 4];8(1):1–10. Available from: https://www.researchgate.net/publication/271012064_The_endocytosis_and_intracellular_fate_of_nanomedicines_Implication_for_rational_design

Krauland AH, Alonso MJ. Chitosan/cyclodextrin nanoparticles as macromolecular drug delivery system. Int J Pharm. Elsevier; 2007 Aug 1;340(1–2):134–42.

Laurent S, Forge D, Port M, Roch A, Robic C, Vander Elst L, et al. Magnetic iron oxide nanoparticles: Synthesis, stabilization, vectorization, physicochemical characterizations, and biological applications. Chem Rev [Internet]. Chem Rev; 2008 Jun [cited 2023 Apr 3];108(6):2064–110. Available from: https://pubmed.ncbi.nlm.nih.gov/18543879/

Leach DG, Dharmaraj N, Piotrowski SL, Lopez-Silva TL, Lei YL, Sikora AG, et al. STINGel: Controlled release of a cyclic dinucleotide for enhanced cancer immunotherapy. Biomaterials. Elsevier; 2018 May 1;163:67–75.

Lee JY, Kapur M, Li M, Choi MC, Choi S, Kim HJ, et al. MFN1 deacetylation activates adaptive mitochondrial fusion and protects metabolically challenged mitochondria. J Cell Sci [Internet]. Company of Biologists Ltd; 2014 Nov 11 [cited 2023 May 1];127(22):4954–63. Available from: /pmc/articles/PMC4231308/

Legge CJ, Colley HE, Lawson MA, Rawlings AE. Targeted magnetic nanoparticle hyperthermia for the treatment of oral cancer. J Oral Pathol Med [Internet]. J Oral Pathol Med; 2019 Oct 1 [cited 2023 Apr 5];48(9):803–9. Available from: https://pubmed.ncbi.nlm.nih.gov/31309616/

Li M, Zhao G, Su WK, Shuai Q. Enzyme-responsive nanoparticles for anti-tumor drug delivery. Front Chem [Internet]. Front Chem; 2020 Jul 30 [cited 2023 Apr 4];8. Available from: https://pubmed.ncbi.nlm.nih.gov/32850662/

Li X, Liu J, Qiu N. Cyclodextrin-based polymeric drug delivery systems for cancer therapy. Polymers (Basel) [Internet]. MDPI AG; 2023 Mar 11 [cited 2023 Apr 5];15(6):1400. Available from: http://www.ncbi.nlm.nih.gov/pubmed/36987181

Li Y, Li Y, Zhang X, Xu X, Zhang Z, Hu C, et al. Supramolecular PEGylated dendritic systems as pH/Redox dual-responsive theranostic nanoplatforms for platinum drug delivery and NIR imaging. Theranostics [Internet]. Ivyspring International Publisher; 2016 [cited 2023 May 1];6(9):1293. Available from: /pmc/articles/PMC4924500/

Li Y, Yang J, Sun X. Reactive oxygen species-based nanomaterials for cancer therapy. Front Chem [Internet]. Front Chem; 2021 Apr 22 [cited 2023 Apr 4];9. Available from: https://pubmed.ncbi.nlm.nih.gov/33968899/

Liu HM, Zhang YF, Xie YD, Cai YF, Li BY, Li W, et al. Hypoxia-responsive ionizable liposome delivery siRNA for glioma therapy. Int J Nanomedicine [Internet]. Int J Nanomedicine; 2017a Feb 8 [cited 2023 May 1];12:1065–83. Available from: https://pubmed.ncbi.nlm.nih.gov/28223799/

Liu J, Liu K, Feng L, Liu Z, Xu L. Comparison of nanomedicine-based chemotherapy, photodynamic therapy and photothermal therapy using reduced graphene oxide for the model system. Biomater Sci [Internet]. R Soc Chem; 2017b Jan 31 [cited 2023 Apr 5];5(2):331–40. Available from: https://pubs.rsc.org/en/content/articlehtml/2017/bm/c6bm00526h

Liu J, Liu Y, Bu W, Bu J, Sun Y, Du J, et al. Ultrasensitive nanosensors based on upconversion nanoparticles for selective hypoxia imaging in vivo upon near-infrared excitation. J Am Chem Soc [Internet]. Am Chem Soc; 2014 Jul 9 [cited 2023 May 1];136(27):9701–9. Available from: https://pubs.acs.org/doi/abs/10.1021/ja5042989

Liu Y, Miyoshi H, Nakamura M. Nanomedicine for drug delivery and imaging: A promising avenue for cancer therapy and diagnosis using targeted functional nanoparticles. Int J Cancer [Internet]. Int J Cancer; 2007 Jun 15 [cited 2023 Apr 5];120(12):2527–37. Available from: https://pubmed.ncbi.nlm.nih.gov/17390371/

Lo ST, Kumar A, Hsieh JT, Sun X. Dendrimer nanoscaffolds for potential theranostics of prostate cancer with a focus on radiochemistry. Mol Pharm [Internet]. NIH Public Access; 2013 Mar 3 [cited 2023 Apr 5];10(3):793. Available from: /pmc/articles/PMC3599782/

Loebrich S. The role of F-actin in modulating clathrin-mediated endocytosis: Lessons from neurons in health and neuropsychiatric disorder. Commun Integr Biol [Internet]. Taylor & Francis; 2014 [cited 2023 May 1];7(4). Available from: /pmc/articles/PMC4091099/

Lu Z, Prouty MD, Quo Z, Golub VO, Kumar CSSR, Lvov YM. Magnetic switch of permeability for polyelectrolyte microcapsules embedded with Co@Au nanoparticles. Langmuir [Internet]. Langmuir; 2005 Mar 1 [cited 2023 Apr 5];21(5):2042–50. Available from: https://pubmed.ncbi.nlm.nih.gov/15723509/

Ma P, Dong X, Swadley CL, Gupte A, Leggas M, Ledebur HC, et al. Development of idarubicin and doxorubicin solid lipid nanoparticles to overcome Pgp-mediated multiple drug resistance in leukemia. J Biomed Nanotechnol [Internet]. J Biomed Nanotechnol; 2009 Apr [cited 2023 Apr 5];5(2):151–61. Available from: https://pubmed.ncbi.nlm.nih.gov/20055093/

Madani SY, Naderi N, Dissanayake O, Tan A, Seifalian AM. A new era of cancer treatment: Carbon nanotubes as drug delivery tools. Int J Nanomedicine [Internet]. Dove Press; 2011 [cited 2023 Apr 5];6:2963. Available from: /pmc/articles/PMC3230565/

Madhusudana Rao K, Krishna Rao KSV, Ramanjaneyulu G, Ha CS. Curcumin encapsulated pH sensitive gelatin based interpenetrating polymeric network nanogels for anti cancer drug delivery. Int J Pharm [Internet]. Int J Pharm; 2015 Jan 30 [cited 2023 May 1];478(2):788–95. Available from: https://pubmed.ncbi.nlm.nih.gov/25528297/

Maeda H, Wu J, Sawa T, Matsumura Y, Hori K. Tumor vascular permeability and the EPR effect in macromolecular therapeutics: A review. J Control Release [Internet]. J Control Release; 2000 Mar 1 [cited 2023 Apr 4];65(1–2):271–84. Available from: https://pubmed.ncbi.nlm.nih.gov/10699287/

Mahato M, Patra S, Gogoi M. Herbal nanocarriers for cancer therapy. 2021;41–75.

Majoros IJ, Thomas TP, Mehta CB, Baker JR. Poly(amidoamine) dendrimer-based multifunctional engineered nanodevice for cancer therapy. J Med Chem [Internet]. Am Chem Soc; 2005 Sep 22 [cited 2023 Apr 5];48(19):5892–9. Available from: https://pubs.acs.org/doi/abs/10.1021/jm0401863

Manzanares D, Ceña V. Endocytosis: The nanoparticle and submicron nanocompounds gateway into the cell. Pharmaceutics [Internet]. Multidisciplinary Digital Publishing Institute (MDPI); 2020 Apr 1 [cited 2023 Apr 4];12(4). Available from: /pmc/articles/PMC7238190/

Martín-Saldaña S, Palao-Suay R, Aguilar MR, García-Fernández L, Arévalo H, Trinidad A, et al. pH-sensitive polymeric nanoparticles with antioxidant and anti-inflammatory properties against cisplatin-induced hearing loss. J Controlled Release. Elsevier; 2018 Jan 28;270:53–64.

Martín-Saldaña S, Palao-Suay R, Aguilar MR, Ramírez-Camacho R, San Román J. Polymeric nanoparticles loaded with dexamethasone or α-tocopheryl succinate to prevent cisplatin-induced ototoxicity. Acta Biomater [Internet]. Acta Biomater; 2017 Apr 15 [cited 2023 Apr 5];53:199–210. Available from: https://pubmed.ncbi.nlm.nih.gov/28213099/

Masuko Y, Tazawa K, Sato H, Viroonchatapan E, Takemori S, Shimizu T, et al. Antitumor activity of selective hyperthermia in tumor-bearing rats using thermosensitive magnetoliposomes as a new hyperthermic material. http://dx.doi.org/10.3109/10717549709033186 [Internet]. Taylor & Francis; 1997 [cited 2023 Apr 5];4(1):37–42. Available from: https://www.tandfonline.com/doi/abs/10.3109/10717549709033186

Mattheolabakis G, Milane L, Singh A, Amiji MM. Hyaluronic acid targeting of CD44 for cancer therapy: From receptor biology to nanomedicine. J Drug Target [Internet]. J Drug Target; 2015 Sep 14 [cited 2023 Apr 4];23(7–8):605–18. Available from: https://pubmed.ncbi.nlm.nih.gov/26453158/

Mehnert W, Mäder K. Solid lipid nanoparticles: Production, characterization and applications. Adv Drug Deliv Rev [Internet]. 2012 Dec [cited 2023 Apr 5];64(SUPPL.):83–101. Available from: https://www.researchgate.net/publication/271580290_Solid_lipid_nanoparticles

Meng J, Fan J, Galiana G, Branca RT, Clasen PL, Ma S, et al. LHRH-functionalized superparamagnetic iron oxide nanoparticles for breast cancer targeting and contrast enhancement in MRI. Materials Science and Engineering: C. Elsevier; 2009 May 5;29(4):1467–79.

Metselaar JM, Lammers T. Challenges in nanomedicine clinical translation. Drug Deliv Transl Res [Internet]. Drug Deliv Transl Res; 2020 Jun 1 [cited 2023 Apr 5];10(3):721–5. Available from: https://pubmed.ncbi.nlm.nih.gov/32166632/

Mi P. Stimuli-responsive nanocarriers for drug delivery, tumor imaging, therapy and theranostics. Theranostics [Internet]. Ivyspring International Publisher; 2020 [cited 2023 Apr 4];10(10):4557. Available from: /pmc/articles/PMC7150471/

Mi P, Wang F, Nishiyama N, Cabral H. Molecular cancer imaging with polymeric nanoassemblies: From tumor detection to theranostics. Macromol Biosci [Internet]. John Wiley & Sons, Ltd; 2017 Jan 1 [cited 2023 Apr 4];17(1):1600305. Available from: https://onlinelibrary.wiley.com/doi/full/10.1002/mabi.201600305

Milton Harris J, Martin NE, Modi M. Pegylation: A novel process for modifying pharmacokinetics. Clin Pharmacokinet [Internet]. Adis International Ltd; 2001 Sep 14 [cited 2023 Apr 4];40(7):539–51. Available from: https://link.springer.com/article/10.2165/00003088-200140070-00005

Mishra B, Patel BB, Tiwari S. Colloidal nanocarriers: A review on formulation technology, types and applications toward targeted drug delivery. Nanomedicine. Elsevier; 2010 Feb 1;6(1):9–24.

Mousa SA, Bharali DJ. Nanotechnology-based detection and targeted therapy in cancer: Nano-bio paradigms and applications. Cancers (Basel) [Internet]. Multidisciplinary Digital Publishing Institute (MDPI); 2011 Sep [cited 2023 Apr 5];3(3):2888. Available from: /pmc/articles/PMC3759178/

Muhamad N, Plengsuriyakarn T, Na-Bangchang K. Application of active targeting nanoparticle delivery system for chemotherapeutic drugs and traditional/herbal medicines in cancer therapy: A systematic review. Int J Nanomedicine [Internet]. Int J Nanomedicine; 2018 Jul 4 [cited 2023 Apr 4];13:3921–35. Available from: https://pubmed.ncbi.nlm.nih.gov/30013345/

Muro S. Alterations in cellular processes involving vesicular trafficking and implications in drug delivery. Biomimetics [Internet]. Multidisciplinary Digital Publishing Institute (MDPI); 2018a Sep 1 [cited 2023 May 1];3(3). Available from: /pmc/articles/PMC6352689/

Muro S. Alterations in cellular processes involving vesicular trafficking and implications in drug delivery. Biomimetics [Internet]. Multidisciplinary Digital Publishing Institute (MDPI); 2018b Sep 1 [cited 2023 May 1];3(3). Available from: /pmc/articles/PMC6352689/

Nakamura H, Maeda H. Cancer chemotherapy. Fundamentals of Pharmaceutical Nanoscience [Internet]. StatPearls Publishing; 2023 Feb 27 [cited 2023 Apr 4];401–27. Available from: https://www.ncbi.nlm.nih.gov/books/NBK564367/

Narayanaswamy R, Torchilin VP. Hydrogels and their applications in targeted drug delivery. Molecules [Internet]. Molecules; 2019 Feb 8 [cited 2023 Apr 5];24(3). Available from: https://pubmed.ncbi.nlm.nih.gov/30744011/

Naseri N, Valizadeh H, Zakeri-Milani P. Solid lipid nanoparticles and nanostructured lipid carriers: Structure, preparation and application. Adv Pharm Bull [Internet]. Tabriz University of Medical Sciences; 2015 [cited 2023 Apr 5];5(3):305. Available from: /pmc/articles/PMC4616893/

Naz S, Wang M, Han Y, Hu B, Teng L, Zhou J, et al. Enzyme-responsive mesoporous silica nanoparticles for tumor cells and mitochondria multistage-targeted drug delivery. Int J Nanomedicine [Internet]. Dove Press; 2019 [cited 2023 Apr 4];14:2533–2542. Available from: /pmc/articles/PMC6497824/

Oerlemans C, Bult W, Bos M, Storm G, Nijsen JFW, Hennink WE. Polymeric micelles in anticancer therapy: Targeting, imaging and triggered release. Pharm Res [Internet]. Pharm Res; 2010 Dec [cited 2023 Apr 5];27(12):2569–89. Available from: https://pubmed.ncbi.nlm.nih.gov/20725771/

Ohulchanskyy TY, Roy I, Goswami LN, Chen Y, Bergey EJ, Pandey RK, et al. Organically modified silica nanoparticles with covalently incorporated photosensitizer for photodynamic therapy of cancer. Nano Lett [Internet]. Nano Lett; 2007 Sep [cited 2023 Apr 5];7(9):2835–42. Available from: https://pubmed.ncbi.nlm.nih.gov/17718587/

Peer D, Karp JM, Hong S, Farokhzad OC, Margalit R, Langer R. Nanocarriers as an emerging platform for cancer therapy. Nat Nanotechnol [Internet]. Nature Publishing Group; 2007 [cited 2023 Apr 4];2(12):751–60. Available from: https://www.nature.com/articles/nnano.2007.387

Phillips W, Willms E, Hill AF. Understanding extracellular vesicle and nanoparticle heterogeneity: Novel methods and considerations. Proteomics [Internet]. Proteomics; 2021 Jul 1 [cited 2023 Apr 5];21(13–14). Available from: https://pubmed.ncbi.nlm.nih.gov/33857352/

Piérard GE, Lachapelle JM, Frentz G, Schopf E, Stolz E. Hydrocortisone 17-butyrate topical emulsion (Locoid Crelo®) in psoriasis. Journal of the European Academy of Dermatology and Venereology. No longer published by Elsevier; 1996 Jan 1;6(1):11–4.

Qin F, Xu C, Hu J, Lei C, Zheng Z, Peng K, et al. Dissecting the cell entry pathway of baculovirus by single-particle tracking and quantitative electron microscopic analysis. J Virol [Internet]. American Society for Microbiology (ASM); 2019 Apr 4 [cited 2023 May 1];93(8). Available from: /pmc/articles/PMC6450101/

Qingnuan L, Yan X, Xiaodong Z, Ruili L, Qieqie D, Xiaoguang S, et al. Preparation of 99mTc-C60(OH)x and its biodistribution studies. Nucl Med Biol. Elsevier; 2002a Aug 1;29(6):707–10.

Qingnuan L, Yan X, Xiaodong Z, Ruili L, Qieqie D, Xiaoguang S, et al. Preparation of 99mTc-C60(OH)x and its biodistribution studies. Nucl Med Biol. Elsevier; 2002b Aug 1;29(6):707–10.

Rak J, Kabesova M, Benes J, Pouckova P, Vetvicka D. Advances in liposome-encapsulated phthalocyanines for photodynamic therapy. Life (Basel) [Internet]. MDPI; 2023 Jan 21 [cited 2023 Apr 5];13(2). Available from: http://www.ncbi.nlm.nih.gov/pubmed/36836662

Rasool M, Malik A, Waquar S, Arooj M, Zahid S, Asif M, et al. New challenges in the use of nanomedicine in cancer therapy. Bioengineered [Internet]. Bioengineered; 2022 [cited 2023 Apr 5];13(1):759–73. Available from: https://pubmed.ncbi.nlm.nih.gov/34856849/

Reza Saboktakin M, Tabatabaie RM, Maharramov A, Ali Ramazanov M. Synthesis and in vitro studies of biodegradable modified chitosan nanoparticles for photodynamic treatment of cancer. Int J Biol Macromol [Internet]. Int J Biol Macromol; 2011 [cited 2023 Apr 5];49(5):1059–65. Available from: https://pubmed.ncbi.nlm.nih.gov/21907233/

Rocca JD, Werner ME, Kramer SA, Huxford-Phillips RC, Sukumar R, Cummings ND, et al. Polysilsesquioxane nanoparticles for triggered release of cisplatin and effective cancer chemoradiotherapy. Nanomedicine [Internet]. Nanomedicine; 2015 Jan 1 [cited 2023 Apr 5];11(1):31–8. Available from: https://pubmed.ncbi.nlm.nih.gov/25038495/

Rommasi F, Esfandiari N. Liposomal nanomedicine: Applications for drug delivery in cancer therapy. Nanoscale Res Lett [Internet]. Nanoscale Res Lett; 2021 [cited 2023 Apr 4];16(1):95–. Available from: https://pubmed.ncbi.nlm.nih.gov/34032937/

Safavi-Sohi R, Maghari S, Raoufi M, Jalali SA, Hajipour MJ, Ghassempour A, et al. Bypassing protein corona issue on active targeting: Zwitterionic coatings dictate specific interactions of targeting moieties and cell receptors. ACS Appl Mater Interfaces [Internet]. Am Chem Soc; 2016 Sep 7 [cited 2023 Apr 4];8(35):22808–18. Available from: https://pubs.acs.org/doi/abs/10.1021/acsami.6b05099

Salústio PJ, Pontes P, Conduto C, Sanches I, Carvalho C, Arrais J, et al. Advanced technologies for oral controlled release: Cyclodextrins for oral controlled release. AAPS PharmSciTech. 2011 Dec;12(4):1276–92.

Sanchez VC, Jachak A, Hurt RH, Kane AB. Biological interactions of graphene-family nanomaterials: An interdisciplinary review. Chem Res Toxicol [Internet]. Chem Res Toxicol; 2012a Jan 13 [cited 2023 Apr 5];25(1):15–34. Available from: https://pubmed.ncbi.nlm.nih.gov/21954945/

Sanchez VC, Jachak A, Hurt RH, Kane AB. Biological interactions of graphene-family nanomaterials: An interdisciplinary review. Chem Res Toxicol [Internet]. Ame Chem Soc; 2012b Jan 13 [cited 2023 May 2];25(1):15–34. Available from: https://pubs.acs.org/doi/abs/10.1021/tx200339h

Sattari S, Adeli M, Beyranvand S, Nemati M. Functionalized graphene platforms for anticancer drug delivery. Int J Nanomed [Internet]. Int J Nanomed; 2021 [cited 2023 Apr 5];16:5955–80. Available from: https://pubmed.ncbi.nlm.nih.gov/34511900/

Schroeder A, Heller DA, Winslow MM, Dahlman JE, Pratt GW, Langer R, et al. Treating metastatic cancer with nanotechnology. Nat Rev Cancer [Internet]. Nat Rev Cancer; 2011 Jan [cited 2023 Apr 5];12(1):39–50. Available from: https://pubmed.ncbi.nlm.nih.gov/22193407/

Shams F, Golchin A, Azari A, Mohammadi Amirabad L, Zarein F, Khosravi A, et al. Nanotechnology-based products for cancer immunotherapy. Mol Biol Rep. Springer Science and Business Media B.V.; 2022 Feb 1;49(2):1389–412.

Shang T, Yu X, Han S, Yang B. Nanomedicine-based tumor photothermal therapy synergized immunotherapy. Biomater Sci [Internet]. R Soc Chem; 2020 Sep 30 [cited 2023 Apr 5];8(19):5241–59. Available from: https://pubs.rsc.org/en/content/articlehtml/2020/bm/d0bm01158d

Sharma G, Parchur AK, Jagtap JM, Hansen CP, Joshi A. Hybrid nanostructures in targeted drug delivery. Hybrid Nanostructures for Cancer Theranostics [Internet]. Elsevier; 2018 Nov 26 [cited 2023 Apr 4];1–10. Available from: https://www.researchgate.net/publication/330056086_Hybrid_Nanostructures_in_Targeted_Drug_Delivery

Shi Y, Liu M, Deng F, Zeng G, Wan Q, Zhang X, et al. Recent progress and development on polymeric nanomaterials for photothermal therapy: A brief overview. J Mater Chem B [Internet]. R Soc Chem; 2017 Jan 4 [cited 2023 Apr 5];5(2):194–206. Available from: https://pubs.rsc.org/en/content/articlehtml/2017/tb/c6tb02249a

Shin WK, Cho J, Kannan AG, Lee YS, Kim DW. Cross-linked composite gel polymer electrolyte using mesoporous methacrylate-functionalized SiO2 nanoparticles for lithium-Ion polymer batteries. Sci Rep [Internet]. Nature Publishing Group; 2016 May 18 [cited 2023 Apr 3];6(1):1–10. Available from: https://www.nature.com/articles/srep26332

Shinkai M, Yanase M, Honda H, Wakabayashi T, Yoshida J, Kobayashi T. Intracellular hyperthermia for cancer using magnetite cationic liposomes: In vitro study. Jpn J Cancer Res [Internet]. Wiley-Blackwell; 1996 [cited 2023 Apr 5];87(11):1179–1183. Available from: /pmc/articles/PMC5921008/

Siram K, Habibur Rahman SM, Balakumar K, Duganath N, Chandrasekar R, Hariprasad R. Pharmaceutical nanotechnology: Brief perspective on lipid drug delivery and its current scenario. Biomedical Applications of Nanoparticles. William Andrew Publishing; 2019 Jan 1;91–115.

Sriraman SK, Aryasomayajula B, & Torchilin VP. Barriers to drug delivery in solid tumors. Tissue Barriers; 2014; 2(3), e29528-1-e29528-10. https://doi.org/10.4161/TISB.29528

Soe HMSH, Maw PD, Loftsson T, Jansook P. A current overview of cyclodextrin-based nanocarriers for enhanced antifungal delivery. Pharmaceuticals (Basel) [Internet]. MDPI; 2022 Nov 22 [cited 2023 Apr 5];15(12). Available from: http://www.ncbi.nlm.nih.gov/pubmed/36558897

Sokolova V, Epple M. Biological and medical applications of calcium phosphate nanoparticles. Chemistry [Internet]. Chemistry; 2021 May 12 [cited 2023 Apr 5];27(27):7471–88. Available from: https://pubmed.ncbi.nlm.nih.gov/33577710/

Sudimack J, Lee RJ. Targeted drug delivery via the folate receptor. Adv Drug Deliv Rev [Internet]. Adv Drug Deliv Rev; 2000 Mar 30 [cited 2023 Apr 4];41(2):147–62. Available from: https://pubmed.ncbi.nlm.nih.gov/10699311/

Tang L, Xiao Q, Mei Y, He S, Zhang Z, Wang R, et al. Insights on functionalized carbon nanotubes for cancer theranostics. J Nanobiotechnol [Internet]. BioMed Central; 2021 Dec 16 [cited 2023 Apr 5];19(1):1–28. Available from: https://jnanobiotechnology.biomedcentral.com/articles/10.1186/s12951-021-01174-y

Thomas J, Beinhorn C, Norton D, Richardson M, Sumler SS, Frenkel M. Managing radiation therapy side effects with complementary medicine. J Soc Integr Oncol [Internet]. 2010 Mar [cited 2023 Apr 4];8(2):65–80. Available from: https://www.researchgate.net/publication/43133525_Managing_radiation_therapy_side_effects_with_complementary_medicine

Thorat ND, Bauer J. Functional smart hybrid nanostructures based nanotheranostic approach for advanced cancer treatment. Appl Surf Sci. Elsevier B.V.; 2020 Oct 15;527.

Tiwari JN, Tiwari RN, Kim KS. Zero-dimensional, one-dimensional, two-dimensional and three-dimensional nanostructured materials for advanced electrochemical energy devices. Prog Mater Sci. Pergamon; 2012 May 1;57(4):724–803.

Tohme S, Simmons RL, Tsung A. Surgery for cancer: A trigger for metastases. Cancer Res [Internet]. American Association for Cancer Research Inc.; 2017 Apr 1 [cited 2023 Apr 4];77(7):1548–52. Available from: https://aacrjournals.org/cancerres/article/77/7/1548/624854/Surgery-for-Cancer-A-Trigger-for-MetastasesSurgery

van der Meel R, Sulheim E, Shi Y, Kiessling F, Mulder WJM, Lammers T. Smart cancer nanomedicine. Nat Nanotechnol 2019 14:11 [Internet]. Nature Publishing Group; 2019 Nov 6 [cited 2023 Apr 4]; 14(11):1007–17. Available from: https://www.nature.com/articles/s41565-019-0567-y

Vijayan V, Reddy KR, Sakthivel S, Swetha C. Optimization and characterization of repaglinide biodegradable polymeric nanoparticle loaded transdermal patchs: In vitro and in vivo studies. Colloids Surf B Biointerfaces [Internet]. Colloids Surf B Biointerfaces; 2013 Nov 1 [cited 2023 Apr 5];111:150–5. Available from: https://pubmed.ncbi.nlm.nih.gov/23792547/

Vila-Caballer M, Codolo G, Munari F, Malfanti A, Fassan M, Rugge M, et al. A pH-sensitive stearoyl-PEG-poly(methacryloyl sulfadimethoxine)-decorated liposome system for protein delivery: An application for bladder cancer treatment. J Control Release [Internet]. J Control Release; 2016 Sep 28 [cited 2023 May 1];238:31–42. Available from: https://pubmed.ncbi.nlm.nih.gov/27444816/

VP S. Non-degradable biocompatible polymers in medicine: Past, present and future. Curr Pharm Biotechnol [Internet]. Curr Pharm Biotechnol; 2003 Mar 25 [cited 2023 Apr 5];4(5):331–7. Available from: https://pubmed.ncbi.nlm.nih.gov/14529423/

Wang AZ, Gu F, Zhang L, Chan JM, Radovic-Moreno A, Shaikh MR, et al. Biofunctionalized targeted nanoparticles for therapeutic applications. Expert Opin Biol Ther. 2008 Aug;8(8):1063–70.

Wang M, Wang Y, Hu K, Shao N, Cheng Y. Tumor extracellular acidity activated "off-on" release of bortezomib from a biocompatible dendrimer. Biomater Sci [Internet]. Biomater Sci; 2015 Mar 1 [cited 2023 May 1]; 3(3):480–9. Available from: https://pubmed.ncbi.nlm.nih.gov/26222291/

Wang Q, Atluri K, Tiwari AK, Babu RJ. Exploring the application of micellar drug delivery systems in cancer nanomedicine. Pharmaceuticals (Basel) [Internet]. MDPI AG; 2023 Mar 12 [cited 2023 Apr 4];16(3):433. Available from: http://www.ncbi.nlm.nih.gov/pubmed/36986532

Wang S, Ni D, Yue H, Luo N, Xi X, Wang Y, et al. Exploration of antigen induced CaCO3 nanoparticles for therapeutic vaccine. Small [Internet]. Small; 2018 Apr 5 [cited 2023 May 1];14(14). Available from: https://pubmed.ncbi.nlm.nih.gov/29468827/

Wang Y, Kohane DS. External triggering and triggered targeting strategies for drug delivery. Nat Rev Mater [Internet]. Springer Nature America, Inc; 2017 May 9 [cited 2023 Apr 4];2. Available from: https://www.scienceopen.com/document?vid=71af8556-4320-4baa-a0c9-1f98f4b0b6d0

Wang Y, Shang W, Niu M, Tian J, Xu K. Hypoxia-active nanoparticles used in tumor theranostic. Int J Nanomedicine [Internet]. Dove Press; 2019 [cited 2023 Apr 4];14:3705. Available from: /pmc/articles/PMC6535445/

Wang Y, Yu L, Han L, Sha X, Fang X. Difunctional pluronic copolymer micelles for paclitaxel delivery: Synergistic effect of folate-mediated targeting and Pluronic-mediated overcoming multidrug resistance in tumor cell lines. Int J Pharm [Internet]. Int J Pharm; 2007 Jun 7 [cited 2023 Apr 5];337(1–2):63–73. Available from: https://pubmed.ncbi.nlm.nih.gov/17289311/

Willms E, Cabañas C, Mäger I, Wood MJA, Vader P. Extracellular vesicle heterogeneity: Subpopulations, isolation techniques, and diverse functions in cancer progression. Front Immunol. Frontiers Media S.A.; 2018 Apr 30;9(APR).

Witwer KW, Wolfram J. Extracellular vesicles versus synthetic nanoparticles for drug delivery. Nature Reviews Materials [Internet]. Nature Publishing Group; 2021 Jan 7 [cited 2023 Apr 5];6(2):103–6. Available from: https://www.nature.com/articles/s41578-020-00277-6

Xiong Y, Schneider J, Ushakova E V., Rogach AL. Influence of molecular fluorophores on the research field of chemically synthesized carbon dots. Nano Today [Internet]. Elsevier B.V.; 2018 Dec 1 [cited 2023 Apr 5];23:124–39. Available from: https://www.researchgate.net/publication/329065841_Influence_of_molecular_fluorophores_on_the_research_field_of_chemically_synthesized_carbon_dots

Xu ZP, Zeng QH, Lu GQ, Yu AB. Inorganic nanoparticles as carriers for efficient cellular delivery. Chem Eng Sci. Pergamon; 2006 Feb 1;61(3):1027–40.

Yang G, Phua SZF, Lim WQ, Zhang R, Feng L, Liu G, et al. A hypoxia-responsive albumin-based nanosystem for deep tumor penetration and excellent therapeutic efficacy. Adv Mater [Internet]. Adv Mater; 2019 Jun 20 [cited 2023 May 1];31(25). Available from: https://pubmed.ncbi.nlm.nih.gov/31069885/

Yang G, Xu L, Chao Y, Xu J, Sun X, Wu Y, et al. Hollow MnO2 as a tumor-microenvironment-responsive biodegradable nano-platform for combination therapy favoring antitumor immune responses. Nature Communications [Internet]. Nature Publishing Group; 2017 Oct 12 [cited 2023 May 1];8(1):1–13. Available from: https://www.nature.com/articles/s41467-017-01050-0

Yao Y, Zhou Y, Liu L, Xu Y, Chen Q, Wang Y, et al. Nanoparticle-based drug delivery in cancer therapy and its role in overcoming drug resistance. Front Mol Biosci. Frontiers Media S.A.; 2020 Aug 20;7:193.

Yeingst TJ, Arrizabalaga JH, Hayes DJ. Ultrasound-induced drug release from stimuli-responsive hydrogels. Gels [Internet]. Multidisciplinary Digital Publishing Institute (MDPI); 2022 Sep 1 [cited 2023 Apr 4];8(9). Available from: /pmc/articles/PMC9498906/

Yi Y, Lin G, Chen S, Liu J, Zhang H, Mi P. Polyester micelles for drug delivery and cancer theranostics: Current achievements, progresses and future perspectives. Mater Sci Eng C Mater Biol Appl [Internet]. Mater Sci Eng C Mater Biol Appl; 2018 Feb 1 [cited 2023 Apr 4];83:218–32. Available from: https://pubmed.ncbi.nlm.nih.gov/29208282/

Yoo Y, Yoon SJ, Kim SY, Lee DW, Um S, Hyun H, et al. A local drug delivery system based on visible light-cured glycol chitosan and doxorubicin hydrochloride for thyroid cancer treatment in vitro and in vivo. Drug Deliv [Internet]. Drug Deliv; 2018 [cited 2023 Apr 5];25(1):1664–71. Available from: https://pubmed.ncbi.nlm.nih.gov/30183420/

Zhan F, Chen W, Wang Z, Lu W, Cheng R, Deng C, et al. Acid-activatable prodrug nanogels for efficient intracellular doxorubicin release. Biomacromolecules [Internet]. Biomacromolecules; 2011 Oct 10 [cited 2023 May 1];12(10):3612–20. Available from: https://pubmed.ncbi.nlm.nih.gov/21905663/

Zhang C, Yan L, Wang X, Zhu S, Chen C, Gu Z, et al. Progress, challenges, and future of nanomedicine. Nano Today. Elsevier; 2020 Dec 1;35:101008.

Zhang X, Xia LY, Chen X, Chen Z, Wu FG. Hydrogel-based phototherapy for fighting cancer and bacterial infection. Sci China Mater [Internet]. Science China Press; 2017a Jun 1 [cited 2023 Apr 4]; 60(6):487–503. Available from: https://www.researchgate.net/publication/317841237_Hydrogel-based_phototherapy_for_fighting_cancer_and_bacterial_infection

Zhang X, Xia LY, Chen X, Chen Z, Wu FG. Hydrogel-based phototherapy for fighting cancer and bacterial infection. Sci China Mater [Internet]. Science China Press; 2017b Jun 1 [cited 2023 Apr 5];60(6): 487–503. Available from: https://link.springer.com/article/10.1007/s40843-017-9025-3

Zhang Y, Li M, Gao X, Chen Y, Liu T. Nanotechnology in cancer diagnosis: Progress, challenges and opportunities. J Hematol Oncol [Internet]. BioMed Central Ltd.; 2019 Dec 17 [cited 2023 May 1];12(1):1–13. Available from: https://jhoonline.biomedcentral.com/articles/10.1186/s13045-019-0833-3

Zhang YS, Khademhosseini A. Advances in engineering hydrogels. Science [Internet]. Science; 2017 May 5 [cited 2023 Apr 4];356(6337). Available from: https://pubmed.ncbi.nlm.nih.gov/28473537/

Zhao X, Bagwe RP, Tan W. Development of organic-dye-doped silica nanoparticles in a reverse microemulsion. Advanced Materials [Internet]. 2004 Jan 16 [cited 2023 Apr 5];16(2):173–6. Available from: https://www.researchgate.net/publication/229935981_Development_of_Organic-Dye-Doped_Silica_Nanoparticles_in_a_Reverse_Microemulsion

Zhao X, Yang L, Li X, Jia X, Liu L, Zeng J, et al. Functionalized graphene oxide nanoparticles for cancer cell-specific delivery of antitumor drug. Bioconjug Chem [Internet]. Bioconjug Chem; 2015 Jan 21 [cited 2023 Apr 5];26(1):128–36. Available from: https://pubmed.ncbi.nlm.nih.gov/25525819/ Full article: Nanoparticles as carriers for drug delivery in cancer [Internet]. [cited 2023 Apr 5]. Available from: https://www.tandfonline.com/doi/full/10.1080/21691401.2018.1457039

2 Computational Modeling of Nano Drug Delivery Systems in Cancer

Kata Krishna Prasad,[1] *Samayaditya Singh*,[1]
Sachin B. Undre,[3] *and Pramod R. Somvanshi*[1,2]
[1]Physiological Systems Engineering and Computational Medicine Laboratory, Department of Systems and Computational Biology, School of Life Sciences, University of Hyderabad, Hyderabad, Telangana, India
[2]Asian Centre for Endocrine Pancreas and Diabetes Research, Asian Healthcare Foundation, Asian Institute of Gastroenterology, Hyderabad, Telangana, India
[3]Department of Chemistry, Institute of Sciences, Silver Oak University, Ahmedabad, Gujrat, India

2.1 INTRODUCTION

The word "nano" originated from the Latin word *nānus*, meaning dwarf, and is frequently used as a prefix for one billionth (10^{-9}) encountered in science. The use of nanotechnology in medicine includes the application of nanomaterials and biological hardware, as well as nanoelectronic biosensors. Nanomedicine was revolutionized by the usage of nanoparticles (NPs) in cancer treatment by targeted delivery, reduced toxicity, and enhancing drug bioavailability. They offer controlled drug release and improved cellular uptake with increased safety and efficacy compared to conventional therapies. Due to the higher drug loading capacity, targeted delivery minimizes side effects on healthy tissues. Despite advancements in cancer nanomedicine, toxicity of nanoscale compounds continues to hinder its clinical translation. NP-based formulations (nanocarriers) transport cargos that are unsafe, insoluble, rapidly removed, or unreliable for delivery as free molecules (e.g., chemotherapeutic drugs, silencing RNAs).

2.2 NANOMEDICINE DRUG DELIVERY IN CANCERS

Through the enhanced permeability and retention (EPR) effect, NPs facilitate improved tissue penetration for tumor targeting. Extravasating through leaky tumor vasculature, NPs can improve drug accumulation [1], thereby solving probable drug-resistance s [2]. Encapsulation within nanoparticles protects drugs from degradation by enzymes or hydrolysis, enhancing stability during transit through harsh environments like the gastrointestinal tract or bloodstream. NPs can be functionalized with ligands or other molecules for targeted delivery, improving specificity and reducing side effects. For instance, PEGylation or antibody conjugation enhances targeting. Both processes—that is, EPR and surface functionalization—have demonstrated that NPs alter the cargo's pharmacokinetics (PK) and increase its half-life in circulation, which promotes delivery to the tumor and lessens collateral harm to healthy cells [3]. There are mother vessels, feeding arteries, glomeruloid

 DOI: 10.1201/9781003799351-2

microvascular proliferations (GMP), capillaries, draining veins, and vascular malformations—distinctly six various forms of tumor blood vessels. On average, a mere 0.7% dose of injected NPs reaches the tumor [4]. NP drug delivery systems come in various forms, broadly categorized into organic and inorganic types. Some of these include liposomes, polymeric NPs, micelles, dendrimers, lipid NPs, gold NPs (AuNPs), mesoporous silica NPs (MSNs), iron oxide NPs (IONPs), quantum dots (QDs), carbon-based NPs (carbon nanotubes, graphene), and hybrid NPs. Table 2.1 lists various types of NP drug delivery systems.

Among various nanocarriers, dendrimers are unique synthetic macromolecules with highly branched, tree-like structures that offer exceptional molecular-level control and versatility. Their defined architecture, functional diversity, and active surface chemistry make them valuable in nanomedicine applications. Dendrimers possess a central core, repetitive branching units, and a functionalized outer surface, enabling precise molecular weight and size control for predictable biological behavior. A novel methodology proposes interchanging the traditional roles of core and branching units, allowing cores to act as branches and vice versa [5]. This dynamic flexibility creates dendrimers with larger internal voids and improved binding capabilities, paving the way for advanced drug delivery systems [6]. The primary advantage of dendritic molecules lies in their large surface area and internal cavities, which are crucial for sustained and targeted drug delivery. By redefining core and branch functionalities, structural flexibility and enhanced performance are introduced, positioning dendrimers as revolutionary platforms in nanomedicine. Dendrimers offer several key advantages in drug delivery systems. Their branched, three-dimensional architecture enables a high drug loading capacity, allowing numerous drug molecules to be encapsulated within their structure or conjugated to their surface. Additionally, dendrimers can be surface-modified with ligands

TABLE 2.1
List of Different Types of NP Drug Delivery Systems Available and Accepted by the U.S. Food and Drug Administration

Sr. No	Type	Example	Drug/Mechanism	Cancer Type	Clinical Trial Stage
1.	Liposomes	Doxil	Doxorubicin	Ovarian, Kaposi's sarcoma	FDA approved
2.	Polymeric NPs	Abraxane	Paclitaxel	Breast, lung, pancreatic	FDA approved
3.	Micelles	Genexol—PM	Paclitaxel	Breast, lung	FDA approved
4.	Dendrimers	PAMAM—methotrexate	methotrexate	Ovarian, lung	Methotrexate is FDA approved but PAMAM-methotrexate is preclinical.
5.	Lipid NPs	mRNA—4157	mRNA (neoantigen vaccine)	Melanoma, HNSCC, solid tumors	Phase 3 ongoing
6.	AuNPs	AuroLase	Photothermal + doxorubicin	Prostate	FDA approved
7.	Silica NPs	MSNs—camptothecin	Camptothecin	Colorectal, breast	Research/Early Preclinical
8.	IONPs	NanoTherm	Hyperthermia + cisplatin	Glioblastoma	Ongoing/recruiting
9.	Quantum Dots	QD—doxorubicin	Doxorubicin	Breast	Preclinical
10.	Carbon-based NPs	SWCNT-cisplatin	Cisplatin	Lung, ovarian	Cisplatin is FDA approved but SWCNT-cisplatin is preclinical

such as peptides, antibodies, or folic acid, which facilitate selective binding to specific cell receptors, thereby improving delivery efficiency and reducing side effects [7]. They also possess stimuli-responsive properties, where engineered functional groups respond to environmental triggers like pH, temperature, or enzymes, enabling controlled and sustained drug release [8]. These material properties provide greater advantage in engineering nano-carrier-based drug delivery systems in cancer for better therapeutic outcomes.

2.3 CHALLENGES OF NANOMEDICINE DELIVERY IN TUMOR MICROENVIRONMENT

There are several biophysical limitations that may hinder tumor accessibility by NPs, necessitating better comprehension of bio-nano interactions. Distinguishing between cancerous and normal cells (target specificity) to reduce peripheral deterioration still remains a challenge in drug delivery. When NPs are administered, they encounter biological fluids like blood plasma and produce a protein corona made up of adsorbed proteins which modifies the surface characteristics, size, and charge of the NP, affecting its clearance and biodistribution. Macroscale drugs mainly dissolve and diffuse, with limited ability to penetrate deep into tissues, however by exploiting a mechanism called endocytosis, NPs get absorbed by the cells rather than just diffusing through cell membranes [9]. NPs mainly diffuse after they enter the tumor interstitium succeeding the capillary extravasation because they are exposed to a damaging microenvironment that reduces fluid transport. This significantly reduces the cargo delivery and penetration distance to malignant cells that are far from the capillaries that feed the tumor. NPs must obtain near-wall access through a process known as margination, which is dependent on size, shape, and hematocrit [10,11]. Therefore, the removal of NPs from the body and their entire biodistribution are defined by an intricate relationship between these small processes within blood capillaries, which has

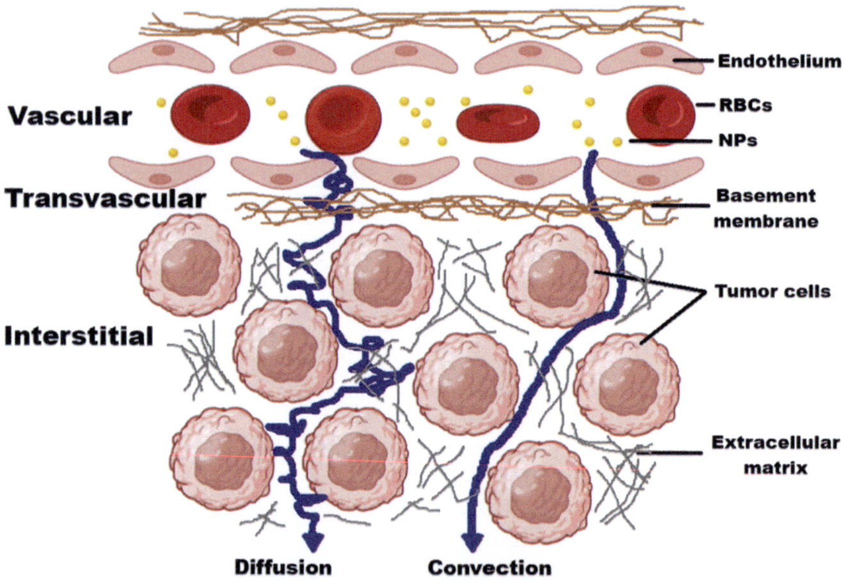

FIGURE 2.1 Macromolecular transport from injection site to target site. NP delivery to the site of action is carried out by perfusion in the vascular region, permeability and hydraulic conductivity in the transvascular region, and diffusion in the interstitial region.

Source: The data are sourced from [20].

a significant impact on the transport of NPs to tumors [12]. Figure 2.1 describes the diffusion of NPs occurring after they enter the tumor interstitium subsequent to capillary extravasation because they are exposed to a hostile microenvironment that reduces convective transport. This severely restricts the cargo delivery and penetration distance to malignant cells that are far from the capillaries [13,14,15,16].

Innovative approaches improvise targeting, getting beyond biological barriers, and disrupting resistance mechanisms thereby enhancing the cancer treatment. Mathematical models that account for the biophysics for the NP drug delivery to the tumor microenvironment serve as the predictive tools to analyze the drug bioavailability. These help in accurate simulations of nanoparticle behavior during therapy as the dynamic models that take into account time-dependent changes in tumor microenvironments and physiology. More precise predictions and effective treatment plans would result from these models' representation of the intricacies of how tumors change, and how the body reacts over time, boosting accuracy of drug delivery and their efficacy in cancer treatment [9,17,18]. Furthermore, organs such as the liver and spleen frequently quickly remove NPs from the bloodstream in vivo, decreasing their capacity to target malignancies. Such effects can be modeled using PKPD modeling framework to determine optimal dosing strategies.

2.4 MATHEMATICAL MODELING FOR CANCER NANOMEDICINE

To enhance tumor delivery and therapeutic efficacy of nanomedicines, the mathematical models take into account the intricate interactions between biological processes (such as transport, absorption, and clearance) and NPs' physicochemical characteristics (such as size, shape, and net surface charge/zeta potential). By conventional methods, comprehending the complex interactions between NPs and protein corona creation, macrophage clearance, and tumor microenvironment barriers are difficult. Iterative clinical studies, which are time-consuming and resource-intensive, are typically used to optimize delivery. Testing multiple NP sizes or shapes experimentally requires synthesizing and evaluating each variant separately. Usage of one-size-fits-all protocols and ignoring inter-patient variability (e.g., tumor vascularity, EPR effect differences) can be erroneous. Traditional approaches struggle to determine the long-term effectiveness or toxicity of NPs and rely on short-term clinical objectives (such as tumor reduction). Barriers such as high interstitial fluid pressure or dense extracellular matrix make it difficult for NPs to penetrate tumors. However, this is difficult to measure or treat experimentally without a lot of imaging or biopsies [19].

To overcome these shortcomings, kinetic models quantify these interactions (e.g., protein binding rates) by offering mechanistic insights into how NP features (size, charge) affect behavior enabling precise NP design (e.g., optimal size <100 nm). Pharmacokinetic (PK) and multiscale models predict NP biodistribution, drug release, tumor cell kill rates and tumor accumulation by simulating variables like circulation half-life and EPR effect, identifying ideal NP characteristics (e.g., PEGylation for prolonged circulation) by pre-screening designs computationally [19]. Individual tumors' high interstitial fluid pressure is considered by tumor deliverability models, thereby personalizing it.

Protein corona formation alters NPs' biological characteristics. Coarse-grained molecular dynamics simulations or kinetic models are best suited to mathematically describe this process. The biochemically changed NPs are delivered to the tumor and other organs by blood after corona formation. At the microscopic or mesoscopic length scales, discrete, hybrid, or continuous models are used to simulate the processes that occur during transit. Discrete modeling techniques are used to simulate cellular absorption of NPs once they reach the wall or flow out into the extravascular region. Pharmacokinetic models describe the whole-body distribution and stripping of NPs resulting from nanoscale biointeractions, while hybrid modeling approaches are used to study particle deliverability to tumors. Lastly, pharmacodynamic models are used to assess the toxicity and effectiveness of nanotherapy.

2.4.1 Overview of Mathematical Modeling

Using mathematical equations, structures, and computer techniques, mathematical modeling is a potent tool used in many different fields to represent, examine, and forecast the behavior of complex systems qualitatively and quantitatively. In order to grasp the underlying dynamics, mathematical modeling reduces reality to straightforward algebraic expressions or to computational systems, depending on the complexity of the task. Various types of mathematical models based on their structure, purpose, and the system they represent are categorized. For example, deterministic, stochastic and continuous models etc.

Ordinary Differential Equations (ODEs) are mathematical equations that relate a function to its derivatives with respect to a single independent variable. Typically, functions represent any physical quantity, and the independent variable is time.

$$\frac{dy}{dt} = f(t, y)$$

Here $y(t)$ is the unknown function (e.g., drug concentration), $\frac{dy}{dt}$ is the derivative of y with respect to time t and $f(t, y)$ is a function that defines how y changes over time. ODEs are deterministic in nature and are used to model dynamic systems. They simulate for a given set of initial conditions and parameters; the outcome is uniquely defined. Key features of ODEs like order (1st or 2nd), linearity/nonlinearity in the simulation etc. govern its quantitative and dynamic behavior. Here we discuss three different scenarios of the applications of the mathematical models to study cancer nanomedicine drug delivery ranging from a PK-PD for plain drug delivery (Case I), bioavailability/PK-PD of NP based drug delivery (Case II) and a detailed physiologically based pharmacokinetic (PBPK) model that accounts for systemic drug distribution and clearance effects (Case III).

2.4.2 Case I: Modeling PK-PD of Cancer Drug Delivery

To get a better understanding of the usage of mathematical models in cancer, we will look at a basic theoretical framework for cisplatin's cellular pharmacodynamics. In the current example, El-Kareh et al. [21] have modeled PK-PD (Pharmacokinetics and Pharmacodynamics) of cisplatin as a whole molecule without NP carrier. Cell absorption and intracellular binding of cisplatin to DNA are considered to predict how survival (in comparison to controls) would depend on the duration of extracellular exposure. When cisplatin reacts both inside and outside of cells, various platinum species are created. Each species has unique kinetics for transport across the nuclear and cellular membranes. It is frequently feasible to combine multiple species to create a usable mathematical model in kinetic systems. The resulting model produces cytotoxicity predictions that align with observations across a variety of exposure scenarios.

Figure 2.2 schematically represents the course of reactions with various rate constants for cisplatin delivery. Intracellular concentration c_i includes aquated platinum that is attached to RNA and other non-DNA proteins as well as hydrolyzed within the nucleus. However, c_k (concentration of DNA-bound cisplatin) and c_i^* (concentration of cisplatin dissociated from DNA as an consequence of DNA repair) are different from c_i. The platinum species that are liberated during DNA repair can no longer bind. In the model proposed in this case, peak intracellular cisplatin levels determine cell death. The peak intracellular level is likewise limited when the extracellular concentration falls below a threshold level irrespective of the exposure time.

Model Structure has two core components, which are pharmacokinetic (PK) model for intracellular drug movement and pharmacodynamic (PD) model for cell survival prediction. A system of two ordinary differential equations (ODEs) are used to describe the free intracellular cisplatin and DNA—bound cisplatin. It is important to note that these equations follow certain assumptions such

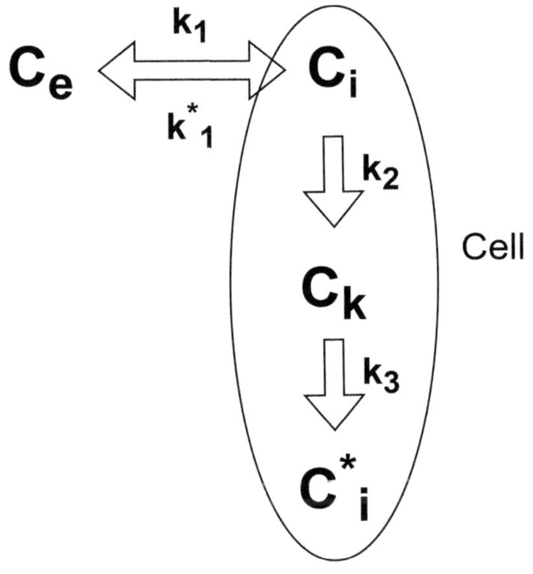

FIGURE 2.2 Reaction Scheme of cisplatin delivery to tumor cells.

as ignoring the spatial effects, considering the intracellular compartment as a well-mixed system, no cisplatin metabolism or degradation taking place, whereas uptake, efflux, binding, and repair follow the first order kinetics. The 2 ODEs are as follows:

$$\frac{dC_i}{dt} = k_1 c_e - k_1^* c_i \tag{1}$$

$$\frac{dC_k}{dt} = k_2 c_i - k_3 c_k \tag{2}$$

The general standard mass balance equation is Input + Generation—Output—Consumption = Accumulation. Both of the ODEs follow the mass action kinetics. Here '$k_1 c_e$' represents the generation term, '$k_1^* c_i$' represents the loss/consumption term and '$\frac{dC_i}{dt}$' represents the accumulation term. Similarly, '$k_2 c_i$' represents the generation term, '$k_3\, c_k$' represents the loss/consumption term and '$\frac{dC_k}{dt}$' represents the accumulation term.

The second core component —pharmacodynamic (PD) model for cell survival prediction—is carried out after computing the peak value of DNA-bound cisplatin; the survival fraction of cells is calculated using a Hill-type equation:

$$S = \frac{1}{1 + Ax^m} \tag{3}$$

Here A represents drug sensitivity scaling constant, S represents fraction of surviving cells (0 to 1), x refers to the area under the curve (AUC), which describes the cytotoxicity, which does not depend on the time of exposure. Few models have described x equal to product of concentration and time of exposure (CT). C^nT is a much more accurate description that follows the Hill equation. Here, in this example, it represents the peak value of DNA-bound cisplatin denoted by $c_{k,max}$. m represents the Hill coefficient.

All these equations are replicated and solved in MATLAB by using the ODE solver ode45. Parameters k_1, k_2, k_1^*, k_3, A and m are taken from experimental cisplatin exposure data from Troger et al. [29]. Table 2.2 lists the model parameters and their effects on the model behavior.

TABLE 2.2
The Set of Parameters Required for Determining the Intracellular Drug Movement and Cell Survival Prediction

S.No	Parameter	Value	Explanation
1	k_1	2.635 h^{-1}	The rate constant for cisplatin absorption from the extracellular media into the cytoplasm. A higher k_1 implies faster accumulation inside the cell leading to more DNA binding which achieves greater cytotoxicity
2	k_2	0.2024 h^{-1}	The rate constant of binding of free intracellular cisplatin to DNA. A higher k_2 means more rapid accumulation of drug, higher $c_{k,max}$ and a greater cytotoxic potential
3	k_1^*	0.1184 h^{-1}	The rate constant describes how quickly free intracellular cisplatin c_i leaves the cell and returns to the extracellular space. A higher value implies less opportunity for DNA binding leading to higher survival
4	k_3	0.4707 h^{-1}	The rate constant for the removal of DNA-bound cisplatin. A higher k_3 implies faster repair leading to lower DNA damage accumulation.
5	A	0.2033	Higher Drug Sensitivity Scaling Factor A means greater sensitivity to cisplatin which implies that a small DNA damage can cause a large number of cells to die.
6.	m	1.229	Hill coefficient is a measure of nonlinearity or steepness of the survival curve. A higher m value means the cell killing response is more switch-like. Survival drops sharply once a threshold DNA damage is reached.

Source: The data are sourced from [29].

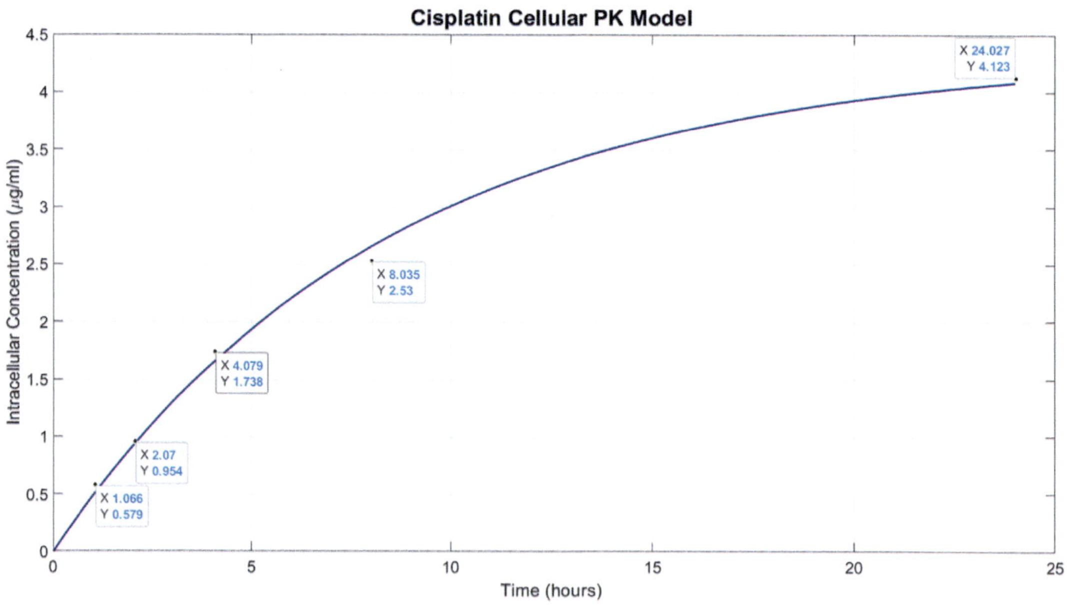

FIGURE 2.3 Cellular pharmacokinetic model simulation (blue line) on in-vitro platinum (cisplatin) uptake by human ovarian carcinoma cells.

Source: Data points are sourced from Andrews et al. [32].

Cellular PK mathematical model simulation was used to predict the intracellular platinum concentration. Figure 2.3 depicts a steady increase of cisplatin inside the cell as time progresses which is explained by the accumulation due to uptake (k_1c_e). The flattening (plateau) reflects a steady-state where uptake and efflux rates balance out. Figure 2.4 shows the cisplatin DNA binding kinetics. Cells were collected at set times after the start of cisplatin exposure and were used

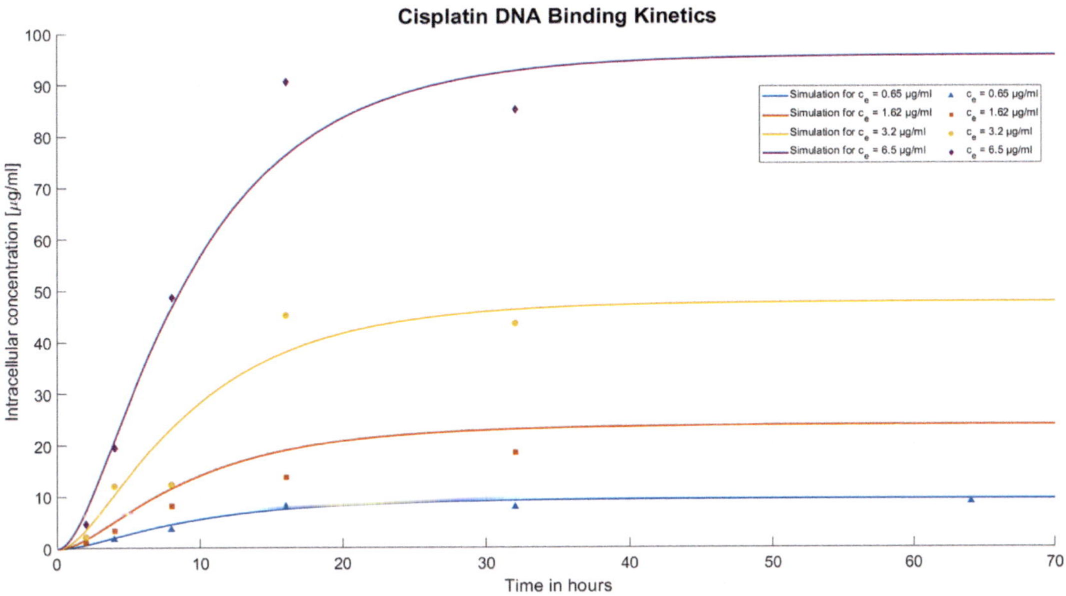

FIGURE 2.4 Intracellular cisplatin at varying extracellular cisplatin concentrations. Cisplatin retention inside the cell helps in binding it to DNA to form adducts and distort its structure.

Source: Data points sourced from Troger et al [31].

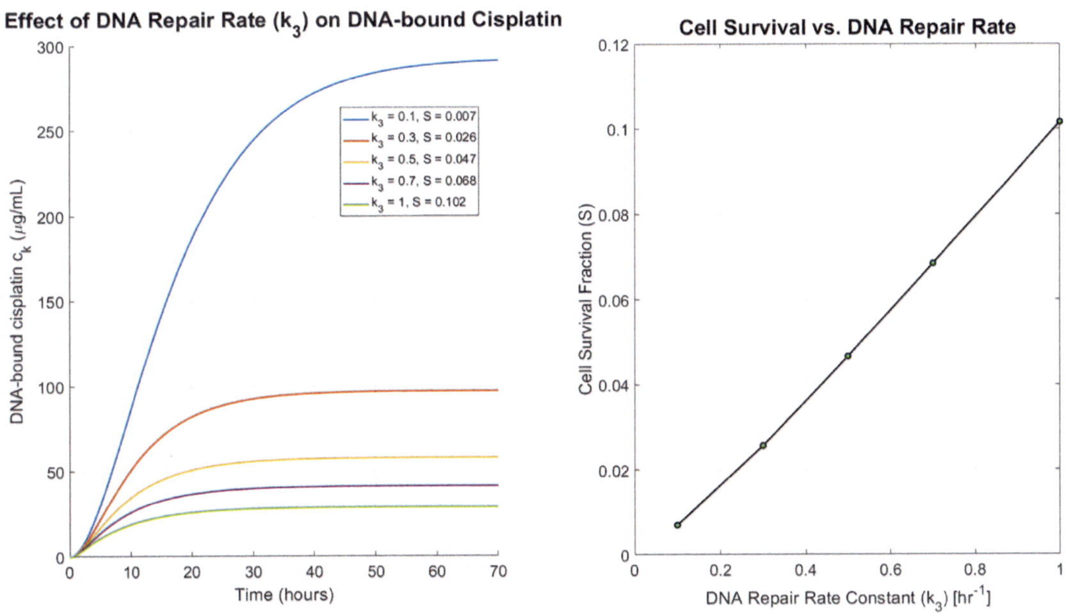

FIGURE 2.5 DNA bound cisplatin at varying DNA repair rate. A higher k_3 implies faster repair and increased survival.

for platinum measurement. As extracellular cisplatin increases, DNA-bound cisplatin increases, and cell death increases. The figure shows different doses of cisplatin and its intracellular concentrations indicate cytotoxicity with respect to period of exposure. Figure 2.5 represents the effect of DNA repair rate —that is, k_3 —on DNA-bound cisplatin. A lower k_3 implies slower repair or persistent adducts and higher toxicity. Again, the plateau is because of the balance between the rate of DNA binding and the rate of DNA repair (unbinding).

2.4.3 Case II: PK-PD Modeling for Nanocarrier-Based Drug Delivery in Cancer

Here we discuss a modeling framework for PK and PD of nanocarrier based cancer drug delivery. Pascal et al., utilized first-principles cell biophysics, drug PK and PD [22] to simulate the transport of doxorubicin (DOX) to hepatocellular carcinoma (HCC) tumor cells with Multiple Drug Resistance (MDR) property and forecast the cytotoxicity data. A perfectly targeted NP drug carrier, or "nanocarrier," should be able to carry large amounts of drugs, siRNAs etc., retain in circulation for longer time without immune clearance or excretion and should only bind to the unhealthy cells (either epithelium or endothelium), avoiding normal cells. They created a versatile, compound nanocarrier "protocell" combining the benefits of porous NPs (stability and a huge capability for simultaneous transport of many cargos) with liposomes (long circulation durations, immunogenicity, and low inherent toxicity) synergistically. They investigated and measured in-vitro tumor drug feedback using a combination of mathematical modeling and experimentation. They created a straightforward yet computational mathematical model from the ground up using experimental cytotoxicity data, connecting the dynamics of the drug and the viable cell number as an indicator of drug concentration and the cells' prior drug uptake[22].

Here we explain a continuous drug-exposure model which is based on the mass conservation of the drug. It has a set of ODEs which are expressed as

$$\frac{d\sigma}{dt} = -\lambda \,.n(t).\sigma \tag{4}$$

$$\sigma(t=0) = \sigma_0$$

Where, $\sigma(t)$ is the local drug concentration at time t with σ_0 as the initial concentration, λ is the specific rate of uptake of drug by the cells, and $n(t)$ is the concentration of the cells.

The conservation of cells is given by

$$\frac{dn}{dt} = -\Lambda_A \,.n \tag{5}$$

$$\frac{dn}{dt} = -\lambda_A \,.n\,.(\sigma_0 - \sigma) \tag{6}$$

where, $\Lambda_A(t) = f\left(-\int_0^t \lambda\,.n(\tau).\sigma(\tau).d\tau\right) = \lambda_A\,.(\sigma_0 - \sigma(t)),\ n(t=0) = n_0$

Here, $\Lambda_A(t)$ is the death rate of the cells and the initial concentration of cells is n_0.

Table 2.3 lists all the parameter values used for various drug and serum concentrations. These parameters have been used in MATLAB using the ode45 solver to simulate the fraction of viable cells at various doses of doxorubicin as a free drug and coupled with protocells.

Here, we approximately predict the effect of the dosage of HCC to DOX administered as free form of a drug or coupled with protocells using a mathematical model which is based on first principles of cell and drug mass conservation, with parameters pertaining to cellular death rates and uptake rates of the drug/NP. We observe an increased efficiency of targeted NP-based distribution in comparison to a free drug. Figure 2.6 shows the plot for the fraction of viable cells (n/n_0) over time, highlighting the higher sensitivity of parental cells compared to MDR cells. Additionally,

TABLE 2.3
The Set of Parameters Required for Determining the Conservation and Cell Survival Prediction.

Sr. No	Drug and serum concentration	Specific death rate λ_A (hr $\cdot\mu$M)$^{-1}$	Uptake rate $\lambda \cdot n_0$ (hr^{-1})
		MDR Cells	
1.	Free Drug, 2.4 μM, 10%	0.025 (hr.μM)$^{-1}$	0.066
2.	DOX Loaded, 2.4 μM, 10%	0.130	0.209
3.	DOX Loaded, 2.4 μM, 50%	0.065	0.130
4.	Free Drug, 9.6 μM, 10%	0.140	0.072
5.	DOX Loaded, 9.6 μM, 10%	0.270	0.171
6.	DOX Loaded, 9.6 μM, 50%	0.210	0.178
		Parental HCC cell lines	
1.	Free Drug, 85.7 nM, 10%	0.708	0.066
2.	DOX Loaded, 85.7 nM, 10%	0.830	0.225
3.	DOX Loaded, 85.7 nM, 500%	0.590	0.178
4.	Free Drug, 286 nM, 10%	0.829	0.072
5.	DOX Loaded, 286 nM, 10%	0.775	0.316
6.	DOX Loaded, 286 nM, 50%	0.460	0.456

Source: The data are sourced from [22].

the simulations for nonlinear response plots for several doses and for both drug delivery methods—that is, free drug and drug-loaded protocells to both drug-sensitive and drug-resistant HCC cell types—are shown in Figure 2.7. The MATLAB code models the time-dependent viability curves over 96 hours for parental HCC cells under continuous doxorubicin (DOX) exposure.

MDR Cell lines subplot consists of 2 curves exhibiting sigmoidal shapes, with viability decreasing as σ_0 increases. MDR free DOX has high viability ($\frac{n}{n_0} \approx 0.8$) across the concentration range, reflecting strong drug resistance due to low λ_A. Even at 15 μM, viability remains above 0.8. MDR DOX-Protocell has lower viability ($\frac{n}{n_0} \approx 0.5$–$0.9$) compared to free DOX, indicating greater efficacy. At 15 μM, viability drops to around 0.5, driven by higher λ_A and λn_0 suggesting proper drug uptake. The protocell curve is consistently below the free DOX curve, demonstrating improved cytotoxicity against MDR cells. Parental HCC Cell lines subplot consists of 2 curves exhibiting steep sigmoids, reflecting high sensitivity of parental cells to DOX. Viability decreases sharply with increasing σ_0. At 0.286 μM and above, it approaches 0, indicating nearly complete cell death. Even at low concentrations, the high $\lambda_A = 0.769$ causes rapid cell death, which is consistent with parental cells' lack of resistance compared to MDR cells.

2.4.4 Case III: A PBPK Model for Cancer Nanomedicine Drug Delivery

To explain the usage of mathematical models in the nanoparticle-based drug delivery, we discuss the Physiologically Based Pharmacokinetics (PBPK) model of P Dogra et al. [19] as the third case example. Dogra and colleagues developed an ODE based mathematical model capable of predicting systemic NP pharmacokinetics and their tumor-specific uptake.

The PBPK model by Dogra et al. is comprised of 35 ODEs that are used for defining the distribution of NPs in the different compartments (vascular and extravascular) of organs (brain, liver, lungs, heart, kidney, gastrointestinal, spleen, lymph node, others, plasma, and excreta) and tumor after an injected NPs dose (ID) of 100%. The PBPK model exclusively defines phagocytic compartments for the spleen and liver as these are major sites of phagocytic cell activity that plays an important role

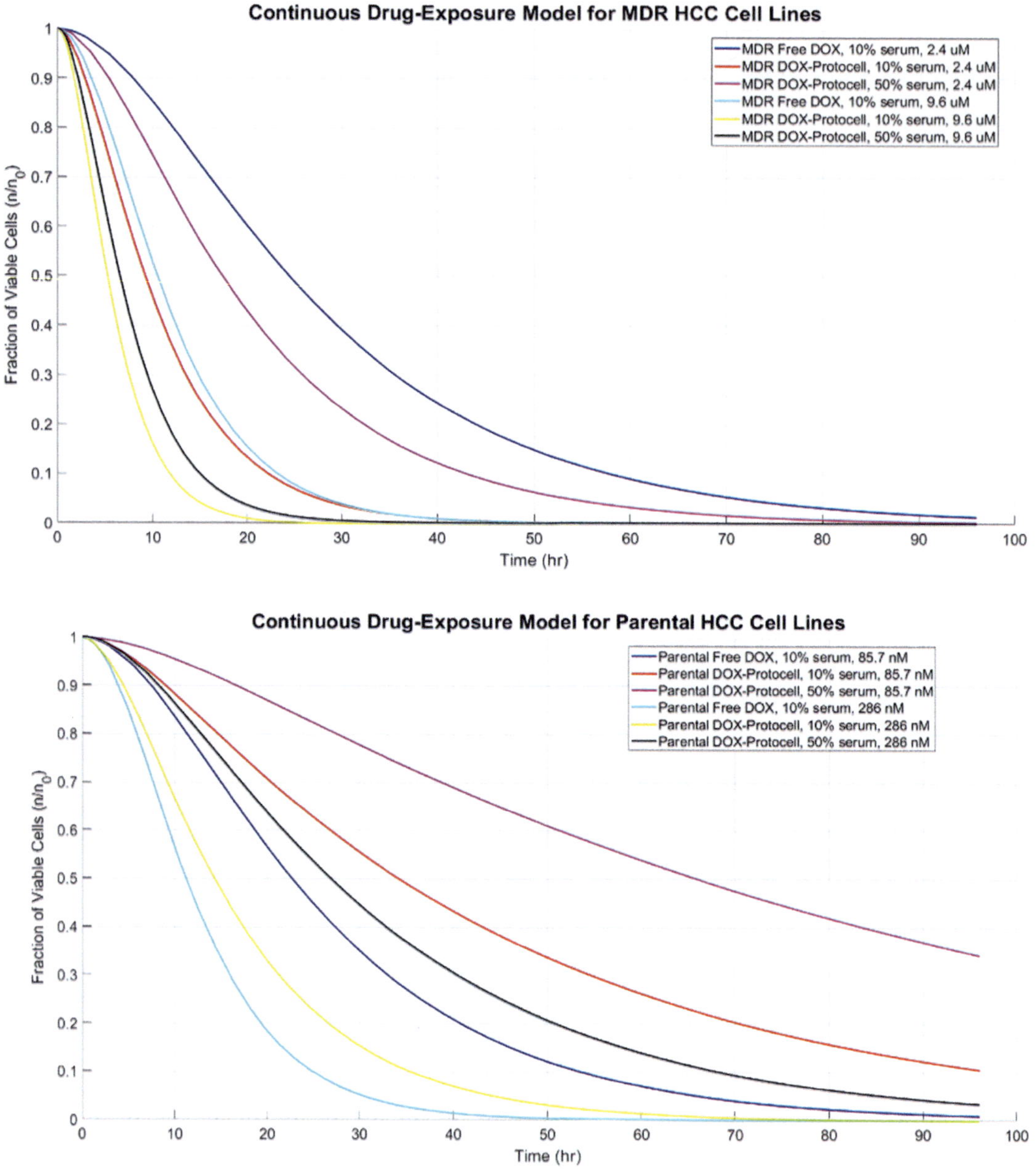

FIGURE 2.6 Sample fits using the continuous drug exposure model to cytotoxicity data at different drug concentrations. Top: MDR cell lines exposed to free DOX and DOX-loaded protocells at various levels of serum and initial drug concentrations ($\sigma_0 = 2.4\ \mu$M and $9.6\ \mu$M). Bottom: parental HCC cell lines exposed to free DOX and DOX-loaded protocells at various levels of serum and initial drug concentrations ($\sigma_0 = 0.0857$ μM and $0.286\ \mu$M).

in clearance of nanoparticles. The lymph and plasma equations represent the effects of circulation on transporting and receiving NPs from the extravascular compartment of organs and tumor. The excreta compartment along with the phagocytic system describes the clearance of NPs with a rate greater than the rate of NP degradation, which is mainly affected by the change in physical parameters (like size, density, shape) of nanoparticles [23, 30]. Table 2.4 lists model variables used for simulations.

They used the following ODEs for determining the levels of free and bound state of NPs in the intravascular compartment,

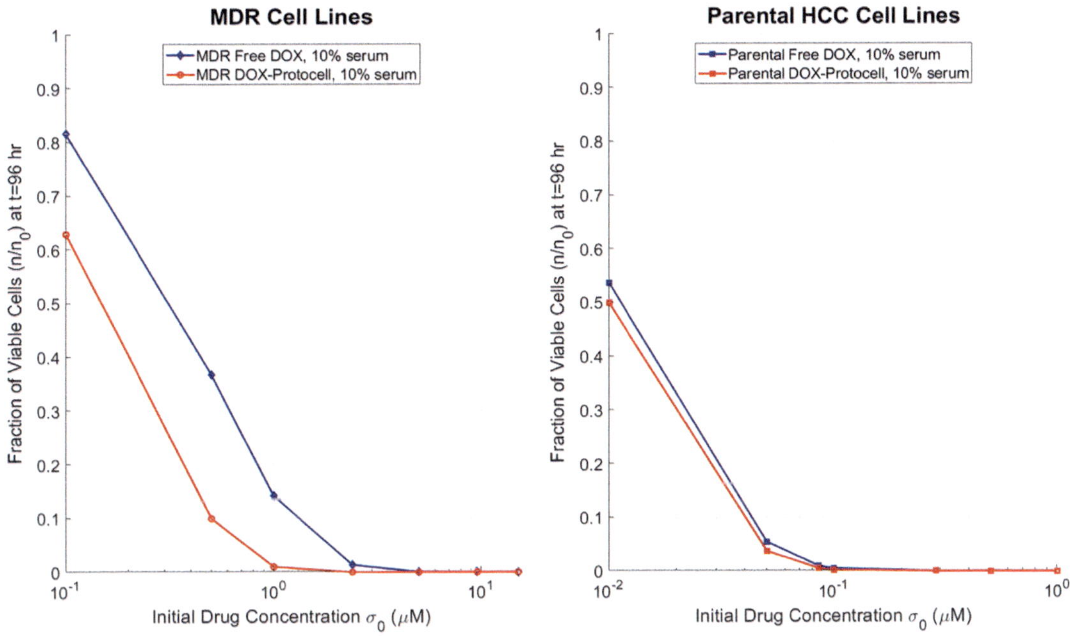

FIGURE 2.7 MDR cells and parental HCC cells, showing the fraction of viable cells ($\frac{n}{n_0}$) at 96 hours as a function of initial drug concentration (σ_0) on a logarithmic scale. MDR Free DOX, 10% serum (blue line): λ_A = 0.025 $hr^{-1}\mu M^{-1}$, λn_0 = 0.069 and σ_0 =[0.1, 0.5, 1, 2.4, 5, 9.6] μM. MDR DOX-Protocell, 10% serum (red line): λ_A = 0.051 $hr^{-1}\mu M^{-1}$, λn_0 = 0.19, same σ_0 as above. Parental Free DOX, 10% serum (blue line): λ_A = 0.769 $hr^{-1}\mu M^{-1}$, λn_0 = 0.069, and σ_0 = [0.01, 0.05, 0.0857, 0.1, 0.286, 0.5, 1] μM. Parental DOX-protocell, 10% serum (red line): λ_A = 0.830 $hr^{-1}\mu M^{-1}$, λn_0 = 0.084, same σ_0 as above.

TABLE 2.4
Variables Used in the Given PBPK Model

Variables	Representing Concentration
$C^f_{v,i}$	Free NPs in vascular compartment of the ith organ ($\%ID\,of\,NPs\,in\,free\,form$)
$C^f_{v,T}$	Free NPs in Tumor vascular compartment ($\%ID\,of\,NPs\,in\,bound\,form$)
$C^b_{v,i}$	Bound NPs in vascular compartment of the ith organ ($\%ID\,of\,NPs\,in\,bound\,form$)
$C^b_{v,T}$	Bound NPs in Tumor vascular compartment ($\%ID\,of\,NPs\,in\,bound\,form\,in\,Tumor$)
$C_{e,i}$	Diffused NPs in the extravascular compartment of the ith organ ($\%ID\,of\,NPs\,in\,Extravascular\,Space$)
$N_{p,i}$	NPs that are phagocytized in ith organ (liver and spleen) ($\%ID\,of\,NPs\,cleared\,by\,macrophages$)
$N_{e,T}$	NPs that are extravasated in the tumor interstitium ($\%ID\,of\,NPs\,in\,excreted$)

Source: The data are sourced from [19].

$$\%ID\,of\,NPs\,in\,free\,form$$

$$NPf = \frac{\left(Q_i C_P - \left(Q_i - L_i\right)C^f_{v,i} - L_i\left(1 - sigma_i\right)C^f_{v,i} - k_{on,i}V_{v,i}C^f_{v,i} + k_{off,i}V_{v,i}C^b_{v,i}\right)}{V_{v,i}} \tag{7}$$

$$\%ID\,of\,NPs\,in\,bound\,form$$

$$NPb = \frac{\left(k_{on,i}C^f_{v,i}V_{v,i} - k_{off,i}V_{v,i}C^b_{v,i} - k_{mac}A_{mac,i}V_{v,i}C^b_{v,i}\right)}{V_{v,i}} \tag{8}$$

Where, i depicts the organ, the $Q_i C_P$ accounts for plasma inflow of NPs, ($-\left(Q_i - L_i\right)C^f_{v,i}$) shows the outflow of NPs in the blood circulation, ($-L_i\left(1 - sigma_i\right)C^f_{v,i}$) defines the movement of NPs into extravascular spaces, $k_{on,i}V_{v,i}C^f_{v,i}\,and\,k_{off,i}V_{v,i}C^b_{v,i}$ represents the amount of bound and unbound NPs in the circulation, respectively. In bound NPs equation the $k_{mac}A_{mac,i}V_{v,i}C^b_{v,i}$ represents the amount of NPs captured by the phagocytic cells.

The following ODE is used for computing the change in NPs levels within the extravascular compartment of organs and tumor.

$$\%ID\,of\,NPs\,in\,Extravascular\,Space = \frac{L_i\left(1 - sigma_i\right)C^f_{v,i} - L_i C_{e,i}}{V_{e,i}} \tag{9}$$

Where, the amount of NPs revert into the circulation by the movement of lymph fluid is depicted by $-L_i C_{e,i}$.

Further, author calculated the amount of NPs phagocytosed by the macrophages by using the following ODE,

$$\%ID\,of\,NPs\,cleared\,by\,macrophages = k_{mac}A_{mac,i}C^b_{v,i} - \frac{\left(k_{Deg}N_{p,i}\right)}{V_{v,i}} \tag{10}$$

Where, the available amount of blood vessel interacted NPs for phagocytosis and the degradation amount of phagocytosed NPs are enumerated by $k_{mac}A_{mac,i}C^b_{v,i}$ and $\left(k_{Deg}N_{p,i}\right)$ respectively.

They describe the non-linear change in the level of NPs in the intravascular compartment of tumor by the following ODE equations,

$$\%ID\,of\,NPs\,in\,free\,form\,in\,Tumor$$

$$NPfT = \frac{\left(Q_T\left(C_P - C^f_{v,T}\right) - PSC^f_{v,T} - k_{on,T}V_{v,T}C^f_{v,T} + k_{off,T}V_{v,T}C^b_{v,T}\right)}{V_{v,T}} \tag{11}$$

$$\%ID\,of\,NPs\,in\,bound\,form\,in\,Tumor$$

$$NPbT = k_{on,T}V_{v,T}C^f_{v,T} - k_{off,T}V_{v,T}C^b_{v,T} \tag{12}$$

Where, the level of free NPs inflow in the tumor blood represented by the $Q_T\left(C_P - C^f_{v,T}\right)$, $PSC^f_{v,T}$ is an amount of NPs extravasated in the tumor interstitium. The amount of free and bounded NPs in the tumor vascular system are given by the $k_{off,T}V_{v,T}C^b_{v,T}$ and $k_{on,T}V_{v,T}C^f_{v,T}$.

Further, Dogra et al calculated the percentage of NPs in the tumor's extravascular compartment by the given equation,

$$\%ID\,of\,NPs\,in\,Tumor\,interstitium = PSC^{f}_{v,T} - k_{Deg}N_{e,T} \tag{13}$$

Where, the $k_{Deg}N_{e,T}$ represents clearance of NPs present in the tumor interstitium.

The amount of NPs getting excreted from the body after administration is calculated by,

$$\%ID\,of\,NPs\,in\,excreted = k_{Deg}N_{p,S} + BC_{e,L} + k_{Deg}N_{p,L} + UC_{e,K} + k_{Deg}N_{e,T} \tag{14}$$

Where, $k_{Deg}N_{p,S}$ or $k_{Deg}N_{p,L}$ or $k_{Deg}N_{e,T}$ represents the clearance of NPs in the spleen/liver/tumor compartment. The excretion/clearance of NPs through the kidney urine and liver bile secretion represented by $UC_{e,K}$ and $BC_{e,L}$, respectively.

Further they determined the physiological parameters based on previous pharmacokinetic studies of NPs to create a baseline working model (Table 2.5). These are further perturbed to analyze the effects on the circulation, distribution, and deposition of NPs in each compartment of organs and tumor. A set of parameters are used for defining the contact of NPs with the blood cells, blood vessels lining, glycocalyx, and macrophages during vascular circulation, which have direct/indirect effect on the sedimentation, distribution, and delivery kinetics of NPs. This causes intravascular partitioning of NPs into a free flowing and bound form, which solely depends on the blood rheology and blood flow dynamics along with the physiological properties of NP. The parameters Db_i (Brownian diffusion) and Ds_i (shear induced-diffusion) are used to define the sedimentation rate of NPs between the vascular periphery (cell-free layer and endothelial wall) and the vascular core (cell-enriched layer) via diffusion after coming in contact with erythrocytes and laminar flow with zero-fluid velocity at the vessel walls [19,24,25]. Further, these are used for calculating the effective diffusivity ($D_i = Db_i + Ds_i$) of NPs and are integrated with the equation of sedimentation rate (due to gravitational and buoyant force) to consider the effect of flow velocity and diffusivity on the NPs deposition ($k_{on,i}$).

They further formulated the rate of NPs dislodging ($k_{off,i}$) by considering the reentering of NPs in the blood circulation due to their back-diffusion from non-specific binding with the glycocalyx layer of endothelium. The mononuclear phagocytic system based clearance of NPs considers the mechanistic wrapping of macrophages with the help of motor proteins (k_{mac}). They considered different sizes of vascular fenestration ($r_{pore,i}$) for the healthy organs and tumor compartments which change the NPs extravasation by the bulk transport or diffusion. In the tumor compartment, diffusion is the only practical way for NPs to extravasate in the interstitium due to impaired neo-angiogenesis (causes larger vascular fenestrations) and lymphatic system [2, 26,27,28]. This leads to heightened interstitial fluid pressure within the tumor, which diminishes the hydrostatic pressure gradient between the vasculature and the interstitium, thereby hindering bulk transport [9,29]. Based on these biophysical scenarios, the rate of NP diffusion was enumerated by considering the product of tumor permeability (P) and micro-vascular surface area (S) of the tumor. Dogra et al. integrated these effects in the PBPK model by using microscopic nano-bio interaction principle, which involves the parameters reporting the concept of NPs deposition/dislodging from the micro-vascular surfaces, phagocytosis by macrophages, diffusion/bulk transport through extravascular spaces as shown in Figure 2.1.

This PBPK model was used to explain the effects of NP size on their extravasation in the interstitium and vascular compartment of the tumor and organs (for discussion kidney is used). The initial NP concentration of different compartments in the model is considered zero, excluding the plasma compartment where NPs concentration is considered 100% (as defined by the Dogra et al. [19]). All

TABLE 2.5
The Set of Parameters for Determining the |Dynamic Distribution of Nanoparticles in the Healthy and Tumor Compartments via Working PBPK

S.No	Parameter	Value			Explanation
1.	u_i	(for tumor state u_T) 30 µm.s^{-1} (for healthy state u_i) 553 µm.s^{-1}			Capillary blood flow velocity (In perfusion, u contributes to the rate of drug delivery to tumor vasculature, governing how quickly nanoparticles are brought to the exchange surface (capillary-tissue interface)
2.	Q_{capi}	0.15 nL.min^{-1}			Capillary blood volumetric flow rate (helps determine the rate of nano drug delivery to the tumor)
3.	$gamma_i$	(for tumor compartment) 16 s^{-1} (for healthy compartment) 116 s^{-1}			Capillary shear rate (Shear rate exerted by blood flow in tumor capillaries)
4.	r_{nano}	50 nm			NP radius (Influences diffusion, EPR effect, Cellular uptake, Clearance, Tumor Penetration, NP distribution, retention, and therapeutic effectiveness in tumors)
5.	$r_{pore,i}$	L= 140 nm S= 2500 nm GI= 2.5 nm	K= 4 nm B= 0.5 nm M= 2.5 nm	LU= 2.5 nm H= 2.5 nm T= 850 nm	Radius of fenestrations in the microvessel wall of various organ compartments (Determines vascular permeability of NPs extravasating from blood vessels into the tissue interstitium. NPs larger than $r_{pore,i}$ will have restricted or no access to the tissue)
6.	r_{tumor}	5 mm			Radius of tumor (useful in computing tumor volume, defines the spatial boundary in diffusion and convection, and allows size-based personalization)
7.	r_{macro}	15 µm			Radius of macrophage helps in defining the geometry for NP–macrophage binding kinetics
8.	R	5000 nm			Radius of capillary (helps in modeling of blood flow, shear stress, and NP transport within capillary networks. Tumor capillaries are wider than normal ones due to abnormal angiogenesis)
9.	l_w	5000 nm			Thickness of tumor microvessel wall inversely affects NP permeability (P)
10.	l	1e6 µm			Length of capillary (influences flow dynamics together with blood velocity u, determines residence time of blood in the capillary. Hence, longer capillary length implies longer interaction time between NPs and vessel walls).
11.	l_g	100 nm			Thickness of glycocalyx (acts as a physical and charge-based filter barrier to extravasation. Its resistance is computed for permeability P or in modifying diffusive flux equations).
12.	ρ_{np}	2 g.cm^{-3}			NP density (vital for linking Concentration, Dosimetry and biodistribution predictions, Hydrodynamic behavior Pharmacokinetic modeling:
13.	rho_P	1 g.cm^{-3}			Plasma density is helpful in momentum balance and NP sedimentation.
14.	k_{Deg}	0.01 h^{-1}			NP degradation rate in tumor and MPS (High k_{Deg} means faster degradation, leading to lower circulating levels of NPs or drugs)
15.	H	0.5			Hematocrit (volume fraction of RBCs in blood)
16.	CO	4217 mL.h^{-1}			Cardiac output (the volume of blood the heart pumps per minute)
17.	μ_T	7.42 cP			Tumor blood viscosity (Blood viscosity is inversely proportional to flow velocity through capillaries. Slower blood flow reduces convective transport, reflects tumor abnormalities like high cell content (hematocrit) etc.

TABLE 2.5 ***(Continued)***

The Set of Parameters for Determining the |Dynamic Distribution of Nanoparticles in the Healthy and Tumor Compartments via Working PBPK

S.No	Parameter	Value	Explanation
18.	μ_i	4 cP	Dynamic viscosity of blood in healthy organs (based on Poiseulle's law. Higher viscosity → greater resistance → lower flow rate → reduced NP transport)
19.	WT	200 gm (rat)	Weight of model organism (here we used rat)
20.	*phi*	0.001	Tumor vascular porosity (fraction of the tumor vascular wall volume that is porous).
21.	$A_{mac,L}$	$\frac{(2827e^{-8} * 2.72e^{8})}{14514}$	Area fraction of hepatic vasculature covered by Kupffer cells
22.	$A_{mac,S}$	0.1	Area fraction of splenic vasculature occupied by macrophages
23.	*GFR*	78.6 mL.h^{-1}	Glomerular filtration rate (flow of plasma filtered from the glomerulus into Bowman's space over a specified period)
24.	*U*	2.0833 mL.h^{-1}	Urine flow rate (volume of urine produced and excreted by the kidneys per unit time)
25.	*B*	0.9375 mL.h^{-1}	Bile flow rate (volume of bile produced by the liver and secreted into the biliary system per unit time)
26.	β	3.6 µm	Radius of erythrocyte is used in shear induced diffusion, lateral margination and blood flow
27.	*P*	10^{-17} W	Power of cellular motor proteins help predict resistance to drag
28.	γ^*	0.06 mN.m^{-1}	Surface tension of cellular membrane governs membrane deformation and NP uptake
29.	K_B	1.38* 10^{-23} J.K^{-1}	Boltzmann constant is used in the Stokes-Einstein equation. K_B relates the average kinetic energy of particles in a system to its temperature.
30.	*T*	310 K	Body temperature
31.	*g*	9.8 m.s^{-2}	Gravitational acceleration constant
32.	V_{LN}	1 mL	Volume of Lymph node compartment
33.	V_P	1.5 mL	Volume of Plasma compartment
34.	*S*	40 mm^2/mm^3	Surface area available for nanoparticle exchange in tumor tissue.
35.	Q_i	(for healthy organs) $f_{CO,i} * CO * (1-H)$ (for tumor Q_T) 0.1 mL.g^{-1}.min^{-1}	The blood flow rate. Tumor blood flow rate (Tumors with higher vascularization will generally have higher Q_T, leading to more efficient and faster drug delivery).
36.	L_i	Q_i/500	Lymph flow rate of organ I (often dysfunctional in tumors, leading to altered NP kinetics)
37.	Q_{HA}	$Q_L - (Q_S - Q_{LS}) - (Q_{GI} - L_{GI})$	Contribution of plasma flow rate into the liver from the hepatic artery
38.	$f_{v,i}$	L=0.21 K=0.16 LU=0.36 S=0.22 B=0.04 H=0.26 GI=0.2 M=0.04 T = 0.1	Vascular fraction of ith organ (for calculating the vascular volume of ith organ)
39.	$f_{WT,i}$	P=0.0589 L=0.05 K=0.015 LU=0.01 S=0.01 B = 0.03 H=0.01 GI=0.04 M = 0.3 O = 0.03	Fractional body weight of organ *i* reflecting the volume of distribution for each organ.
40.	*porgan*	1 g.cm^{-3}	Density for all organs

(Continued)

TABLE 2.5 ***(Continued)***

The Set of Parameters for Determining the |Dynamic Distribution of Nanoparticles in the Healthy and Tumor Compartments via Working PBPK

S.No	Parameter	Value	Explanation
41.	$f_{CO,i}$	L=0.021 K=0.141 LU=1 S=0.02 B=0.02 H=0.051 GI=0.133 M=0.278	Fractional cardiac output to ith organ (for calculation of plasma flow rate Q_i to the ith organ)
42.	f_{cap}	0.55	Capillary volume fraction (fraction of tissue volume that is made up of capillaries, higher capillary volume fraction refers to greater surface area, more vascular access for NPs to enter tissues via transvascular transport).
43.	Vv_i	$f_{v,i} * \left(f_{WT,i} * \frac{WT}{porgan} \right)$ (for tumor Vv_T) 0.0524 ml	Volume of the vascular sub-compartment of organ i
44.	Ve_i	$f_{v,i} * \left(f_{WT,i} * \frac{WT}{porgan} \right) - Vv_i$	Volume of the extravascular space in each compartment
45.	α_i	$\frac{r_{nano}}{r_{pore,i}}$ Where, "i" represents different organ and tumor compartments.	The ratio of nano-particle size to vascular pore size of a compartment aid in determining an optimum size of NPs which can readily diffuse
46.	F_i	$1-2.1*\alpha_i+2*\alpha_i^3-0.9*\alpha_i^5$ $-1.3*\alpha_i^6+3.8*\alpha_i^8-4.1*\alpha_i^9$	A dimensionless variable for modulating the hydrodynamic function based on the size of NPs size
47.	G_i	$\frac{\left(1-0.667*\alpha_i^2-0.2*\alpha_i^5\right)}{\left(1-0.7*\alpha_i^5\right)}$	A dimensionless variable for modulating the hydrodynamic function based on the size of NPs size
48.	P	$1e^{28} * phi * (1-\alpha_T) * F_T * \frac{Db_T}{lw}$	Permeability across the leaky vasculature of tumor compartment
49.	$sigma_i$	$1-\left(1-\left(1-(1-\alpha_i)^2\right)^2\right)*G_i$ $+\frac{16}{9}\alpha_i^2(1-\alpha_i)^2 F_i$	Reflection coefficient shows the reflection of a wave by an interface of vessel wall and blood with NPs, crucial for understanding the potential of NP in diagnosis or drug delivery. The value fluctuates between 0 (free passage) and 1 (no passage) based on the size of NPs
50.	Ds_i	$0.39 * \beta^2 * gamma_i * H^2$	Shear induced diffusion is caused by interactions with shear gradients (velocity differences) and collisions with red blood cells which enhances lateral transport and margination
51.	Db_i	$\frac{\left(K_B * T * Cslip\right)}{\left(6\pi * \mu_i * r_{nano}\right)}$	Stokes-Einstein equation for determining the NPs diffusivity through Brownian motion in blood vessels near surfaces. The equation shows relation between the diffusion coefficient of a particle in a fluid to the particle's size, fluid viscosity, and body temperature
52.	D_i	$Ds_i + Db_i$	Effective diffusivity of nanoparticles in the ith organ and tumor
53.	$k_{on,i}$	$\frac{2}{9}\left(\frac{\rho_{np}-\rho_p}{\mu_i}\right) * \frac{g\, r_{nano}{}^2 D.l}{u_T R^3}$	Nanoparticle microvascular wall depositioning rate, which is calculated by dividing the sedimentation velocity of nanoparticles by the characteristic sedimentation length.
54.	$k_{off,i}$	$\frac{D_b}{l_g^2}$	$k_{off,i}$ quantifies the dissociation of NPs from endothelial receptors, ECM, or cell surfaces in organ *i*. It gives an idea about how long NPs stay bound. Higher $k_{off,i}$ means NPs detach quickly leading to short residence time.

TABLE 2.5 *(Continued)*
The Set of Parameters for Determining the |Dynamic Distribution of Nanoparticles in the Healthy and Tumor Compartments via Working PBPK

S.No	Parameter	Value	Explanation
55.	k_{mac}	$\frac{p}{4 * \pi * r_{nano2} * gamma}$	NP interaction rate with macrophages.

Source: Some of the data are sourced from the literature, while others are estimated by parameter estimation methods.

these equations are solved and results generated on MATLAB by using the ODE solver ode45. The distribution dynamics of NPs (dia. size ~ 5 nm, 20 nm, 100 nm) are calculated and further used for estimating the effect of NP size on their distribution in the extravascular and vascular compartments. The change in nanoparticle size (5 nm→20 nm→100 nm) will perturb different parameters of the model *viz* pore-to-particle ratio (defines the degree of NPs extravasation), hydrodynamic functioning (accounts for change in flow resistance and permeability), reflection coefficient (degree of hindrance for NPs extravasation), effective diffusivity (diffusion of NPs during circulation based on size), and binding and dislodging of NPs from vascular walls (defines the retention and extravasation of NPs). These changes are reflected in the circulation (via plasma), deposition, and clearance dynamics of NPs in the tumor vascular/interstitium compartment, as shown in Figure 2.8. The pharmacokinetic simulation shows the better retention of 20 nm size NP in the tumor interstitium in comparison to 5 nm and 100 nm size NPs, which is due to the better permeability, increased plasma circulation, and improved diffusion at the region of interest (ROI). The NPs retention in the tumor interstitium is also increased and remains stable in comparison to deposition in the (healthy) kidney extravascular compartment, indicating the efficacy of NPs drug delivery due to improvement in nanoparticle accumulation at ROI based on their change in size compared to non-targeted sites. The increase in NPs size changes the reflection coefficient of the kidney to ~1 in comparison to the tumor, which reduces the extravasation and retention of NPs in the kidney interstitium. Moreover, the smaller size NPs (diameter ≤ 5 nm) showed lower distribution dynamics due to increased renal clearance and reduced NPs plasma concentration, which directly lowered their retention in other compartments. The data shows the importance of this mathematical model for studying the pharmacokinetic dynamics, deposition, and retention of NPs based on change in the biophysical, physiological, and physicochemical parameters of blood vessels, lymphatic system, organ/tumor compartment, and NPs. It helps to understand the NPs retention in the ROI by studying different parameters that are challenging and time consuming at the laboratory scale.

In the next case scenario, we perturb the tumor vasculature pore size ($r_{pore,T}$ = 0.39 μm → 1.7 μm) to study the retention and distribution of two NP sizes (100 nm and 20 nm dia.) in the tumor compartment as observed in the distribution dynamics in Figure 2.9. A perturbation in tumor vasculature pore size causes changes in the respective parameters of tumor compartment *viz* vascular permeability (rate of transvascular transport of NPs), pore-to-particle ratio, and hydrodynamic functioning. The comparative analysis in NP size 20 nm, showed that as the vasculature pore size increases the distribution and retention of the tumor interstitium NPs and vascular compartment remain almost the same. Whereas, in the case of NP size 100 nm the effective accumulation of NPs in tumor interstitium compartment lowers down as the vasculature pore size reduces (1.7 μm→0.39 μm). The simulation data infers that the perturbed vasculature pore size of tumor will reduce permeability of tumor at small fenestration size, and interrupt the effective extravasation of NPs. This advocates for an optimal NP size for their effective interstitium retention and distribution to deal with tumor

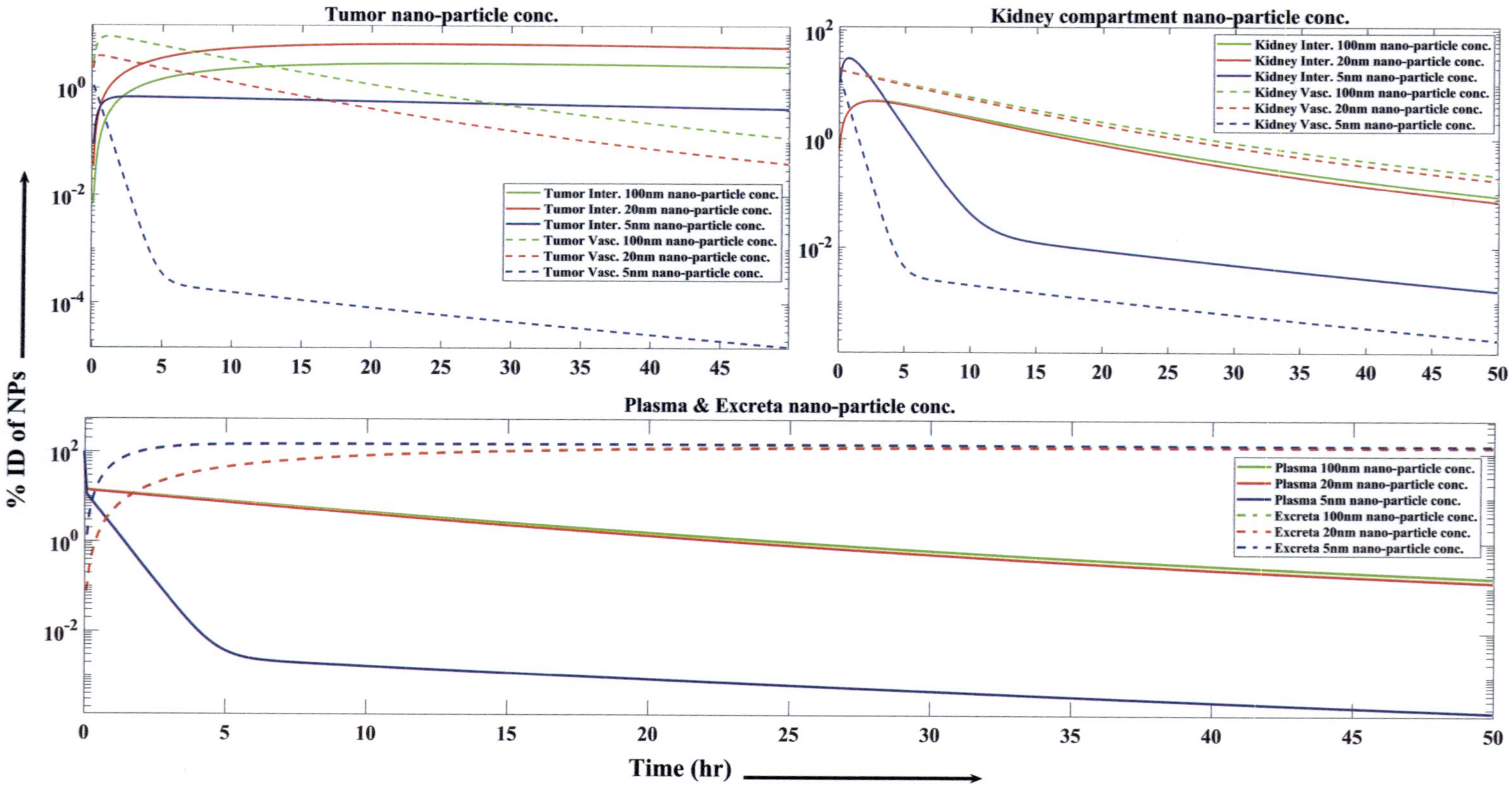

FIGURE 2.8 The dynamic distribution of different size diameter of NPs (100 nm, 20 nm, 5 nm) within kidney (Vascular "- - - -" and Interstitium "—"), tumor (Vascular "- - - -" and Interstitium "—"), plasma (—), and excreta (—) compartment. The delivery efficiency of NPs increases in the tumor interstitium for the diameter of 20 nm and 100 nm in comparison to the 5 nm diameter NPs. Whereas, the 100 nm size NPs showed lowering of distribution in interstitium than the 20 nm size NPs due to lowering of NPs diffusivity from vascular compartment to interstitium. In comparison to healthy organs (i.e., kidney compartment) the NPs (size 100 nm and 20 nm) deposition is found more in the tumor compartment, which infers the size dependent increase in efficacy of NPs deposition in the tumor compartment.

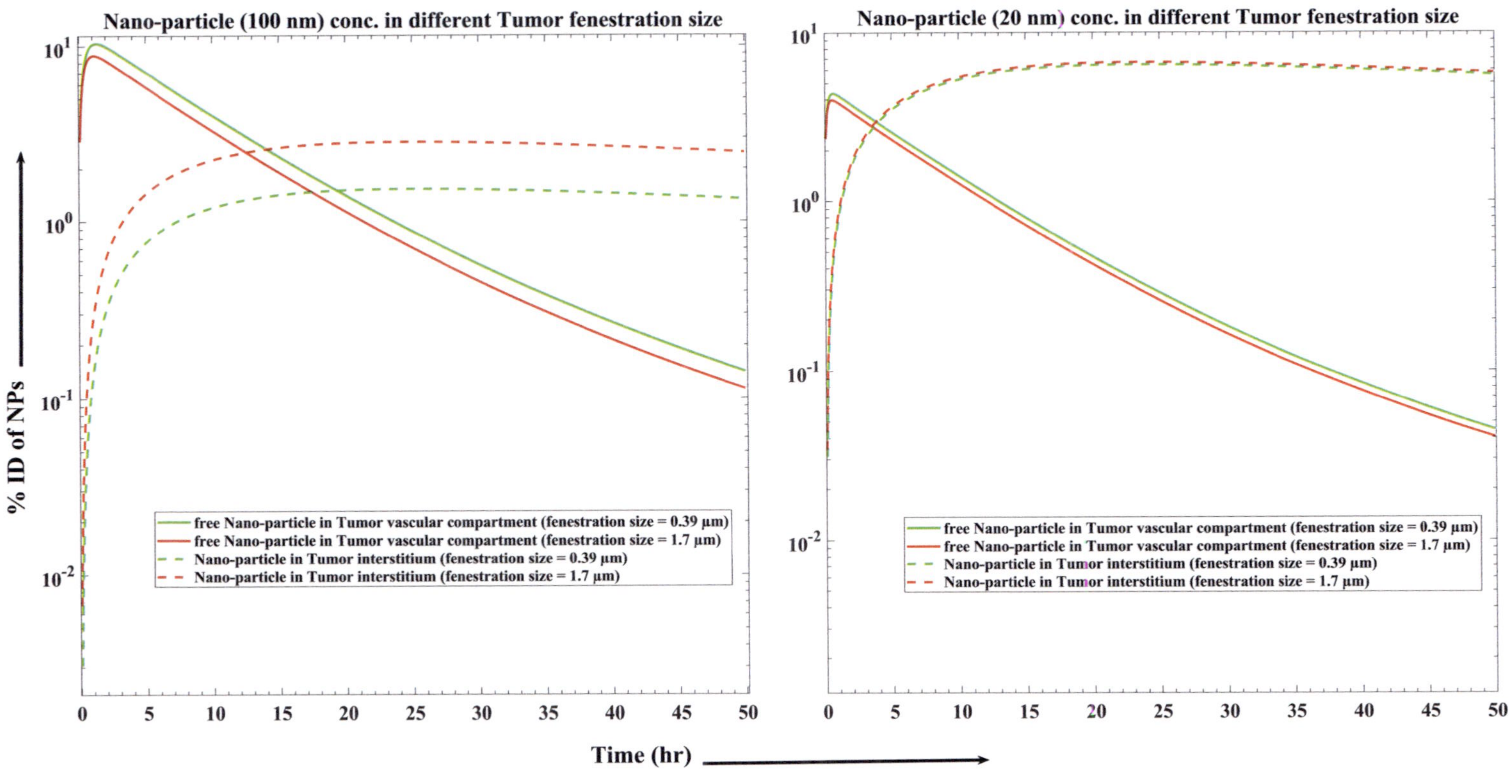

FIGURE 2.9 The dynamic distribution of NPs (100 nm and 20 nm dia.) in the tumor vascular pore size of 0.39 μm dia. (Vascular "—" and Interstitium "—") and 1.7 μm dia. (Vascular "—" and Interstitium "—") is represented by the graph. As the size of tumor vascular pore size increases (0.39 μm→1.7 μm) the vessel permeability and effective diffusivity of NPs increase for the 100 nm size NP, however, the diffusivity remain same in both case scenario of tumor for 20 nm size of NP. In the case of 100 nm size NP, this will reduce their effective deposition or transportation in the Tumor interstitium and increase vascular level of NPs. This indicates a requirement of adjusting the NPs size according to the changing physical parameters of the tumor for increasing their treatment efficacy.

vasculature of different pore size. The pharmacokinetic studies also showed the efficacy (regarding delivery, retention, and distribution) of nanoparticles within a size range of ~10–50 nm diameter at the ROI more in comparison to the non-targeted regions. Similarly, the PBPK model of Dogra et al also depicts the effectiveness of NPs (size ~20 nm) in leaking within the tumor interstitium from the vascular compartment of different pore size (0.39 μm or 1.7 μm).

2.5 LIMITATIONS AND CHALLENGES

Various factors limit the scope of assumptions in nanomedicine-based mathematical models. These include the lack of sufficient research for proper parameterization, inadequate or biased optimization of models, and challenges in model creation and execution. Additionally, extracting accurate parameter values and initial conditions for both diseased and healthy states rely heavily on existing literature, which may not always be comprehensive or up to date. Key parameters like vascular permeability, interstitial diffusivity, or macrophage uptake rates are difficult to measure directly. Also, getting these parametric values in a diseased condition might vary individual wise. This can generate a biased prediction of the diseased stages in the individuals which can be rectified by selecting a diverse cohort of disease data for optimizing the parameters of mathematical models. The system of ODEs is based on the law of mass action. It assumes reactants (e.g., nanoparticles and receptors) are uniformly distributed in space. But in natural system cells, receptors, biomolecules, and NPs differ in their distribution by spatially and temporally, which affect or limit their interaction, localization, and diffusion/advection for accessing the targeted region in the body.

Most MMs of nanomedicine, also assume the occurrence of binding and unbinding based on concentrations and rate constants without considering the stochastic or discrete nature of rare events (important at low concentrations or with low receptor density). Cellular membranes, ECM, and nanoparticle corona create crowding and steric effects, thereby overestimating reaction rates. Many of these models don't usually account for any inhibitor kinetics unless specified. Also, the systems biology approach assumes that the product will definitely be forming until the substrates exhaust, which is untrue occasionally. There is no account for any intermediary products formed. Predictive power is reduced by complex models with many parameters which may overfit limited datasets. The model prediction shows that all the NPs (% Injected Dose) are excreted out of the system as time progresses. But there is a possibility that few NPs are still retained/accumulated. Moreover, models validated in mice often don't scale well to humans due to differences in metabolism, tumor physiology, and immune response.

2.6 CONCLUSION

Computational modeling provides a theoretical framework to simulate and mitigate several biophysical and pharmacological difficulties that occur in cancer nanomedicine. Traditionally, empirical "one-size-fits-all" techniques do not essentially account for the complex bio-nano interactions inside the varied tumor microenvironment, such as protein corona development, high interstitial fluid pressure, and individual patient vascular variance. Hence, computational modelling helps in tailoring the physiologically based PK-PD scenarios. The three comparative case scenarios show that mathematical models offer a non-invasive, provident framework to methodically disintegrate these processes. As seen across the three case studies, moving from plain, unencapsulated cisplatin kinetics to a mass-conserving nanocarrier framework, and finally to a detailed 35-compartment physiologically based pharmacokinetic (PBPK) model, it reveals that capillary blood flow velocity, vascular pore size, and nanoparticle radius govern a drug's therapeutic window. These in-silico techniques effectively predict drug biodistribution, cellular uptake history, and tumor accumulation by switching from free-drug cellular kinetics to PBPK models.

Importantly, these models grant us predictive insights into how changes in nanoparticle characteristics affect various parameters. For instance, a range of 10–50 nm size NP is ideal for vascular permeability, diffusion, and renal clearance in healthy and diseased tissues when compared to >50 nm size counterpart. Mathematical modeling is still crucial despite current constraints in spatial parameterization, nonuniform receptor distribution, and the difficulties of clinical scaling from animal data. Therefore, incorporating computational oncology into the development process speeds up the clinical translation of highly focused, safer nanotherapeutics, while balancing efficacy and systemic toxicity.

REFERENCES

1. Sykes, E. A., J. Chen, G. Zheng, and W. C. W. Chan. "Investigating the Impact of Nanoparticle Size on Active and Passive Tumor Targeting Efficiency." *ACS Nano* 8, no. 6 (2014): 5696–5706. https://doi.org/10.1021/nn500299p.
2. Brocato, T., P. Dogra, E. J. Koay, A. Day, Y. L. Chuang, Z. Wang, and V. Cristini. "Understanding Drug Resistance in Breast Cancer with Mathematical Oncology." *Current Breast Cancer Reports* 6, no. 2 (June 1, 2014): 110–120. https://doi.org/10.1007/s12609-014-0143-2.
3. Chow, E. K. et al. "Nanodiamond Therapeutic Delivery Agents Mediate Enhanced Chemoresistant Tumor Treatment." *Science Translational Medicine* 3, no. 73 (2011): 73ra21–73ra21. https://doi.org/10.1126/scitranslmed.3001713.
4. Wilhelm, S., A. J. Tavares, Q. Dai, et al. "Analysis of Nanoparticle Delivery to Tumours." *Nature Reviews Materials* 1 (2016): 16014. https://doi.org/10.1038/natrevmats.2016.14.
5. Jiang, D., Z. Ge, M. Imran, G. Zhang, and Q. Yin. "Reversible Dendrimer Self-Assembly By Dynamic Core-Branch Interchange for Drug Delivery." *Advanced Materials* 30, no. 18 (2018): 1705550. https://doi.org/10.1002/adma.201705550
6. Ghosh, S., and S. Mukherjee. "Dendrimers: A Versatile Nanocarrier for Drug Delivery and Targeting." *Drug Delivery* 22, no. 6 (2015): 646–659. https://doi.org/10.3109/10717544.2013.841735
7. Kukowska-Latallo, J. F., and J. R. Baker. "Targeted Drug Delivery Using Dendrimer Conjugates." *Nanomedicine* 5, no. 6 (2010): 837–844. https://doi.org/10.2217/nnm.10.64
8. Kesharwani, P., and N. K. Jain. "Stimuli-Responsive Dendrimers for Drug Delivery." *Current Drug Delivery* 11, no. 4 (2014): 386–400. https://doi.org/10.2174/156
9. Nichols, J. W., and Y. H. Bae. "Odyssey of a Cancer Nanoparticle: From Injection Site to Site of Action." *Nano Today* 7, no. 6 (December 1, 2012): 606–618. https://doi.org/10.1016/j.nantod.2012.10.010
10. Lee, T. R., M. Choi, A. Kopacz, et al. "On the Near-Wall Accumulation of Injectable Particles in the Microcirculation: Smaller Is Not Better." *Scientific Reports* 3 (2013): 2079. https://doi.org/10.1038/srep02079
11. Müller, K., D. Fedosov, and G. Gompper. "Margination of micro- and nano-particles in blood flow and its effect on drug delivery." *Scientific Reports* 4 (2014): 4871. https://doi.org/10.1038/srep04871
12. Dogra, P., N. L. Adolphi, Z. Wang, et al. "Establishing the Effects of Mesoporous Silica Nanoparticle Properties on In Vivo Disposition Using Imaging-Based Pharmacokinetics." *Nature Communications* 9 (2018): 4551. https://doi.org/10.1038/s41467-018-06730-z
13. Deisboeck, T. S., Z. Wang, P. Macklin, and V. Cristini. "Multiscale Cancer Modeling." *Annual Review of Biomedical Engineering* 13 (2011): 127–155. https://doi.org/10.1146/annurev-bioeng-071910-124729
14. Pascal, J., C. E. Ashley, Z. Wang, T. A. Brocato, J. D. Butner, E. C. Carnes, E. J. Koay, C. J. Brinker, and V. Cristini. "Mechanistic Modeling Identifies Drug-Uptake History as Predictor of Tumor Drug Resistance and Nano-Carrier-Mediated Response." *ACS Nano* 7, no. 12 (2013): 11174–11182. https://doi.org/10.1021/nn4048974.
15. Wang, Z., R. Kerketta, Y. Chuang, P. Dogra, J. D. Butner, T. A. Brocato, A. Day, et al. "Theory and Experimental Validation of a Spatio-Temporal Model of Chemotherapy Transport to Enhance Tumor Cell Kill." *PLoS Computational Biology* 12, no. 6 (2016): e1004969. https://pmc.ncbi.nlm.nih.gov/articles/PMC4902302/
16. Cristini, V., E. J. Koay, and Z. Wang. *An Introduction to Physical Oncology: How Mechanistic Mathematical Modeling Can Improve Cancer Therapy Outcomes.* Elsevier, 2017. https://mdanderson.elsevierpure.com/en/publications/an-introduction-to-physical-oncology-how-mechanistic-mathematical
17. Joseph, J. F., L. Gronbach, J. García-Miller, L. M. Cruz, B. Wuest, U. Keilholz, C. Zoschke, and M. K. Parr. Automated real-time tumor pharmacokinetic profiling in 3D models: A novel approach for personalized medicine. *Pharmaceutics* 12, no. 413 (2020). https://doi.org/10.3390/pharmaceutics12050413

18. Gutmann, D. H., J. S. Boehm, E. K. Karlsson, E. Padron, M. Seshadri, D. Wallis, and J. C. Snyder. Precision preclinical modeling to advance cancer treatment. *Journal of the National Cancer Institute* (2024): djae249. https://doi.org/10.1093/jnci/djae249
19. Dogra, P., J. D. Butner, J. R. Ramírez, Y. Chuang, A. Noureddine, C. J. Brinker, V. Cristini, and Z. Wang. "A Mathematical Model to Predict Nanomedicine Pharmacokinetics and Tumor Delivery." *Computational and Structural Biotechnology Journal* 18 (2020): 518–531. https://doi.org/10.1016/j.csbj.2020.02.014.
20. Dogra, P., J. D. Butner, S. Nizzero, J. R. Ramírez, A. Noureddine, M. J. Peláez, D. Elganainy, Z. Yang, A. K. El-Naggar, S. Goel, H. S. Leong, E. J. Koay, C. Jeffrey Brinker, V. Cristini, and Z. Wang. "Image-Guided Mathematical Modeling for Pharmacological Evaluation of Nanomaterials and Monoclonal Antibodies." *Wiley Interdisciplinary Reviews: Nanomedicine and Nanobiotechnology* 12, no. 5 (September 2020): e1628. https://doi.org/10.1002/wnan.1628.
21. El-Kareh AW, Secomb TW. A mathematical model for cisplatin cellular pharmacodynamics. *Neoplasia* 5, no. 2 (2003 Mar-Apr): 161–169. https://doi.org/10.1016/s1476-5586(03)80008-8. PMID: 12659689; PMCID: PMC1502402.
22. Pascal J, Ashley CE, Wang Z, Brocato TA, Butner JD, Carnes EC, Koay EJ, Brinker CJ, Cristini V. Mechanistic modeling identifies drug-uptake history as predictor of tumor drug resistance and nano-carrier-mediated response. *ACS Nano* 7, no. 12 (2013 Dec 23): 11174–11182. https://doi.org/10.1021/nn4048974. Epub 2013 Nov 11. PMID: 24187963; PMCID: PMC3891887.
23. Dogra, P., J. D. Butner, Y.-L. Chuang, and others. "Mathematical Modeling in Cancer Nanomedicine: A Review." *Biomedical Microdevices* 21, no. 40 (2019). https://doi.org/10.1007/s10544-019-0380-2.
24. Fang, J., H. Nakamura, and H. Maeda. "The EPR Effect: Unique Features of Tumor Blood Vessels for Drug Delivery, Factors Involved, and Limitations and Augmentation of the Effect." *Advanced Drug Delivery Reviews* 63, no. 3 (March 18, 2011): 136–151. https://doi.org/10.1016/j.addr.2010.04.009.
25. Hashizume, H., P. Baluk, S. Morikawa, J. W. McLean, G. Thurston, S. Roberge, R. K. Jain, and D. M. McDonald. "Openings between Defective Endothelial Cells Explain Tumor Vessel Leakiness." *The American Journal of Pathology* 156, no. 4 (April 2000): 1363–1380. https://doi.org/10.1016/S0002-9440(10)65006-7.
26. Wang, Z., J. D. Butner, R. Kerketta, V. Cristini, and T. S. Deisboeck. "Simulating Cancer Growth with Multiscale Agent-Based Modeling." *Seminars in Cancer Biology* 30 (February 2015): 70–78. https://doi.org/10.1016/j.semcancer.2014.04.001.
27. Brocato, T. A., U. Brown-Glaberman, Z. Wang, R. G. Selwyn, C. Matthew Wilson, E. F. Wyckoff, L. C. Lomo, J. L. Saline, A. Hooda-Nehra, R. Pasqualini, W. Arap, C. Jeffrey Brinker, and V. Cristini. "Predicting Breast Cancer Response to Neoadjuvant Chemotherapy Based on Tumor Vascular Features in Needle Biopsies." *JCI Insight* 5, no. 8 (March 5, 2019): e126518. https://doi.org/10.1172/jci.insight.126518.
28. Stylianopoulos, T., and R. K. Jain. "The Solid Mechanics of Cancer and Strategies for Improved Therapy." *Journal of Biomechanical Engineering* 139, no. 2 (2017): 021004. https://doi.org/10.1115/1.4035695.
29. Jain, R. K., and T. Stylianopoulos. "Delivering Nanomedicine to Solid Tumors." *Nature Reviews Clinical Oncology* 7 (2010): 653–664. https://doi.org/10.1038/nrclinonc.2010.139.
30. Alexis, F., E. Pridgen, L. K. Molnar, and O. C. Farokhzad. "Factors Affecting the Clearance and Biodistribution of Polymeric Nanoparticles." *Molecular Pharmaceutics* 5, no. 4 (2008): 505–515. https://doi.org/10.1021/mp800051m.
31. Troger, V., J. L. Fischel, P. Formento, J. Gioanni, and G. Milano. "Effects of Prolonged Exposure to Cisplatin on Cytotoxicity and Intracellular Drug Concentration." *European Journal of Cancer* 28: 82–86.
32. Andrews, P. A., S. Velury, S. C. Mann, and S. B. Howell. "cis-Diamminedichloroplatinum(II) Accumulation in Sensitive and Resistant Human Ovarian Carcinoma Cells." *Cancer Research* 48, no. 1 (1988 Jan 1): 68–73. PMID: 3335000.

3 Functionalized Lipid Nanoparticles for Cancer Therapy

Sujith M. Subrahmanian,[1] Suchona Ghosh,[1] Vibha Choudhary,[1] Megha M. Unnimaya,[1] Poonam Dogra,[1] Pratik Katare,[1] Ratul Dutta,[1] Vaishali Makwana,[2] and Jyotsnendu Giri[1]
[1]Department of Biomedical Engineering, Indian Institute of Technology Hyderabad, Kandi, Telangana, India
[2]Centre for Interdisciplinary Programs, Indian Institute of Technology Hyderabad, Kandi, Telangana, India

3.1 INTRODUCTION

Cancer continues to be one of the leading causes of death worldwide, affecting millions of people each year and placing a significant burden on healthcare systems. Although considerable progress has been made in cancer diagnosis and treatment, many therapeutic approaches still face challenges such as poor tumor specificity, severe side effects, drug resistance, and disease recurrence. These limitations have prompted the search for more effective and targeted treatment strategies.

In recent years, nanotechnology has emerged as a promising tool for improving cancer therapy. Among the various nanocarrier systems, lipid nanoparticles have gained particular attention because of their biocompatibility, ability to carry a wide range of therapeutic agents, and potential for clinical translation. The incorporation of functional components, such as targeting ligands, stimuli-responsive materials, and biomimetic coatings, has further enhanced their ability to selectively deliver therapeutic payloads to tumor sites while minimizing off-target effects.

As a result, functionalized lipid nanoparticles have become an important platform for the delivery of anticancer drugs, genes, proteins, and immunotherapeutic agents. This chapter explores the development and application of functionalized lipid nanoparticles in cancer therapy, with a focus on their design strategies, therapeutic advantages, and potential to address the limitations of conventional cancer treatments.

3.1.1 Global Burden of Cancer and Limitations of Current Therapies

Cancer is a lingering threat to worldwide health and is still one of the significant causes of death worldwide, with around 19.3 million fresh cases and almost 10 million fatalities in 2020 alone (1). Cancer's worldwide burden is still on the rise due to aging populations, lifestyle factors, and genetic predispositions. It brings significant socioeconomic and healthcare burdens, especially in low- and middle-income countries. Despite significant developments in surgical interventions, chemotherapy, radiotherapy, targeted therapies, and immunotherapy, many problems persist. Conventional chemotherapeutic agents are commonly characterized by low tumor selectivity and thus result in a lot of system-wide toxicity, drug resistance, and relapse of disease. Similarly, although radiotherapy and surgery are effective in localized tumors, they are rarely effective when metastasis occurs. Moreover, even newer therapies such as immune checkpoint inhibitors and CAR-T therapy face

DOI: 10.1201/9781003799351-3

setbacks in the form of immune-related side effects, restrictive use in specific types of cancer, and skyrocketing costs. These issues attest to a pressing need for novel therapy approaches that combine efficacy, safety, and specificity.

3.1.2 Emergence of Nanotechnology in Oncology

Nanotechnology has transformed biomedical research by providing unprecedented possibilities for breaking away from limitations in traditional cancer therapies. Nanoparticles (NPs), which range in size between 10 and 200 nm in diameter, display favorable pharmacokinetics, superior tumor accumulation attributed to the enhanced permeability and retention (EPR) effect, and potential for directed delivery by virtue of design. Lipid-structured nanoparticles (LNPs), polymeric nanoparticles, inorganic nanocarriers (gold, silicon dioxide, iron oxide nanoparticles), and hybrid nanostructures have been studied for cancer diagnostics, drug delivery, imaging, and theranostics (2).

Lipid nanoparticles are today a rising force in medicine for their exceptional biocompatibility, structural adaptability, and clinical translatability. Historic approval in 2018 for lipid nanoparticle–structured siRNA drug patisiran (Onpattro®) and their contribution toward mRNA vaccine delivery in the COVID-19 pandemic further boosted enthusiasm for their use in cancer therapies. Consequently, nanotechnology, in general, and lipid nanoparticles, in particular, are leading next-generation cancer therapies.

3.1.3 Advantages of Lipid-Based Nanoparticles in Cancer Therapy

Lipid nanoparticles possess several benefits over inorganic or polymeric nanocarriers. Because their lipid bilayer composition is structurally close to cell membranes, effective entrapment is achievable for a variety of compounds, ranging from hydrophilic to hydrophobic drugs, nucleic acids, as well as imaging agents. Lipid nanoparticles confer protection to therapeutic agents against enzymatic cleavage, thereby enhancing their circulating half-life and biodistribution. Moreover, a variety of functionalization schemes, ranging from PEGylation to ligand conjugation, enable improved tumor targetability while simultaneously reducing clearance by the reticuloendothelial system.

Further, LNPs are rationally engineered as pH-responsive/carbohydrate-responsive/oxidation-responsive/heat-responsive carriers for delivering their cargo in synchronization with pH gradients, enzyme activity, redox state, or temperature in the tumor microenvironment. Combination therapies are administered simultaneously by simultaneous delivery of photothermal or photodynamic agents in combination with chemotherapeutic agents or nucleic acids to maximize synergistic anticancer effects. Less toxic, mass producible, and clinically acceptable compared with polymeric nanoparticles or inorganic nanocarriers, are LNPs (Pattni et al., 2015).

3.1.4 Scope and Objectives of the Chapter

This chapter provides an in-depth analysis of functionalized lipid nanoparticles (LNPs) for cancer therapy applications based on their design, functionalization strategies, therapeutic agents, and translatability to clinical applications. The discussion begins with the categorization and physicochemical properties of different LNPs. It explores advanced techniques for artificial engineering, including surface manipulation, stimuli-responsive materials, and hybrid nanostructures, to enhance therapeutic effectiveness. The chapter further explores a wide range of therapeutics suitable for LNP integration, encompassing small molecules, nucleic acids, immunotherapeutic entities, and chemicals for photothermal or sonodynamic treatments. Moreover, it addresses developments in both preclinical and clinical arenas, focusing on functionalized LNPs for improved cancer therapy outcomes. Finally, issues concerning mass production, stability, approval for clinical use, and future direction in line with personalized nanomedicine are critically analyzed.

The ultimate aim is for scientists, doctors, and practitioners in industry to acquire a contemporary understanding of how functionalized LNPs can be mobilized in the pursuit of meeting today's therapeutic needs, enhancing patient outcomes, and shaping tomorrow's cancer nanomedicines.

The ultimate goal is to provide scientists, doctors, and industry experts with an up-to-date account of how functionalized LNPs can be leveraged to overcome current therapeutic hurdles, improve patient outcomes, and shape tomorrow's cancer nanomedicine.

3.2 OVERVIEW OF LIPID-BASED NANOPARTICLES

A dynamic and incredibly adaptable family of nanocarriers, lipid-based nanoparticles (LNPs) have been the subject of extensive cancer research due to their distinct physicochemical characteristics, biocompatibility, and capacity to overcome several drawbacks of traditional chemotherapeutics. Due to their structural adaptability, hydrophilic and hydrophobic compounds, nucleic acids, and biomacromolecules can be encapsulated, thereby increasing solubility, enhancing pharmacokinetics, and reducing systemic toxicity. LNPs allow for the preferential accumulation of nanoscale carriers in tumor tissues by taking advantage of the enhanced permeability and retention (EPR) effect, which is a characteristic of tumor vasculature marked by leaky capillaries and inadequate lymphatic outflow. Additionally, LNP surface engineering enables the integration of stimuli-responsive features and active targeting using ligands (such as antibodies, peptides, and small molecules) to provide spatiotemporally controlled drug release. LNP-based formulations are now being used in clinical settings, such as in RNA vaccines and liposomal doxorubicin (Doxil) for the treatment of breast cancer. These advances show promise for personalized cancer treatments. However, there are still challenges to address, like stability, production scale-up, and differences in patient tumor physiology (4).

3.2.1 Classification and Types

LNPs are categorized according to their intended medicinal use, lipid phase composition, and structural arrangement. In oncology, each type has unique benefits for medication delivery, stability, and targeting. These are divided into four categories: Liposomes, solid lipid nanoparticles (SLNs), nanostructured lipid carriers (NLCs), and hybrid lipid–polymer nanoparticles (5).

3.2.1.1 Liposomes

Liposomes are tiny, round structures made up of water surrounded by one or more layers of phospholipids (6). They are naturally biocompatible and adaptable for drug delivery applications because of their architecture, which closely resembles biological membranes. A variety of therapeutic molecules, including small-molecule chemotherapeutics, peptides, nucleic acids, and imaging agents, can be incorporated into liposomes due to their amphiphilic nature, which allows for the simultaneous incorporation of hydrophilic drugs within the aqueous interior and hydrophobic agents within the lipid bilayer. Natural or synthesized phospholipids (such as phosphatidylcholine and phosphatidylethanolamine) and stabilizing substances like cholesterol, which alter bilayer rigidity and permeability, are commonly found in liposome composition (Figure 3.1) (5). Liposomes have shown promise in oncology as a means of addressing the main drawbacks of traditional chemotherapy, namely its quick clearance, poor solubility, and systemic toxicity. Drugs encapsulated in liposomes are protected from early breakdown, their pharmacokinetic characteristics are altered, and weakly water-soluble medicines like paclitaxel become more soluble (7). The creation of long-circulating liposomes by surface modification with polyethylene glycol (PEG), or PEGylation, is one of the key developments in liposomal design. By reducing detection and clearance by the mononuclear phagocyte system (MPS), PEGylation confers a "stealth" property that prolongs plasma half-life and permits increased accumulation in tumors through the enhanced permeability and retention (EPR) effect. Through the functionalization of their surface with ligands like folic acid, transferrin, antibodies, aptamers, or peptides that bind to receptors overexpressed on cancer cells, actively

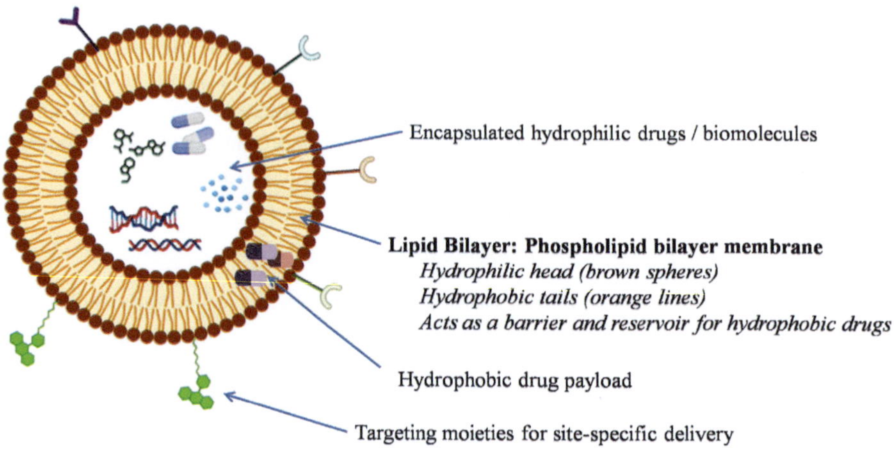

FIGURE 3.1 Schematic representation of a multifunctional liposome for targeted drug delivery. The liposome consists of a phospholipid bilayer encapsulating hydrophilic drugs, nucleic acids, or proteins in its aqueous core, while hydrophobic drugs are embedded within the bilayer. Surface ligands, such as antibodies, peptides, or aptamers, enable targeted delivery, while PEGylation enhances stability and prolongs circulation time.

targeted liposomes have been developed to attain better selectivity beyond passive accumulation (8). By targeting cytotoxic medicines to the tumor location and minimizing off-target effects, these strategies enhance therapeutic indices.

The successful entry of several liposomal formulations into clinical practice highlights their potential for translation. The first FDA-approved liposomal anticancer medication was Doxil® (liposomal doxorubicin), which showed notable cardiotoxicity reductions in comparison to traditional doxorubicin while retaining antitumor activity in ovarian and breast malignancies. In a similar vein, Onivyde® (liposomal irinotecan), which offers enhanced treatment response and extended circulation, has been approved for metastatic pancreatic cancer. Liposomal vincristine (Marqibo®) and liposomal cytarabine (DepoCyt®) are two further clinically tested formulations that have expanded their use in both solid tumors and hematological malignancies.

Liposomes face difficulties despite their progress as medicines and potential drug. Lipid oxidation, hydrolysis, and aggregation are examples of physical and chemical instability that can shorten a product's shelf life during storage (6). Drug leakage is still an issue, especially for tiny hydrophilic compounds; thus, production processes and lipid composition must be optimized. Furthermore, the "accelerated blood clearance" (ABC) phenomenon, in which anti-PEG antibodies cause rapid clearance after consecutive doses, may be triggered by the repeated administration of PEGylated liposomes. Investigating new stabilizing lipids, stimuli-responsive systems (such as pH- or enzyme-sensitive liposomes), and stealth coatings other than PEG are necessary to overcome these constraints. All things considered, liposomes are a fundamental component of oncology nanomedicine, providing a clinically proven and versatile delivery system for biologics and chemotherapeutics. Ongoing design advancements have the potential to improve tumor targeting even more, get past resistance mechanisms, and make combo therapy possible for better cancer control (10).

3.2.1.2 Solid Lipid Nanoparticles

Solid lipid nanoparticles (SLNs) are submicron colloidal carriers with a lipid core stabilized by surfactants that stay solid at room temperature and physiological temperatures. Usually between 10 and 1000 nm in size, they are made with physiologically appropriate lipids, including waxes, fatty acids (like stearic and palmitic acids), and triglycerides (like glyceryl behenate). With improved stability, protection of labile medicines, and regulated release patterns, the solid lipid matrix offers a distinct advantage over liquid lipid-based carriers (Figure 3.2) (11).

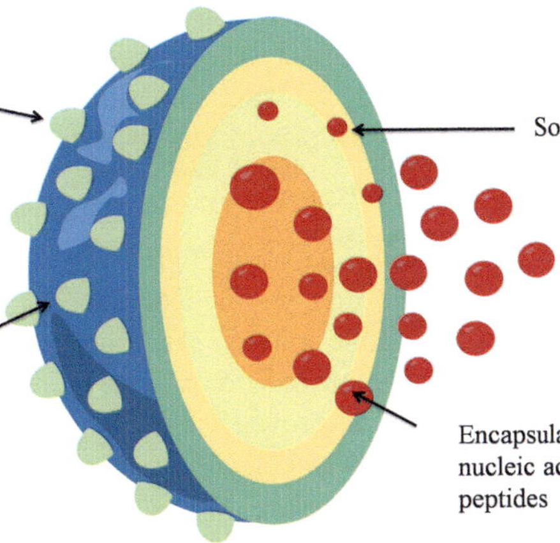

FIGURE 3.2 Schematic illustration of a solid lipid nanoparticle (SLN). The system consists of a solid lipid matrix that encapsulates hydrophobic drugs or biomolecules, surrounded by surfactants or polymers for stabilization. Surface functionalization with targeting ligands or PEG enhances specificity, stability, and therapeutic performance through controlled drug release.

SLNs have shown great potential as delivery systems for hydrophobic phytochemicals and chemotherapeutics in the field of oncology. Poorly soluble anticancer drugs like paclitaxel, docetaxel, curcumin, and quercetin can be encapsulated within SLNs to improve their water dispersibility, shield them from early metabolic breakdown, and enable long-term therapeutic concentrations at the tumor site. Additionally, SLNs' stiff lipid matrix offers a diffusion-controlled release mechanism that can limit systemic side effects and reduce the frequency of dose administration. Additionally, studies have demonstrated that SLNs can be designed for active targeting by surface modification with ligands such as folic acid or transferrin, promoting receptor-mediated uptake by cancer cells, as well as for passive tumor targeting through the enhanced permeability and retention (EPR) effect.

The use of paclitaxel in SLNs is one noteworthy application; in comparison to more traditional formulations such as Cremophor EL-based Taxol, it has demonstrated enhanced tumor inhibition and less systemic toxicity. In preclinical breast and colon cancer models, curcumin-loaded SLNs have also demonstrated improved bioavailability and higher antitumor activity, highlighting the promise of SLNs in delivering bioactive natural chemicals. Notwithstanding these benefits, SLNs have intrinsic drawbacks. Due to polymorphic transitions caused by their high degree of crystallinity, drugs may be expelled during storage, thereby decreasing their long-term stability and loading capacity. Furthermore, they often exhibit poor encapsulation efficiency for highly hydrophilic medications. Strategies like using lipid blends to lessen crystallinity, incorporating liquid lipids to create nanostructured lipid carriers (NLCs), and implementing advanced manufacturing techniques (like high-pressure homogenization and microemulsion techniques) have all been used to get past these obstacles. All things considered, SLNs are a cutting-edge platform in lipid nanotechnology for cancer treatment, providing a harmony of functionality, scalability, and safety. In order to treat cancer more precisely and successfully, ongoing research attempts to improve their composition, create targeted SLNs, and incorporate stimuli-responsive properties (14).

3.2.1.3 Nanostructured Lipid Carriers

Innovative second-generation lipid-based drug delivery systems called nanostructured lipid carriers (NLCs) were created to overcome the intrinsic drawbacks of solid lipid nanoparticles (SLNs), including limited drug loading and drug ejection during storage. An imperfect crystalline or amorphous lipid matrix is produced by the special mix of solid and liquid lipids in NLCs, typically in ratios ranging from 70:30 to 99.9:0.1 (solid:liquid). By creating gaps in the matrix, this structural alteration disrupts the densely packed arrangement of lipid molecules present in SLNs, thereby improving long-term stability, minimizing drug leakage, and enhancing drug uptake. Glyceryl behenate, cetyl palmitate, and stearic acid are examples of common solid lipids. In contrast, medium-chain triglycerides (MCTs), oleic acid, and isopropyl myristate are examples of liquid lipids that help create matrix flexibility (Figure 3.3) (16).

NLCs have shown great promise in oncology as delivery vehicles for combination treatments, hydrophobic chemotherapeutic drugs, and phytochemicals. Multiple medications can be encapsulated simultaneously in their adaptable matrix, resulting in synergistic therapeutic effects. For example, in preclinical models of breast and colon cancer, resveratrol-loaded NLCs have demonstrated enhanced chemical stability, improved bioavailability, and increased anticancer activity. Additionally, by taking use of curcumin's capacity to alter drug resistance pathways, co-delivery systems that employ NLCs—such as temozolomide-curcumin NLCs—have demonstrated improved therapeutic outcomes in glioblastoma by amplifying the effects of temozolomide. The therapeutic potential of NLCs is further enhanced by surface modification. While conjugation with targeting ligands, such as transferrin, folic acid, or antibodies, enables active tumor targeting through receptor-mediated endocytosis, functionalization with biopolymers like chitosan enhances mucoadhesion and extends the residence duration at tumor locations. Furthermore, by avoiding immune recognition, stealth coatings made of polyethylene glycol (PEG) or zwitterionic polymers prolong circulation times. Stimuli-responsive NLCs are another recent invention that enhances site-specific delivery and reduces systemic toxicity by selectively releasing their payload in response to tumor-associated triggers, such as acidic pH, increased reactive oxygen species (ROS), or enzymatic activity. NLCs are among the most promising nanocarrier systems for future cancer treatments due to their exceptional encapsulation efficiency, controlled release characteristics, and multifunctionality. However, even with their potential, issues persist with reproducibility, large-scale manufacture, and regulatory approval. It is anticipated that further research, concentrating on refining formulation characteristics, including precision targeting, and verifying clinical performance, will hasten the use of NLC-based treatments in clinical cancer (18).

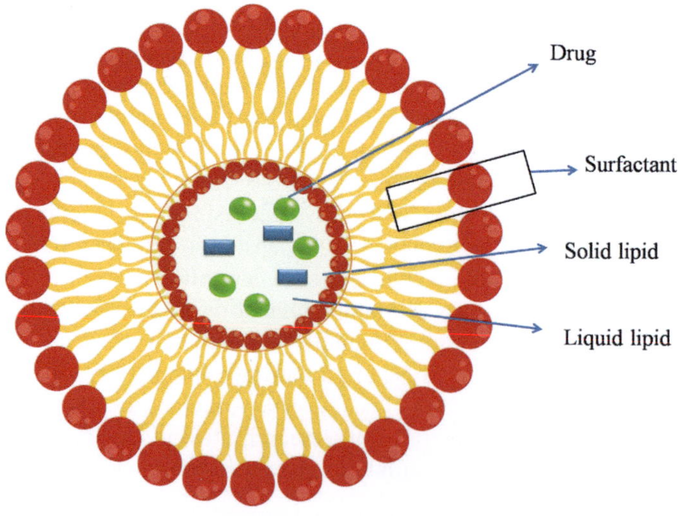

FIGURE 3.3 Nanostructured lipid carriers (NLCs): The NLC consists of a solid–liquid lipid matrix stabilized by surfactants. The small spheres represent the hydrophilic head groups of lipids, while the yellow tails depict the hydrophobic fatty acid chains forming the disordered lipid matrix. This mixed matrix allows incorporation of both hydrophobic and amphiphilic drugs, enhancing stability and controlled drug release.

3.2.1.4 Hybrid Lipid–Polymer Nanoparticles

Hybrid lipid–polymer nanoparticles (HLPNs) are a next-generation class of nanocarriers that combine the advantages of lipid-based and polymer-based delivery systems into a single multifunctional platform. These hybrid systems typically consist of a polymeric core—commonly formed using biodegradable and biocompatible polymers such as poly (lactic-co-glycolic acid) (PLGA), polycaprolactone (PCL), or chitosan—surrounded by a stabilizing lipid shell made of phospholipids, cholesterol, or other amphiphilic lipids. This core–shell structure integrates the structural robustness, tunable drug release, and high loading capacity of polymeric nanoparticles with the excellent biocompatibility, reduced immunogenicity, and membrane-mimicking properties of lipid-based systems. A new family of nanocarriers known as hybrid lipid–polymer nanoparticles (HLPNs) combine the benefits of polymer-based and lipid-based delivery systems into a single, multipurpose platform. A stabilizing lipid shell composed of phospholipids, cholesterol, or other amphiphilic lipids usually envelops a polymeric core, which is often made of biodegradable and biocompatible polymers like poly (lactic-co-glycolic acid) (PLGA), polycaprolactone (PCL), or chitosan. This core-shell structure combines the superior biocompatibility, decreased immunogenicity, and membrane-mimicking capabilities of lipid-based systems with the structural stability, adjustable drug release, and high loading capacity of polymeric nanoparticles (Figure 3.4) (19).

The lipid layer prolongs systemic circulation by preventing the polymeric core from opsonizing, preventing premature drug leakage, protecting sensitive cargo from degradation, and improving colloidal stability. In the meantime, the polymeric core provides a flexible space that can accommodate both hydrophilic and hydrophobic substances, such as therapeutic peptides, nucleic acids (including DNA, siRNA, and mRNA), and small-molecule medications. Furthermore, the co-delivery of several therapeutic drugs is made possible by the modular construction of HLPNs, allowing combination therapies that can target many cancer hallmarks at once (19).

HLPNs have demonstrated great potential in oncology as carriers for nucleic acid-based treatments as well as chemotherapeutic medications. In breast and ovarian cancer models, for instance, PLGA-lipid hybrid nanoparticles co-loaded with doxorubicin and siRNA have shown strong

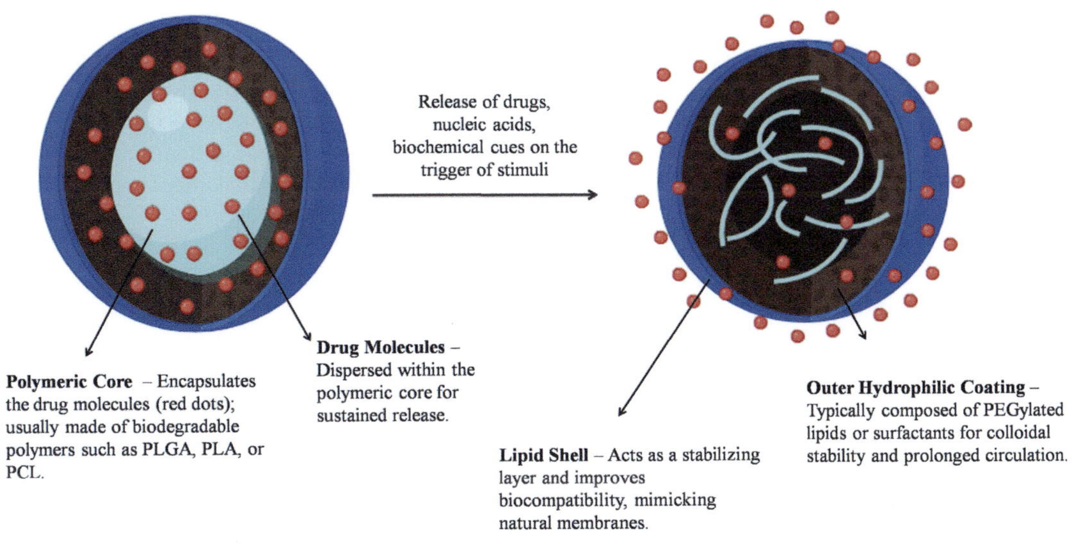

FIGURE 3.4 Schematic representation of hybrid lipid–polymer nanoparticles (HLPNs). The figure shows two structural models: (left) core–shell type, consisting of a polymeric core encapsulating the drug and coated with a lipid shell, and (right) matrix type, in which lipids and polymers are uniformly blended to form a hybrid matrix. Both structures combine the advantages of polymeric nanoparticles (mechanical stability and controlled release) with lipid nanoparticles (biocompatibility and enhanced cellular uptake)

synergistic effects, defeating multidrug resistance by delivering lethal drugs directly to tumor cells and silencing resistance-associated genes. Similarly, the rapid release of drugs in the acidic tumor microenvironment is facilitated by pH-responsive HLPNs with acid-labile linkers in the lipid shell, which maximizes therapeutic efficacy while minimizing systemic side effects (20).

The usefulness of HLPNs has been further enhanced by targeting tactics. Through receptor-mediated endocytosis, surface modification with ligands such as monoclonal antibodies, folic acid, and RGD peptides (which target integrins and folate receptors) improves tumor-specific uptake. Utilizing the enhanced permeability and retention (EPR) effect in solid tumors requires longer circulation durations, which are ensured by stealth coatings such as polyethylene glycol (PEG) and zwitterionic lipids, which decrease clearance by the mononuclear phagocyte system (MPS). The promise of HLPNs for cancer immunotherapy has also been highlighted by recent research; therapeutic cancer vaccines have been made possible by the strong immune responses elicited by lipid-coated polymeric nanoparticles loaded with tumor antigens and adjuvants (13).

Despite its many benefits, the complexity of their core–shell structure makes it difficult for HLPNs to be produced on a large scale, obtain regulatory approval, and ensure batch-to-batch reproducibility. To overcome these difficulties, sophisticated production methods have been developed that provide exact control over particle size, composition, and surface functionality, including microfluidics and nanoprecipitation. It is expected that further research would expedite the transition of HLPNs from bench to bedside by refining their formulations, incorporating stimuli-responsive and biomimetic designs (such as cell membrane-coated HLPNs), and confirming their clinical efficacy. All things considered, HLPNs are a strong and adaptable nanoplatform that can combine several therapeutic modalities into a single delivery system, offering enormous promise for enhancing the effectiveness, safety, and specificity of cancer therapies (21).

Several lipid-based nanocarrier systems have been developed for cancer therapy, each exhibiting distinct structural features, drug-loading capacities, stability profiles, and targeting capabilities. A comparative overview of the key properties of SLNs, NLCs, HLPNs, and liposomes is presented in Table 3.1.

3.2.2 Physicochemical Characteristics and Design Parameters

The in vivo behavior, therapeutic efficacy, and translational potential of lipid-based nanoparticles (LNPs) are all significantly influenced by their physicochemical properties. Biodistribution, cellular uptake, drug loading, release kinetics, and stability are all influenced by several factors, including particle size, surface charge, morphology, lipid content, and surface modifications. Creating therapeutically effective nanocarriers requires a logical design process that incorporates these elements (13).

- **Particle Size:** When it comes to the pharmacokinetics and biodistribution of LNPs, particle size is crucial. Because they can extravasate through leaky tumor vasculature without being opsonized by the mononuclear phagocyte system (MPS) (>200 nm) or rapidly cleared by the kidneys (<10 nm), nanoparticles in the 10–200 nm size range are perfect for passive tumor targeting through the enhanced permeability and retention (EPR) effect. Size also affects cellular uptake mechanisms; for example, particles with a diameter of 100 nm tend to favor clathrin-mediated endocytosis, which improves intracellular drug delivery. Using methods such as extrusion, microfluidics, or high-pressure homogenization to control size ensures therapeutic repeatability and batch-to-batch consistency (5).
- **Surface Charge (Zeta Potential):** The surface charge of LNPs, often represented as zeta potential, affects cellular interactions, circulation time, and colloidal stability. Due to electrostatic repulsion, highly charged particles (>+30 mV or <–30 mV) have exceptional physical stability; yet, interactions with serum proteins may cause them to be cleared quickly. Polyethylene glycol (PEG) coating is frequently used to achieve near-neutral or

TABLE 3.1
Comparison of the Properties of NLCs, HLPNs, SLNs, and Liposomes in Oncology Applications

Feature	Liposomes	Solid Lipid Nanoparticles (SLNs)	Nanostructured Lipid Carriers (NLCs)	Hybrid Lipid–Polymer Nanoparticles (HLPNs)
Structure	spherical vesicles with an aqueous core encircled by one or more phospholipid bilayers.	stiff crystalline matrix with a solid lipid core stabilized by surfactants.	combination of liquid and solid lipids that creates an amorphous or defective matrix.	PLGA and PCL are polymeric cores covered with lipid shells (cholesterol, phospholipids).
Drug Loading	Drugs that are hydrophilic in the aqueous core and hydrophobic in the bilayer.	mostly lipophilic medications distributed in a solid substrate.	Lipophilic medicines have a high loading because of structural flaws.	High loading of hydrophilic and hydrophobic medications; appropriate for co-administration.
Release Mechanism	PEGylation and lipid composition regulate diffusion across the bilayer.	diffusion and gradual degradation of the lipid matrix.	matrix disorganization for sustained release; gradual reduction in drug ejection.	Lipid permeability and polymer breakdown control the release.
Stability	PEGylation improves this oxidation and leakage sensitivity.	Although it has good physical stability, it is susceptible to polymorphic changes while being stored.	decreased crystallinity, which results in improved stability over SLNs.	Outstanding stability; the polymer core adds strength, and the lipid shell inhibits aggregation.
Targeting Potential	Both active (ligand/antibody conjugation) and passive (EPR impact).	mainly passive, though it can be changed to target actively.	improved drug retention at tumor locations; passive and active targeting.	High adaptability; targeting can be done passively, actively, or in response to inputs.
Clinical Status	a number of FDA-approved formulations (such as Onivyde and Doxil).	Most are in preclinical phases, with a few numbers in clinical evaluation.	new technology; a number of encouraging preclinical investigations.	expanding research quickly; several are undergoing cancer treatment clinical trials in their early stages.
Advantages	dual drug loading, biocompatibility, and clinical validation.	dual drug loading, biocompatibility, and clinical validation.	enhanced bioavailability, prolonged release, and high drug loading.	combines the advantages of polymers and lipids; it is versatile and multipurpose.
Limitations	rapid blood clearance with repeated dosage and storage instability.	restricted drug loading and polymorphism changes.	difficult formulation optimization and scalability issues.	complicated production, difficult regulations, and increased expenses.

slightly negative zeta potential, which is desirable for extended systemic circulation and less immune recognition. On the other hand, positively charged LNPs may increase toxicity and activate complement, but they can also improve cellular absorption by electrostatically attracting negatively charged cell membranes (22).

- **Morphology and Structure:** The majority of LNPs have spherical morphology, which is often preferred for consistent distribution and predictable biodistribution. However, in specific investigations, different forms, including rod-like or discoidal nanoparticles, have demonstrated improved tumor penetration and vascular margination, suggesting that morphology may be deliberately altered to enhance therapeutic outcomes. Structural characteristics, such as crystallinity in solid lipid carriers or bilayer integrity in liposomes, directly impact drug retention and release kinetics (5).
- **Lipid Composition:** The selection of lipids is crucial for LNP activity. While cholesterol improves bilayer stability by lowering permeability, natural phospholipids (such as phosphatidylcholine and phosphatidylethanolamine) offer biocompatibility and membrane-mimicking qualities. Matrix stiffness, drug loading capacity, and release behavior for SLNs and NLCs are determined by the kind and proportion of solid to liquid lipids (18). Lipids' phase transition temperature (Tm) and other thermodynamic characteristics are crucial. Lipids with a high Tm provide more rigid carriers that reduce leakage but may impede drug release, whereas lipids with a lower Tm increase flexibility and enhance release rates.
- **Surfactants and Stabilizers:** To stabilize LNPs by reducing interfacial tension and inhibiting aggregation, surfactants such as lecithin, Poloxamer 188, and Tween 80 are employed. Particle size, stability, and cytocompatibility are strongly influenced by the kind and concentration of surfactant. To guarantee stability without causing cytotoxic consequences, the ideal equilibrium must be struck (24).
- **Surface Functionalization:** By reducing opsonization and clearance through a "stealth" effect, surface engineering LNPs with hydrophilic polymers (like PEG) extends circulation time (25). Additionally, active targeting to tumor-specific receptors is made possible by conjugating targeting ligands (antibodies, peptides, aptamers, and small molecules like folic acid), which enhances absorption and the therapeutic index. Biomimetic coatings that use cell membranes (such as those of cancer cells or immune cells) to improve tumor homing and immune evasion are examples of emerging techniques.
- **Encapsulation Efficiency and Drug Loading:** Achieving therapeutic efficacy at clinically relevant doses requires effective drug encapsulation and a large loading capacity. For lipophilic pharmaceuticals in NLCs and hybrids, encapsulation efficiency (EE) frequently exceeds 80–90%. In contrast, hydrophilic medications in liposomes may require the refinement of preparation techniques, such as ethanol injection, thin-film hydration, or microfluidics. In addition to guaranteeing appropriate dosage, high EE also reduces the toxicity associated with excipients (26).
- **Stability and Scalability:** One important factor influencing LNPs' therapeutic utility is their stability in biological fluids and during storage (13). Performance can be hampered by problems such lipid oxidation, aggregation, and polymorphic transitions. Using antioxidants, lyophilizing with cryoprotectants, and optimizing lipid compositions are some methods to improve stability. The scalability of the production process is also crucial; techniques like high-pressure homogenization, microfluidics, and supercritical fluid technology are favored due to their industrial compatibility and reproducibility. Creating successful LNP-based treatments requires a thorough grasp of these physicochemical properties and design factors. LNPs' function in precision oncology can be advanced by carefully adjusting their size, charge, composition, and surface characteristics. This will increase tumor selectivity, control drug release, and lessen systemic toxicity (13).

3.2.3 Mechanisms of Drug Encapsulation and Release

The therapeutic efficacy of lipid-based nanoparticles (LNPs) is mainly dependent on the mechanisms underlying drug encapsulation and release. The drug's physicochemical characteristics, the carrier's makeup and structure, and the environmental factors present in biological systems all influence these processes. LNPs can increase tumor-specific targeting, controlled delivery, and drug stability by refining their encapsulating techniques and release patterns (27).

- **Drug Encapsulation Mechanisms:** The drug's hydrophobicity, molecular weight, and solubility profile, in addition to the kind of nanoparticle, determine how well the drug loads into LNPs:
  - **Liposomes:** Amphiphilic and hydrophobic substances intercalate inside the lipid bilayer, whilst hydrophilic medications are trapped within the watery core. Lipid composition, cholesterol concentration (for membrane stability), and preparation techniques like thin-film hydration, ethanol injection, and microfluidics all affect encapsulation efficiency (EE). Active loading methods, such as remote loading with pH or ion gradients, can achieve >90% entrapment and significantly boost the EE of weakly basic medications like doxorubicin (16).
  - **SLNs:** Depending on the formulation model (homogeneous, drug-enriched shell, or drug-enriched core), drugs are either molecularly disseminated or dissolved inside the solid lipid matrix. To ensure uniform distribution and trapping of lipophilic substances, high-pressure homogenization and microemulsion methods are commonly employed.
  - **NLCs, or nanostructured lipid carriers**: When liquid lipids are incorporated into the solid matrix, structural flaws are created that improve medication accommodation and reduce expulsion while being stored. Because of this, NLCs are exceptionally well-suited for anticancer drugs that are weakly soluble, like docetaxel, curcumin, and paclitaxel. Drugs can be co-loaded in both compartments, incorporated in the lipid shell, or enclosed within the polymeric core of hybrid lipid–polymer nanoparticles (HLPNs). This architecture supports combination therapy meant to overcome malignancies' multidrug resistance by allowing the simultaneous delivery of chemotherapeutics and nucleic acids (such as siRNA and miRNA) (29).
- **Drug Release Mechanisms:** The type of nanoparticle, matrix composition, and physiological stimuli all affect the several pathways through which medicines are released from LNPs. In SLNs/NLCs, release occurs through diffusion within the lipid matrix, whereas in liposomes, drug molecules progressively diffuse through the lipid bilayer. The ratio of saturated to unsaturated lipids, for example, affects permeability and, consequently, release kinetics. In SLNs and NLCs, the lipid matrix gradually breaks down enzymatically in vivo, resulting in prolonged drug release. Polymer degradation, such as PLGA hydrolysis, is crucial to HLPNs because it yields consistent, often zero-order release patterns over extended periods. To accomplish site-specific release, advanced LNPs use environmental triggers. Examples include: pH-sensitive liposomes that cause fast drug unloading by destabilizing in acidic tumor microenvironments or endosomes. SLNs/NLCs that respond to enzymes and break down when tumor-associated lipases are present, Redox-responsive HLPNs that break down in cancer cells' high glutathione environments. To accomplish site-specific release, advanced LNPs use environmental triggers. Examples include: pH-sensitive liposomes that cause fast drug unloading by destabilizing in acidic tumor microenvironments or endosomes (26). SLNs/NLCs that respond to enzymes and break down when tumor-associated lipases are present. Redox-responsive HLPNs that break down in cancer cells' high glutathione environments. In conclusion, the success of LNPs in oncology is largely dependent on the design of the encapsulation and release mechanisms.

To advance precision nanomedicine, future directions include combining multi-stimuli-responsive devices, refining combination treatments, and utilizing real-time imaging to track drug release in vivo.

3.3 FUNCTIONALIZATION STRATEGIES

While lipid nanoparticles possess several inherent advantages as drug delivery systems, their therapeutic performance can be further enhanced through surface functionalization. Functionalization strategies involve the incorporation of targeting ligands, stealth polymers, stimuli-responsive moieties, or biomimetic components to improve nanoparticle stability, prolong circulation time, enhance tumor-specific accumulation, and facilitate efficient cellular uptake. These modifications have significantly increased the potential of lipid-based nanocarriers for precision cancer therapy.

3.3.1 Surface Modification Techniques

Researchers are actively evaluating lipid-based nanoparticles, liposomes, solid lipid nanoparticles, and nanostructured lipid carriers for drug delivery, focusing on their biocompatibility, ability to carry both hydrophilic and hydrophobic drugs, and structural flexibility. Surface modification is one way to improve their therapeutic potential and efficacy. Surface engineering refers to the modification of a nanoparticle's surface by attaching ligands or biomimetic molecules, which enhances the nanoparticle's stability, cell targeting, and cellular uptake following injection. A technique commonly employed in surface engineering is the use of polymer-based coatings termed PEGylation. PEGylation is the process of attaching a layer of PEG to the particle's surface, which serves to hide it from the immune system and results in a longer time in circulation. Surface engineering could also involve ligands conjugated to small molecules, such as antibodies, peptides, aptamers, or folic acid, and attaching these to a surface to direct accumulation to specific cells that express those receptors in greater quantities. Furthermore, other examples of charge modification or biomimetic coatings similar to the cell membrane (that can improve nanoparticle-cell interaction and/or targeted delivery) have been explored (33).

Overall, surface modifications can lead to several advantages, including: longer half-life, improved accumulation of drug in target diseased tissue with better biodistribution, and sustained release of therapeutic drug payloads. Targeting can be passive, utilizing the enhanced permeability and retention (EPR) effect in tumor tissues, or active, where the surface is functionalized with ligands that bind selectively to cellular receptors. In terms of uptake, lipid-based nanoparticles primarily enter cells through endocytic pathways, such as clathrin-mediated or caveolae-mediated endocytosis, macropinocytosis, or direct fusion with the plasma membrane (34). This allows for efficient drug delivery to the target cells. Overall, surface modification transforms lipid nanoparticles from simple carriers into advanced drug delivery platforms, providing enhanced selectivity, reduced side effects, and improved therapeutic efficacy in various biomedical applications (Figure 3.5).

3.3.1.1 PEGylation for Stealth Properties

PEG is a synthetic polymer whose distinct physical, chemical, and biological properties make it extremely popular, and thus very valuable in research fields, biomedical research, and nanomedicine. The process of matching PEG to nanoparticles, proteins, peptides, or other therapeutic agents is known as PEGylation and represents an important means of engineering "stealth" drug delivery systems. "Stealth" refers to the ability of PEGylated systems to avoid the immune surveillance mechanisms of the body, specifically rapid recognition and clearance by the MPS, or the reticuloendothelial system (RES) (35). Foreign particles (drug-loaded nanoparticles, liposomes, protein therapeutics), when in the circulation, are quickly recognized by plasma proteins (immunoglobulins,

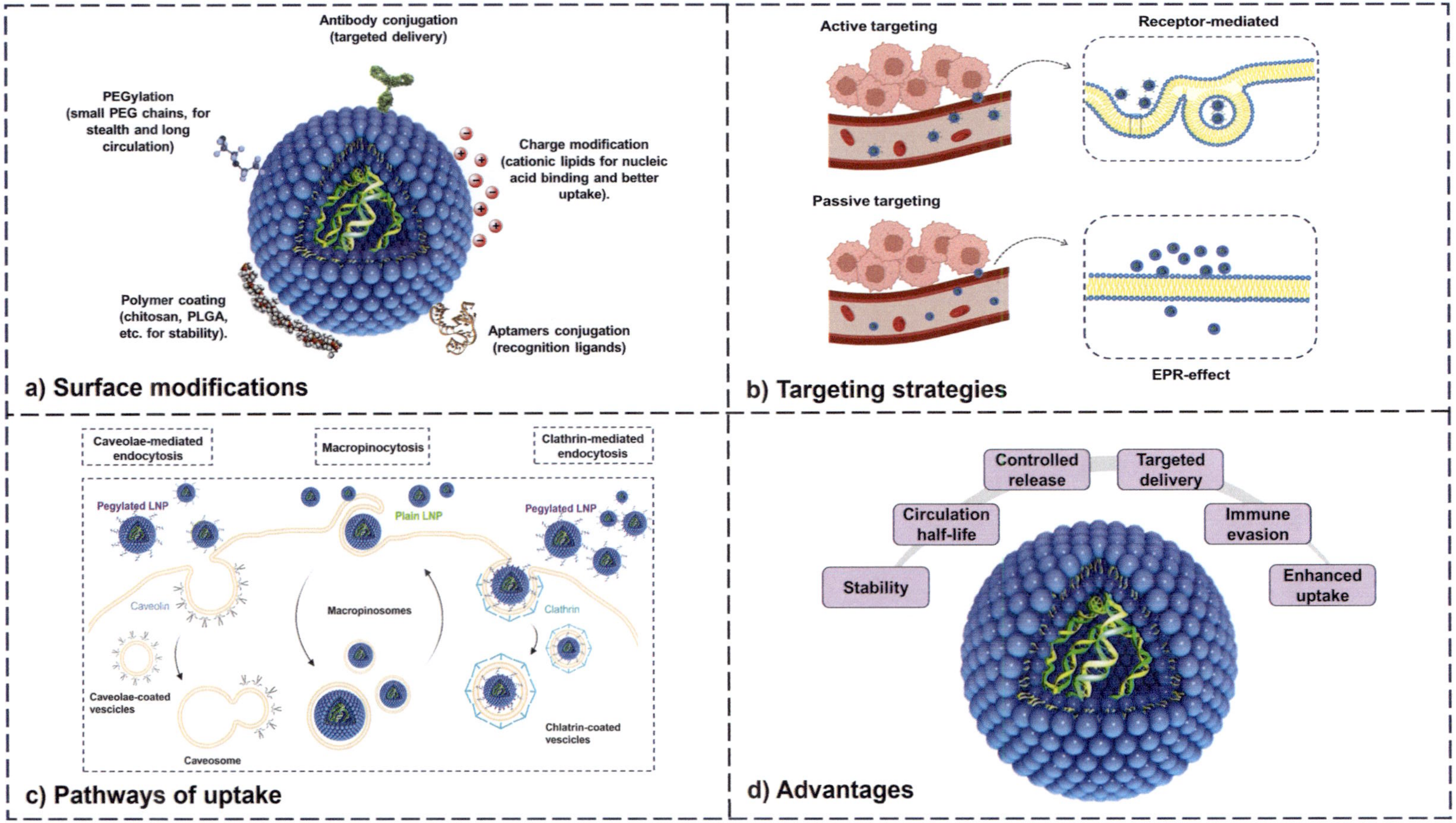

FIGURE 3.5 Schematic illustration of lipid nanoparticle (LNP)-based drug delivery: (a) structural design of surface-modified lipid nanoparticle (LNP), (b) passive versus active tumor targeting, (c) endocytosis pathways (clathrin, caveolin, and micropinocytosis, (d) the associated advantages, including prolonged circulation half-life, controlled release, and improved cellular uptake.

complement factors, and so on) via a process called opsonization. The result is that the drug-loaded nanoparticles are captured and consequently driven into the liver, spleen and other immune organs and eliminated from circulation. In short, this results in a low half-life and eventually reduces the therapeutic effect.

To address these shortcomings, PEGylation has been proposed as a surface modification approach that creates a hydrophilic barrier around the particle or biomolecule. The stealth property of PEGylation primarily results from the formation of a dense, hydrated corona surrounding the nanoparticle. PEG is highly hydrophilic and can accommodate large amounts of water to form a hydrated shell around the particle. This hydrated shell imposes substantial physical and energetic barriers to the adsorption of serum proteins, and this type of resistance or stealth property avoids opsonization and subsequent phagocyte uptake. In addition to hydrophilicity, PEG provides steric hindrance due to its long and flexible polymer chains. These chains will extend outward around the nanoparticles, creating a physical barrier that allows biomolecules or immune receptors to access and bind to the particle. As a result, PEGylation affords stealth to nanoparticles due to barriers from hydrophobic interactions and steric hindrance by using (Veronese & Pasut, 2008).

Another key advantage that PEGylation confers to nanoparticles is their effective colloidal stabilization. Naked nanoparticles do not last long in physiological fluids due to aggregation. Nanoparticles aggregate in physiological fluids mainly due to van der Waals attractions or due to electrostatic interaction with serum proteins. PEG chains minimize specific interactions by acting as a neutral, non-fouling interface, ultimately increasing the dispersion and stability of nanoparticles during circulation. Thus, PEGylated nanoparticles have long half-lives, and while unmodified carriers will only last a few minutes, the time can be approximated to range from hours to several days depending on the PEG molecular weight and density. Longer systemic circulation allows for increased drug bioavailability, and in the case of solid tumors, enhanced passive targeting would occur as a result of the EPR effect (38). The EPR effect occurs due to leaky vasculature and impaired lymphatic drainage, which is a result of the tumor tissue's structure, thereby priming long-circulating nanocarriers for accumulation in the tumor microenvironment. PEGylation can significantly enhance the passive targeting mechanism by prolonging the circulation time of nanoparticles.

PEGylation also reduces the immunogenicity and antigenicity of therapeutic agents. For example, protein or peptide-based drugs are often highly immunogenic, leading to the formation of neutralizing antibodies that limit their therapeutic potential. Conjugation of these biomolecules to PEG hides their antigenic epitopes, thereby protecting them from immune recognition and enzymatic degradation. This is why many biopharmaceuticals, such as PEG-interferon and PEG-asparaginase, are already in clinical use. Similarly, PEGylated liposomal doxorubicin (Doxil) was the first FDA-approved nanomedicine that enhanced systemic circulation and reduced off-target toxicity using PEGylation (40). These successful examples clearly show how clinical translation of PEGylation for stealth applications has been established.

Despite its widespread success, PEGylation is not free of challenges, often referred to as the PEG dilemma. Although PEG increases circulation and decreases clearance, it can also sometimes inhibit cellular uptake and intracellular drug release. The same steric barrier that inhibits immune recognition can also limit interactions between nanoparticles and target cells, resulting in reduced therapeutic efficiency even after reaching the desired locations. Additionally, the production of anti-PEG antibodies has been observed in some patients from repeated administration of PEGylated drugs. The antibodies accelerate the blood clearance of PEGylated nanoparticles, a phenomenon known as the ABC phenomenon. Such an ABC phenomenon not only diminishes therapeutic effectiveness but can also initiate undesirable aspects of immune responses. These concerns have led to the development of alternative stealth modalities, with several biomimetic tools available, including zwitterionic polymers such as poly(carboxybetaine) and poly(sulfobetaine), polysarcosine, and cell membrane camouflaging. These are examples of options toward mimicking or enhancing the PEG stealth effect and negating its drawbacks (Nogueira et al., 2020).

Several design factors, including the molecular weight of the PEG polymer, the density of PEG grafting, and the method of conjugation, influence the effectiveness of PEGylation. In general, high-molecular-weight PEG (5–20 kDa) and dense surface coverage provide the highest steric stabilization against surfactants and opsonization. However, high-density PEGylation reduces the reach of targeting ligands to the nanoparticle surface, possibly impacting active targeting approaches. A compromise between stealth targeting and targeting can also be achieved with cleavable PEG linkers that disassemble in response to tumor microenvironment stimuli, such as pH, redox gradients, or enzymatic activity. This sheddable PEG strategy keeps the nanoparticles stealthy during circulation, but exposes their functional groups or ligands at the target site, thereby maximizing therapeutic efficacy.

In conclusion, PEGylation remains one of the most effective and widely adopted strategies for imparting stealth properties to nanoparticles and therapeutic biomolecules. By providing a hydrophilic and sterically protective envelope, PEGylation inhibits opsonization, prolongs systemic circulation, reduces immunogenicity, and enhances tumor accumulation through the EPR effect. These benefits have been translated into many successful clinical applications and remain a cornerstone of nanomedicine and drug delivery design. However, the emergence of challenges such as the PEG dilemma, anti-PEG immunity, and the ABC effect highlights the need for continuous innovation. Future stealth nanomedicine will likely be based on hybrid strategies, where PEGylation will be combined with other smart modifications such as cleavable linkers, biomimetic coatings, or alternative polymers to overcome the limitations of PEG while maintaining its benefits. Overall, PEGylation has fundamentally changed the design of drug delivery systems and will continue to serve as a benchmark in the development of next-generation stealth nano-carriers.

At the molecular level, PEGylated becomes interlinked in LNPs through their hydrophobic regions, extending the hydrophilic and hydrophobic PEG chains toward the surrounding aqueous environment. These PEG chains create a dynamic hydration shell, generating steric repulsion that inhibits the adsorption of plasma proteins. This results in the formation of a dense protein corona from immunoglobulins, fibrinogen, complement proteins, and apolipoproteins. Due to this limitation of opsonization, the complement cascade's activation is also reduced, particularly the deposition of C3 and C3b on the nanoparticle surface, which typically acts as a molecular tag for immune recognition. PEGylation also modifies the surface charge of LNPs; newly modified encapsulated LNPs become shielded from necessary cations, causing a shift toward potential neutralization and significantly reducing unwanted electrostatic interactions with serum proteins and negatively charged cells. All these molecular transformations maintain the physical and chemical profile of LNPs in the bloodstream and reduce aggregation or clearance over time (Mohamed et al., 2019).

At the cellular level, PEGylation prevents the recognition of LNPs and their uptake by the MPS, primarily involving Kupffer cells in the liver, macrophages in the spleen, and resident phagocytes. In unmodified LNPs, opsonins, such as IgG and complement proteins, act as ligands for phagocytic receptors, including Fc receptors, complement receptors (CR1 and CR3), and scavenger receptors (SR-A and MARCO). PEGylation reduces the binding and activity of these opsonins, leading to decreased receptor engagement and receptor-mediated endocytosis. As a result, phagocytosis and subsequent lysosomal degradation are significantly reduced. Consequently, PEG chains effectively shield the LNPs from being recognized by endothelial or immune cells, thereby reducing unnecessary membrane fusion. The net effect is a notable decrease in clearance from the bloodstream by the MPS, an increase in half-life, and enhanced distribution in pathological tissues, particularly through the EPR) effect. PEGylation acts as a sequential barrier: first, by inhibiting molecular tagging through protein corona suppression and complement activation, and second, by reducing receptor-mediated clearance at the cellular level (M. Liu, Su, et al., 2022) (Figure 3.6).

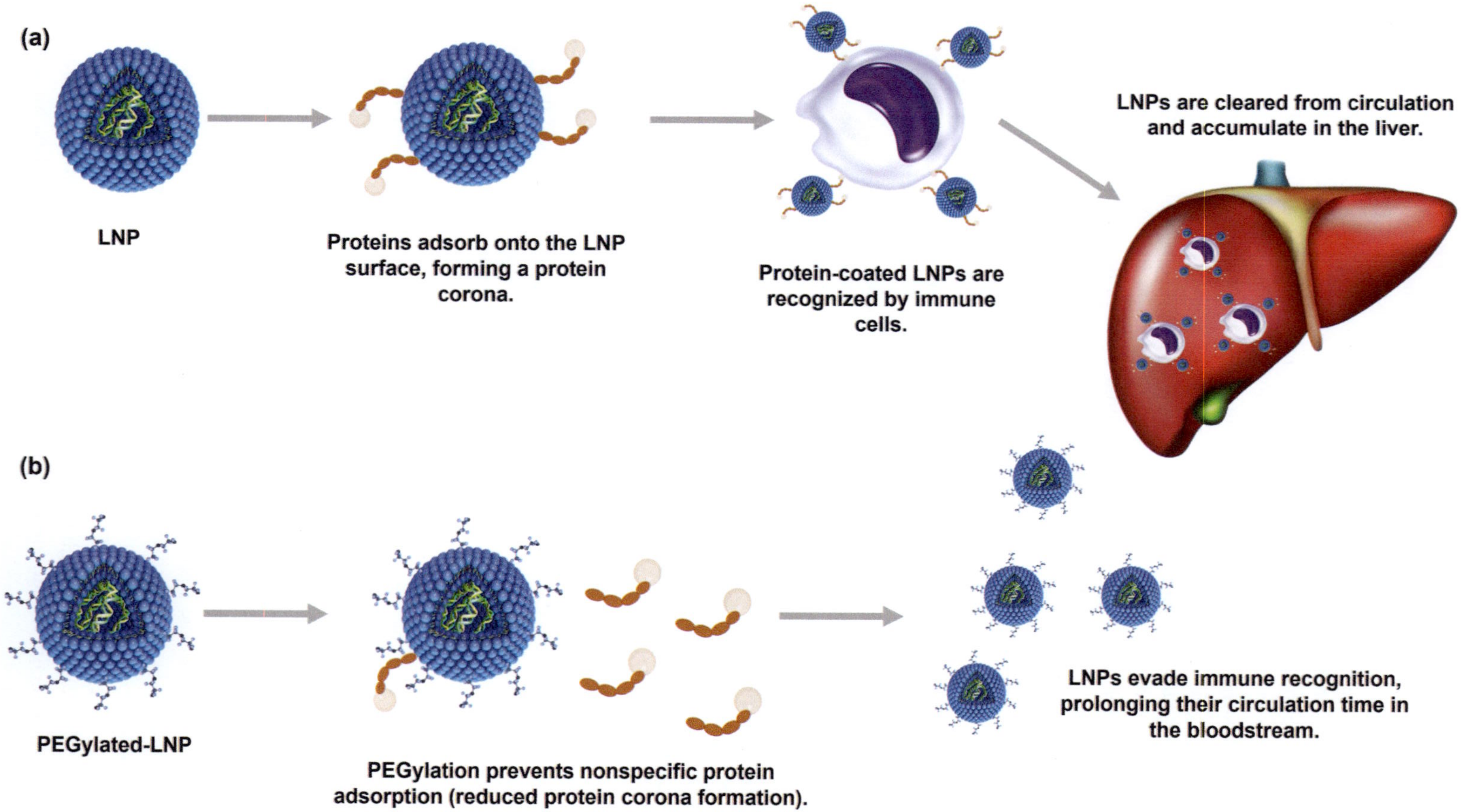

FIGURE 3.6 Schematic illustration showing the impact of PEGylation on nanoparticle fate in vivo. (a) Non-PEGylated nanoparticles adsorb plasma proteins, form a protein corona, and are rapidly recognized and cleared by immune cells, leading to liver accumulation. (b) PEGylated nanoparticles resist protein corona formation, evade immune clearance, and exhibit prolonged circulation for improved therapeutic delivery.

3.3.1.2 Ligand Conjugation (Antibodies, Aptamers, Peptides, Folic Acid, RGD)

PEGylation and other stealth strategies increase the circulation time of nanoparticles into the bloodstream, but they alone cannot guarantee the selective delivery of therapeutic agents to diseased tissues. To achieve true precision, it is necessary to direct the drug carriers specifically to the target cells or microenvironment, such as cancer cells, inflammatory tissue or angiogenic vasculature. This is achieved through ligand conjugation, in which bio-recognition molecules, such as antibodies, aptamers, peptides, or small motifs like folic acid or RGD sequences, are added to the nanoparticle surface in a covalent or non-covalent manner. These ligands can recognize and bind to cell-surface receptors that are expressed either exclusively or in excessive amounts on diseased cells, enabling active targeting through receptor-mediated endocytosis. Unlike passive targeting, which relies on non-specific processes such as the EPR effect, ligand conjugation provides a high degree of specificity, ensuring that nanoparticles preferentially assemble at diseased sites and minimize off-target distribution. This approach significantly increases therapeutic efficacy and reduces systemic toxicity, making it a foundational pillar of modern nanomedicine design (49). Of the various types of targeting ligands, antibodies are one of the most studied and clinically proven options. Their inherent ability to bind antigens with high specificity and affinity makes them ideal for recognizing cancer-related markers such as HER2, EGFR, and CD20. Nanoparticles equipped with monoclonal antibodies or antibody fragments can selectively recognize tumor cells, thereby promote internalization and improve localized drug release. A notable example of this is the development of immunoliposomes, where antibodies are conjugated to PEGylated liposomes to combine stealth properties with active targeting (51). However, antibodies also present some challenges, such as large size, high cost of production, and potential immunogenicity, which has prompted the search for smaller and more versatile alternatives. Aptamers have emerged as an attractive alternative or complement to antibodies. Aptamers are small, single-stranded DNA or RNA sequences that fold into unique three-dimensional structures capable of binding with high affinity to specific targets. They are commonly referred to as chemical antibodies due to their ability to perform a recognition function similar to that of antibodies and have some unique advantages. Aptamers can be synthesized chemically in a way that is highly reproducible, are less immunogenic, and can also be simply modified for conjugation to nanoparticles. One common aptamer that has been studied in detail is the AS1411 aptamer, which binds to nucleolin, a receptor that is often overexpressed on many cancer cells, and has been to functionalize gold nanoparticles and liposomes for tumor-targeted drug delivery (53). It is the chemical stability and versatility of aptamers that provide a great deal of utility for applications where antibody-based targeting may not be effective.

Peptides are certainly a class of targeting ligands that can be utilized in various ways. Peptides, due to their small size and ease of synthesis, can penetrate tissues more effectively than larger biomolecules and are often conjugated to nanoparticles to enhance tumor accumulation and uptake. One of the most frequently used peptides in nanomedicine is the RGD (arginine-glycine-aspartic acid) motif, due to its ability to bind to integrin receptors (e.g., $\alpha v\beta 3$) that are overexpressed in angiogenic endothelial cells, particularly during tumor growth stages. RGD-functionalized nanoparticles have considerable potential for selectively targeting tumor vasculature to inhibit angiogenesis and improve drug delivery to tumors (55). In addition to RGD, there are several tumor-homing and penetrating peptides (e.g., TAT [trans-activator of transcription] or iRGD [internalizing RGD]) already developed for not only targeting, but also enhanced cellular uptake (Arduino et al., 2021). Likewise, peptide ligands can also be rationally designed or sourced from phage display libraries, giving access to a relatively complete toolkit for disease-based targeting.

Small molecules, such as folic acid, are also commonly used because they are small, stable, and have good receptor-binding capability. The folate receptor is abundantly expressed in various cancers, including ovarian, breast, lung, and colorectal cancers, whereas it has low expression in most normal tissues. This makes folic acid an effective ligand for tumor-targeted delivery of drugs. Folic acid can easily be conjugated to the surface of various LY, micelles, polymeric nanoparticles, or dendrimers, and its small size means that its addition should not interfere significantly with the physico-chemical properties of the carrier (59). Animal and clinical studies have demonstrated that folate-conjugated nanoparticles can enhance therapeutic efficacy and mitigate off-target toxicity by facilitating selective uptake by cancer cells.

Several factors can influence the efficiency of ligand conjugation, including the density of ligand on the nanoparticle surface, the orientation of binding, and the binding affinity to the target receptor. Generally, the higher the ligand density, the greater the binding avidity, a phenomenon known as the multivalency effect. However, high ligand density can also influence non-specific binding due to steric hindrance or acute withdrawal by the immune system. The type of ligand conjugation method is also important. Covalent coupling, particularly via stable linkers, ensures stability in circulation, while cleavable linkers responsive to stimuli (pH, enzyme gradient, or redox) release ligands in the target microenvironment, such as cancer, thereby focusing on site-specific distribution (60). Another key aspect is the heterogeneity of receptor expression; tumors often show variations in receptor levels between patients or within the same tumor, which can limit the efficiency of single-ligand targeting. To address this, researchers are increasingly exploring bi or multi-ligand conjugation strategies, where the nanoparticle is functionalized with two or more dissimilar ligands to target multiple receptors simultaneously. This multi-targeted approach increases the likelihood of binding, stimulates cellular absorption, and removes. Despite its promise, ligand conjugation faces some limitations. Antibodies, although highly specific, can increase the size and complexity of nanoparticles, thereby reducing stability and circulation time. Aptamers can be sensitive to nuclease degradation in the body, although chemical modifications, such as 2'-fluoro or 2'-O-methyl substitutions, can improve their stability (61). To maintain a balance between stealth and targeting, bright designs often employ cleavable or stimuli-responsive PEG layers, which shield ligands in circulation but expose them to the target site, thereby combining long circulation times with effective targeting.

In passive targeting, antibody-functionalized LNPs initially behave similarly to un-conjugated or only PEGylated LNPs. Their biodistribution is primarily controlled by the Enhanced Permeability and Retention (EPR) effect, where leaky blood vessels of tumors or inflamed tissues allow nanoparticles of approximately 50–150 nm size to enter the interstitium. The PEGylated lipid layer prolongs the presence of LNPs in the bloodstream and reduces the binding of opsonin proteins, thereby reducing the chances of premature clearance by the MPS. At the molecular level, these LNPs accumulate in tissues mainly independently of antibody-receptor interactions; Hemodynamic forces, interstitial fluid pressure, and non-specific physico-chemical interactions with the cell membrane determine their pathway. When they approach cells, their absorption occurs by non-specific endocytosis such as macropinocytosis or clathrin-dependent pathways, where cationic or fusogenic lipids further promote endosomal fusion and escape. Thus, the conjugated antibody in passive targeting does not yet act actively; rather, nanoparticles depend on their structural and physicochemical characteristics, as well as blood vessel abnormalities (Suzuki et al., 2025).

In contrast, active targeting occurs when the antibody on the LNP surface binds to its cognate antigen. At the molecular level, the Fab region of the conjugated antibody maintains structural specificity to its epitope. It establishes high-affinity binding to receptors (such as HER2, EGFR, or CEA) present on the cell surface. This bonding is possible due to hydrogen bonding, hydrophobic complementarity, and shape-based interactions. The correct orientation of the antibody is very important because incorrect association can prevent antigen recognition. The association of multiple antibody molecules with receptor clustering produces an avidity effect, making the surface association of the nanoparticle even stronger, even when serum proteins are present in the vicinity (Attia et al., 2019).

At the cellular level, antibody-receptor binding activates receptor-mediated endocytosis, a process that differs from passive absorption. For example, antibody binding to HER2 or EGFR induces receptor dimerization, leading to the formation of clathrin-coated pits, followed by invagination and vesicle formation. In immune-targeting, anti-CD20 or anti-PD-L1 antibodies carry Ab-LNPs to specific immune cells through Fc receptor-dependent internalization or receptor crosslinking. Once introduced into the cell, the fate of Ab-LNPs depends on the biology of that receptor: Some receptors quickly return to the surface and release LNPs into the early endosome, while others move them toward the lysosomal pathway (Kim et al., 2024). To avoid lysosomal degradation, fusogenic lipids or pH-sensitive linkers present in the LNP bilayer destabilize the endosomal membrane in an acidic environment, allowing for the release of the drug or nucleic acid into the cytosol (Figure 3.7). Thus, while passive targeting is primarily based on vascular permeability and non-specific uptake, active targeting is driven by the molecular accuracy of antibody-antigen binding and the cellular consequences of receptor-mediated internalization. The conjugated antibody not only provides specificity but also alters the intracellular entry pathway of nanoparticles, making drug delivery more selective, effective, and biologically relevant.

The ligand conjugation represents a fundamental advance in the design of targeted nanocarrier systems. By decorating nanoparticles with antibodies, aptamers, peptides, folic acid, RGD

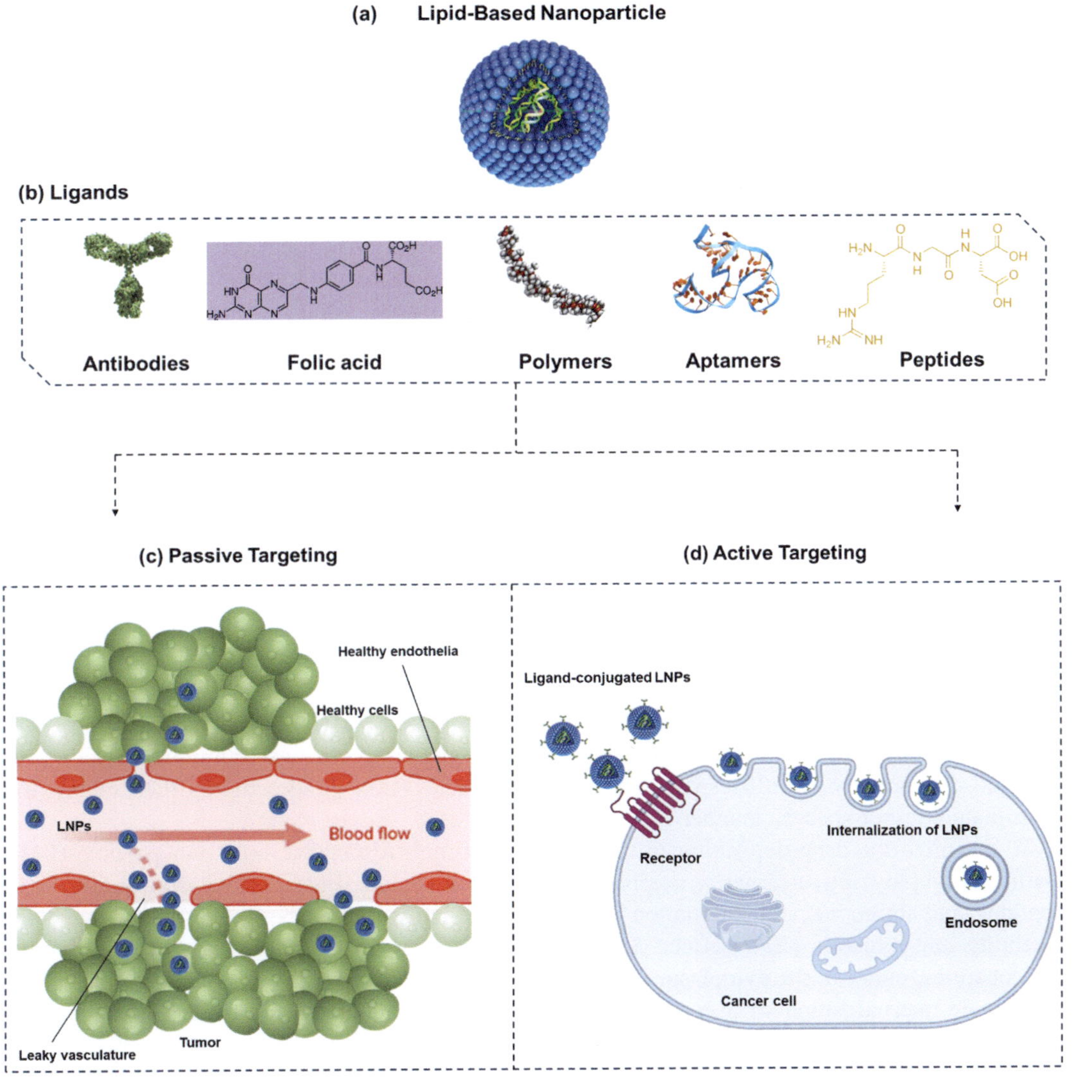

FIGURE 3.7 Schematic representation of functionalized LNPs for targeted cancer therapy. (a) Lipid-based nanoparticle (b) LNPs can be engineered with various ligands such as antibodies, small molecules, polymers, peptides, and aptamers for targeted delivery. Following systemic administration, (c) LNPs circulate through the bloodstream, accumulate in the tumor microenvironment, (d) internalize into cancer cells via receptor-mediated endocytosis, enabling efficient intracellular delivery of therapeutic cargo.

sequences, or other biomolecules, the molecular signatures of diseased cells can be harnessed, allowing for precise drug delivery. This approach not only increases therapeutic efficacy but also reduces systemic toxicity, paving the way for safer and more effective treatments. With continuous innovations such as multi-ligand conjugation, stimuli-responsive linkers, and biomimetic modifications, ligand-targeted nanomedicine holds immense potential in the development of personalized therapies, where nanocarriers can be customized according to the molecular profile of individual patients. As research progresses, ligand conjugation is expected to remain at the forefront of strategies bridging the gap between nanotechnology and precision medicine.

3.3.2 Stimuli-Responsive Functionalization

Stimuli-responsive functionalization is the most sophisticated and effective method for designing lipid-based nanoparticle (LNP)-based drug delivery systems in oncological applications, where drug delivery can be adjusted in a spatiotemporal setting in response to specific biological stimuli or external stimuli. Stimuli-responsive carriers are carefully designed for stability in systemic circulation while allowing for selective activation at the tumor microenvironmental level, in contrast to conventional nanocarriers that rely on passive targeting. These carriers are effective in overcoming major problems, including early drug leakage, off-site cytotoxicity, and inadequate drug efficacy. The tumor microenvironment (TME) is distinctly different from normal tissues in terms of pH, enzymatic activity, redox potential, and thermal characteristics. For this reason, the stimuli-responsiveness model can benefit from these distinctive attributes. In tumors and even subcellular compartments, such as endosomes and lysosomes, endogenous stimuli, including acidic pH gradients, overexpressed proteolytic enzymes, and increased intracellular glutathione (GSH) levels, serve as intrinsic triggers for the controlled release mechanisms. At the same time, it is possible to carefully employ external stimuli, such as heat, light, magnetic fields, and ultrasound, to support the release of medication at specific locations and times. The combination of external control and the dual targeting of intrinsic tumor features makes stimuli-responsive lipid nanoparticles (LNPs) particularly well-suited for precision oncology (66).

There are several advantages of Stimuli-Responsive Functional, such as enhanced selectivity and safety, which effectively diminish systemic toxicity and alter adverse effects through the activation of preventive medication tailored to tumor-specific environments, better therapeutic index by increasing the drug's local concentration, the controlled release mechanism allows for better tumor eradication with fewer systemic dosages; overcoming biological barriers where endosomal release, penetration through dense stroma within tumors, as well as evading multidrug resistance (MDR) mechanisms are key functions promoted by reactions initiated by stimuli (69), compatibility with combination therapies: where chemotherapeutic drugs, nucleic acids, and immunomodulators can all be co-delivered by stimuli-responsive lipid nanoparticles (LNPs), allowing for their release in a coordinated, tumor-specific manner.

To optimize the drug deposition in tumors, most stimuli-responsive lipid nanoparticle (LNP) platforms employ active targeting approaches based on surface ligands, including folate, RGD peptides, and antibodies, in combination with passive targeting approaches based on enhanced permeability and retention (EPR) effect. Such delivery vehicles are engineered for release at optimal locations, either in the cytoplasm of cancer cells or within tumors in the extracellular matrix, upon their internalization in a commonly receptor-mediated endocytosis manner. Due to their exceptional flexibility, stimuli-responsive LNPs are increasingly being studied in both preclinical and clinical settings. Promising examples include pH-responsive mRNA vaccines prepared for melanoma, enzyme-sensitive doxorubicin-loaded liposomes for hepatocellular carcinoma, redox-responsive siRNA delivery systems for liver and colon cancer treatment, and thermosensitive liposomes combined with treatments for liver and breast cancer involving hyperthermia. Altogether, such developments showcase stimuli-responsive functionalization's promise for repackaging cancer nanomedicine toward delivering tumor-specific as well as on-demand therapies (64) (Figure 3.8).

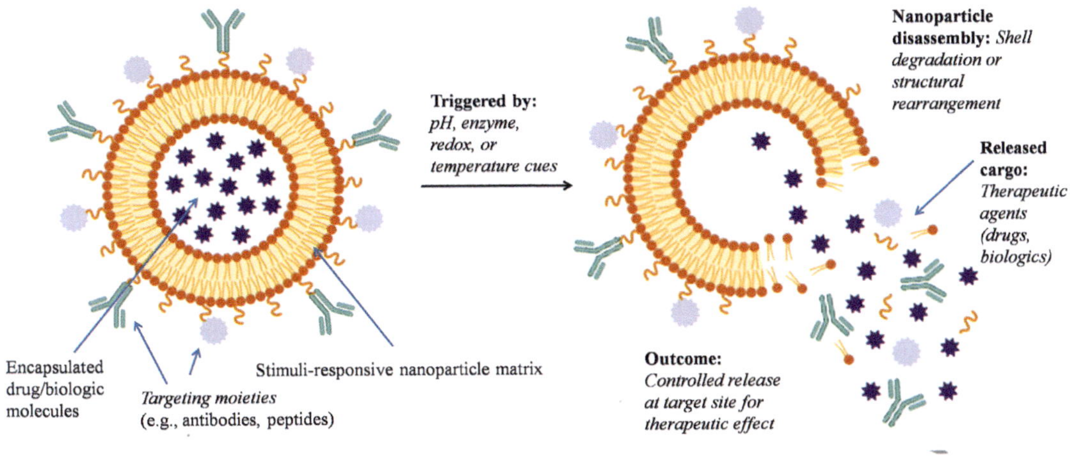

FIGURE 3.8 Stimuli-responsive release of therapeutics from nanoparticles. Under physiological or disease-specific triggers such as changes in pH, enzymatic activity, redox potential, or temperature, the nanoparticle shell disassembles, releasing the encapsulated drugs or biologics at the target site to achieve enhanced therapeutic efficacy.

3.3.2.1 pH-Sensitive Systems

pH-responsive lipid nanoparticles (LNPs) enable site-specific drug delivery and increased therapy effectiveness. These nanoparticles are carefully constructed, taking advantage of solid tumors' acidic microenvironments and those within cell organelles. Extracellular tumor microenvironments (TMEs) are generally mildly acidic in nature, with a pH ranging between 6.5 and 7.2. That is in sharp contrast with the close to normal pH 7.4 found in normal tissues. Acidic nature in TME is a result of cancer cells' abnormal metabolism, specifically aerobic glycolysis, also known as the Warburg effect, leading to lactic acid deposits. Other acidic stimuli for releasing payloads within cell organelles include lysosomes, whose pH ranges from 4.5 to 5.5, and endosomes, whose pH is approximately 5.5 to 6.0. With those pH gradients in mind, one can improve drug stability in the circulatory system while allowing specific activation at cancer sites (17).

Mechanism of Action: Ionizable lipids or acid-labile linkers are commonly used in the design of pH-responsive LNPs. Ionizable lipids like dioleoylphosphatidylethanolamine (DOPE) and cholesteryl hemisuccinate (CHEMS) destabilize the structure of nanoparticles and release payloads when they shift from a stable lamellar form at physiological pH to a fusogenic hexagonal form in acidic media. Acid-labile linkages, such as hydrazone, acetal, imine, and orthoester linkages, are commonly employed in polymer-lipid hybrids and liposomes for covalently linking drugs or target groups that cleave in acidic environments. This facilitates the controlled release of drugs within cells. The proton sponge effect observed in cationic polymers in LNPs causes osmotic swelling, which destabilizes the endosomal membrane. It further enhances endosomal escape and enhances the distribution of materials in the cytoplasm. pH-responsive LNPs commonly contain actively targetable ligands like RGD peptides, hyaluronic acid, or even folate. These ligands bind to overexpressing receptors found on cancer cells, such as CD44 in breast cancer or even the folate receptor in ovarian cancer (71). Internalization primarily occurs by clathrin-mediated endocytosis. Acidification in endosomes also initiates the release of the payload. The second-generation pH-responsive systems are anticipated to target dual and multi-stimuli responsiveness. Such integration would entail adding pH-responsive stimuli with enzymatic or redox-responsive mechanisms for enhanced specificity. There are still problems involving scalability for achieving long-term stability and handling tunability issues in tumor pH, which may hinder universal applicability. Nonetheless, advancements in microfluidic production processes and applications in visualizing in real-time with imaging agents may permit rapid clinical applications (28).

3.3.2.2 Enzyme-Responsive Systems

Enzyme-responsive lipid-based nanoparticles (LNPs) capitalize on the overexpression of enzymes in the tumor microenvironment (TME) and in neoplastic cells for controlled, site-specific drug release. These enzymes, like matrix metalloproteinases (MMPs), cathepsins (B, D, L), phospholipases (PLA2), and esterases are commonly upregulated in a wide range of cancer types. These enzymes are crucial for tumor growth, expansion, invasion, and the metastasis process. Through harnessing such enzymatic functionalities, it is feasible to activate therapies within disease sites while protecting normal tissue specifically. Such an approach optimizes the therapeutic index with reduced system toxicity (73).

- **Mode of Action:** Enzyme-responsive LNPs are usually designed with enzyme-cleavable linkers, peptide substrates, or prodrug conjugates built into their structure (74). In numerous designs, enzymatic cleavage serves the dual purpose of liberating the drug and potentially unveiling concealed targeting ligands or diminishing size, thereby enhancing tumor penetration. A pertinent example includes "sheddable coatings" that react to MMPs, which eliminate a protective PEG layer at the tumor location (75). This modification facilitates cellular uptake without compromising the stability of systemic circulation.

Enzyme-responsive materials offer several notable advantages, including higher specificity, Controlled Release within the Cell, and Potential for Combination Therapy. Some examples include MMP-responsive micelles for enhancing drug penetration in desmoplastic pancreatic tumors and cathepsin B-cleavable doxorubicin liposomes for increased anticancer activity in hepatocellular carcinoma models. Targeted chemotherapy with enzyme-activatable prodrug-loaded LNPs is also a focus of research for reducing undesirable drug exposure for much of the rest of the body (73). Prior to undergoing enzymatic activation, enzyme-responsive lipid nanoparticles typically incorporate active targeting ligands to enhance tumor accumulation. Examples include scenarios rich in matrix metalloproteinases (MMP), where MMP-sensitive coatings of PEG in combination with RGD peptides allow for localized activation, tumor targeting based on integrin binding, and longer-lasting circulations. cells internalize nanoparticles mainly by receptor-mediated endocytosis, which is followed by enzymatic degradation either at or within lysosomes at the tumor site for release of the therapeutic agent. Dual or multi-enzyme targeting utilizes substrates for multiple tumor-associated enzymes in an effort to overcome tumor heterogeneity. Furthermore, theranostic enzyme-responsive devices, consisting of MMP-activatable fluorescent probes, couple drug delivery with imaging. Such devices permit real-time visualization of drug release and tumor response. Nonetheless, clinical utility is compromised by issues such as patient-specific variation in enzyme levels, as well as the need for scalable and reproducible production. Future developments in high-throughput screening of enzyme substrates coupled with microfluidic fabrication technologies should eliminate such issues while allowing for patient-specific, enzyme-actuated cancer nanotherapies.

3.3.2.3 Redox-Responsive Systems

The redox potential differences between cancer cells and normal tissues enable the site-specific release of therapeutic agents from redox-sensitive lipid nanoparticles (LNPs), resulting in improved efficacy in treatment. Concentrations of reducing agents, in particular glutathione (GSH; 2–10 mM), are 100–1000 times higher in the cytosol and nucleus of cancer cells relative to their extrinsic fluids and normal tissues (2–20 μM). Such a redox imbalance arising as a result of adaptation toward oxidative stress and deranged metabolic pathways is a hallmark feature in cancer biology. Scientists can trigger the release of therapeutics specifically in cancer cells through the design of nanocarriers sensitive toward such increased reducing milieus, when needed for improved efficacy at reduced system toxicity (77).

- **Mode of Action:** Mostly, cleavable chemical bonds such as disulfide (-S-S-) and diselenide (-Se-Se-) are employed in the construction of redox-sensitive lipid nanoparticles (LNPs). These bonds are stable at external oxidation conditions but are rapidly cleaved in the reducing intracellular medium (78). Once endocytosed into cancer cells and in response to an increased concentration of glutathione (GSH), the following events unfold: Dissipation of nanoparticles, Prodrug activation, and Co-delivery are triggered. For instance, disulfide-crosslinked lipid-polymer hybrid nanoparticles have been demonstrated to deliver doxorubicin and siRNA efficiently. It leads to the killing of tumor cells through treatment as well as gene knockdown (80). In a similar vein, diselenide-mediated approaches enhance oxidation-specific selectivity within tumor microenvironments by raising ROS sensitivity. Redox-switching systems offer several advantages in cancer therapies, including tumor selectivity and overcoming multidrug resistance (MDR). Some examples include redox-activated paclitaxel prodrug liposomes for enhanced tumor inhibition in colon cancer xenografts, disulfide-stabilized micelles for the delivery of doxorubicin in a chemotherapy- and redox-mediated cell death-ferroptosis regimen for breast cancer, and others (80). Redox-responsive LNPs have also boosted immunotherapy by allowing cytosolic mRNA delivery of cancer vaccines.

Active target ligands are commonly used in conjunction with redox-sensitive LNPs for target-specific accumulation before redox activation (9). These include such nanoparticles as those for mitochondria drug delivery in solid tumors, using triphenylphosphonium-modified nanoparticles, or GLUT transporter-targeted delivery in gliomas with glucose-functionalized carriers. Uptake is typically clathrin- or caveolae-mediated endocytosis with endosomal escape by fusogenic lipids and disassembly within the cytoplasm by GSH. Prospective Vision: New research includes dual redox/pH-responsive systems that take advantage of both reducing intracellular environments and acidic environments for greater specificity. Another promising method is to take advantage of self-amplifying redox-responsive systems, which lower intracellular concentrations of GSH to induce cell death through oxidative stress in combination with immunotherapy or chemotherapy. Challenges include patient-to-patient variations in the amount of GSH within a cell, a need for non-toxic, biodegradable linkers, and the development of scalable manufacturing methods. However, further advancements in microfluidic Assembly and click chemistry make redox-responsive nanocarriers an integral candidate for next-generation personalized cancer therapies (9).

3.3.2.4 Temperature-Sensitive Systems

The ability to raise the temperature of neoplastic tissues in response to internal or external stimuli is exploited by temperature-sensitive lipid-based nanoparticles (LNPs). Such nanoparticles are developed to release their drug cargoes in response to controlled heat. The rationale for temperature-sensitive systems is supported by evidence that mild hyperthermia (40–43°C) enhances the cell uptake of drugs, improves tumor-vasculature permeability, and generates phase transitions in temperature-sensitive carriers, resulting in consequent drug release. Such a method ensures drug release only at the tumor site, controls for systemic toxicity, and functions in concert with heat-mediated sensitization of cancer cells to chemotherapy or radiation (81).

Temperature-responsive lipid nanoparticles (LNPs) comprise thermosensitive polymers or lipids whose structure changes upon exposure to elevated temperatures. As an illustration, dipalmitoylphosphatidylcholine (DPPC)-induced liposomes display a phase transition temperature close to 41°C, thus producing thermosensitive liposomes (TSLs). At 37°C, which is a normal body temperature, the lipid bilayer is stable, thus safeguarding an encapsulated drug agent. Temperature-sensitive liposomes hold great promise in clinical applications. For example, ThermoDox®, a lysolipid-encapsulated doxorubicin liposome, has demonstrated superior results in clinical trials for hepatocellular carcinoma when used in combination with radiofrequency ablation. It releases its drug in a heat-dependent local environment. Magnetoliposomes loaded with superparamagnetic nanoparticles have made MRI-controlled, hyperthermia-actuated drug delivery a possibility in preclinical applications, offering both therapeutic and diagnostic advantages. The enhanced permeability and retention (EPR) effect associated with passive targeting facilitates the accumulation of agents in primary tumors. Active targeting strategies utilize ligands such as folate, RGD sequences, or antibodies to enhance cellular uptake prior to heat activation. Most drugs enter cells through endocytosis. When the tumor is locally heated, drugs are rapidly released from lipid nanoparticles into the surrounding space, allowing them to enter cancer cells more easily. Heat also makes cell membranes more fluid, which facilitates the entry of drugs (81).

3.3.3 Hybridization with Other Nanomaterials for Multifunctionality

A novel strategy to address the shortcomings of conventional nanocarriers and allow for multifunctional cancer therapies is by the hybridization of lipid-based nanoparticles (LNPs) with other nanomaterials. Although conventional LNPs are biocompatible and excellent at drug dissolution, they tend to suffer from issues like premature drug leakage, limited circulation lifetimes, and a lack of ability to impart other features such as imaging, immune regulation, or responsiveness to external stimuli. Scientists have developed hybrid nanoplatforms that combine the biological benefits of lipids with the convenience of man-made materials by combining other nanomaterials, such as polymers, inorganic nanoparticles, or biological membranes, into lipid-based systems. These hybrids, in addition to enhancing the stability and pharmacokinetics of the encapsulated cargo, also provide opportunities for theranostic uses. This innovation results in a new age of targeted oncology through the ability to diagnose and treat in a single formulation (84) (Figure 3.9).

- **Lipid-Polymer Hybrid Nanoparticles (LPHNs):** LPHNs are among the most extensively studied hybrid systems. They are a stabilizing lipid monolayer or bilayer encapsulating a biodegradable polymer core, such as poly (lactic-co-glycolic acid) [PLGA] or polycaprolactone

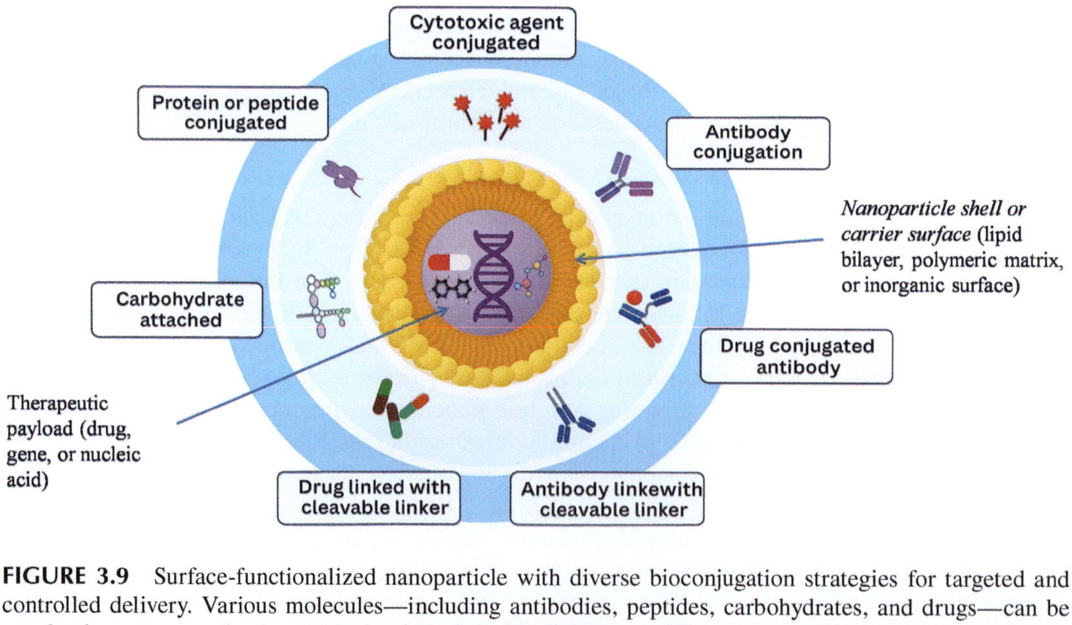

FIGURE 3.9 Surface-functionalized nanoparticle with diverse bioconjugation strategies for targeted and controlled delivery. Various molecules—including antibodies, peptides, carbohydrates, and drugs—can be covalently or noncovalently attached using cleavable linkers, enabling site-specific delivery and stimuli-triggered release of therapeutic agents.

[PCL]. The lipid shell provides enhanced biocompatibility, reduces opsonization, and enables surface modifications with targeted ligands, such as folate, antibodies, and peptides. The polymer core offers enhanced mechanical strength and increased drug loading capability. For instance, PLGA-lipid hybrids co-loading paclitaxel and siRNA have demonstrated robust anticancer activity in multidrug-resistant breast cancer models through the delivery of cytotoxic payloads and the silencing of resistance genes. Gene therapy potential is also remarkable, as they can shield delicate macromolecules such as mRNA and CRISPR/Cas9 elements (85).

- **Magnetoliposomes:** Superparamagnetic iron oxide nanoparticles (SPIONs) are incorporated into LNPs to confer contrast for magnetic resonance imaging (MRI). This permits non-invasive monitoring, magnetic field-directed delivery, and magnetic hyperthermia. Magnetoliposomes can enhance the accumulation of specific drugs in tumors and reduce exposure to the rest of the body by targeting deep-seated tumors using external magnetic fields. SPIONs produce localized heat upon irradiation with an alternating magnetic field (AMF) and induce the release of temperature-sensitive drugs from the lipid matrix. When used in conjunction with AMF-induced hyperthermia, folate-modified magnetic SLNs have demonstrated enhanced efficacy and increased tumor accumulation in clinical tests. Magnetoliposomes promise to be helpful agents for real-time image-guided cancer therapy based on their dual imaging and therapeutic ability (87).
- **Gold-Lipid Hybrids:** The combination of gold nanoparticles (AuNPs) with LNPs has enhanced photothermal treatment (PTT) and photodynamic therapy (PDT) through the optical properties of gold. AuNPs generate localized heat or reactive oxygen species (ROS) upon exposure to near-infrared (NIR) radiation. This action facilitates the ablation of the tumor and induces the release of drugs from the lipid coating, allowing for controlled therapy on demand can be achieved. Preclinical trials show that gold-lipid hybrids with doxorubicin and photosensitizers can entirely eradicate tumors in breast cancer and melanoma upon treatment with chemotherapy and photothermal therapy. AuNPs can also be used as CT imaging contrast agents, providing therapeutic carriers with further diagnostic capabilities (90).

To enhance the therapeutic efficacy of lipid-based nanoparticles, various functionalization approaches have been developed, including stimuli-responsive and hybrid strategies. These modifications enable controlled drug release, improved tumor targeting, enhanced cellular uptake, and better adaptation to the complex tumor microenvironment. A comparative overview of the major stimuli-responsive and hybrid functionalization strategies employed in lipid-based nanoparticles for oncology is presented in Table 3.2.

Hybrid nanoplatforms have numerous benefits, such as enhanced pharmacokinetics, which means increased half-life, enhanced stability, and sustained drug release; Multimodal therapy, which means the capability of delivering immunotherapies, gene therapies, and chemotherapy concurrently; Theranostics, which means targeted therapy with real-time imaging (MRI, CT, and optical) in conjunction with therapy. Penetrating tumor barriers, which means improved access via the extracellular matrix (ECM) of tumors, with evasion of biological clearance systems (92). The future of hybrid LNPs is in multi-stimuli-responsive theranostic systems that are capable of integrating immune modulation, diagnostic imaging, and other triggers such as pH, redox, magnetic, and thermal factors.

3.4 THERAPEUTIC PAYLOADS IN FUNCTIONALIZED LNPS

The versatility of functionalized lipid nanoparticles lies in their ability to accommodate diverse therapeutic payloads, ranging from conventional anticancer drugs to advanced biological molecules. The nature of the encapsulated cargo plays a crucial role in determining the therapeutic outcome, biodistribution, and clinical applicability of these nanocarrier systems. The major classes

TABLE 3.2
Comparative Overview of Stimuli-Responsive and Hybrid Functionalization Strategies for Lipid-Based Nanoparticles in Oncology

Representative Applications	Targeting and Uptake Pathway	Advantages	Key Materials and Examples	Mechanism of Trigger	Strategy
DOX-loaded pH-sensitive liposomes for breast and lung cancer	EPR effect, folate/HA targeting, clathrin-mediated endocytosis.	Minimizes premature release. Improves endosomal escape. Bypasses MDR.	DOPE, CHEMS, hydrazone bonds, BNT122 (mRNA vaccine)	Acidic TME (pH 6.5, 7.2) and endosomes/lysosomes (pH 4.5, 6.5) lead to the protonation of ionizable lipids or the cleavage of acid-labile bonds.	**pH-Sensitive Systems**
Cathepsin B-cleavable DOX liposomes for hepatoma	RGD or antibody-targeted uptake, endocytosis, and lysosomal cleavage.	High specificity, controlled activation inside cells, and synergy with other stimuli.	MMP-cleavable peptides, GPLGVRG, and Val-Cit linkers.	Overexpressed enzymes in TME, including MMPs, cathepsins, and PLA2, lead to the cleavage of peptide linkers or prodrugs.	**Enzyme-Responsive Systems**
DOX-siRNA disulfide hybrids for breast cancer, mRNA vaccines	GLUT or TPP targeting; endocytosis + cytoplasmic disassembly	Tumor-selective release, overcomes MDR, ideal for gene therapy	Disulfide-crosslinked LPHNs, GSH-sensitive prodrugs	High intracellular GSH (2–10 mM); cleavage of disulfide/diselenide bonds	**Redox-Responsive Systems**
Thermosensitive liposomes in liver/breast cancer	EPR + ligand targeting; endocytosis + heat-induced release	Site-specific on-demand release, synergizes with hyperthermia/radiotherapy	DPPC, PNIPAM, ThermoDox®	Hyperthermia (40–43°C); lipid phase transition or polymer collapse	**Temperature-Sensitive Systems**
Folate-targeted magnetoliposomes, cancer cell membrane-coated LNPs	Active ligand targeting, magnetic guidance, homotypic recognition	High stability, multimodal therapy, theranostics, immune evasion	PLGA-lipid hybrids, SPION-liposomes, RBC-coated LNPs	combination of multiple functionalities (polymeric, magnetic, gold, biomimetic)	**Hybrid Systems**

of therapeutic payloads employed in functionalized lipid nanoparticles for cancer therapy are discussed in this section.

3.4.1 Small-Molecule Chemotherapeutics

Small-molecule drugs have long been the mainstay of cancer treatment due to their distinct architectures, reliable pharmacokinetics, and broad range of cytotoxic effects. However, their therapeutic effectiveness is often limited by their short systemic half-lives, substantial off-target toxicity, rapid renal clearance, and poor water solubility, particularly in highly proliferative healthy tissues such as the gastrointestinal tract and bone marrow. Furthermore, recurrent treatment of small-molecule chemotherapeutics frequently leads to MDR due to efflux pump overexpression, modifications in drug metabolism, or mutations in drug targets (94).

Functionalized LNPs have emerged as a powerful nanoplatform to overcome these challenges. By encapsulating hydrophobic drugs, such as doxorubicin, docetaxel, or paclitaxel, in their lipid bilayers or cores, LNPs significantly enhance the solubility and stability of these drugs in the bloodstream. By protecting chemotherapeutics from early metabolism and removal, encapsulation also extends their plasma half-life. Importantly, LNPs passively accumulate in tumor tissues by exploiting the enhanced EPR effect, in which impaired lymphatic outflow and leaky vasculature facilitate selective drug deposition (95).

Surface functionalization with tumor-specific ligands (e.g., aptamers, peptides, antibodies, or folic acid) that precisely target malignant cells enables both active and passive targeting. This approach reduces systemic toxicity, enhances the therapeutic index, and gets around resistance mechanisms by bypassing drug efflux pumps. Additionally, stimuli-responsive functionalization (e.g., pH-sensitive lipids, redox-responsive linkers, or enzyme-cleavable coatings) enables controlled and site-specific drug release inside the intracellular compartments or TME.

The potential of LNPs in co-delivery systems, which combine genetic payloads (e.g., siRNA targeting resistance-related genes) with small-molecule drugs, has also been highlighted by recent investigations. Together, these strategies can suppress MDR pathways and ensure effective chemotherapeutic activity. Furthermore, customized lipid compositions and PEGylation methods increase circulation duration and decrease immunogenicity, enhancing therapeutic outcomes.

3.4.1.1 Recent Advancements in LNP-Based Therapies

To address MDR in glioblastoma (GBM) and glioblastoma stem cells (GSCs), researchers created a system by combining the P-glycoprotein (P-gp) inhibitor Reversan (RV) with curcumin (CMN) and regorafenib (RF) in nanostructure hybrid lipid capsules (nHLCs). This strategy sought to address the resistance mechanisms behind glioblastoma's poor prognosis (96). Lipid nanocapsules (LNCs) were used to co-deliver salinomycin (SAL) and paclitaxel (PTX) to target cancer stem cells as well as bulk breast cancer cells. The dual-drug LNCs demonstrated high encapsulation efficiency and storage stability. A significant obstacle in the therapy of breast cancer was overcome when they were successfully internalized by both cell types, resulting in apoptosis and a synergistic cytotoxic effect that prevented the creation of tumor mammospheres. As well as research groups examined the cytotoxicity and cellular absorption mechanism of paclitaxel-loaded lipid nanocapsules (LNCs-PTX) in three breast cancer cells.

Magnetic, temperature-sensitive liposomes were created by Pradhan, Giri, et al. in 2010 by combining biological targeting with magnetic field targeting with folate receptor-based biological targeting. Doxorubicin and magnetic nanoparticles were enclosed in these liposomes, which enabled magnetically driven drug release when heated to 43°C. This dual-targeting strategy improved drug delivery and cellular absorption in HeLa and KB cancer cell lines that express folate receptors. The system showed a synergistic increase in cytotoxicity when paired with magnetic hyperthermia (97).

Due to problems with limited solubility, poor systemic half-life, off-target toxicity, and multidrug resistance, small-molecule chemotherapeutics provide substantial obstacles in the treatment of cancer. One significant step toward getting beyond these restrictions is the development of lipid nanoparticles, or LNPs. LNPs improve medication stability and solubility, prolong circulation durations, and increase drug accumulation in tumor tissues through the increased EPR effect by encapsulating small-molecule medicines.

Additionally, LNP technology has advanced beyond passive targeting due to research and development. By using tumor-specific ligands to target malignant cells actively, advances in surface functionalization enable better therapeutic indices and get around drug resistance mechanisms. Co-delivery systems, which encapsulate several therapeutic drugs or combine chemotherapy with gene-based payloads like siRNA, have also been shown in recent research to have the potential to inhibit multidrug resistance pathways simultaneously.

3.4.2 Nucleic Acids (siRNA, mRNA, miRNA, CRISPR Components)

Using nucleic acids for medicinal purposes has ushered in a new era of biomedicine, particularly in precision medicine. By directly modifying gene expression at the transcriptional or translational level, nucleic acids offer unparalleled specificity and versatility compared to conventional small-molecule drugs or protein-based biologics. This class of treatments includes siRNAs, mRNAs, miRNAs, and genome-editing tools such as CRISPR-Cas systems. Although each modality operates through distinct molecular pathways, they all encounter the same challenges: low cellular absorption because of hydrophilicity and negative charge, instability in the systemic circulation, susceptibility to nuclease-mediated degradation, and the need for efficient intracellular release.

Functionalized LNPs have emerged as a significant solution to these issues. By encasing nucleic acids in protective nanostructures. LNPs not only shield them from enzyme degradation but also facilitate coordinated cytosolic release, efficient cellular absorption, and tailored transport to specific tissues. pH-responsive lipids, stimuli-sensitive modifications, and ligand decoration are other functionalization strategies that reduce off-target effects while permitting accurate delivery to sick regions. Further details are discussed in the following subsections about the therapeutic potential and delivery issues for siRNA, mRNA, miRNA, and CRISPR components.

3.4.2.1 Small Interfering RNAs (siRNAs)

siRNAs are among the most well-established and extensively studied classes of nucleic acid therapeutics. These double-stranded RNA molecules shut genes by selectively breaking down complementary messenger RNAs via the RNA interference (RNAi) pathway. In oncology, siRNAs can silence oncogenes, drug resistance genes, and other genetic drivers of tumor growth. Nevertheless, siRNAs have significant serum instability and are subject to quick renal elimination. To overcome these limitations, functionalized LNPs enhance siRNA transport to target tissues and stabilize them. Ionizable lipids in LNPs that promote endosomal escape are used by RNA-induced silencing complexes (RISCs) to distribute siRNAs in the cytoplasm.

- **Patisiran (Onpattro):** Approved to treat the polyneuropathy of hereditary transthyretin-mediated amyloidosis (hATTR), Patisiran is a prime example of a therapeutically effective siRNA-LNP. An ionizable lipid (DLin-MC3-DMA) functionalizes this LNP-siRNA, enabling targeted distribution to hepatocytes (liver cells). When the siRNA enters the hepatocyte, it attaches itself to the transthyretin (TTR) mRNA, breaks it down, and lowers the amount of the harmful TTR protein that is produced (98).
- **T-Lyp1-functionalized LNPs:** T-Lyp1-functionalized LNPs were created to deliver anti-KRAS siRNA in preclinical cancer research. Silencing the expression of KRAS, a common oncogene, is a promising cancer therapy. When coupled with gemcitabine, the T-Lyp1 peptide functions as a targeting ligand, increasing the accumulation of siRNA-LNP in tumors and demonstrating efficacy against pancreatic cancer in mouse models (99).

- **Folate-tagged LNPs:** Scientists have employed folate-tagged LNPs to transfer siRNA to prostate cancer cells exhibiting excessive folate receptor expression. By increasing the siRNA's cellular absorption, the folate functionalization decreased non-specific toxicity and raised the therapeutic index.

3.4.2.2 Messenger RNAs (mRNAs)

Instead of mutating genes like siRNAs do, mRNA treatments act as templates for protein production. This process makes it possible to produce tumor-associated antigens for cancer immunotherapy, inject therapeutic cytokines, or replace or repair damaged proteins. mRNA's non-integrative nature eliminates the potential for insertional mutagenesis, which is a major advantage over DNA-based techniques.

On the other hand, unmodified mRNA is inherently unstable and immunogenic. Functionalized LNPs tackle these issues by ensuring efficient cellular absorption, enhancing endosomal escape, and protecting mRNA from nucleases. Moreover, chemical nucleotide modification and LNP composition modification improve translational efficiency while reducing innate immune detection. The rapid development of COVID-19 mRNA vaccines (e.g., Pfizer-BioNTech and Moderna) demonstrated the scalability and therapeutic potential of LNP–mRNA formulations, laying a strong foundation for cancer immunotherapy and protein replacement therapy. In the future, LNPs might be organ-specifically functionalized to restore tumor suppressors in cancer cells or transport therapeutic enzymes to metabolic tissues.

Some of the Recent Advancements in LNP-based mRNA Delivery are as follows. The most well-known example of COVID-19 mRNA vaccines is the effectiveness of the Moderna (Spikevax®) and Pfizer-BioNTech (Comirnaty®) COVID-19 vaccines. These vaccines transfer mRNA encoding the SARS-CoV-2 spike protein to host cells via functionalized LNPs. After shielding the mRNA from deterioration, the LNP transports it to antigen-presenting cells, generating the spike protein to initiate a robust immune response.

- **Pfizer-BioNTech: Polack et al., 2020 (NEJM) (BNT162b2/Comirnaty®):** The New England Journal of Medicine published this historic Phase 3 study report. It describes the BNT162b2 vaccine's safety and effectiveness, demonstrating that after two doses, it provided 95% protection against COVID-19 in those 16 years of age or older. Additionally, the study details the mild-to-moderate short-term adverse effects that were noted.
- **Personalized cancer vaccines:** Organizations like Moderna have created mRNA vaccines based on LNP targeting specific neoantigens in melanoma. For instance, in high-risk melanoma patients, a Phase II trial (NCT03897881) combining mRNA-4157 with pembrolizumab demonstrated encouraging outcomes. By directing the production of several tumor-specific antigens by the patient's cells, the mRNA trains the immune system to identify and combat the cancer cells.
- **Protein replacement therapy:** In preclinical research, LNPs were utilized to transfer mRNA for protein replacement, including encoding factor IX for hemophilia B treatment. These examples demonstrate how LNPs may be used to deliver therapeutic proteins for genetic illnesses, even though it is still early (100).

3.4.2.3 MicroRNAs (miRNAs)

MicroRNAs are short, non-coding RNAs that post-transcriptionally regulate gene expression by binding to complementary sequences in target mRNAs. Aberrant expression of miRNA influences a number of pathogenic processes, including metastasis, oncogenesis, and chemoresistance. The two forms of therapeutic modulation are miRNA mimics to restore tumor-suppressive miRNAs or anti-miRs to block oncogenic miRNAs.

Delivery is still a significant problem, though, because miRNAs require precise intracellular location and are prone to degradation. A versatile platform for miRNA administration is provided by functionalized LNPs, which stabilize these small molecules and direct them to the diseased tissue. To reduce systemic toxicity, for instance, surface-functionalized LNPs coupled with tumor-homing ligands or antibodies can specifically deliver miRNA mimics to malignant cells. To achieve synergistic effects, such as tumor cell sensitization to conventional drugs, multifunctional LNPs that co-deliver miRNAs and chemotherapeutics can be developed. Therefore, the combination of miRNA treatments with functionalized nanocarriers is a feasible strategy to decrease treatment resistance in oncology.

- **Delivery of miR-122 to liver cancer:** Cationic LNPs (LNP-DP1) are designed to give hepatocellular carcinoma (HCC) cells a miR-122 mimic. Intrathecal injection of LNP-DP1 containing miR-122 mimics reduced tumor growth by almost 50% in a mouse model of HCC, indicating its potential as a treatment.
- **Multi-component delivery for breast cancer:** Research has looked into multifunctional LNPs that transport a miRNA mimic (such as miR-200c) and a chemotherapeutic medication like paclitaxel together. With this strategy, the medication can kill cancer cells, and the miRNA mimic can reverse chemoresistance, producing synergistic effects.
- **Hyaluronic acid-coated LNPs:** HA-coated LNPs were created by Hayward et al. to deliver miRNA-125a-5p to breast cancer cells that overexpress the CD44 receptor, which is HA's known target. As a result of this functionalization, the HER2 oncogene was effectively silenced, and targeting was improved (101).

3.4.2.4 CRISPR-Cas Components

The CRISPR-Cas system, particularly CRISPR-Cas9, has revolutionized genome editing by enabling precise and programmable modification of nearly any genomic region. Therapeutic applications include genetic mutation correction, oncogene knockdown, and tumor suppressor activation. However, the distribution of CRISPR components, such as the Cas nuclease (protein or mRNA) and the guide RNA, poses unique challenges due to their size, negative charge, and requirement for many components to be given simultaneously.

In this regard, functionalized LNPs have shown a lot of promise. By encapsulating Cas9 mRNA and single-guide RNAs, LNPs can facilitate the temporary production of editing machinery while reducing the possibility of off-target consequences associated with prolonged Cas9 activity. Chemical functionalization, such as tissue-specific ligands or stimuli-responsive lipids, increases distribution accuracy. Targeting polo-like kinase 1 (PLK1) in glioblastoma is one example of the notable advancement of employing LNP-delivered CRISPR systems to alter disease-causing genes in vivo in preclinical cancer models. Even if clinical translation is still in its early stages, the revolutionary significance of LNP-based delivery is highlighted by the possibility of long-lasting medicines through one-time genome editing therapy.

A safe and effective LNP formulation to deliver CRISPR-Cas9 components for targeted cancer therapy was created by Rosenblum et al. in their 2020 Science Advances paper. Cas9 mRNA and sgRNAs targeting the PLK1 gene are co-encapsulated in LNPs, which were specifically designed with a new amino-ionizable lipid to ensure transient expression and minimize off-target effects. An orthotopic glioblastoma mouse model showed up to 70% gene editing after a single intracerebral injection of these LNPs, which markedly reduced tumor growth by 50% and increased survival by 30% (103).

In their 2019 *Journal of Controlled Release* paper, Li et al. developed a tumor-targeted lipid-based delivery system for CRISPR-Cas9 to knock down hypoxia-inducible factor-1α (HIF-1α) in pancreatic cancer. Their system featured cationic liposomes modified with the R8-dGR peptide, which significantly enhanced cellular uptake and tumor penetration by targeting integrin αvβ3 and neuropilin-1 receptors. Co-encapsulating a HIF-1α CRISPR-Cas9 plasmid with paclitaxel, the researchers demonstrated that this targeted delivery system successfully suppressed HIF-1α and its downstream pro-metastatic molecules, leading to enhanced anti-tumor and anti-metastatic effects in a mouse model. This dual-action approach, combining genetic knockdown with chemotherapy, not only improved the therapeutic efficacy against primary tumor growth but also significantly inhibited metastasis and prolonged survival without causing major toxicity (104).

In a 2020 *Journal of Controlled Release* paper, Liu et al. developed a virus-like nanoparticle (VLN) system for co-delivering CRISPR/Cas9 and a small molecule drug to treat melanoma. The core-shell VLN was engineered to encapsulate Cas9 RNP targeting the PD-L1 gene and the tyrosine kinase inhibitor axitinib within a mesoporous silica core further enclosed by a lipid shell. This design protected the payload during circulation and ensured its release in the tumor's reductive microenvironment. In a melanoma mouse model, the combination therapy synergistically inhibited tumor growth by achieving PD-L1 knockout in cancer cells, which reversed T-cell exhaustion, and delivering axitinib, which reduced immunosuppressive regulatory T cells (Tregs) in the tumor microenvironment. This multi-pronged approach successfully enhanced anti-tumor immunity and demonstrated the VLN's potential as a versatile platform for advanced combination therapies (105).

The use of functionalized LNPs in conjunction with nucleic acid therapies has created a new avenue for personalized treatment. Long-lasting genomic modifications are made possible by CRISPR components, siRNAs inhibit oncogenic drivers, mRNAs add or restore therapeutic proteins, and miRNAs adjust gene regulatory networks. Even with remarkable progress, some difficulties remain, including immunogenicity, the efficiency of distribution in extrahepatic tissues, and long-term safety. Combinatorial designs, biodegradable polymers, stimuli-responsive lipids, and other functionalization approaches are expected to enhance the therapeutic potential of nucleic acids.

Ultimately, the use of functionalized LNPs in conjunction with nucleic acid techniques has the potential to transform the management of genetic disorders, cancer, and infectious diseases, advancing medicine toward genuinely tailored and curative treatments.

3.4.3 Photothermal Therapeutics

Photothermal therapy (PTT) is a minimally invasive therapeutic technique that generates localized thermal energy from light, often near-infrared (NIR) radiation, using photo-absorbing materials. PTT, as opposed to conventional systemic treatments, allows for spatiotemporal control over therapeutic action, minimizing collateral injury to adjacent healthy tissues. When used as delivery vehicles, functionalized LNPs address long-standing problems in PTT, including limited solubility, rapid clearance, and off-target accumulation. It's vital to delve into the unique biological and molecular processes to elaborate on the mechanisms of PTT, especially the many cellular outcomes impacted by temperature. The precise concentration of this thermal energy at the tumor location is made possible by functionalized LNPs, which provide precisely controlled therapeutic effects.

3.4.3.1 The Temperature-Dependent Spectrum of Cellular Response

The temperature and length of exposure have a significant impact on the biological consequences of heat, which are not consistent. From subtle, synergistic, low-temperature hyperthermia to focused, high-temperature thermal ablation, this spectrum enables different treatment approaches. Tumor cells experience necrosis (T>45–48°C), an uncontrollable cell death process marked by swift and significant damage, when heated to high temperatures.

- **Rapid and Severe Damage:** The integrity of the cell is almost immediately jeopardized when the local temperature rises above 45–48°C. Important cellular components are quickly degraded.
- **Protein Denaturation:** Enzymes and structural proteins, which are essential for cellular function, lose their native shape and aggregate. This halts all vital cellular processes and leads to cell death.

- **Membrane Disruption:** The cell membrane becomes permeable and irreversibly disrupted by high heat. This involves harm to the membranes of organelles, such as mitochondria and the plasma membrane.
- **DAMP Release and Inflammation:** Intracellular materials, such as damage-associated molecular patterns (DAMPs), are released into the surrounding tissue when the cell membrane ruptures. In addition to occasionally inciting an immune response against the tumor, this sets off a potent and frequently harmful inflammatory response that may inadvertently cause harm to adjacent healthy tissue. A moderate temperature range that preferentially triggers apoptosis, or programmed cell death, can be attained by carefully regulating the concentration of the photothermal agent and the NIR dose. Since apoptosis is a highly controlled and non-inflammatory process, it is a more desirable result for targeted cancer therapy than necrosis.
- **Mitochondrial Pathway Activation:** When mitochondria are subjected to moderate heat stress, the outer membrane of the mitochondria becomes permeable. Pro-apoptotic proteins, particularly cytochrome c, are released into the cytoplasm as a result. **Apoptosome formation:** Cytochrome C forms the apoptosome in the cytoplasm by binding with other proteins. The main executors of apoptosis, caspase-9 and caspase-3, are among the cascade of caspases (cysteine-aspartic proteases) that are activated by this combination. **Caspase Cascade:** By cleaving structural proteins and DNA repair enzymes, the activated caspases, Hyperthermia Induces Apoptosis through the endoplasmic methodically destroy the cell from within. This leads to the creation of membrane-bound apoptotic bodies by regulated nuclear fragmentation and cell shrinkage (106).
- **Immunologically "Silent" Cell Clearance:** Phagocytes identify and eliminate these apoptotic bodies without inflaming the surrounding milieu, reducing harm. LNPs can be made especially to encourage this type of cell death that is beneficial to the immune system. Mild or sub-lethal hyperthermia makes cancer cells more sensitive to other therapies rather than killing them directly. This tactic works especially well when paired with conventional immunotherapy, radiation, or chemotherapy.

3.4.3.2 Mechanisms for Enhanced Chemosensitivity

- **Increased Membrane Permeability:** Chemotherapeutic medications are more readily absorbed intracellularly when cell membranes are more fluid due to mild heat. For instance, research on liver cancer cells revealed that, in comparison to either treatment alone, sublethal hyperthermia increased the uptake of doxorubicin and increased cell death. **DNA Repair Inhibition:** Radiation or chemotherapy-induced DNA damage can be difficult to repair when a person is too hot. These medicines increase their cytotoxic effects by blocking DNA repair pathways. **Increased Oxygenation and Blood Flow:** In the case of PTT, modest hyperthermia may cause the tumor's oxygen and blood flow to increase. Given that hypoxic cancers frequently resist radiation and several chemotherapies, this is particularly crucial. **Improved medication Release from Nano-carriers:** When combined with thermosensitive LNPs, mild hyperthermia can cause a controlled, prolonged release of the medication that is encapsulated right at the tumor site, increasing the concentration of the drug locally. The use of thermosensitive liposomes in conjunction with hyperthermia to improve the delivery of chemotherapeutic medications to solid tumors. **Immunomodulatory Effects Immunomodulatory Effects:** An immunologically "cold" tumor may become "hot" and vulnerable to immune attack as a result of LNP-mediated PTT's ability to affect the body's immune system (108). **Immunogenic Cell Death (ICD):** ICD is triggered by PTT and results in an immunological response that fights the tumor. When tumor cells die, they emit particular "eat me" signals and antigens that the immune system can encounter. **Heat Shock Protein (HSP) Release:** When tumor cells experience heat stress, they release HSPs (such as HSP70 and HSP90). Antigen-presenting cells (APCs), including dendritic cells (DCs), are drawn to and activated by these proteins, which function as danger signals. Toll-like receptor 4 (TLR4) on dendritic cells is activated and matured by extracellular HSP70. This promotes adaptive immune responses and improves antigen presentation. Overall, the results show that HSP70 is a crucial mediator that connects stress brought on by hyperthermia to efficient immune activation against malignancies. **Immune Checkpoint Sensitization:** The tumor may become more sensitive to immunotherapy, particularly immune checkpoint inhibitors, as a result of heat-induced immunomodulation. A synergistic therapeutic impact can result from immune system activation and tumor antigen release, which can prime T cells to react more effectively to checkpoint inhibition. An immunologically "cold" tumor may become "hot" and vulnerable to immune attack as a result of LNP-mediated PTT's ability to affect the body's immune system. Immunogenic Cell Death (ICD): ICD is triggered by PTT and results in an immunological response that fights the tumor. When tumor cells die, they emit particular "eat me" signals and antigens that the immune system can encounter. Immuno-adjuvant nanoparticles containing imiquimod (R837) as an immune stimulant and indocyanine green (ICG) for photothermal therapy were created by Chen et al. R837 stimulated dendritic cells to improve immune priming, and local tumor ablation brought about by near-infrared irradiation released tumor antigens. The treatment eliminated initial tumors, inhibited metastasis, and created long-term immunological memory in animal models when paired with anti-CTLA-4 checkpoint inhibition. The study shows that immune checkpoint inhibition and photothermal therapy work together to produce long-lasting, systemic anti-tumor immunity. Immuno-adjuvant nanoparticles containing imiquimod (R837) as an immune stimulant and indocyanine green (ICG) for photothermal therapy were created in this 2016 work by Chen et al. R837 stimulated dendritic cells to improve immune priming, and local tumor ablation brought about by near-infrared irradiation released tumor antigens. The treatment eliminated initial tumors, inhibited metastasis, and created long-term immunological memory in animal models when paired with anti-CTLA-4 checkpoint inhibition. The study shows that immune checkpoint inhibition and photothermal therapy work together to produce long-lasting, systemic anti-tumor immunity (Q. Chen et al. 2016).

3.4.3.3 Photothermal Agents in LNPs

For a variety of photothermal material classes, functionalized LNPs act as flexible carriers.

- **Organic Dyes:** ICG, despite being FDA-approved, has problems with photobleaching and instability. Encapsulation in LNPs improves tumor accumulation, stabilizes fluorescence, and prolongs circulation. Theranostic nanoplatform BSA@ICG-DOX was created by Ma et al. (2021) to treat cervical cancer by combining PTT and chemotherapy under the guidance of NIR fluorescence imaging. The technique enhances the stability and tumor-targeting potential of indocyanine green (ICG) by encapsulating it in bovine serum albumin (BSA). Co-loading doxorubicin (DOX) allows for the synergistic destruction of cancer cells. Strong NIR-I fluorescence, effective photothermal conversion, and biocompatibility are all displayed by the nanoparticles. Effective tumor suppression was demonstrated in xenograft mice models used in in vivo investigations. This strategy demonstrates how LNP-based chemo-PTT platforms can be used to improve targeted therapy (110). **Metallic Nanostructures:** Both gold nanostars (AuNSs) and nanourchins (AuNUs) have anisotropic geometries that boost electromagnetic field effects and local electron density, resulting in increased PTT efficiency. The significant absorption of these nanoparticles in the NIR-I and NIR-II windows allows for deep tissue heating. The enhancement of biocompatibility, cellular uptake, and regulated biodistribution can be achieved through surface conjugation with LNPs or other carriers. Additionally, AuNSs and AuNUs combine PTT with bioimaging and synergistic cancer therapies to provide multifunctional theranostic capabilities. **Metallic Nanostructures:** Both gold nanostars (AuNSs) and nanourchins (AuNUs) have anisotropic geometries that boost electromagnetic field effects and local electron density, resulting in increased PTT efficiency. The significant absorption of these nanoparticles in the NIR-I and NIR-II windows allows for deep tissue heating. The enhancement of biocompatibility, cellular uptake, and regulated biodistribution can be achieved through surface conjugation with LNPs or other carriers. Additionally, AuNSs and AuNUs combine PTT with bioimaging and synergistic cancer therapies to provide multifunctional theranostic capabilities. Because of their high NIR absorption, gold nano-shells can transform light into localized heat inside tumor tissues. The hyperthermia produced by NIR laser irradiation causes selective tumor cell death, reducing harm to nearby healthy tissues. The study showed that gold nano-shells could effectively accumulate in prostate cancers, indicating that they could be used for targeted, less invasive therapy. This approach offers a promising alternative to conventional therapies, improving treatment specificity and reducing systemic side effects. Furthermore, deeper tissue penetration may be optimized because to the nanoshells' adjustable optical characteristics. The findings support the broader application of nanoparticle-mediated photothermal therapy in oncology (111).

- **Carbon-Based Nanomaterials:** Because of their high optical absorbance, graphene oxide, carbon nanotubes, and carbon dots can all be used to co-load drugs into LNPs. **Polymer-Based Photothermal Agents:** Semiconducting polymer nanoparticles and π-conjugated polymers are being researched as biocompatible substitutes with adjustable optical properties. The impact of biocompatible semiconducting polymer nanoparticles (SPNs) with different donor-acceptor topologies on photothermal and photoacoustic performance was investigated by Zhang et al. 52.6% photothermal conversion efficiency was attained by the SPN with the longest π-conjugation and the best donor–acceptor balance. The nanoparticles were appropriate for use in biomedical applications because of their strong size stability, water dispersibility, and biocompatibility. The SPNs produced heat when exposed to NIR radiation, which allowed for both considerable tumor reduction in vivo and efficient tumor cell death in vitro. The study showed that the photothermal and photoacoustic characteristics of polymeric nanoparticles are significantly influenced by their chemical structure. All things considered, these SPNs offer a potential foundation for theranostic applications, fusing therapy with imaging in the fight against cancer (112).

3.4.3.4 Advantages of LNP-Mediated PTT

Pharmacokinetics and Stability: As demonstrated by the enhanced stability of ICG when encapsulated, LNP encapsulation reduces renal clearance and shields photothermal agents from degradation.

- **Enhanced stability of photothermal agents:** Because LNPs shield photothermal agents (PTAs) from environmental deterioration and the body's clearance processes, they perform noticeably better. Zein–phosphatidylcholine hybrid nanoparticles were created by Lee et al. to contain ICG for use in cancer phototherapy. In watery conditions, encapsulation reduced aggregation and photobleaching while greatly increasing ICG stability. In order to enable successful phototherapy, the hybrid nanoparticles maintained the photo-cytotoxic activity of ICG against oral cancer cells. The organic color is structurally protected by the nanoparticles' lipid–protein makeup. Studies conducted in vitro showed enhanced cellular absorption and a long-lasting photothermal impact when exposed to radiation. Overall, this study shows that LNPs are a good way to deliver and preserve photothermal drugs for the treatment of cancer (113).
- **Decreased renal and immunological clearance:** LNPs' ideal size, which is usually between 100 and 200 nm, enables them to avoid the body's quick immune clearance by the RES and kidney filtration. PEG surface functionalization intensifies this "stealth" action and extends circulation time. **Defense against deterioration:** By encapsulating organic dyes, such as ICG, in LNPs, the agent is kept available and functional at the target site by preventing photobleaching and enzymatic breakdown in the bloodstream. **Control over release kinetics:** Scientists can create systems that release their payload in a controlled or prolonged way by modifying the lipid composition of the LNP. This maximizes efficacy

by extending the treatment window and can be triggered by particular stimuli at the tumor location. **Improved Targeting for Selective Action**: LNPs can be specifically designed for active targeting, which greatly improves therapeutic selectivity and reduces harm to healthy tissues, in addition to passive accumulation through the EPR effect. **Active targeting with ligands:** with receptor-mediated endocytosis, surface functionalization with ligands that bind selectively to receptors overexpressed on cancer cells enhances tumor selectivity. To improve cellular absorption and lessen non-specific toxicity in prostate cancer, folate-tagged LNPs have been created to target tumors that express the folate receptor. **Drug efflux pump blockage:** Active targeting can also get around resistance mechanisms such as drug efflux pumps. LNPs can carry PTAs and co-loaded medications into the cell by encouraging direct cellular internalization, avoiding these pumps and overcoming MDR.

- **Optimized and Controlled Heating:** LNPs enable carefully regulated, localized heating that can be adjusted for a variety of therapeutic outcomes. Precise, localized heating, by active targeting and the EPR effect, LNPs selectively accumulate in tumors, guaranteeing that the heat produced by NIR irradiation is focused at the tumor location. This reduces collateral harm to healthy tissues in the vicinity. **Hyperthermia-induced synergy:** LNP-PTT-induced mild, controlled hyperthermia can enhance the way other medicinal drugs are delivered. Heat enhances the permeability of cell membranes and tumor vasculature, which promotes the intracellular uptake and accumulation of medicines that are delivered together. In breast cancer models, moderate hyperthermia has been found to boost the cellular absorption of chemotherapeutic medicines by multiple times. **Modifiable cell death mechanisms:** The mechanism of cell death can be controlled by varying the PTT parameters. Low-energy PTT can encourage a more regulated apoptosis, but high-energy irradiation can cause fast necrosis. Synergistic combination therapy can then be implemented using the selected mechanisms.

3.4.3.5 Advanced Theranostic and Combination Applications

LNPs are flexible platforms that can be used to combine various therapeutic activities with diagnostic imaging, allowing for individualized and very successful treatment plans.

- **Monitoring and direction in real time:** Real-time monitoring of LNP biodistribution and treatment response is made possible by the intrinsic imaging capabilities of several PTAs, such as the fluorescence of ICG or the photoacoustic qualities of gold nanostructures. Treatment is administered at the appropriate time and place thanks to this image-guided method.
- **Combination with chemotherapy (Chemo-PTT):** PTAs and chemotherapy medications can be co-encapsulated using LNPs. While the LNP shields and transports both chemicals, the PTT-induced heat amplifies the drug's cytotoxic action. For instance, doxorubicin (DOX) is delivered via the PDA-modified ultrasmall UGO platform for synergistic chemo-PTT in breast cancer.
- **Immunotherapy in combination (Immuno-PTT):** PTT can cause immunogenic cell death, which releases heat shock proteins and antigens linked to tumors. To target distant metastases and boost the anti-tumor immune response, LNPs can be engineered to co-deliver PTAs with immunoadjuvants or checkpoint inhibitors.
- **Combination with gene therapy (Gene-PTT):** LNPs can deliver gene-modulating agents like siRNA and PTAs at the same time, enabling gene silencing and local ablation to get beyond resistance mechanisms.

3.4.3.6 Increased Biocompatibility and Reduced Immunogenicity

LNPs lower the possibility of negative responses linked to free PTAs by offering a biocompatible and safe PTT delivery method. **Decreased systemic toxicity:** The PTA is contained within LNPs, limiting its exposure to healthy tissues and reducing systemic toxicity and adverse effects. **Immune**

system protection: The structure of the LNP, particularly when PEGylation is present, protects the therapeutic payload against unintended immunological responses. This lessens immunogenicity and stops anti-LNP antibodies from forming, which could hasten clearance with repeated dosing. **Personalized medicine:** LNPs can be highly customized in terms of composition, targeting ligands, and payloads due to their modular construction. This adaptability has enormous potential for the development of personalized medicine strategies for PTT, in which the course of treatment is customized to the unique features of each patient's tumor.

3.4.3.7 Chemo-Photothermal Therapy (Chemo-PTT)

Combining photothermal therapy and chemotherapy has a synergistic effect that is very successful at fighting cancer and frequently overcomes the drawbacks of either treatment alone. Because LNP-based platforms can co-encapsulate a photothermal agent and a chemotherapeutic medication, allowing for precision co-delivery and localized activity, they are perfect for this strategy. The process is based on PTT-induced hyperthermia, which improves the uptake and lethal effects of the co-delivered chemotherapeutic drug by increasing the permeability of cell membranes and the tumor vasculature.

3.4.3.8 Immuno-Photothermal Therapy (Immuno-PTT)

By causing ICD, releasing tumor-associated antigens (TAAs), and releasing DAMPs, PTT can initiate an immune response against tumors. By stimulating APCs and triggering a systemic immune response, this functions as an in-situ vaccination. Immuno-checkpoint blockage (ICB) therapy, which enables T-cells to target both the original tumor and metastases, works in perfect harmony with this strategy. In order to improve anti-tumor immunity, Chen et al. (2016) presented a nanoparticle-based method for Immuno-Photothermal Therapy (Immuno-PTT) in Nature Communications. This method combines ICB with PTT. PLGA, imiquimod (R837), an immune adjuvant, and ICG, a photothermal agent, make up the nanoparticles. Tumor-associated antigens (TAAs) and DAMPs are released when the system causes photothermal ablation of tumors under NIR laser irradiation. R837 acts as an in-situ vaccination by stimulating APCs, which in turn sets off a systemic immune response. Primary and metastatic tumor T-cell targeting is improved when combined with anti-CTLA-4 therapy. This approach fosters long-term immunity and successfully defeats tumor immune evasion. The findings demonstrate the possibility of immuno-PTT mediated by nanoparticles for synergistic cancer treatment. All things considered, it offers a strong foundation for integrating PTT and immunotherapy to enhance therapeutic results (Q. Chen et al. 2016).

3.4.3.9 Gene-Photothermal Therapy (Gene-PTT)

PTT and gene therapy together enable simultaneous thermal ablation and the modification of genes linked to malignancy. LNPs can deliver gene payloads such as siRNA or mRNA along with photothermal agents. PTT can also improve gene therapy by encouraging endosomal escape and absorption. Chuan et al. co-delivered PD-L1 siRNA with IR780, a photothermal agent, to create lipid–polymer hybrid nanoparticles for tumor photothermal immunotherapy. Dopamine-modified polyethylenimine (PEI) is used in the nanoparticles' construction to allow for both agents' stable encapsulation and effective distribution. The device produces mild hyperthermia when exposed to NIR light, which promotes the release of PD-L1 siRNA and causes ICD. This dual effect promotes anti-tumor immunity while also blocking the PD-L1 immune checkpoint pathway. Experiments conducted both in vitro and in vivo showed that the nanoparticles successfully inhibited tumor development while triggering systemic immune responses. A synergistic therapeutic effect is produced when PD-L1 knockdown and photothermal therapy are combined. The study emphasizes how this multipurpose platform may improve cancer immunotherapy. All things considered, the method presents a viable way to combine immunological checkpoint modification and photothermal therapy to enhance therapeutic results (114).

3.4.3.10 Photo- and Sonodynamic Synergy

PTT can be used in conjunction with sonodynamic therapy (SDT) or PDT to enhance therapeutic results and tackle issues such as treating deeper tumors or tumor hypoxia.

Using cerium oxide (CeO_2) and ICG-loaded up-conversion nanoparticles (UCNPs) researchers created a multifunctional LNP platform for improved PDT and PTT. The UCNPs imitate the effects of SDT under NIR irradiation by converting NIR light into higher-energy emissions that activate ICG to produce ROS for tumor cell death. CeO_2 increases the effectiveness of PDT/PTT by modifying the TME by lowering hypoxia and regulating ROS levels. The limits of single-modality therapy are overcome by the dual-action system, which produces mutually reinforced photothermal and photodynamic effects. Studies conducted in vivo and in vitro revealed low off-target damage and significant tumor inhibition. Additionally, the platform increased systemic anti-tumor effects by enhancing immunogenic responses. This approach shows how to use LNPs for precise, NIR-triggered PTT/SDT combination therapy.

Multimodal therapy mediated by functionalized LNP represents a major breakthrough in the treatment of cancer. In order to fight tumors from multiple angles, researchers are combining PTT with other modalities including as immunotherapy, chemotherapy, and gene therapy. With the help of these nanoparticles, cancer treatments can become more individualized and efficient by enabling precise delivery, spatiotemporal control, and resistance removal. The preclinical data from the referenced research shows how promising this technology is and how it is evolving toward clinical translation.

The low penetration depth of NIR light, the possibility of searing adjacent healthy tissues, and the uneven heat distribution in large or heterogeneous tumors are some of the disadvantages of LNP-mediated PTT, despite its considerable promise. Additionally, by overexpressing HSPs, tumor cells can become thermoresistant. Numerous tactics are being developed to overcome these issues.

Stimuli-Responsive LNPs improve chemo- and photothermal therapy by releasing payloads in response to tumor-specific signals, such as pH shifts or photothermal triggers, which decreases off-target damage and improves treatment precision. PTT with Image Guidance (Theranostics) integrates imaging modalities like as MRI, CT, and fluorescence to guide precise tumor ablation, enabling real-time monitoring of nanoparticle biodistribution and therapeutic response. Deeper tissue penetration and less scattering are two benefits of NIR-II photothermal agents that allow for controlled photothermal therapy and supplementary imaging, such as photoacoustic imaging. Advanced LNP Design ensures effective cytosolic delivery of nucleic acids and medicines by enhancing organ-specific targeting, biodistribution, and endosomal escape using techniques such helper lipid optimization, selective organ targeting, and new ionizable lipids.

Future directions for LNP-mediated PTT development point to theranostic platforms that are incredibly accurate, customized, and multipurpose. Important prospects consist of:

- **Clinical translation:** More research and manufacturing process standardization are required to get additional LNP-PTT systems into clinical trials and receive regulatory approval. **Combined therapeutic approaches:** To overcome tumor resistance and enhance treatment results, researchers will keep looking into how PTT can work in concert with immunotherapy, gene therapy, chemotherapy, and other cutting-edge modalities.
- **Advanced materials:** To improve tissue penetration, increase biocompatibility, and facilitate more accurate drug release, new biodegradable PTAs, NIR-II agents, and stimuli-responsive materials will be developed further. PTT has been transformed into an extremely effective and tailored cancer treatment by the clever fusion of functionalized LNPs with photothermal agents. By enhancing the stability, circulation time, and tumor-specific concentration of photothermal agents, LNPs get around some of PTT's main drawbacks. PTT is changing from a stand-alone treatment to a vital part of all-encompassing cancer management when combined with developments in multimodal therapy. Future studies that

concentrate on resolving enduring issues like as heat distribution and tissue penetration will further develop LNP-mediated PTT's potential, advancing it toward broad clinical use and providing cancer patients with a more accurate, minimally intrusive treatment alternative.

3.4.4 Sonodynamic Therapeutics

Low-intensity ultrasound (US) is used in SDT, a novel non-invasive treatment technique, to activate sonosensitizers. These substances subsequently emit ROS, such as singlet oxygen and hydroxyl radicals, which induce oxidative stress in cancer cells and lead to necrosis, apoptosis, and autophagic cell death. The potential of SDT to treat hypoxic and deep-seated cancers is increased since it can reach deeper tissues than PDT because of ultrasound's deep tissue penetration. Functionalized LNPs significantly expand the therapeutic potential of SDT when used as delivery vehicles. Conventional sonosensitizers frequently suffer from weak solubility, rapid systemic clearance, and low tumor accumulation. These limitations are circumvented via LNP encapsulation by the following:

Improving Pharmacokinetics and Biodistribution—encapsulation extends the duration of sonosensitizer circulation by shielding them from enzymatic and renal elimination.

Improving Tumor Accumulation—LNPs can be functionalized with targeted ligands for active delivery or use passive accumulation through the increased EPR effect. Co-encapsulating sonosensitizers with various therapeutic payloads allows LNPs to facilitate synergistic treatment regimens. Mechanistically, ultrasound causes sonic cavitation, or the rapid formation and burst of microbubbles, which improves medication penetration, oxygen transport, and tumor cell membrane permeability. Because of its dual purpose, ultrasound directly produces cytotoxic ROS and improves therapeutic delivery at the tumor site.

3.4.4.1 Sonosensitizers Delivered by LNPs

In order to overcome their inherent constraints, LNPs can be used as flexible delivery systems for a variety of sonosensitizers.

- **Natural Dyes:** To increase its solubility and tumor accumulation, LNPs can supply the well-researched organic sonosensitizer chlorin e6 (Ce6). For instance, research has demonstrated that Ce6-loaded nanocarriers can improve the formation of singlet oxygen following ultrasonic activation and increase intracellular sonosensitizer accumulation, hence increasing the efficacy of SDT. The sonosensitizer Ce6 and manganese dioxide (MnO_2), which have catalase-like activity to break down tumor-abundant H_2O_2 into oxygen, were co-loaded into oxygen-generating polymer vesicles (PVs) by Wei et al. (2023). These Ce6-MnO_2-PVs greatly increased the formation of ROS during ultrasonic irradiation by alleviating hypoxia in the tumor microenvironment, which increased the effectiveness of SDT. Studies conducted both in vitro and in vivo verified that Ce6-MnO_2-PVs and ultrasound together produced better tumor suppression than either treatment alone. Furthermore, the system changed how hypoxia-responsive proteins were expressed, suggesting that tumor hypoxia was effectively modulated. All things considered, the study shows that oxygen-generating polymer vesicles offer a potent way to get beyond hypoxia-induced restrictions and improve SDT results (115).
- **Inorganic Nanomaterials:** Titanium dioxide (TiO_2) and other inorganic nanoparticles are also efficient SDT agents. As a new sonosensitizer, Tian et al. created a Pt–TiO_2 heterostructure with an oxygen-deficient layer. Oxygen vacancies increased ROS production and ultrasonic sensitivity, while Pt nanoparticles improved charge separation. Stronger anticancer effects were made possible by this method through synergistic chemo-sonodynamic treatment (CDT + SDT). Significant tumor growth suppression, increased ROS generation, and increased tumor cell death were demonstrated in both in vitro and in vivo studies.

- **Nanozymes:** Under ultrasonic irradiation, tiny iron-platinum (FePt) nanoparticles can function as nanozymes, stimulating the breakdown of hydrogen peroxide to produce oxygen while also generating singlet oxygen. This offers a two-pronged strategy to combat tumor hypoxia. Dong et al. used thermal reduction to create ultra-small FePt nanoparticles (~3.22 nm) and verified their crystalline nature and steady dispersion. By breaking down hydrogen peroxide to liberate oxygen, these nanoparticles demonstrated peroxidase-like activity, reducing tumor hypoxia. FePt produced singlet oxygen under ultrasonic irradiation in both normoxic and hypoxic circumstances (with H_2O_2), significantly increasing the formation of reactive oxygen species. Their safety without ultrasonic activation was confirmed by toxicity experiments that showed negligible dark toxicity. FePt with ultrasound effectively reduced the survival of MCF-7 breast cancer cells in sonodynamic therapy trials; it was more effective in normoxia but still effective in hypoxia. All things considered, the study emphasizes FePt nanoparticles as oxygen-enhanced sonosensitizers that have a great chance of overcoming hypoxia-related cancer treatment constraints (116).

3.4.4.2 Advanced LNP Functionalization for Sonodynamic Therapy (SDT)

By regulating particle biodistribution and initiating therapy at the tumor site, sophisticated LNP functionalization techniques can be employed in addition to straightforward encapsulation to increase SDT accuracy and efficacy.

- **Folate receptors:** A novel albumin-based nanodelivery system intended for improved immunological and sonodynamic combined anticancer therapy. Targeting folate receptors on tumor cells, this approach co-loads the STING agonist manganese oxide (MnOx) with the sonosensitizer ICG. ICG produces ROS when ultrasound is activated, and MnOx releases Mn^{2+} ions that trigger the cGAS-STING pathway, causing ICD and encouraging T-cell proliferation. Combining immune modulation with sonodynamic therapy provides a synergistic way to increase therapeutic efficacy. This approach offers a promising way to treat cancer by addressing issues, including tumor hypoxia and immune evasion (117).
- **RGD-targeted polypeptide nano-micelles for SDT:** An inventive method of using SDT to treat breast cancer is presented in the paper "Integrin $\alpha v\beta 3$-targeted self-assembled polypeptide nanomicelles for efficacious sonodynamic therapy against breast cancer". In order to create nanomicelles that can encapsulate the sonosensitizer rose bengal (RB), researchers created amphiphilic polypeptides that self-assemble. To improve tumor-specific accumulation, these RB-loaded nanomicelles (REPNs) were functionalized with an integrin $\alpha v\beta 3$-targeting peptide. The REPNs produced ROS when exposed to ultrasonic radiation, which caused tumor cells to undergo apoptosis. They also demonstrated strong anticancer activity in vivo with no discernible adverse effects. The potential of REPNs as a promising platform for targeted SDT in breast cancer therapy is demonstrated by this study (118).

3.4.4.3 Microenvironment-Responsive Release

Because the TME is characterized by circumstances including low pH, high GSH levels, and oxidative stress, LNPs can be designed to release their payload only in the TME.

- **pH-sensitive lipids:** Since they become cationic in the acidic endosome and rupture the membrane to liberate the cargo, ionizable lipids that promote endosomal escape are an example of pH-responsive functionalization. Zhang et al.'s (2020) study offers a novel way to improve SDT for breast cancer by using pH-responsive liposomal nanocarriers to address tumor hypoxia. To increase SDT efficacy in the acidic TME, our liposomes co-encapsulate the oxygen-consumption reducer metformin and the sonosensitizer IR780. By using pH-sensitive phospholipids that promote drug release in the acidic TME and take advantage of the increased EPR effect, the liposomal formulation, known as MI-PEOz-lip, allows for tailored delivery. ROS are produced by the released IR780 upon ultrasonic activation, but metformin lowers oxygen consumption, hence reducing hypoxia-induced resistance to SDT. By boosting oxygen availability and ROS production, this tactic successfully improves SDT and produces better therapeutic results when treating breast cancer (119).

3.4.4.4 Oxygen Generation and Delivery

Tumor hypoxia is a serious challenge since SDT relies on oxygen to generate ROS. LNPs can be designed to overcome this limitation.

- **Moieties that carry oxygen:** Lipid coatings have the ability to trap perfluorocarbon (PFC) gases, creating nano-emulsions or microbubbles that transport and supply oxygen to the tumor site. Ultrasound can melt phase-shift nano-emulsions in particular to release their oxygen load locally.
- The paper "Alleviating tumor hypoxia with perfluorocarbon-based oxygen carriers" by Krafft et al. (2020) offers a thorough analysis of PFC-based oxygen carriers and how they might be used to improve cancer treatments, such as SDT. This review, the technologies, explores how PFC-based carriers can reduce tumor hypoxia and enhance the effectiveness of SDT and other therapies. The authors list many PFC formulations that can be designed for regulated oxygen delivery in tumor tissues, including nanoemulsions and microbubbles. To improve treatment results, these carriers can be further functionalized with imaging agents, targeted ligands, and stimuli-responsive components. The review highlights how PFC-based oxygen carriers may be able to help cancer treatment overcome the difficulties caused by tumor hypoxia (120).
- **Nanozymes that generate oxygen**: In order to improve SDT, Gong et al. created BSA-CAT-Ir nanoparticles, a nanozyme-based system that combines BSA, catalase (CAT), and iridium (Ir) complexes. As a nanozyme, the catalase component breaks down hydrogen peroxide (H_2O_2) that is common in tumors into oxygen and water, reducing tumor hypoxia, a major barrier to successful SDT. The oxygen produced during ultrasonography increases the generation of reactive oxygen species (ROS), which improves the destruction of tumor cells. This nanozyme-assisted SDT approach showed a considerable reduction of tumor growth in both in vitro and in vivo tests. All things considered, our study shows how catalase-based nanozymes may increase SDT effectiveness in hypoxic tumor microenvironments (121). **Acoustic cavitation enhancement**: Through engineering, LNPs can reduce the cavitation threshold, increase microbubble generation and amplify the SDT impact upon ultrasonic exposure.
- **PFC-loaded nanodroplets:** The use of oxygen-loaded PFC nanodroplets to improve SDT in the brain is examined in the article "Ultrasound-triggered oxygen-loaded nanodroplets enhance and monitor cerebral damage from sonodynamic therapy" by Lea-Banks et al. By injecting these nanodroplets intravenously and then activating them with ultrasound, the researchers showed that they considerably exacerbated the localized tissue damage that the sonosensitizer 5-ALA caused in rats. Because the oxygen in the nanodroplets reduced tumor hypoxia, more ROS were produced during SDT. The study also used acoustic emissions from the nanodroplets' vaporization to track the degree of tissue damage in real time. This strategy not only increased SDT's therapeutic effectiveness but also offered a way to track treatment results without invasive procedures. According to the results, oxygen-loaded PFC nanodroplets may be a viable method for improving and tracking SDT in brain applications (122).
- **Surface modification for enhanced cavitation:** In order to stabilize nanobubbles on their rough, hydrophobic surfaces, Yildirim et al. (2017) created phospholipid-capped, hydrophobically functionalized mesoporous silica nanoparticles. Under high-intensity focused

ultrasound (HIFU), these stabilized nanobubbles serve as inertial cavitation nucleation sites. Without ultrasound, the nanoparticles demonstrated minimal cytotoxicity; but, with ultrasound, cavitation-induced mechanical breakdown caused the nanoparticles to significantly kill cancer cells. Crucially, just a little amount of warmth was seen, indicating that the damage mechanism was mechanical rather than thermal. The phospholipid-coated silica core system illustrates how surface chemistry increases cavitation activity, even though it is not a typical LNP. Despite not using a sonosensitizer, the work offers mechanistic information useful for designing SDT nanocarriers (123).

3.4.4.5 Combination SDT Approaches with LNPs

LNP delivery methods greatly increase the effectiveness of SDT in treating cancer by making it easier to combine SDT with other therapeutic techniques. Synergistic therapeutic effects are possible when multiple medicines are co-encapsulated within a single LNP, which is not possible with single-agent therapy.

- **Chemo-SDT:** LNP-mediated co-administration of chemotherapeutic medications and sonosensitizers enables a synergistic strategy that capitalizes on the mechanisms of both therapies. 5-ALA, a precursor to the sonosensitizer PpIX, and cationic liposomal hydroxycamptothecin (CLH) were used in study by Xiao et al. The formulation, characterization, and in vitro and in vivo assessment of this combination medication are all examined in this study. According to the findings, the cationic liposomal formulation improves the stability and bioavailability of 5-ALA and HCPT, which leads in increased therapeutic efficacy. With 5-ALA boosting sonodynamic therapy by producing reactive oxygen species during sonication and HCPT offering chemotherapeutic action, the combined therapy exhibits synergistic results. By more precisely targeting tumor cells, this method presents a viable treatment option for metastatic lung cancer that may enhance patient outcomes (124).
- **Immuno-SDT:** TAAs are released and an anti-tumor immune response is activated when SDT triggers ICD. A novel nanomedicine approach to cancer treatment is presented in the research "Albumin-based co-loaded sonosensitizer and STING agonist nanodelivery system for enhanced sonodynamic and immune combination antitumor therapy" FA-ICG&MnOx@HSA is an albumin-based nanodelivery system that co-loads the STING agonist manganese oxide (MnOx) and the sonosensitizer ICG. By concurrently triggering the STING pathway to activate the immune system and producing reactive oxygen species during ultrasound activation, this approach seeks to improve SDT. Immune modulation and SDT together provide a synergistic approach to increase antitumor activity. The study demonstrates the potential of this nanodelivery system in overcoming tumor hypoxia and enhancing the therapeutic response through both direct tumor cell killing and immune activation (125).
- **SDT theranostics:** A "see-and-treat" strategy is made possible by LNPs, which combine imaging agents and sonosensitizers to allow for real-time surveillance of SDT efficacy.

3.4.4.6 Imaging-Guided Liposomal Nanobubbles

Using nanobubbles that experience a phase transition when exposed to ultrasound, the study "Ultrasound-Augmented Phase Transition Nanobubbles for Targeted Cancer Therapy" offers a novel method of treating cancer. When activated by ultrasound, these nanobubbles are designed to precisely release therapeutic chemicals from their encapsulation at tumor locations. The phase shift improves the payload's stability and controlled release, increasing therapy effectiveness while reducing adverse effects on healthy tissues. This method uses ultrasound and the special qualities of nanobubbles to provide effective and targeted cancer treatment. The study shows how this technology can be used to improve the accuracy and efficacy of cancer therapies.

3.4.4.7 Lipid Nanoparticle-Based Sonodynamic Therapy: Obstacles and Opportunities

Although LNP-based sonodynamic therapy (LNP-SDT) has several benefits as a minimally invasive treatment for resistant, deep-seated malignancies, a number of issues need to be resolved before it can be widely used in clinical settings. The goal of ongoing research is to overcome these challenges by improving medicinal approaches and nanoparticle design. **Tumor hypoxia:** Since hypoxia reduces the generation of deadly ROS, it is a major obstacle to efficient SDT. Hypoxia is a state of low oxygen that is frequently present in solid tumors. To increase the effectiveness of SDT, advanced LNPs are being designed to carry oxygen-generating devices, which will reoxygenate the tumor microenvironment. Sonosensitizers, which need enough oxygen to produce cell-damaging ROS when activated by ultrasound, are less effective in hypoxic environments. **Penetration depth and tumor heterogeneity:** SDT has trouble treating bigger, more varied tumors. The distribution and efficacy of LNPs can be impacted by the diverse microenvironment within a single tumor, and ultrasonic penetration can vary depending on the kind of tissue. **Acoustic cavitation control:** The effectiveness and security of SDT are associated with the management of acoustic cavitation, which is the ultrasound-induced process of microbubble creation and collapse. For targeted LNP payload release, it is essential to maximize the energy released by this action while reducing the possibility of high-energy inertial cavitation side effects.

- **Clinical translation hurdles—Safety and toxicity:** Although LNPs have shown promise in other fields (such as mRNA vaccines), bringing LNP-SDT to the clinic has special safety and efficacy challenges. Concerns include inflammatory reactions, possible systemic toxicity from LNP components such as ionizable lipids, and uneven efficacy in humans in contrast to preclinical models. Reducing possible toxicities from the SDT procedure, as well as the LNP components, is necessary to guarantee the safety of LNP-SDT. For instance, high ROS production and unchecked cavitation can damage healthy tissues, whereas some LNP lipids might cause an inflammatory immunological response.
- **Overcoming tumor hypoxia:** Oxygen-generating LNPs are being used in advanced ways to overcome tumor hypoxia and improve the effectiveness of SDT. Among these are LNPs that have been modified to contain catalase, a naturally occurring enzyme that raises intratumoral oxygen levels by converting the hydrogen peroxide that is common in tumors into oxygen and water. FePt nanozyme systems are another strategy that significantly reduces hypoxia-induced resistance to SDT by catalyzing the generation of oxygen in the tumor microenvironment.
- **Enhancing treatment precision and control:** In order to combine SDT with cutting-edge imaging techniques like Positron Emission Tomography (PET), Computed Tomography (c), and Magnetic Resonance Imaging (MRI), theranostic LNPs are being developed. This will allow for precise treatment planning, real-time tumor visualization, and therapeutic response monitoring. Simultaneously, LNP engineering and ultrasonic parameter optimization are being used to control nanobubble stability, guarantee regulated payload release at the tumor location, and minimize off-target effects in order to improve control over sonic cavitation. Some nanoplatforms have been developed to combine SDT with cuproptosis or starvation therapy, which depletes intracellular glutathione and glucose to further promote cancer cell death. Combination therapies, which pair LNP-SDT with treatments like chemotherapy or immunotherapy, are also being investigated to achieve synergistic effects.

3.4.4.8 Improving Clinical Translation and Safety

LNPs' composition and formulation are being improved to increase biocompatibility and decrease immunogenicity. This includes the use of new, less toxic lipid components and improved targeting techniques. The goal is to increase the safety and clinical translation of LNPs. With the use of ligands that selectively bind tumor cells, targeted LNPs can enhance drug accumulation at the site of disease, increasing therapeutic efficacy while reducing exposure and harm to healthy tissues. Furthermore, the deliberate development and assessment of LNPs seeks to regulate immune responses, striking a balance between preventing detrimental inflammation and the immunological activation required for therapeutic benefit.

Although there are still issues with tumor heterogeneity, hypoxia, cavitation control, and LNP safety in clinical translation, these issues should be resolved with continued advancements in targeted delivery and nanoparticle engineering. By fusing therapeutic adaptability with mechanistic sophistication, LNP-SDT is a versatile, next-generation nanomedicine technology that has the potential to improve cancer treatment.

3.4.5 Immunotherapeutics

LNPs are very adaptable carriers for a variety of immunomodulatory payloads, successfully addressing the primary problem of immunotherapy, evoking robust antigen-specific T-cell activation while reducing systemic damage. They are especially well-suited for immunological regulation because of their biocompatibility, potential for regulated intracellular distribution, and ability to shield labile nucleic acids from destruction. LNPs' modular construction is a crucial component that enables the co-delivery of several payloads, including adjuvants and antigens, inside a single particle, fostering synergistic immune activation.

Overcoming the drawbacks of traditional methods, such as the immunogenicity of viral vectors and the instability of naked nucleic acids, is essential to the success of LNP-based immunotherapy. Although viral vectors are good at spreading genetic material, they can also cause unintended immune reactions and pose safety risks. Conversely, naked nucleic acids have trouble passing through cell membranes and are quickly broken down by nucleases. By protecting the cargo, promoting cellular absorption, and mediating endosomal egress, LNPs get beyond these barriers. Because of its modular design, the LNP's components may be precisely controlled.

Ionizable lipids are essential for the development and operation of LNPs. They are neutral at physiological pH to lessen toxicity, but positively charged at acidic pH to facilitate effective encapsulation of negatively charged nucleic acids. By encouraging membrane fusion in the acidic endosome, this pH-dependent charge also makes endosomal escape easier (126)

Helper lipids are phospholipids such as DOPE and DSPC (1,2-distearoyl-sn-glycero-3-phosphocholine), which impact membrane fluidity and stiffness, affect endosomal escape characteristics and LNP stability. Cholesterol, this element improves the compactness of the LNP core and modifies membrane fluidity to increase particle stability. Lipids conjugated to PEG, are PEGylated lipids, have a hydrophilic surface coat that decreases non-specific protein binding, delays circulation, and stops LNP aggregation. PEG chain length and concentration selection are essential for striking a balance between delivery effectiveness and stability. LNPs can be tailored for certain uses by adjusting the makeup of these constituents, allowing for more precise, safe, and efficient immunotherapy techniques.

3.4.5.1 Rational Design of Functionalized LNPs

The goal of active targeting of functionalized LNPs in immunotherapy is to precisely distribute therapeutic payloads by using certain ligands to decorate the LNP surface. By optimizing the payload concentration at the targeted location and reducing systemic exposure and off-target effects, this approach raises the therapeutic index.

3.4.5.2 Active Targeting Strategies for Immune Cells and Tumors

Active targeting strategies have emerged as an effective approach to enhance the specificity and therapeutic efficacy of functionalized lipid nanoparticles in cancer treatment. By incorporating ligands that recognize overexpressed receptors on tumor cells or specific immune cell populations, these nanocarriers can achieve selective accumulation at the target site, improve cellular uptake, and minimize off-target effects. Such strategies have shown considerable promise in both direct tumor targeting and the modulation of antitumor immune responses.

3.4.5.2.1 Targeting Immune Cells

Effective regulation of particular immune cell subsets is necessary for immunotherapy. By delivering cargo straight to these cells, functionalized LNPs can expedite the therapeutic process and boost the immune response.

- **Targeting DCs:** DCs are essential for triggering T-cell responses.
- **Mannosylated LNPs:** These APCs enhance antigen presentation and T-cell priming by increasing LNP uptake by ligands such as mannose, which are recognized by mannose receptors on DCs (127).
- **LNPs modified with sialic acid (SA):** Tang et al. created an mRNA vaccine that was altered with SA, which caused DCs to absorb LNPs twice as much. This led to improved mRNA transfection efficiency in DCs and more effective endosomal escape (128).
- **Targeting lymph nodes:** LNPs can be administered locally, such as by subcutaneous injection, to lymph nodes, which are abundant in immune cells. In a melanoma model, Chen et al. 2022's lymph-node-targeting mRNA vaccination produced a strong CD8+ T-cell response. LNPs coated with anti-CD4 antibodies were used to target human T-cells. They found that the binding affinity and reporter gene expression of CD4+ T-cells were higher than those of non-targeted LNPs. Off-the-shelf CAR-T cell therapies may be possible because of the utilization of LNPs functionalized with anti-CD3 antibodies to transfer CAR-encoding mRNA to T-cells in vivo.

3.4.5.2.2 Targeting Tumor-Associated Macrophages (TAMs)

One intriguing tactic is to rewire immunosuppressive TAMs to exhibit pro-inflammatory traits. Immunomodulators such as siRNA can be delivered using LNPs functionalized with mannose to alter the TME.

3.4.5.2.3 Targeting Tumors

Active targeting can also be used to deliver immunomodulatory payloads directly to tumor cells.

- **Antibody-drug conjugates:** LNPs can be surface-modified with antibodies against tumor-specific antigens, like HER2, to direct therapeutic cargo to cancer cells. Rybakova et al. showed that LNPs encoding trastuzumab (anti-HER2 antibody) led to sustained antibody production and significant tumor suppression in HER2-positive breast cancer models (130).
- **Peptides:** RGD and other peptides can be joined to LNPs to target integrin receptors, which are overexpressed on some cancer cells and tumor vasculature. At the tumor location, this encourages the buildup of LNP. Certain tumor xenografts have been demonstrated to accumulate more when functionalized with cRGD peptide.
- **Single-stranded DNA or RNA**: Molecules known as aptamers can be modified to attach to particular cancer cell receptors. The delivery of tumor suppressor mRNA to prostate cancer cells via aptamer-conjugated LNPs has been demonstrated to improve treatment efficacy.
- **Tiny molecules:** Targeting ligands can be demonstrated by some small compounds. Folate is a popular small-molecule ligand that targets folate receptors that are overexpressed in many cancer cells. LNPs conjugated with folic acid have shown improved drug delivery to cancer cells that express the folate receptor.

3.4.5.2.4 Stimuli-Responsive and Surface Modulation Strategies

- **pH-responsive LNPs:** To accomplish targeted and regulated payload release, pH-responsive LNPs take advantage of the acidic conditions of endosomes and the TME. The mechanisms are explained in further detail in this section, along with particular instances drawn from current research.

- **Enhanced endosomal escape via ionizable lipids:** The most popular pH-responsive ingredient in LNPs, ionizable lipids, are designed to have a pKa that falls between the bloodstream's neutral pH (pH ~7.4) and endosomes' acidic pH (pH ~5.0–6) (132).
- **Mechanism:** The tertiary amines in an LNP containing ionizable lipids become protonated upon endocytosis due to the endosome's dropping pH. The lipid's positive charge is increased by this protonation, which facilitates its contact with the negatively charged endosomal membrane. Before being broken down by lysosomal enzymes, the encapsulated cargo (such as RNA/DNA) can escape into the cytoplasm thanks to the electrostatic contact that promotes membrane fusion and disintegration. A common term for this phenomenon is the "proton sponge effect".
- **Significance:** A rate-limiting step in the transport of mRNA is effective endosomal escape. Researchers can balance stability in the bloodstream with effective release within the target cell by adjusting the ionizable lipid's pKa.
- **TME-specific payload release:** In addition to endosomal escape, LNPs can be engineered to react to the extracellular TME's somewhat acidic pH, allowing for localized drug release before cellular absorption.
- **Mechanism:** This tactic frequently entails adding components or linkers to the LNP structure that are sensitive to pH. Lipids having pH-sensitive cleavage sites, for example, can destabilize the LNP structure at the TME pH, which results in the extracellular release of the payload. This is especially helpful for administering antigens or small-molecule medications that must be given to adjacent immune cells.
- **Significance:** TME-specific release reduces off-target toxicity by minimizing systemic exposure. Additionally, by concentrating the therapeutic payload where it is most required, it may be able to overcome LNPs' low penetration into dense tumor tissues.

3.4.5.3 Dual-Responsive LNPs

Advanced delivery systems called dual-responsive LNPs are made to get beyond biological obstacles in targeted therapy, especially for diseases with distinct microenvironments like cancers. Dual-responsive systems have a complex, sequential activation process, in contrast to conventional LNPs, which could have a low endosomal escape efficiency. This procedure reacts to the low pH of the TME initially, then goes through a secondary change inside the cell's endosomes to release the cargo, ensuring accurate intracellular delivery of therapeutic payloads such as nucleic acids. By reducing off-target effects and preventing payload degradation before it reaches its targeted location within the cell, this process increases the therapeutic efficacy. **Mechanism:** Upon cellular absorption, these LNPs frequently feature a surface coating or a component that cleaves at the TME pH, revealing a second component (such as an ionizable lipid) that facilitates endosomal escape. This method guarantees that the LNP delivers its payload inside the cell after being "activated" by the TME. **Significance:** Dual-responsive LNPs offer a potent platform for the delivery of immune-therapeutics with high specificity and potency by combining the advantages of TME targeting with effective intracellular transport.

3.4.5.4 Enzyme-Responsive LNPs

The zinc-dependent endopeptidases known as MMPs are often overexpressed in the TME and play a role in tumor invasion, extracellular matrix remodeling, and metastasis. LNPs can be made to react to these enzymatic cues by integrating particular peptide sequences that are selectively cleaved by MMPs. This allows for the regulated and targeted release of payloads at the tumor location. This approach provides a very selective trigger for therapeutic activation, reduces systemic exposure, and improves medication accumulation within the tumor. **Targeting Matrix Metalloproteinases (MMPs):** MMP-sensitive peptide sequences are incorporated into the structure of MMP-responsive LNPs to create them. Until they are broken down by overexpressed MMPs in the TME, these peptide substrates serve as molecular switches that keep the LNP in a steady, inactive state. The cleavage can trigger several processes for payload release. **Removal of surface shielding:** An

MMP-cleavable peptide connects the protective layer, which is frequently PEG, to the LNP surface. The PEG shield prolongs circulation time by reducing non-specific absorption and offering stealth qualities while in circulation. When MMPs get to the TME, they cleave the peptide linker, releasing the PEG shield and allowing cells to absorb the LNP. **Structural destabilization:** Peptides that are cleavable by MMP can cross-link the LNP. The encapsulated payload is released when the LNP disintegrates as a result of MMPs cleaving these peptides. **Masked targeting ligand activation:** It is possible to construct an LNP with a masked targeting ligand. It is possible to position the MMP-cleavable peptide linker between the LNP surface and the targeted ligand. The targeting ligand is revealed by the peptide's cleavage by MMPs in the TME, which enables the LNP to bind and be internalized by cancer cells.

One notable example involves the development of MMP-9-activatable lipid nanoparticles (LNPs) for targeted delivery in pancreatic cancer. **MMP-9 activatable nanocarriers for pancreatic cancer:** Studies have shown that MMP-9 activatable LNPs may be delivered to pancreatic tumors with precision. A PEG shield is attached to these nanocarriers by an MMP-9-cleavable peptide linker. The peptide is broken in the TME of pancreatic cancer, which frequently overexpresses MMP-9. This unshields the nanocarrier and encourages its uptake into cancer cells. This improves the delivery of drugs to the tumor location selectively.

- **Advantages and challenges:** Because MMPs are overexpressed in the TME, MMP-responsive LNPs have a high specificity for tumors while causing the least amount of harm to healthy tissues. **Tunable release:** By creating peptides with varying cleavage sensitivities to particular MMPs, the rate of drug release can be adjusted. **Synergistic therapy:** MMP-responsive LNPs can have more potent therapeutic effects when combined with other treatments like immunotherapy or pH-sensitive release. **Variability in MMP expression:** The expression of particular MMPs might differ between patients, as well as based on the kind and stage of cancer. This necessitates thorough patient categorization and may affect the effectiveness of MMP-responsive LNPs. **Non-specific cleavage:** Despite MMPs' great specificity, the peptide linker may occasionally cleave off-target in other tissues, which could cause an early drug release. **Clinical translation:** To guarantee the security, stability, and effectiveness of MMP-responsive LNPs in people, further investigation is required.

3.4.5.5 Surface Optimization: Enhancing LNP Performance for Immunotherapy

- **Reduced PEGylation and alternatives:** A key tactic for getting beyond biological barriers and raising LNPs' therapeutic index in immunotherapy is to optimize their surface characteristics. Researchers can regulate interactions with the immune system, affect biodistribution, and accomplish targeted delivery to particular cell types by altering the LNP surface. PEG has long been employed as a "stealth" coating to prolong the duration that LNP circulates by blocking the RES opsonization and clearance. High PEGylation, on the other hand, can prevent cellular absorption and, more importantly, during repeated administration, result in the ABC effect. The succeeding LNP doses are cleared quickly as a result of this process, which is mediated by anti-PEG antibodies. There are new functionalization strategies being explored to overcome these restrictions. **Polysarcosine (pSar):** A biocompatible and non-immunogenic polymer that has demonstrated potential in prolonging the circulation period of nanoparticles, pSar is an alternative to PEG. LNPs modified with pSar are appropriate for repeat-dose immunotherapy regimens because they have stealth characteristics comparable to PEGylated LNPs without inducing the ABC effect (134). **Including "self" indicators:** Using peptides that resemble "self" signals, like the CD47 peptide, can tell phagocytic cells, including macrophages, not to take up the LNP. This tactic prolongs the life of the LNP in circulation by utilizing the CD47-SIRPα signaling pathway, which red blood cells naturally exploit to evade macrophage clearance. **Cleavable PEG:** Cleavable PEG linkers can be employed to overcome the trade-off between prolonged circulation and effective cellular absorption. The PEG coating is lost, and effective cellular uptake is made possible by these linkers' ability to be broken at the target spot by particular triggers (such as pH or enzymes). This tactic combines the high absorption efficiency of non-PEGylated LNPs with the covert qualities of PEG. **Surface charge reversal:** The stability, circulation time, and cellular interactions of LNPs are all significantly influenced by their surface charge. To improve tumor accumulation and retention, charge-reversible LNPs are made to alter their surface charge in response to the acidic TME.

- **Mechanism**: To minimize non-specific interactions and extend circulation, charge-reversible LNPs are usually constructed with pH-sensitive components that are negatively or neutrally charged at physiological pH (pH ~7.4). These components experience a conformational shift or protonation in the acidic TME (pH < 7.0), which reverses the surface charge to positive. The resultant positive charge promotes uptake and local retention by strengthening electrostatic interactions with the negatively charged surface of cancer cells. **Benefits**: By encouraging targeted accumulation at the tumor site, this approach reduces off-target interactions in the bloodstream. The delivery of therapeutic payloads, like mRNA or small-molecule medications, can be improved by the increased cellular absorption at the target site.

Surface-optimized lipid nanoparticles (LNPs) have been engineered to improve immunotherapy by enhancing immune cell targeting, enabling repeated dosing, and increasing tumor uptake. **CD47 peptide-conjugated Polysarcosine-modified LNPs:** Studies demonstrated that pSar-modified LNPs could be used for repeated delivery of siRNA, showing no evidence of the (accelerated blood clearance) ABC effect. This highlights the potential of pSar as a superior alternative to PEG for repeated-dose immunotherapy (134).

3.4.5.6 Combination Therapies Enabled by Functionalized LNPs

To provide synergistic effects, functionalized LNPs are being used more and more in multimodal therapy to co-deliver various therapeutic drugs. By focusing on several pathways at once, including immune system regulation and tumor cell death, this strategy tackles the complex character of cancer.

- **Immunochemotherapy**: The drawbacks of single-agent treatment can be addressed by combining immunotherapy and chemotherapy. ICD brought on by chemotherapy releases DAMPs and TAAs, which APCs can absorb. By administering chemotherapy and an immunomodulator simultaneously, LNP-based chemo-immunotherapy takes advantage of this effect. **Mechanism:** Dual-responsive LNPs are used in cancer treatment to co-deliver immunomodulators like mRNA or siRNA with chemotherapeutic medications like doxorubicin, which releases tumor antigens to cause ICD. By reprogramming the local immune environment, possibly by delivering immunostimulatory cytokine mRNA or silencing immune checkpoint genes (like PD-L1), the immunomodulator improves the anti-tumor immune response while chemotherapy lowers the tumor burden.
- **For instance, chemotherapy with photodynamic treatment (PDT):** Chemotherapy combined with photodynamic therapy (PDT) has been demonstrated using nanoscale coordination polymer lipid nanoparticles that incorporate a chemotherapeutic agent in the core and a photosensitizer in the lipid shell. This dual-modality system induces immunogenic cell death (ICD), leading to the release of tumor-associated antigens (TAAs) and the creation of a pro-inflammatory tumor microenvironment. As a result, such formulations are capable of driving local tumor regression and, when paired with immunomodulatory strategies, can also promote a systemic anti-tumor immune response capable of targeting distant malignancies.

Similarly, other nanoparticle-based strategies have explored the co-delivery of chemotherapy together with immunological adjuvants such as CpG oligodeoxynucleotides or STING agonists. This approach aims to enhance tumor cell death, amplify ICD-mediated antigen release, and simultaneously activate antigen-presenting cells. By promoting dendritic cell maturation and efficient cross-priming, these systems help generate a strong cytotoxic T-cell response against the liberated TAAs, ultimately improving systemic anti-tumor immunity.

- **Blockade of immune checkpoints (ICB):** Cancer treatment has been transformed by ICB, which targets immunological checkpoint proteins like CTLA-4 and PD-1. ICB monotherapy does have several drawbacks, though, including immune-related side effects and a lack of response in many individuals. These difficulties can be solved by combining ICB with treatments delivered by LNP. **Mechanism:** ICB increases the activity of these T-cells by removing the "brakes" on the immune system, while LNPs can deliver mRNA vaccines that produce T-cells that target certain tumor antigens. One benefit of functionalized LNPs is that they enable controlled and localized distribution, which may lessen the systemic toxicity linked to monoclonal antibodies. **Personalized mRNA vaccine and pembrolizumab, for instance**: In high-risk melanoma patients, the KEYNOTE-942 trial showed that an LNP-based tailored mRNA vaccine (mRNA-4157/V940) in conjunction with pembrolizumab significantly decreased the risk of mortality or disease recurrence when compared to pembrolizumab alone. The trial validated the safety and synergistic impact of ICB in combination with a customized mRNA neoantigen vaccination (135).
- **Toxicological and off-target impact:** There are still a number of obstacles to overcome before functionalized LNPs may be turned into immunotherapies that are clinically successful, despite the encouraging developments. In order to prevent toxicity and unintended immunological reactions, great specificity must be attained. Side effects could result from targeted LNPs building up in off-target organs, such as the liver and spleen. In the future, sophisticated functionalization techniques, such as multi-responsive systems and sophisticated targeting ligands, will be used to increase selectivity and reduce off-target accumulation.
- **Overcoming the immunosuppressive TME Obstacle:** It can be challenging for functionalized LNPs to produce successful therapy since the TME is a complex environment that can dampen immune responses. Research aims to create LNPs that can efficiently enter and circumvent the TME's immunosuppressive properties, for example, by delivering substances that rewire immunosuppressive cells such as myeloid-derived suppressor cells (MDSCs) or regulatory T cells (Tregs). **Manufacturing complexity and cost:** Personalized treatments, especially vaccinations based on neoantigens, require intricate production procedures that can be expensive and time-consuming. Personalized LNP-based immunotherapies may become more affordable and accessible with the use of computational design in conjunction with developments in microfluidic mixing and other scalable production processes.
- **High-throughput screening and computational design:** Designing and optimizing functionalized LNPs will be accelerated by combining high-throughput screening with computational techniques. While high-throughput screening can experimentally test these designs, computational modeling can forecast the behavior of LNP components, assisting in the identification of appropriate formulations for particular applications.
- **Clinical translation challenge:** Safety and regulatory barriers make it difficult to translate sophisticated functionalized LNP platforms into clinical practice, even with encouraging preclinical and early clinical outcomes. Building on the KEYNOTE-942 study's success, ongoing and upcoming clinical trials will confirm the safety and effectiveness of functionalized LNPs and open the door for their wider clinical use (Weber et al., 2024b).

The creation of functionalized lipid nanoparticles marks a revolutionary advancement in immunotherapy, enabling active therapeutic payload direction with previously unheard-of precision, surpassing passive delivery. Researchers can get around some of the main biological obstacles and restrictions of traditional immunotherapy by logically constructing LNPs to include targeted ligands, stimuli-responsive components, and tailored surface features. Because of these platforms' modularity, numerous agents can be delivered simultaneously, opening the door to the possibility of synergistic multi-modal therapies that might effectively address the intricate and multidimensional character of cancer.

A potent strategy for enhancing vaccination efficacy and simplifying the immune response is the neoantigen vaccines. These responses, when paired with immune checkpoint inhibition, result in better clinical outcomes for patients with high-risk melanoma. Additionally, a viable method of avoiding the difficult and expensive ex vivo manufacturing process is the development of in vivo CAR-T production utilizing targeted LNPs, which could democratize access to this ground-breaking treatment.

Therapeutic precision is further improved by techniques to modify the LNP surface and add reactivity to microenvironmental stimuli. For instance, pH-responsive LNPs maximize intracellular delivery efficiency and minimize systemic toxicity by utilizing the acidic TME and endosomes to accomplish regulated, localized payload release (138). In a similar vein, enzyme-responsive LNPs provide a highly selective trigger for therapeutic activation at the tumor site by reacting to over-expressed MMPs in the TME. To ensure that the LNP reaches its target, innovations in surface optimization—such as substitutes for PEGylation and the addition of "self" identifiers like CD47—are essential for prolonging circulation duration and avoiding immune clearance.

There are still difficulties despite these noteworthy developments. Future research must focus on overcoming the immunosuppressive TME, achieving universally high specificity, and tackling the expense and complexity of manufacturing customized medicines. The next generation of functionalized LNPs will be much more sophisticated, providing specialized and multifunctional platforms for precisely manipulating the immune system, as researchers increasingly use high-throughput screening and powerful computational techniques. The ultimate objective is to get past proof-of-concept and fully utilize these cutting-edge nanomedicines, opening the door to cancer immunotherapies that are safer, more efficient, and really customized.

3.5 PRECLINICAL AND CLINICAL APPLICATIONS

Lipid nanoparticles, or LNPs, are acknowledged as a flexible and physiologically applicable delivery system for small-molecule medicines and nucleic acids. An ionizable or cationic lipid for complexation with nucleic acids, helper lipids for structural stability, cholesterol for membrane rigidity, and PEG-lipids for "stealth" qualities that extend circulation are all common components of their modular architecture. The capacity to precisely adjust particle size, surface charge, and stability to suit a variety of therapeutic needs is made possible by this compositional flexibility. LNPs are very useful for gene editing, gene silencing, and vaccination applications because of their capacity to encapsulate and shield delicate nucleic acids like siRNA, mRNA, and microRNA from nuclease-mediated destruction. By means of the EPR effect, LNPs provide the benefit of passive accumulation in tumors in oncology. Additionally, their surface can be functionalized with ligands to allow active targeting of receptors specific to tumors, offering a two-pronged strategy for treating cancer. Beyond modularity, another feature that has accelerated the clinical translation of is their tunable pharmacokinetics and biodistribution. Adjusting the ratio of ionizable lipids to PEG-lipids can significantly alter the circulation half-life, immune recognition, and organ selectivity of the particles. For instance, modifying the chemical structure of lipids has been shown in preclinical studies to redirect LNP accumulation away from the liver toward other tissues, including tumors, expanding their therapeutic potential beyond hepatic diseases. Furthermore, incorporating biodegradable lipids, which are rapidly metabolized and cleared, helps mitigate long-term toxicity, addressing a key safety concern associated with earlier-generation, non-degradable cationic lipid carriers.

LNPs are now generally regarded as a clinically verified delivery technology from a translational perspective. The effectiveness of LNP-formulated siRNA (patisiran for ATTR amyloidosis) (139) and mRNA vaccines against COVID-19 (140) has shown their acceptable safety profile in both human subjects and animal models. These medicines' regulatory approvals have demonstrated their large-scale manufacturing feasibility, repeatability, and regulatory acceptability, laying a strong basis for cancer applications. Furthermore, the capacity to scale up LNP synthesis through the use of microfluidic mixing and other high-throughput techniques guarantees that laboratory achievements may be effectively and consistently transferred to the clinic.

In the context of cancer, LNPs possess several distinct advantages. First, they enable the efficient delivery of highly negatively charged nucleic acids, which are poorly transported by conventional drug formulations. Second, LNPs facilitate combination strategies, including the co-delivery of siRNA with chemotherapeutic drugs or immune adjuvants. This approach helps overcome tumor heterogeneity and drug resistance mechanisms by simultaneously targeting multiple pathways. Finally, functionalization strategies are being actively investigated to enhance tumor-specific accumulation and minimize systemic side effects. By decorating the LNP surface with ligands such as antibodies, aptamers, or peptides, researchers can promote active targeting of tumor-specific receptors.

All of these traits put LNPs in a position to revolutionize contemporary oncology as a next-generation treatment platform. As a result, this chapter will concentrate on three important areas: (i) preclinical studies that show proof-of-concept efficacy, (ii) clinical trials using functionalized LNPs for cancer therapy, and (iii) approved LNP-based therapeutics that, although not specifically targeting cancer, offer important evidence for their potential future integration into oncology treatment paradigms.

3.5.1 Highlights from Preclinical Studies

LNP preclinical studies have shown that they are adaptable as delivery vehicles for a variety of cancer treatments, going much beyond their original application for nucleic acids. LNPs have been designed to transport agents for cutting-edge modalities like photodynamic and photothermal therapy, proteins, gene-editing systems, and small compounds. All of these investigations point to LNPs as a versatile platform that can overcome significant obstacles in the delivery of cancer treatments, including off-target effects, systemic clearance, low solubility of hydrophobic medications, and nucleic acid instability.

Early advances in LNP research centered on nucleic acids, including siRNA and mRNA delivery. Once inside cells, LNPs facilitate endosomal escape by encasing and shielding siRNA and mRNA from enzymatic destruction by the incorporation of ionizable or cationic lipids. Oncogenes such as vascular endothelial growth factor (VEGF) and KRAS were effectively suppressed by siRNA-LNPs in murine tumor models, which resulted in decreased angiogenesis and notable tumor regression (141).

- **Targeted formulations:** Preclinical research has demonstrated that functionalizing LNPs with ligands such as transferrin, folate, peptides, or antibodies greatly increases tumor selectivity on top of passive tumor accumulation through the EPR effect. Such ligand-directed formulations demonstrate the versatility of LNPs for precision oncology by increasing tumor absorption while reducing systemic dispersion. Studies have demonstrated, for instance, that EGFR-targeted LNPs enhanced delivery and effectiveness in models of glioblastoma.
- Small-molecule chemotherapeutics: Docetaxel, paclitaxel, and doxorubicin are examples of conventional anticancer medications that have been effectively encapsulated in LNPs to enhance their pharmacological characteristics. Doxorubicin-induced cardiotoxicity is one of the dose-limiting toxicities that are decreased by encapsulation, which also increases solubility and prolongs systemic circulation. Compared to free-drug administration, LNP-based formulations have sustained greater drug concentrations within tumors in rodent tumor models, resulting in stronger tumor suppression and fewer systemic side effects.

- **Combination therapy**: Co-encapsulation techniques have taken advantage of LNPs' modularity to administer several medicines at once. One example is the combination of siRNA and chemotherapy, in which the siRNA inhibits genes that are resistant to drugs while the chemotherapy exerts cytotoxic pressure. These dual-action strategies have postponed the establishment of resistant cancer cell populations and produced synergistic tumor shrinkage.

Delivery of proteins, peptides, and gene editing: LNPs have also been employed to stabilize and transport therapeutically promising proteins and peptides. Notably, in xenograft models, it has been demonstrated that encapsulating p53 protein fragments restores tumor-suppressor function. LNPs have more recently been modified for genome editing, delivering CRISPR–Cas9 systems as ribonucleoprotein complexes or Cas9 mRNA with guide RNAs. These systems have effectively disrupted oncogenes like as MYC and KRAS in preclinical animals, demonstrating the potential of LNPs for next-generation precision oncology (Bender, Fahrioglu Yamaci, and Taneri 2021).

Applications in immunotherapy: mRNA-LNPs that encode tumor-associated antigens or neoantigens unique to a patient have been studied as potential cancer vaccines. These vaccinations produced robust $CD8^+$ T-cell responses, inhibited tumor growth, and occasionally resulted in total remission in animal experiments. In addition, LNPs have been employed to deliver immune adjuvants such as TLR agonists or STING agonists, amplifying dendritic cell activation and boosting anti-tumor immunity.

In addition to molecular medications, LNPs have been developed for energy-based treatments such as PDT and PTT. Photosensitizers, like indocyanine green or chlorin e6, can be encapsulated to increase their solubility, stability, and tumor localization. PDT produces reactive oxygen species when light is activated, which kills tumor cells. In the same manner, LNPs functionalized with photothermal agents enable specific tumor ablation in PTT by converting NIR light into localized heat. By upsetting tumor cells and promoting intracellular drug release, phototherapies in combination with chemotherapy or siRNA delivery have improved therapeutic efficacy in both situations.

Drug synergistic treatment (DST) and platforms that use many modalities: Expanding upon these approaches, scientists have created "theranostic" LNPs that combine medication administration, imaging, and multimodal therapies. For instance, formulations that combine PDT or PTT with chemotherapy have been shown to achieve higher tumor suppression than those that use either technique alone. These systems demonstrate how LNPs can be used as platforms for integrated cancer therapy in addition to acting as drug carriers.

When combined, these preclinical investigations unequivocally demonstrate that LNPs are more than RNA carriers. Most other nanocarriers cannot match their unique breadth in delivering nucleic acids, proteins, small chemicals, gene-editing tools, immunomodulators, and phototherapeutic agents. This adaptability offers a solid basis for their subsequent development into clinical trials and their eventual function as a key component of contemporary cancer treatment.

3.5.2 Functionalized LNPs in Clinical Trials

LNPs are being developed into clinical oncology by utilizing sophisticated functionalization techniques that increase stability, specificity, and therapeutic efficacy, building on their preclinical promise. Key methods and illustrative trial examples that show how these nano-formulations are developing through human investigations are provided below:

- **Stealth PEGylated LNPs:** Through the creation of a hydrophilic barrier that lowers immune clearance and enhances biocompatibility, the addition of PEG extends systemic circulation. PEGylation may cause anti-PEG antibody reactions after repeated doses, despite being commonly utilized to improve pharmacokinetics. To combat this, researchers are looking into methods such as employing cleavable PEG lipids.

- **Ligand-Targeted LNPs:** Clinical prospects investigating receptor-mediated targeting in addition to passive accumulation through the EPR effect include: LNPs adorned with transferrin. These are being studied to improve the uptake of particular tumor cells in malignancies such as hepatocellular carcinoma, which overexpress transferrin receptors. Folate-modified LNPs: These improve delivery and reduce off-target exposure by targeting the folate receptor, which is frequently overexpressed in ovarian and other malignancies.
- **mRNA-LNP Vaccines for Cancer:** Numerous trials are being conducted to assess customized mRNA-LNP vaccines. These vaccines produce a strong anti-tumor immune response by encoding tumor-specific neoantigens. Combining pembrolizumab with mRNA-4157 (V940) (KEYNOTE-942), this customized vaccine decreased the chance of mortality or recurrence in patients with high-risk melanoma. There are ongoing phase III trials (137). After surgery, patients with pancreatic cancer can get another customized mRNA vaccination called Autogene cevumeran (BioNTech/Genentech). According to phase I data, it produced strong, enduring immune responses against neoantigens and was safe and well-tolerated. Phase II studies are being recruited internationally.
- **RNA-LP for glioblastoma (GBM):** Researchers evaluated the safety and immunological response of a neoantigen-targeting RNA-LP vaccine in patients with newly diagnosed GBM in a Phase I trial (NCT04573140). There is also a recurrent GBM trial (NCT06389591) in progress.
- **Additional mRNA immunomodulatory experiments:** Phase I/II trials (e.g., NCT03323398 and NCT03739931) have assessed the intratumoral delivery of mRNAs encoding immune activators such as OX40L, IL-23, and IL-36γ for solid tumors and lymphomas. The goal of these experiments is to directly stimulate the immune system in the tumor microenvironment.
- **Programmable mRNA therapy (Strand Therapeutics):** This method encodes interleukin-12 (IL-12) using mRNA and incorporates safety features. By limiting systemic toxicity, these systems guarantee that the powerful cytokine is only expressed within the tumor. Promising effects have been observed in early human trials.

3.5.2.1 siRNA-LNPs in Oncology

- **KRAS Mutations:** mRNA-5671 (now V941) and other therapies target the KRAS and other members of the Ras protein family are proto-oncogenes that are frequently mutated in malignancies such as colorectal, pancreatic, and non-small-cell lung cancer (NSCLC). In order to suppress KRAS expression in animal models of pancreatic cancer, early attempts used siRNA-LNP delivery. When paired with chemotherapy, such as gemcitabine, these attempts frequently demonstrated synergistic results.
- **Clinical translation:** To target four prevalent KRAS mutations (G12D, G12V, G13D, and G12C), mRNA-5671 (now V941), an mRNA-based cancer vaccine developed by LNP, was created. A Phase I study (NCT03948763) evaluated V941 as monotherapy and in combination with pembrolizumab in patients with KRAS-mutant advanced or metastatic NSCLC, colorectal cancer, or pancreatic adenocarcinoma. However, this trial has concluded, and further progress has not been announced as of May 2024.

3.5.2.2 Combination and Theranostic LNP Trials

LNPs are being investigated in more intricate clinical trials for combination and theranostic applications, leveraging their adaptability as multimodal platforms, in addition to single-agent delivery.

- **Combination Treatment:** Combining nucleic acids and chemotherapy, getting beyond medication resistance. Co-administration of siRNA and chemotherapy can improve anti-tumor synergy and get past drug resistance mechanisms. The co-administration of the chemotherapy drug DOX and the anti-apoptotic siRNA against B-cell lymphoma 2 (BCL2) was one preclinical example. This method demonstrated its ability to overcome medication resistance in a preclinical lymphoma model by entirely inhibiting tumor growth and causing a synergistic increase in apoptosis.

Restoring tumor suppressors and silencing oncogenes: A preclinical study on prostate cancer showed that LNP delivery of siRNA to silence the oncogene androgen receptor (AR) and mRNA to restore the tumor suppressor PTEN produced synergistic therapeutic effects in prostate cancer cells that were AR-positive and PTEN-null. Because it simultaneously regulated important survival pathways, the combination dramatically boosted apoptosis when compared to either drug alone.

Improving both effectiveness and safety: Co-formulation of various RNA types, such as siRNA and mRNA, in a single LNP can enhance synergistic effects and increase therapeutic results and delivery efficiency when compared to independent LNPs.

Although combination and theranostic LNPs have made great strides in preclinical research, a number of obstacles still need to be addressed before they can be widely used in clinical settings. Formulating and optimizing systems with various components is still quite hard, and thorough validation is necessary to guarantee the safety of all encapsulated components. Additionally, standardizing manufacturing for large-scale production remains a challenge, and the exorbitant expense of creating such intricate nano systems is a serious obstacle to commercialization. However, continued developments in LNP technology and encouraging preclinical findings imply that these adaptable platforms could transform cancer treatment via image-guided, targeted, and combination therapies. As summarized in Table 3.3, several RNA-based and liposomal nanotherapeutic candidates—ranging from personalized mRNA vaccines to theranostic LNPs—are advancing through clinical and translational stages, underscoring the significant progress and future potential of these technologies in precision oncology.

3.5.2.3 Approved LNP-Based Therapeutics Relevant to Cancer

There is currently no oncology-specific regulatory approval for an LNP-based treatment; the clinical achievements of LNPs in other illnesses have created a solid basis for their application in cancer treatment. The platform's safety, scalability, and efficacy have all been confirmed by these approvals, giving assurance that oncology applications are both possible and impending.

3.5.2.4 Onpattro® (patisiran)

The first siRNA medication administered using LNPs, Patisiran, was licensed by the U.S. Food and Drug Administration (FDA) in 2018 to treat hereditary hATTR (Adams et al., 2018).**Significance and Translatability:** This historic approval demonstrated that LNPs can effectively silence genes, deliver siRNA to hepatocytes safely, and produce long-lasting therapeutic benefits. Although not an oncology medication, its approval showed that pharmacokinetic challenges may be solved by systemically administering LNPs. Cancer treatments that target the oncogenic drivers of solid tumors can directly apply this lesson.

3.5.2.5 COVID-19 mRNA-LNP Vaccines

A second revolutionary milestone for LNPs was made possible by the quick development, licensure, and distribution of the COVID-19 vaccines produced by Moderna (mRNA-1273) and Pfizer–BioNTech (BNT162b2). **Safety, scalability and immunological parallels:** These vaccines confirmed the safety of repeated dosing in millions of people globally and demonstrated the scalability of LNP production in emergencies. They showed how LNPs can carry mRNA encoding viral antigens and elicit robust immune responses. This process is similar to how they might be used to deliver patient-specific neoantigens in cancer immunotherapy.

TABLE 3.3
Summary of Selected Clinical and Translational Trials Involving RNA-Based and Liposomal Nanotherapeutics in Cancer Treatment

Trial/Agent	Cargo Type	Cancer Type	Status/Phase	Notes and References
mRNA-4157 (V940) + Pembrolizumab	Personalized mRNA	High-risk Melanoma	Phase II → Phase III (NCT05933577)	Phase II KEYNOTE-942 showed a significant reduction in recurrence or death risk with the combination (~44%) compared to pembrolizumab alone. Phase III trials are underway. (NCT05933577)
mRNA-4157 (V940) + Pembrolizumab	Personalized mRNA	Non-Small Cell Lung Cancer (NSCLC)	Phase III (NCT06077760)	Conducted by Merck and Moderna for patients with NSCLC and an incomplete response to neoadjuvant chemo-immunotherapy (NCT06077760).
Autogene Cevumeran (BNT122) + Atezolizumab	Personalized mRNA	Resected Pancreatic Ductal Adenocarcinoma (PDAC)	Phase I → Phase II (NCT05968326)	Phase I showed that durable T-cell responses correlated with delayed recurrence. Phase II is ongoing to confirm findings (NCT05968326).
Autogene Cevumeran (BNT122)	Personalized mRNA	Colorectal Cancer (CRC)	Phase II (NCT04486378)	Investigates efficacy versus watchful waiting in ctDNA-positive patients after adjuvant chemotherapy (NCT04486378).
RNA-LP (GBM trials)	mRNA (CMV pp65, neoantigens)	Glioblastoma (GBM)	Phase I (NCT04573140, NCT06389591)	Evaluates safety and immune response of neoantigen-targeted RNA-LP vaccines in newly diagnosed and recurrent GBM (NCT06389591).
OX40L/IL-23/IL-36γ LNPs (mRNA-2752)	Immune-activating mRNA	Advanced Solid Tumors/ Lymphoma	Phase I/II (e.g., NCT03739931)	Intratumoral delivery to locally activate immune responses and limit systemic toxicity (NCT03739931).
Programmable IL-12 mRNA (STX-001)	Tumor-activated self-replicating mRNA	Advanced Solid Tumors	Early Human Trial (NCT06249048)	Engineered for tumor-specific IL-12 expression to minimize toxicity. Early Phase I data showed clinical activity and immune activation (NCT06249048).
siRNA-LNPs (e.g., ALN-VSP02, Atu027)	siRNA (e.g., against VEGF, KSP, PKN3)	Various Solid Tumors	Early Phase Trials	Demonstrate proof-of-concept for gene silencing and show acceptable safety profiles, though some trials were terminated early (143).
Theranostic LNPs	Therapeutic + Imaging Agents	Various	Early Translational Stage	Combines therapy with diagnostic imaging. Preclinical examples include MRI-compatible and multimodal systems for guided therapy (144).
Doxorubicin (DOX) Liposomes (DOXIL)	Doxorubicin	Advanced Ovarian Cancer, Multiple Myeloma, etc.	Clinically Approved	An approved liposomal drug that uses the EPR effect to reduce cardiotoxicity and improve safety (145).

3.5.2.6 Progress in the Oncology Pipeline

Although LNP medications with an oncology emphasis have not yet received approval, a number of candidates are making headway in late-stage clinical evaluation. **Customized mRNA cancer vaccines:** Phase II/III trials are underway for melanoma, pancreatic cancer, and other solid tumors using Moderna's mRNA-4157 (V940) (137) and BioNTech's autogene cevumeran (BNT122) (146). **siRNA-LNP formulations:** In Phase I/II trials, candidates that target important oncogenic drivers such as VEGF-driven angiogenesis, KRAS mutations, or anti-apoptotic pathways are making progress against a range of malignancies, including ovarian, lung, and hepatocellular carcinoma. The goal of combination platforms is to maximize cytotoxicity while circumventing resistance mechanisms by co-delivering chemotherapeutic drugs and nucleic acids.

3.5.2.7 Implications for Oncology

The success of the mRNA and Onpattro® COVID-19 vaccines shows that LNPs are now clinically validated platforms rather than experimental ones. **Basis for approval:** These achievements reassure patients, physicians, and regulators about the scalability, safety, and adaptability of LNPs. This implies that, in the case of oncology, current expedited routes may be appropriate, and regulatory approval may come quickly after efficacy is proven in late-phase trials.

Despite significant progress in the development of nanoparticle-based drug delivery systems, many challenges remain before their widespread clinical use. A major obstacle is the complex biological environment, where nanoparticles face conditions such as rapid clearance, protein corona formation, and variable receptor expression, which can affect target efficiency and therapeutic outcomes. Toxicity and long-term safety also remain concerns, especially for inorganic or hybrid nanomaterials, which can accumulate in tissues and not be cleared effectively. Additionally, problems associated with extensibility, reproducibility, and regulatory approval limit access from laboratory prototypes to clinically approved structures.

3.6 CHALLENGES AND FUTURE DIRECTIONS

Despite the remarkable progress achieved in the development of functionalized lipid nanoparticles for cancer therapy, several challenges continue to hinder their widespread clinical translation. Issues related to biological barriers, manufacturing scalability, long-term safety, regulatory approval, and tumor heterogeneity remain significant concerns. Addressing these limitations through innovative design strategies, advanced manufacturing technologies, and personalized therapeutic approaches will be crucial for realizing the full potential of lipid-based nanomedicines in oncology.

3.6.1 Scale-Up and Manufacturing Hurdles

One of the most serious challenges of bringing nanocarrier systems from laboratory research to clinical application is the problem of scale-up and manufacturing. While nanoparticles can be reproducibly synthesized in the laboratory on a small scale, making them with uniform quality on a large, industrially relevant scale is still a daunting task. Complexity arises from the fact that properties of nanoparticles, such as size, shape, surface charge, and ligand density, directly affect their biological behavior, including biodistribution, target-directed efficiency, and clearance. Even small differences during mass production can lead to batch-to-batch variations, raising questions about safety and therapeutic reliability. Unlike traditional small-molecule drugs, which are chemically clearly defined and can be easily prepared on a large scale, nanocarriers are multi-component systems that often include polymers, lipids, surfactants, ligands, and medicinal cargoes. Regeneratively controlling the assembly of these diverse components is particularly challenging, especially when processes are scaled up from the milligram to the kilogram scale. A further layer of complexity involves the strict regulatory and quality control requirements of nanomedicines. Because the therapeutic efficacy of nanocarriers is dependent on the drug molecule and the physicochemical characteristics of the carrier, the regulatory agencies require proper characterization of several parameters such as the particle size distribution, surface chemistry, drug loading, release kinetics and temperature/condition stability during storage. There is an additional challenge in meeting these requirements during scale-up because traditional analytical tools are not optimized to evaluate the subtle differences that can exist between batches that are thousands of times larger than the initial formulation. These limitations can significantly raise the cost of production and the challenges to meet GMP (Good Manufacturing Practice) compliance, sterilization and guaranteed absence of endotoxins. Sterilization methods such as irradiating, filtration, or autoclaving can alter as well as destroy the fabrication and the drug stability of the nanoparticles (147).

Production costs also serve as a tremendous barrier. Just that to generate nanoparticles at scale, especially if they are going to involve complex surface modifications that may involve an antibody or an aptamer attached or a biomimetic coating, will require costly intellectual property, raw materials, reagents, and purification steps that can really raise the final price of nanomedicines and impact procurement in resource-limited health systems. Hybrid or multi-functional nanoplatforms are very common in such nanoparticles, but many also include precious metals (e.g., gold, platinum) or rare materials (e.g., quantum dots, lanthanide) that further inflate production costs. Thus, cost-effective, scalable and environmentally sustainable manufacturing processes are required to encourage clinical uptake. Recent developments designed to overcome these barriers have primarily been in microfluidics, sustainable production, and modular assembly systems, which are starting to serve as alternatives to batch processes. Microfluidic platforms offer a level of control over mixtures, temperatures, and flow rates that allows for the control of particle shape and properties. Microfluidic systems are also scalable based on parallelism and have more reproducibility than manually-made laboratory nanoparticles (149). Like microfluidics, sustainable production has the potential for nanoparticles to be produced in a continuous stream and therefore not have as much diversity in nanoparticle characteristics, while also improving process efficiency. One last avenue we see as promising is the development of standardizable and modular nanocarrier platforms. The idea is that you have interchangeable components (core material, targeting ligand, stealth coating, and therapeutic cargo) that can all be assembled in controlled conditions to simplify lot testing and approval from regulatory authorities. Not only would they become more reproducible, but the process could be better equipped with a Process Analytical Technologies (PAT) to measure characteristics of the particle when made in real time.

3.6.2 Stability and Storage Issues

Furthermore, one of the other major problems restricting the clinical translation of nanomedicine is the problem of stability and storage. Nanocarriers are structured forms of polymers, lipids, proteins or inorganic materials that interact in complex ways, and their performance as a therapeutic will greatly depend on whether they have maintained their structure upon storage and transportation. Though small-molecule drugs are conventionally much simpler with generally greater chemical stability, such that they can be stored as solid powders or tablets, nanocarriers are much more prone to problems with aggregation, leakage of drug prior to being administered, hydrolysis, oxidation, and dissociation of surface ligands. This can result in even very small changes in humidity, ionic strength, temperature or pH during storage can result in significant changes to their physicochemical properties (i.e., particle size, surface charge, composition, and drug release kinetics). This type of instability not only reduces therapeutic effectiveness but also raises safety concerns, as nanocarriers can alter their biodistribution or cause unexpected immune responses when they are introduced into the body. For example, liposomes can be affected by fusion, aggregation, or leakage of attached drugs, while polymeric nanoparticles can withstand hydrolytic dissolution or crystallization of the polymer matrix. Similarly, antibody- or peptide-conjugated nanoparticles often lose their activity due to denaturation or proteolysis of biomolecules, making stability one of the most important factors in product development (152).

The storage environment also presents additional difficulties. Many nanocarrier structures require refrigeration or freezing to maintain stability, which complicates mass distribution and patient access, especially in areas where cold-chain infrastructure is limited. Lyophilization (freeze-drying) is often used to improve shelf-life, but the process itself can produce structural stress, leading to loss of functional activity. These problems can be partially mitigated by adding cryoprotectants such as trehalose, sucrose or mannitol, but universal protocols that work identically on different nanocarrier platforms have yet to be established. In addition, some nanocarriers, especially lipid-based and protein-based systems, are inherently sensitive to oxidation and microbial contamination, requiring antioxidants, stabilizers, and sterile production conditions. Another complicating factor is that some nanocarriers are designed to be stimuli-responsive (such as pH-sensitive, redox-sensitive or enzyme-sensitive). While this design is beneficial for drug release in the body, it makes them even more unstable during long-term storage (153). Batch-to-batch reproducibility is also a concern in sustainability studies. Regulatory agencies for clinical approval demand comprehensive data on long-term and accelerated stability, including parameters such as drug quantity, encapsulation efficiency, particle size distribution, and release kinetics over time. Achieving the same stability profile across different production lots is challenging because of the inherent diversity in nanoparticle synthesis and the sensitivity of the structures to environmental fluctuations. This problem is particularly severe for multi-functional or hybrid nanocarriers, where many components (drug payloads, stealth coatings, targeting ligands, imaging agents) must remain stable without reacting with each other or disintegrating. Ensuring that these components do not interact chemically during long storage is often complex and requires careful formulation design.

To solve these problems, researchers are exploring new stabilization techniques. Lyophilization with optimized cryo and lyoprotectants remains the most widely adopted method, but alternative approaches such as spray drying, vacuum drying, and supercritical fluid processing are being explored for more robust and scalable solutions (154). Encapsulation of lipid nanoparticles within protective matrices such as hydrogels or polymer films can also increase stability and facilitate controlled release upon rehydration. Advances in materials science are leading to the design of more stable polymers, lipid analogues, and biomimetic coatings that can resist dissolution under storage conditions. Inorganic nanomaterials such as silica or gold, which are less sensitive to hydrolysis and oxidation, are also being used to increase stability by hybridizing with organic carriers. On the regulatory front, harmonized guidelines for nanocarrier stability testing are being developed, with emphasis on accelerated stability studies, predictive shelf-life models, and real-time monitoring techniques.

3.6.3 Regulatory and Safety Considerations

One of the most persistent challenges in the clinical translation of nanomedicine is the lack of clear and universally harmonized regulatory frameworks that can adequately evaluate the safety, effectiveness, and quality of nanocarrier-based therapies. Unlike conventional drugs, which are usually clearly defined chemical units, nanocarriers are complex, multi-component systems whose properties depend not only on their chemical composition but also on their shape, surface charge, coating, and their dynamic behavior in biological systems. These physicochemical characteristics can profoundly affect biodistribution, clearance, immune recognition, and therapeutic outcome, but traditional regulatory protocols are often not able to capture such complex interactions. As a result, many promising nanomedicine structures are stuck during late-stage development because they do not fully meet existing safety and effectiveness requirements. This regulatory uncertainty related to nanomedicine creates a gap between laboratory success and clinical approval, slowing innovation and discouraging investment in commercialization.

Safety evaluation is particularly complex because nanocarriers can have unique interactions with biological systems that are different from bulk materials or small molecules. For example, nanoparticles can cross biological barriers (e.g., blood-brain barrier, placental barrier) that conventional drugs cannot cross, raising concerns of off-target effects. The response of the immune system is also a major concern, as nanoparticle surfaces can activate complement cascades, release cytokines, or produce hypersensitivity reactions. For example, lipid-based nanoparticles have been linked to complement activation-related pseudo allergy (CARPA), while some inorganic nanoparticles (such as gold, quantum dots, silica) can accumulate in organs such as the liver, spleen, and kidney, causing long-term toxicity. In addition, multi-functional nanocarriers carrying imaging agents, targeting ligands or adjuvants present additional complexity, as each component has to be evaluated separately for safety, as well as considering possible synergistic or antagonistic interactions in the structure. Another important regulatory concern is long-term toxicity and biodegradability. Many nanocarriers are designed to remain in the body long enough until they achieve therapeutic effectiveness, but incomplete clearance or slow degradation can cause bioaccumulation. Inorganic nanoparticles (such as gold, quantum dots, silica) are particularly scrutinized for the possibility that they can remain in tissues and produce long-term toxicity, while polymeric and lipid systems are also required to exhibit predictable decomposition and safe metabolite profiles. Conventional toxicology studies, which are well established for small molecules, are often inadequate for nanomedicine, as nanoparticle toxicity can be dose-dependent, size-dependent, and context-specific. Therefore, regulatory agencies demand comprehensive preclinical characterization, including studies on pharmacokinetics, biodistribution, immunotoxicity, genotoxicity, and reproductive toxicity. Meeting these requirements is resource-intensive, time-consuming, and often varies across jurisdictions, further complicating the path to approval (157).

Regulatory agencies such as the U.S. FDA (Food and Drug Administration) and EMA (European Medicines Agency) have begun issuing guidance documents on nanomedicine, but these are still evolving and not universally harmonized. For example, there are no standardized protocols for nanoparticle characterization, stability testing, or in vivo behavior, leading to inconsistencies in data reporting and difficulty in comparisons between studies. The lack of predictive in-vitro models that accurately reflect human physiology also limits the reliability of preclinical data, leading regulators to be cautious in approving new nanomedicines (Clogston et al., 2024). To address these concerns, agencies are encouraging the adoption of advanced analytical techniques (such as high-resolution imaging, nanoparticle tracking analysis, and omics-based toxicity profiling) and computational modeling to better predict nanoparticle interactions and safety profiles. Ethical and social considerations also play a role in regulatory decision-making. Public perception of nanomedicine safety can influence regulatory policies, as concerns about nanotoxicity and unknown long-term risks can create resistance to adoption. Therefore, reporting transparently, standardized labelling and clear risk-benefit communication will be key to earning public trust. At the same time, the cost of regulatory compliance—including large-scale toxicology studies, sustainability testing, and manufacturing quality assurance—can be extremely expensive for academic groups and startups, creating barriers to entry and potentially limiting innovation to only large pharmaceutical companies.

3.6.4 Next-Generation LNPs and Personalized Cancer Therapy

The rapid development of lipid-based nanocarriers has brought next-generation LNPs to the center of cancer nanomedicine, providing unprecedented opportunities for precision oncology and personalized therapy. Traditional LNPs, such as those used in siRNA delivery and mRNA vaccines, have already demonstrated clinical feasibility, but their design has been based primarily on generalized formulations that were developed for a wider population. In contrast, next-generation LNPs are being developed with a standardized lipid composition, surface modification, and modular structure, also with regard to the genetic, epigenetic, and microenvironmental characteristics of the specific patient and the tumor heterogeneity. This paradigm has been driven by the general trend toward personalized cancer therapies seeking to optimize therapeutic modalities based on patient-specific biomarkers, mutational landscape, and immune condition to yield maximum efficacy with minimum systemic toxicity.

A defining characteristic of next-generation LNPs is their adaptable and programmable architecture. As a result of high-throughput lipid development and computational screening, researchers now have the capacity to create libraries of ionizable and helper lipids that exhibit controlled physicochemical properties such as pKa, hydrophobicity, and membrane fluidic properties, allowing for optimization toward specific cancers or delivery routes. Next-generation LNPs can also deliver passenger therapeutics with surface functionalities that can be altered with specific ligands—for example, antibodies, peptides, aptamers or small molecules to target tumor-specific antigens or receptors. When developed properly, this targeted delivery results in high payload concentration in malignant tissues and reduced exposure to normal cells. This selective payload toxicity is important for cancers that demonstrate a high difference between in-patient and out-patient therapy, as delivery of the therapeutic, including siRNA, mRNA, CRISPR-Cas components or small molecule drugs, delivers the therapeutic to the tumor subpopulations responsible for driving the disease. Also, a number of cancers have been identified as "cancer stem cell" (CSC) malignancies. These cancers rely on multisystem complexities as the tumor nodes strictly adhere to a mosaic of genetic and phenotypic characteristics. When various cancers develop, they usually gain a basis of initial molecular malignancy, benefiting a patient population that often heavily relies on patient-specific secondary omics-based therapy.

Next-generation LNPs allow for the ability to deliver multiple and combinatorial passenger therapeutic payloads for a designed/engineered therapeutic. LNPs can be co-loaded with chemotherapeutics and immune-modulators that allow for a directed disease-modifying effect (synergistic chemo-immunotherapy), delivery of nucleic acid therapeutics that silence oncogenes and express tumor-suppressor proteins simultaneously. This range of targeting is specifically important within cancers that commonly are non-responsive to single-moiety therapy, due to the tumor escape phenomena observed in the patient-specific CSCs and drug-resistant tumor cells. Using LNPs significantly enables these formulations to be developed, since there is a patient-specific range of omics channels to direct the respective individual therapeutic payload. This patient-specific aspect is to incorporate the patients-specific omics phenotype and predilections for mutational signatures, transcriptomic profiling and immune cell infiltrations so that a custom LNP therapeutic is uniquely designed to address the exactness of the molecular biologics at risk within the tumor populations of each patient. Advances in artificial intelligence and machine learning support this personalization, as they are able to predict lipid-payload interactions, biodistribution, and therapeutic outcomes (162).

Another transformative avenue is the creation of stimulus-responsive and microenvironment-adaptive LNPs. Tumor tissues exhibit unique features, such as hypoxia, acidic PH, increased ROS, and over-expressed enzymes, that can be used for the controlled release of a payload. Next-generation LNPs are being developed to leverage these signals with the aim of achieving spatio-temporality of drug release to increase effectiveness while reducing off-target exposure. In addition, if immunomodulating lipids are incorporated or adjuvant molecules are included, LNPs can be modified to alter the TIME to improve antigen presentation and/or reduce T-cell exhaustion, thereby promote long-lasting anti-tumor immunity. Such designs that target the immune system complement personalized cancer immunotherapy strategies when treatments are based on the immune signatures of individual patients.

Nonetheless, the clinical implementation of next-generation LNPs for personalized cancer therapy will experience challenges. Mass delivery of patient-specific formulations will require adaptable, modular manufacturing platforms that are flexible enough to account for patient-specific lipid ratios, target ligands, and payload combinations. Additionally, regulatory approvals will require new approaches for evaluating patient-specific formulations for safety and efficacy, as unique patient-specific formulations run contrary to the typical one size fits all clinical trial design. Lastly, while it is likely that individualized LNP systems may generate greater individual costs, the health care systems to adopt a precision medicine reimbursement model. Despite these challenges, the combination of nanotechnology, genomics, bioinformatics, and immunology places next-generation

LNPs and they may be foundational for the next generation of cancer treatment paradigms. By enabling the tailored delivery of therapeutic payloads that fit each patient's molecular and immunology profile, these platforms will address the shortcomings of traditional therapy, comply with tumor heterogeneity, and ultimately enhance long-term survival. In the near future, next-generation LNPs are set to be centerpiece for advanced personalized cancer therapy and ultimately improve oncology as more predictive, prevention based, patient specific.

3.7 CONCLUSION

Functionalized LNPs have emerged as one of the most innovative and clinically significant nanoplatforms within the field of oncology. Their inherent advantages—biocompatibility, adjustable physicochemical characteristics, and the capacity to encapsulate a diverse range of therapeutic agents—position them prominently in the realm of cancer nanomedicine. By utilizing both passive targeting mechanisms through the EPR effect and active targeting strategies via ligand conjugation, LNPs possess the ability to enhance intratumoral drug delivery while reducing systemic toxicity. Additionally, functionalization techniques such as PEGylation, conjugation with aptamers or antibodies, and the implementation of stimuli-responsive designs have notably prolonged circulation half-life, facilitated spatiotemporal control of release, and improved selectivity. Collectively, these features signify a transformative shift from non-specific chemotherapies toward precision-engineered therapeutics.

The translational success of LNPs, as exemplified by drugs that have attained clinical approval such as liposomal doxorubicin (Doxil®), liposomal irinotecan (Onivyde®), and siRNA therapeutics like patisiran, highlights their promise in bridging laboratory progress with patient benefit. Nevertheless, the field also faces challenges that need close investigation. Instabilities upon storage, the problem of drug leakage, immunity clearance mechanisms such as the ABC phenomenon, as well as lot-to-lot batch variability in manufacturing, create significant challenges. Of equal urgency are the issues of scalability, the need for harmonized regulation, as well as the high costs that accompany complex-formulation drugs, factors that hamper the widescale clinical use of such therapies. The next-generation development of functionalized LNPs will thus require a multidimensional approach. New technologies such as hybrid lipid–polymer NPs, multi-stimuli-sensitive carriers, as well as cell membrane biomimetic coating offer avenues toward breaking such constraints. Meanwhile, computer modeling, artificial intelligence/machine learning, as well as high-throughput screening will facilitate accelerating rationally designed LNPs specific to the heterogeneity of the tumor as well as patient-specificity. Of importance, compatibility with immunotherapies as well as gene editing strategies holds promise toward delivering a series of synergistic therapies beyond the traditional scope of chemotherapy.

In the long run, the future of functionalized LNPs mirrors an increasing trend toward precision and personalized nanomedicine more broadly. Their promise is not just that they might enhance therapeutic indices but that they could fundamentally change the way cancer therapy is thought about—away from shotgun cytotoxicity toward targeted, variable, patient-specific interventions. Should scale-up, regulation, and affordability challenges be successfully overcome, then functionalized LNPs could revolutionize oncology by providing safer, smarter, more enduring methods of therapy. In so doing, they could bring closer the long-held promise of nanotechnology: that cancer therapies might be more effective, less toxic, and better tailored to the patient as an individual.

ACKNOWLEDGMENT

This work was supported by the Department of Biotechnology, Ministry of Science and Technology, India (BT/PR36505/NNT/28/1818/2022), Department of Science and Technology, DST-Science and Engineering Research Board (SB/S3/CE/048/2015), CRG/2020/005244 and IMPRINT (DST/IMP/2018/000687), Abdul Kalam Technology Innovation National Fellowship, Indian National

Academy of Engineering, India (INAE/121/AKF/37), Higher Education Financing Agency (HEFA/CSR/IITH/01/2024-25), University of Grants Commissions for fellowship of Author Megha M Unnimaya and Vibha Choudhary and Ministry of education for Prime Minister Research Fellowship (PMRF) of author Vaishali Makwana.

CONFLICT OF INTEREST

The authors declare no conflict of interest.

LIST OF ABBREVIATIONS

5-ALA—5-aminolevulinic acid
ABC—Accelerated blood clearance
AMF—Alternating magnetic field
APCs—Antigen Presenting Cells
AuNCs—Gold nanoclusters
AuNRs—Gold nanorods
AuNPs—Gold nanoparticles
AuNSs—Gold nanostars
AuNUs—Gold nanourchins
BCL2—B-cell lymphoma 2
BSA—Bovine Serum Albumin
CAR-T—Chimeric Antigen Receptor T cells
CARPA—Complement activation-related pseudoallergy
CAT—Catalase
Ce6—Chlorin e6
CeO_2—Cerium Oxide
CHEMS—Cholesteryl hemisuccinate
CLH—Cationic Liposomal hydroxycamptothecin
CMN—Curcumin
CPNs—Conjugated polymer nanoparticles
CSCs—Cancer stem cells
CT—Computed Tomography
DAMPs—Damage associated molecular patterns
DCs—Dendritic Cells
DNA—Deoxyribonucleic Acid
DNR—Daunorubicin
DOPE—Dioleoylphosphatidylethanolamine
DOX—Doxorubicin
DPPC—Dipalmitoylphosphatidylcholine
DST—Drug synergistic treatment
ECM—Extracellular matrix
EE—Encapsulation efficiency
EGFR—Epidermal Growth Factor Receptor
EMA—European Medicines Agency
EPR—Enhanced Permeation and Retention
FDA—Food and Drug Administration
FePt—Iron-platinum
GBM—Glioblastoma
GNCs—Gold nanoclusters
GO—Graphene oxide

GSCs—Glioblastoma stem cells
GSH—Glutathione
H2O$_2$—Hydrogen peroxide
HA—Hyaluronic Acid
HCPT—Hydroxycamptothecin
HER2—Human Epidermal Growth Factor Receptor
HIF-1α—Hypoxia-inducible factor-1α
HIFU—High-intensity focused ultrasound
HIFUT—High-intensity focused ultrasound therapy
HLPNs—Hybrid lipid–polymer nanoparticles
HMME—Hematoporphyrin Monomethyl Ether
HSP—Heat shock protein
hATTR—Hereditary transthyretin-mediated amyloidosis
ICB—Immune checkpoint blockage
ICD—Immunogenic cell death
ICG—Indocyanine green
IL-12—Interleukin-12
Ir—Iridium
LBL—Layer by layer
LNCs—Lipid Nanocapsules
LNPs—Lipid Nanoparticles
MCTs—Medium-chain triglycerides
MDR—Multidrug resistance
miRNA—Micro RNA
MMPs—Matrix Metalloproteinases
MnO$_2$—Manganese dioxide
MPS—Mononuclear phagocyte system
MRI—Magnetic Resonance Imaging
mRNA—Messenger RNA
MTX—Mitoxantrone
NIR—Near-infrared
nHLCs—Nanostructure hybrid lipid capsules
NLCs—Nanostructured lipid carriers
NPs—Nanoparticles
NSCLC—Non-small-cell lung cancer
PCL—Polycaprolactone
PDA—Polydopamine
PDT—Photodynamic therapy
PEG—Polyethylene Glycol
PEI—Polyethylenimine
PFC—Perfluorocarbon
PET—Positron Emission Tomography
PLGA—Poly(lactic-co-glycolic acid)
PLK1—Polo-like kinase 1
PLA—Phospholipases
PNIPAM—Poly(N-isopropylacrylamide)
pSar—Polysarcosine
PTA—Photothermal agents
PTT—Photothermal treatment
PTX—Paclitaxel
PVs—Polymer vesicles

RES—Reticuloendothelial system
REPNs—RB-loaded nanomicelles AA
RF—Regorafenib
RGD—Arginine-glycine-aspartic acid
RNA—Ribonucleic Acid
RNAi—RNA interference
RISCs—RNA-induced silencing complexes
ROS—Reactive oxygen species
RV—Reversan
RB—Rose Bengal
SA—Sialic Acid
SAL—Salinomycin
SLNs—Solid lipid nanoparticles
SPNs—Semiconducting polymer nanoparticles
TAAs—Tumor Associated Antigens
TAMs—Tumor-Associated Macrophages
Tregs—Regulatory T cells
TiO_2—Titanium dioxide
TLR—Toll like Receptor
Tm—Phase transition temperature
TME—Tumor Microenvironment
TSLs—Thermosensitive liposomes
TTR—Transthyretin
UCNPs—Upconversion nanoparticles
UGO—Ultra small graphene oxide
US—Ultrasound
VEGF—Vascular endothelial Growth Factor
VLN—Virus like nanoparticle

REFERENCES

1. Sung H, Ferlay J, Siegel RL, Laversanne M, Soerjomataram I, Jemal A, et al. Global cancer statistics 2020: GLOBOCAN estimates of incidence and mortality worldwide for 36 cancers in 185 countries. CA Cancer J Clin. 2021 May;71(3):209–49.
2. Peer D, Karp JM, Hong S, Farokhzad OC, Margalit R, Langer R. Nanocarriers as an emerging platform for cancer therapy. Nat Nanotechnol. 2007 Dec;2(12):751–60.
3. Pattni BS, Chupin V V., Torchilin VP. New developments in liposomal drug delivery. Chem Rev. 2015 Oct 14;115(19):10938–66.
4. Chuprun SS, Kantin G, Krasavin M. Synthesis and medicinal applications of N-Aryl-C-nitroazoles. Mini-Reviews in Medicinal Chemistry. 2018 Nov 12;18(20):1733–52.
5. Mehta M, Bui TA, Yang X, Aksoy Y, Goldys EM, Deng W. Lipid-based nanoparticles for drug/gene delivery: An overview of the production techniques and difficulties encountered in their industrial development. ACS Materials Au. 2023 Nov 8;3(6):600–19.
6. Lombardo D, Kiselev MA. Methods of liposomes preparation: Formation and control factors of versatile nanocarriers for biomedical and nanomedicine application. Pharmaceutics. 2022 Feb 28; 14(3):543.
7. Guimarães D, Cavaco-Paulo A, Nogueira E. Design of liposomes as drug delivery system for therapeutic applications. Int J Pharm. 2021 May;601:120571.
8. Pande S. Liposomes for drug delivery: Review of vesicular composition, factors affecting drug release and drug loading in liposomes. Artif Cells Nanomed Biotechnol. 2023 Dec 31;51(1):428–40.
9. Chen M, Hu J, Wang L, Li Y, Zhu C, Chen C, et al. Targeted and redox-responsive drug delivery systems based on carbonic anhydrase IX-decorated mesoporous silica nanoparticles for cancer therapy. Sci Rep. 2020 Sep 2;10(1):14447.
10. Advances in liposome-based delivery of RNA therapeutics for cancer treatment. (2024): 177–218.

11. Queiroz M de CV, Muehlmann LA. Characteristics and preparation of solid lipid nanoparticles and nanostructured lipid carriers. Journal of Nanotheranostics. 2024 Nov 25;5(4):188–211.
12. Viegas C, Patrício AB, Prata JM, Nadhman A, Chintamaneni PK, Fonte P. Solid lipid nanoparticles vs. nanostructured lipid carriers: A comparative review. Pharmaceutics. 2023 May 25;15(6):1593.
13. Dave V, Tak K, Sohgaura A, Gupta A, Sadhu V, Reddy KR. Lipid-polymer hybrid nanoparticles: Synthesis strategies and biomedical applications. J Microbiol Methods. 2019 May;160:130–42.
14. Elmowafy M, Al-Sanea MM. Nanostructured lipid carriers (NLCs) as drug delivery platform: Advances in formulation and delivery strategies. Saudi Pharmaceutical Journal. 2021 Sep;29(9):999–1012.
15. Tekade AR, Mittha PS, Pisal CS. Nanostructured lipid carriers for nose to brain delivery targeting CNS: Diversified role of liquid lipids for synergistic action. Adv Pharm Bull. 2021 Oct 4.
16. Chauhan AS, Chand P, Parashar T. Lipid-based nanoparticles: Strategy for targeted cancer therapy. BIO Integration. 2025;6(1).
17. Bose RJC, Ravikumar R, Karuppagounder V, Bennet D, Rangasamy S, Thandavarayan RA. Lipid–polymer hybrid nanoparticle-mediated therapeutics delivery: Advances and challenges. Drug Discov Today. 2017 Aug;22(8):1258–65.
18. Zeng SQ, Chen YZ, Chen Y, Liu H. Lipid–polymer hybrid nanoparticles for synergistic drug delivery to overcome cancer drug resistance. New J Chem. 2017;41(4):1518–25.
19. Lüdtke FL, Silva TJ, da Silva MG, Hashimoto JC, Ribeiro APB. Lipid nanoparticles: Formulation, production methods and characterization protocols. Foods. 2025 Mar 12;14(6):973.
20. Alsaidan OA, Elmowafy M, Shalaby K, Alzarea SI, Massoud D, Kassem AM, et al. Hydrocortisone-loaded lipid–polymer hybrid nanoparticles for controlled topical delivery: Formulation design optimization and in vitro and in vivo appraisal. ACS Omega. 2023 May 30;8(21):18714–25.
21. Khater D, Nsairat H, Odeh F, Saleh M, Jaber A, Alshaer W, et al. Design, preparation, and characterization of effective dermal and transdermal lipid nanoparticles: A review. Cosmetics. 2021 May 18;8(2):39.
22. Jain S, Kumar M, Kumar P, Verma J, Rosenholm JM, Bansal KK, et al. Lipid–polymer hybrid nanosystems: A rational fusion for advanced therapeutic delivery. J Funct Biomater. 2023 Aug 23;14(9):437.
23. Chang D, Ma Y, Xu X, Xie J, Ju S. Stimuli-responsive polymeric nanoplatforms for cancer therapy. Front Bioeng Biotechnol. 2021 Jun 25;9.
24. Yuan Z, Yan R, Fu Z, Wu T, Ren C. Impact of physicochemical properties on biological effects of lipid nanoparticles: Are they completely safe. Sci Total Environ. 2024 Jun;927:172240.
25. Xu L, Wang X, Liu Y, Yang G, Falconer RJ, Zhao CX. Lipid nanoparticles for drug delivery. Adv Nanobiomed Res. 2022 Feb 25;2(2).
26. Rehman M, Tahir N, Sohail MF, Qadri MU, Duarte SOD, Brandão P, et al. Lipid-based nanoformulations for drug delivery: An ongoing perspective. Pharmaceutics. 2024 Oct 26;16(11):1376.
27. Aditya NP, Aditya S, Yang H, Kim HW, Park SO, Ko S. Co-delivery of hydrophobic curcumin and hydrophilic catechin by a water-in-oil-in-water double emulsion. Food Chem. 2015 Apr;173:7–13.
28. Kumar R, Dkhar DS, Kumari R, Divya, Mahapatra S, Srivastava A, et al. Ligand conjugated lipid-based nanocarriers for cancer theranostics. Biotechnol Bioeng. 2022 Nov 10;119(11):3022–43.
29. Kulkarni JA, Darjuan MM, Mercer JE, Chen S, van der Meel R, Thewalt JL, et al. On the formation and morphology of lipid nanoparticles containing ionizable cationic lipids and siRNA. ACS Nano. 2018 May 22;12(5):4787–95.
30. Neves AR, Queiroz JF, Costa Lima SA, Figueiredo F, Fernandes R, Reis S. Cellular uptake and transcytosis of lipid-based nanoparticles across the intestinal barrier: Relevance for oral drug delivery. J Colloid Interface Sci. 2016 Feb;463:258–65.
31. Zelepukin I V., Shevchenko KG, Deyev SM. Rediscovery of mononuclear phagocyte system blockade for nanoparticle drug delivery. Nat Commun. 2024 May 22;15(1):4366.
32. Veronese FM, Pasut G. PEGylation: Posttranslational bioengineering of protein biotherapeutics. Drug Discov Today Technol. 2008 Sep;5(2–3):e57–64.
33. Zhdanov VP. Nanoparticles without and with protein corona: Van der Waals and hydration interaction. J Biol Phys. 2019 Sep 15;45(3):307–16.
34. Xu FJ. Deciphering the impact of PEG antifouling layer on surface attached functional peptides in regulating cell behaviors. Chin Chem Lett. 2019 Dec;30(12):2051–2.
35. Gonçalves J, Caliceti P. Optimizing pharmacological and immunological properties of therapeutic proteins through PEGylation: Investigating key parameters and their impact. Drug Des Devel Ther. 2024 Nov;18:5041–62.
36. Barenholz Y (Chezy). Doxil®—The first FDA-approved nano-drug: Lessons learned. J Controlled Release. 2012 Jun;160(2):117–34.
37. Zalba S, ten Hagen TLM, Burgui C, Garrido MJ. Stealth nanoparticles in oncology: Facing the PEG dilemma. J Controlled Release. 2022 Nov;351:22–36.

38. Sung Y, Guo H, Ghasemizadeh A, Shen X, Chintrakulchai W, Kobayashi M, et al. Cancerous pH-responsive polycarboxybetaine-coated lipid nanoparticle for smart delivery of siRNA against subcutaneous tumor model in mice. Cancer Sci. 2022 Dec 3;113(12):4339–49.
39. Zhao Z, Ding R, Wang Y, Yuan R, Zhang H, Li T, et al. Sulfobetaine modification of poly (D, L-lactide-co-glycolic acid) nanoparticles enhances mucus permeability and improves bioavailability of orally delivered liraglutide. J Drug Deliv Sci Technol. 2024 Mar;93:105437.
40. Nogueira SS, Schlegel A, Maxeiner K, Weber B, Barz M, Schroer MA, et al. Polysarcosine-functionalized lipid nanoparticles for therapeutic mRNA delivery. ACS Appl Nano Mater. 2020 Nov 25;3(11):10634–45.
41. Shimizu T, Awata M, Abu Lila AS, Yoshioka C, Kawaguchi Y, Ando H, et al. Complement activation induced by PEG enhances humoral immune responses against antigens encapsulated in PEG-modified liposomes. J Controlled Release. 2021 Jan;329:1046–53.
42. Mohamed M, Abu Lila AS, Shimizu T, Alaaeldin E, Hussein A, Sarhan HA, et al. PEGylated liposomes: Immunological responses. Sci Technol Adv Mater. 2019 Dec 31;20(1):710–24.
43. Tian K, Pan F, Qiu W, Ma Y, Guo Z, Qian J, et al. Dissociable PEGylation alleviates Kupffer cells capture of PEGylated liposomal doxorubicin. Int J Pharm. 2025 Oct;683:126092.
44. Liu M, Su Y, Chen M, Wang J, Liu M, Dai Y, et al. A preliminary study of the innate immune memory of Kupffer cells induced by PEGylated nanoemulsions. J Controlled Release. 2022 Mar;343:657–71.
45. Dilliard SA, Siegwart DJ. Passive, active and endogenous organ-targeted lipid and polymer nanoparticles for delivery of genetic drugs. Nat Rev Mater. 2023 Jan 19;8(4):282–300.
46. Vaidyanathan K, Vasudevan DM. Organ specific tumor markers: What's new? Indian J Clin Biochem. 2012 Apr 8;27(2):110–20.
47. Huwyler J, Wu D, Pardridge WM. Brain drug delivery of small molecules using immunoliposomes. Proc Natl Acad Sci. 1996 Nov 26;93(24):14164–9.
48. Zhou G, Wilson G, Hebbard L, Duan W, Liddle C, George J, et al. Aptamers: A promising chemical antibody for cancer therapy. Oncotarget. 2016 Mar 22;7(12):13446–63.
49. Carvalho J, Paiva A, Cabral Campello MP, Paulo A, Mergny JL, Salgado GF, et al. Aptamer-based targeted delivery of a G-quadruplex Ligand in cervical cancer cells. Sci Rep. 2019 May 28;9(1):7945.
50. Yu HT, Meng D, Feng MX, Ruan KY, Dong JJ, Bin-Shen, et al. RGD-modified solid lipid nanoparticles improve oral doxorubicin absorption: In vitro and in vivo study. J Drug Deliv Sci Technol. 2024 Jan;91:105293.
51. Lorenzoni S, Rodríguez-Nogales C, Blanco-Prieto MJ. Targeting tumor microenvironment with RGD-functionalized nanoparticles for precision cancer therapy. Cancer Lett. 2025 Apr;614:217536.
52. Hernando S, Nikolakopoulou P, Voulgaris D, Hernandez RM, Igartua M, Herland A. Dual effect of TAT functionalized DHAH lipid nanoparticles with neurotrophic factors in human BBB and microglia cultures. Fluids Barriers CNS. 2022 Dec 17;19(1):22.
53. Arduino I, Liu Z, Iacobazzi RM, Lopedota AA, Lopalco A, Cutrignelli A, et al. Microfluidic preparation and in vitro evaluation of iRGD-functionalized solid lipid nanoparticles for targeted delivery of paclitaxel to tumor cells. Int J Pharm. 2021 Dec;610:121246.
54. Young O, Ngo N, Lin L, Stanbery L, Creeden JF, Hamouda D, et al. Folate receptor as a biomarker and therapeutic target in solid tumors. Curr Probl Cancer. 2023 Feb;47(1):100917.
55. Narmani A, Rezvani M, Farhood B, Darkhor P, Mohammadnejad J, Amini B, et al. Folic acid functionalized nanoparticles as pharmaceutical carriers in drug delivery systems. Drug Dev Res. 2019 Jun 29;80(4):404–24.
56. McCombs JR, Owen SC. Antibody drug conjugates: Design and selection of linker, payload and conjugation chemistry. AAPS J. 2015 Mar 22;17(2):339–51.
57. Kratschmer C, Levy M. Effect of chemical modifications on aptamer stability in serum. Nucleic Acid Ther. 2017 Dec;27(6):335–44.
58. Suzuki Y, Yakuwa M, Sato M, Samaridou E, Beck-Broichsitter M, Maeki M, et al. Splenic B cell-targeting lipid nanoparticles for safe and effective mRNA vaccine delivery. J Controlled Release. 2025 Jun;382:113687.
59. Dilliard SA, Siegwart DJ. Passive, active and endogenous organ-targeted lipid and polymer nanoparticles for delivery of genetic drugs. Nat Rev Mater. 2023 Jan 19;8(4):282–300.
60. Waheed I, Ali A, Tabassum H, Khatoon N, Lai WF, Zhou X. Lipid-based nanoparticles as drug delivery carriers for cancer therapy. Front Oncol. 2024 Apr 10;14.
61. Zhou W, Jia Y, Liu Y, Chen Y, Zhao P. Tumor microenvironment-based stimuli-responsive nanoparticles for controlled release of drugs in cancer therapy. Pharmaceutics. 2022 Oct 31;14(11):2346.
62. Ashrafizadeh M, Delfi M, Zarrabi A, Bigham A, Sharifi E, Rabiee N, et al. Stimuli-responsive liposomal nanoformulations in cancer therapy: Pre-clinical & clinical approaches. J Controlled Release. 2022 Nov;351:50–80.

63. Advances in liposome-based delivery of RNA therapeutics for cancer treatment. 2024:177–218.
64. Mahmoudzadeh M, Magarkar A, Koivuniemi A, Róg T, Bunker A. Mechanistic insight into how PEGylation reduces the efficacy of pH-sensitive liposomes from molecular dynamics simulations. Mol Pharm. 2021 Jul 5;18(7):2612–21.
65. Elsayed N. Selective imaging, gene, and therapeutic delivery using PEGylated and pH-Sensitive nanoparticles for enhanced lung disorder treatment. Int J Pharm. 2024 Dec;666:124819.
66. Liu H, Yang F, Chen W, Gong T, Zhou Y, Dai X, et al. Enzyme-responsive materials as carriers for improving photodynamic therapy. Front Chem. 2021 Nov 2;9.
67. Sun L, Liu H, Ye Y, Lei Y, Islam R, Tan S, et al. Smart nanoparticles for cancer therapy. Signal Transduct Target Ther. 2023 Nov 3;8(1):418.
68. Li Y, Zhang C, Li G, Deng G, Zhang H, Sun Y, et al. Protease-triggered bioresponsive drug delivery for the targeted theranostics of malignancy. Acta Pharm Sin B. 2021 Aug;11(8):2220–42.
69. Fouladi F, Steffen KJ, Mallik S. Enzyme-responsive liposomes for the delivery of anticancer drugs. Bioconjug Chem. 2017 Apr 19;28(4):857–68.
70. Guo X, Cheng Y, Zhao X, Luo Y, Chen J, Yuan WE. Advances in redox-responsive drug delivery systems of tumor microenvironment. J Nanobiotechnol. 2018 Dec 22;16(1):74.
71. Sun B, Luo C, Yu H, Zhang X, Chen Q, Yang W, et al. Disulfide Bond-driven oxidation- and reduction-responsive prodrug nanoassemblies for cancer therapy. Nano Lett. 2018 Jun 13;18(6):3643–50.
72. Chaudhry M, Lyon P, Coussios C, Carlisle R. Thermosensitive liposomes: A promising step toward localised chemotherapy. Expert Opin Drug Deliv. 2022 Aug 3;19(8):899–912.
73. Majerník M, Jendželovský R, Vargová J, Jendželovská Z, Fedoročko P. Multifunctional nanoplatforms as a novel effective approach in photodynamic therapy and chemotherapy, to overcome multidrug resistance in cancer. Pharmaceutics. 2022 May 17;14(5):1075.
74. Parveen S, Gupta P, Kumar S, Banerjee M. Lipid polymer hybrid nanoparticles as potent vehicles for drug delivery in cancer therapeutics. Med Drug Discov. 2023 Dec;20:100165.
75. Shahsavari S, Rad MB, Hajiaghajani A, Rostami M, Hakimian F, Jafarzadeh S, et al. Magnetoresponsive liposomes applications in nanomedicine: A comprehensive review. Biomed Pharmacother. 2024 Dec; 181:117665.
76. Zhigaltsev I V., Tam YYC, Kulkarni JA, Cullis PR. Synthesis and characterization of hybrid lipid nanoparticles containing gold nanoparticles and a weak base drug. Langmuir. 2022 Jun 28;38(25):7858–66.
77. Liu WS, Wu LL, Chen CM, Zheng H, Gao J, Lu ZM, et al. Lipid-hybrid cell-derived biomimetic functional materials: A state-of-the-art multifunctional weapon against tumors. Mater Today Bio. 2023 Oct;22:100751.
78. Siafaka PI, Okur NÜ, Karantas ID, Okur ME, Gündoğdu EA. Current update on nanoplatforms as therapeutic and diagnostic tools: A review for the materials used as nanotheranostics and imaging modalities. Asian J Pharm Sci. 2021 Jan;16(1):24–46.
79. Luiz MT, Dutra JAP, Viegas JSR, de Araújo JTC, Tavares Junior AG, Chorilli M. Hybrid magnetic lipid-based nanoparticles for cancer therapy. Pharmaceutics. 2023 Feb 23;15(3):751.
80. Duan C, Yu M, Xu J, Li BY, Zhao Y, Kankala RK. Overcoming cancer multi-drug resistance (MDR): Reasons, mechanisms, nanotherapeutic solutions, and challenges. Biomedicine and Pharmacotherapy. Elsevier Masson s.r.l.; 2023;162.
81. Vagena IA, Malapani C, Gatou MA, Lagopati N, Pavlatou EA. Enhancement of EPR effect for passive tumor targeting: Current status and future perspectives. Applied Sciences. 2025 Mar 14;15(6):3189.
82. Hasan U, Chauhan M, Basu SM, Jayakumar R, Giri J. Overcoming multidrug resistance by reversan and exterminating glioblastoma and glioblastoma stem cells by delivering drug-loaded nanostructure hybrid lipid capsules (nHLCs). Drug Deliv Transl Res. 2024 Feb 1;14(2):342–59.
83. Pradhan P, Giri J, Rieken F, Koch C, Mykhaylyk O, Döblinger M, et al. Targeted temperature sensitive magnetic liposomes for thermo-chemotherapy. J Controlled Release. 2010 Feb;142(1):108–21.
84. Kulkarni JA, Witzigmann D, Chen S, Cullis PR, van der Meel R. Lipid nanoparticle technology for clinical translation of siRNA therapeutics. Acc Chem Res. 2019 Sep 17;52(9):2435–44.
85. Anthiya S, Öztürk SC, Yanik H, Tavukcuoglu E, Şahin A, Datta D, et al. Targeted siRNA lipid nanoparticles for the treatment of KRAS-mutant tumors. J Controlled Release. 2023 May;357:67–83.
86. Ramaswamy S, Tonnu N, Tachikawa K, Limphong P, Vega JB, Karmali PP, et al. Systemic delivery of factor IX messenger RNA for protein replacement therapy. Proc Natl Acad Sci. 2017 Mar 7;114(10).
87. Hayward SL, Francis DM, Kholmatov P, Kidambi S. Targeted delivery of MicroRNA125a-5p by engineered lipid nanoparticles for the treatment of HER2 positive metastatic breast cancer. J Biomed Nanotechnol. 2016 Mar 1;12(3):554–68.
88. Kazemian P, Yu SY, Thomson SB, Birkenshaw A, Leavitt BR, Ross CJD. Lipid-nanoparticle-based delivery of CRISPR/Cas9 genome-editing components. Mol Pharm. 2022 Jun 6;19(6):1669–86.

89. Rosenblum D, Gutkin A, Kedmi R, Ramishetti S, Veiga N, Jacobi AM, et al. CRISPR-Cas9 genome editing using targeted lipid nanoparticles for cancer therapy. Sci Adv. 2020 Nov 20;6(47).
90. Li M, Xie H, Liu Y, Xia C, Cun X, Long Y, et al. Knockdown of hypoxia-inducible factor-1 alpha by tumor targeted delivery of CRISPR/Cas9 system suppressed the metastasis of pancreatic cancer. J Controlled Release. 2019 Jun;304:204–15.
91. Liu Q, Wang C, Zheng Y, Zhao Y, Wang Y, Hao J, et al. Virus-like nanoparticle as a co-delivery system to enhance efficacy of CRISPR/Cas9-based cancer immunotherapy. Biomaterials. 2020 Nov;258:120275.
92. Parrish AB, Freel CD, Kornbluth S. Cellular mechanisms controlling caspase activation and function. Cold Spring Harb Perspect Biol. 2013 Jun;5(6).
93. Koning GA, Eggermont AMM, Lindner LH, Ten Hagen TLM. Hyperthermia and thermosensitive liposomes for improved delivery of chemotherapeutic drugs to solid tumors. Pharmaceutical Research. 2010;27:1750–4.
94. Chen L, Zhang H, Hou Y, Yunlong W, Feng X. Immunomodulatory effects of photothermal therapy in breast cancer: Advances and challenges. Frontiers in Immunology. Frontiers Media SA;2025;16.
95. Chen Q, Xu L, Liang C, Wang C, Peng R, Liu Z. Photothermal therapy with immune-adjuvant nanoparticles together with checkpoint blockade for effective cancer immunotherapy. Nat Commun. 2016 Oct 21;7.
96. Ma R, Alifu N, Du Z, Chen S, Heng Y, Wang J, et al. Indocyanine green-based theranostic nanoplatform for nir fluorescence image-guided chemo/photothermal therapy of cervical cancer. Int J Nanomedicine. 2021;16:4847–61.
97. Rastinehad AR, Anastos H, Wajswol E, Winoker JS, Sfakianos JP, Doppalapudi SK, et al. Gold nanoshell-localized photothermal ablation of prostate tumors in a clinical pilot device study. Proc Natl Acad Sci U S A. 2019 Sep 10;116(37):18590–6.
98. Zhang J, Chen J, Ren J, Guo W, Li X, Chen R, et al. Biocompatible semiconducting polymer nanoparticles as robust photoacoustic and photothermal agents revealing the effects of chemical structure on high photothermal conversion efficiency. Biomaterials. 2018 Oct 1;181:92–102.
99. Lee EH, Lee MK, Lim SJ. Enhanced stability of indocyanine green by encapsulation in zein-phosphatidylcholine hybrid nanoparticles for use in the phototherapy of cancer. Pharmaceutics. 2021 Mar 1;13(3):1–10.
100. Chuan D, Fan R, Chen B, Ren Y, Mu M, Chen H, et al. Lipid-polymer hybrid nanoparticles with both PD-L1 knockdown and mild photothermal effect for tumor photothermal immunotherapy. ACS Appl Mater Interfaces. 2023 Sep 13;15(36):42209–26.
101. Wei P, Chen S, Shi J, Du J. Oxygen-generating polymer vesicles for enhanced sonodynamic tumor therapy. J Controlled Release. 2023 Jan 1;353:975–87.
102. Dong Q, Jiang Z. Platinum–iron nanoparticles for oxygen-enhanced sonodynamic tumor cell suppression. Inorganics (Basel). 2024 Dec 1;12(12).
103. Huang H, Du L, Su R, Li Z, Shao Y, Yuan Y, et al. Albumin-based co-loaded sonosensitizer and STING agonist nanodelivery system for enhanced sonodynamic and immune combination antitumor therapy. J Controlled Release. 2024 Nov 1;375:524–36.
104. Ren X, Yang Y, Kong X, Liu Z. Integrin αvβ3-targeted self-assembled polypeptide nanomicelles for efficacious sonodynamic therapy against breast cancer. Nanoscale. 2024 Apr 19;16(20):9953–65.
105. Zhang N, Tan Y, Yan L, Zhang C, Xu M, Guo H, et al. Modulation of tumor hypoxia by pH-responsive liposomes to inhibit mitochondrial respiration for enhancing sonodynamic therapy. Int J Nanomedicine. 2020;15:5687–700.
106. Krafft MP. Alleviating tumor hypoxia with perfluorocarbon-based oxygen carriers. Current Opinion in Pharmacology. Elsevier Ltd; 2020;53:117–25.
107. Gong Q, Huo L, Xiong S, Han Y, Zhao X, Wen L, et al. Engineering BSA-CAT-Ir nanoparticles for enhanced sonodynamic therapy via alleviating tumor hypoxia. Nanoscale Adv. 2025 Jul 22;7(15):4559–62.
108. Lea-Banks H, Wu SK, Lee H, Hynynen K. Ultrasound-triggered oxygen-loaded nanodroplets enhance and monitor cerebral damage from sonodynamic therapy. Nanotheranostics. 2022;6(4):376–87.
109. Yildirim A, Chattaraj R, Blum NT, Shi D, Kumar K, Goodwin AP. Phospholipid capped mesoporous nanoparticles for targeted high intensity focused ultrasound ablation. Adv Healthc Mater. 2017 Sep 20;6(18).
110. Xiao Z, Zhuang B, Zhang G, Li M, Jin Y. Pulmonary delivery of cationic liposomal hydroxycamptothecin and 5-aminolevulinic acid for chemo-sonodynamic therapy of metastatic lung cancer. Int J Pharm. 2021 May 15;601.
111. Huang H, Du L, Su R, Li Z, Shao Y, Yuan Y, et al. Albumin-based co-loaded sonosensitizer and STING agonist nanodelivery system for enhanced sonodynamic and immune combination antitumor therapy. J Controlled Release. 2024 Nov 1;375:524–36.

112. Hald Albertsen C, Kulkarni JA, Witzigmann D, Lind M, Petersson K, Simonsen JB. The role of lipid components in lipid nanoparticles for vaccines and gene therapy. Advanced Drug Delivery Reviews. Elsevier B.V. 2022;188.
113. Goswami R, Chatzikleanthous D, Lou G, Giusti F, Bonci A, Taccone M, et al. Mannosylation of LNP results in improved potency for self-amplifying RNA (SAM) vaccines. ACS Infect Dis. 2019 Sep 13;5(9):1546–58.
114. Tang X, Zhang J, Sui D, Yang Q, Wang T, Xu Z, et al. Simultaneous dendritic cells targeting and effective endosomal escape enhance sialic acid-modified mRNA vaccine efficacy and reduce side effects. J Controlled Release. 2023 Dec 1;364:529–45.
115. Chen J, Ye Z, Huang C, Qiu M, Song D, Li Y, et al. Lipid nanoparticle-mediated lymph node-targeting delivery of mRNA cancer vaccine elicits robust CD8 + T cell response. 2022; Available from: https://doi.org/10.1073/pnas.2207841119
116. Rybakova Y, Kowalski PS, Huang Y, Gonzalez JT, Heartlein MW, DeRosa F, et al. mRNA delivery for therapeutic anti-HER2 antibody expression in vivo. Molecular Therapy. 2019 Aug 7;27(8):1415–23.
117. Shinn J, Kwon N, Lee SA, Lee Y. Smart pH-responsive nanomedicines for disease therapy. Journal of Pharmaceutical Investigation. Springer 2022;52:427–41.
118. Tang X, Zhang Y, Han X. Ionizable lipid nanoparticles for mRNA delivery. Advanced NanoBiomed Research. John Wiley and Sons Inc 2023;3.
119. Grünwald B, Vandooren J, Locatelli E, Fiten P, Opdenakker G, Proost P, et al. Matrix metalloproteinase-9 (MMP-9) as an activator of nanosystems for targeted drug delivery in pancreatic cancer. J Controlled Release. 2016 Oct 10;239:39–48.
120. Wilhelmy C, Keil IS, Uebbing L, Schroer MA, Franke D, Nawroth T, et al. Polysarcosine-functionalized mRNA lipid nanoparticles tailored for immunotherapy. Pharmaceutics. 2023 Aug 1;15(8).
121. Weber JS, Carlino MS, Khattak A, Meniawy T, Ansstas G, Taylor MH, et al. Individualised neoantigen therapy mRNA-4157 (V940) plus pembrolizumab versus pembrolizumab monotherapy in resected melanoma (KEYNOTE-942): A randomised, phase 2b study. The Lancet. 2024 Feb 17;403(10427):632–44.
122. Haque MA, Shrestha A, Mikelis CM, Mattheolabakis G. Comprehensive analysis of lipid nanoparticle formulation and preparation for RNA delivery. International Journal of Pharmaceutics: X. Elsevier B.V. 2024;8.
123. Weber JS, Carlino MS, Khattak A, Meniawy T, Ansstas G, Taylor MH, et al. Individualised neoantigen therapy mRNA-4157 (V940) plus pembrolizumab versus pembrolizumab monotherapy in resected melanoma (KEYNOTE-942): A randomised, phase 2b study. The Lancet. 2024 Feb 17;403(10427):632–44.
124. Shinn J, Kwon N, Lee SA, Lee Y. Smart pH-responsive nanomedicines for disease therapy. 52, Journal of Pharmaceutical Investigation. Springer 2022;52:427–41.
125. Adams D, Gonzalez-Duarte A, O'Riordan WD, Yang CC, Ueda M, Kristen A V., et al. Patisiran, an RNAi therapeutic, for hereditary transthyretin amyloidosis. New England Journal of Medicine. 2018 Jul 5;379(1):11–21.
126. Wilson B, Geetha KM. Lipid nanoparticles in the development of mRNA vaccines for COVID-19. Journal of Drug Delivery Science and Technology. Editions de Sante 2022;74.
127. Chen J, Sun X, Shao R, Xu Y, Gao J, Liang W. VEGF siRNA delivered by polycation liposome-encapsulated calcium phosphate nanoparticles for tumor angiogenesis inhibition in breast cancer. Int J Nanomedicine. 2017 Aug 21;12:6075–88.
128. Bender G, Fahrioglu Yamaci R, Taneri B. CRISPR and KRAS: A match yet to be made. Journal of Biomedical Science. BioMed Central Ltd 2021;28.
129. Schultheis B, Strumberg D, Santel A, Vank C, Gebhardt F, Keil O, et al. First-in-human phase I study of the liposomal RNA interference therapeutic Atu027 in patients with advanced solid tumors. Journal of Clinical Oncology [Internet]. 2014;32(36):4141–8. Available from: https://ascopubs.org/doi/abs/10.1200/JCO.2013.55.0376
130. Yen TYC, Abbasi AZ, He C, Lip HY, Park E, Amini MA, et al. Biocompatible and bioactivable terpolymer-lipid-MnO2 Nanoparticle-based MRI contrast agent for improving tumor detection and delineation. Mater Today Bio. 2024 Apr 1;25.
131. Pisano C, Cecere SC, Di Napoli M, Cavaliere C, Tambaro R, Facchini G, et al. Clinical trials with pegylated liposomal doxorubicin in the treatment of ovarian cancer. J Drug Deliv. 2013 Mar 14;2013:1–12.
132. Lopez J, Powles T, Braiteh F, Siu LL, LoRusso P, Friedman CF, et al. Autogene cevumeran with or without atezolizumab in advanced solid tumors: A phase 1 trial. Nat Med. 2025 Jan 1;31(1):152–64.
133. Mehta M, Bui TA, Yang X, Aksoy Y, Goldys EM, Deng W. Lipid-based nanoparticles for drug/gene delivery: An overview of the production techniques and difficulties encountered in their industrial development. ACS Materials Au. 2023 Nov 8;3(6):600–19.

134. Hu C, Qian A, Wang Q, Xu F, He Y, Xu J, et al. Industrialization of lipid nanoparticles: From laboratory-scale to large-scale production line. European Journal of Pharmaceutics and Biopharmaceutics. 2016 Dec;109:206–13.
135. Roces CB, Lou G, Jain N, Abraham S, Thomas A, Halbert GW, et al. Manufacturing considerations for the development of lipid nanoparticles using microfluidics. Pharmaceutics. 2020 Nov 15;12(11):1095.
136. VandenBerg MA, Dong X, Smith WC, Tian G, Stephens O, O'Connor TF, et al. Learning from the future: Towards continuous manufacturing of nanomaterials. AAPS Open. 2025 Mar 17;11(1):7.
137. Ball R, Bajaj P, Whitehead K. Achieving long-term stability of lipid nanoparticles: Examining the effect of pH, temperature, and lyophilization. Int J Nanomedicine. 2016 Dec;12:305–15.
138. Gomes-da-Silva LC, Fonseca NA, Moura V, Pedroso de Lima MC, Simões S, Moreira JN. Lipid-based nanoparticles for siRNA delivery in cancer therapy: Paradigms and challenges. Acc Chem Res. 2012 Jul 17;45(7):1163–71.
139. del Pozo-Rodríguez A, Solinís MA, Gascón AR, Pedraz JL. Short- and long-term stability study of lyophilized solid lipid nanoparticles for gene therapy. European Journal of Pharmaceutics and Biopharmaceutics. 2009 Feb;71(2):181–9.
140. Sheth P, Sandhu H, Singhal D, Malick W, Shah N, Serpil Kislalioglu M. Nanoparticles in the pharmaceutical industry and the use of supercritical fluid technologies for nanoparticle production. Curr Drug Deliv. 2012 Apr 1;9(3):269–84.
141. Isibor PO. Regulations and policy considerations for nanoparticle safety. In: Environmental Nanotoxicology. Cham: Springer Nature Switzerland; 2024. p. 295–316.
142. Szebeni J, Storm G. Complement activation as a bioequivalence issue relevant to the development of generic liposomes and other nanoparticulate drugs. Biochem Biophys Res Commun. 2015 Dec; 468(3):490–7.
143. Souto EB, Martins-Lopes P, Lopes CM, Gaivão I, Silva AM, Guedes-Pinto H. A note on regulatory concerns and toxicity assessment in lipid-based delivery systems (LDS). J Biomed Nanotechnol. 2009 Aug 1;5(4):317–22.
144. Sharifi S, Mahmoud NN, Voke E, Landry MP, Mahmoudi M. Importance of standardizing analytical characterization methodology for improved reliability of the nanomedicine literature. Nanomicro Lett. 2022 Dec 20;14(1):172.
145. Clogston JD, Foss W, Harris D, Oberoi H, Pan J, Pu E, et al. Current state of nanomedicine drug products: An industry perspective. J Pharm Sci. 2024 Dec;113(12):3395–405.
146. Cui L, Pereira S, Sonzini S, van Pelt S, Romanelli SM, Liang L, et al. Development of a high-throughput platform for screening lipid nanoparticles for mRNA delivery. Nanoscale. 2022;14(4):1480–91.
147. Chan C, Du S, Dong Y, Cheng X. Computational and experimental approaches to investigate lipid nanoparticles as drug and gene delivery systems. Curr Top Med Chem. 2021 Jan 11;21(2):92–114.
148. Bhujel R, Enkmann V, Burgstaller H, Maharjan R. Artificial intelligence-driven strategies for targeted delivery and enhanced stability of RNA-based lipid nanoparticle cancer vaccines. Pharmaceutics. 2025 Jul 30;17(8):992.

4 Polymeric-Nanoparticles for Cancer Therapy

Priyanka Tyagi,[1] Megha Gupta,[2] Rakshita Yadav,[2] Khushboo,[2] Shaheen,[2] Nilay Solanki,[3] and Rachana R.[4]
[1]Department of Botany, Maitreyi College, University of Delhi, Chanakyapuri, New Delhi, India
[2]Department of Basic and Applied Sciences, School of Engineering and Sciences, G D Goenka University, Gurugram, Haryana, India
[3]Ramanbhai Patel College of Pharmacy, Charotar University of Science and Technology, CHARUSAT Campus, Changa, Gujarat, India
[4]Department of Biotechnology, Jaypee Institute of Information Technology, Noida, Uttar Pradesh, India

4.1 INTRODUCTION

Cancer is one of the most important challenges faced by the world today, with an urgent need for an efficient and safe treatment approach. Commonly used anticancer medications, such as paclitaxel, docetaxel, cisplatin, methotrexate, carboplatin, and bleomycin, suffer from low aqueous solubility and toxicity, leading to inappropriate action, which has raised a crucial demand to create innovative delivery methods (Nazir et al., 2014). Nanotechnology has transformed the field of drug delivery in oncology by offering innovative strategies for cancer therapy. In recent years, polymeric nanoparticles (PNPs) have surfaced as a promising platform for targeted delivery of anticancer drugs (Parveen & Sahoo, 2008), as shown in Table 4.1. These nano-sized materials minimize systemic toxicity while enabling targeted drug delivery, extended circulation durations, and improved therapeutic efficacy through encapsulation of therapeutic chemicals within a polymeric matrix (Smith & Jones, 2006). PNPs improve the efficacy of cancer treatment by facilitating targeted delivery of drugs to the action site. They are tailored for cancer therapy using various approaches such as micellar synthesis, polymer-drug conjugation, and surface functionalization for improved biocompatibility (Kedar et al., 2010). The present chapter gives special attention to the incorporation of targeting ligands, such as antibodies and peptides, which enable specific recognition of cancer cells and tissues (Jin et al., 2020).

PNPs improve the solubility, stability, and bioavailability of anticancer agents, enabling their precise delivery into tumor sites while minimizing side effects on the healthy tissues. A variety of biocompatible and biodegradable polymers are utilized for designing PNPs, including poly (lactic-co-glycolic acid) (PLGA), polyethylene glycol (PEG), and chitosan (Prabhu et al., 2015) etc. Engineered PNPs have successfully solved many difficulties associated with conventional chemotherapy, such as limited drug accumulation into tumor tissues, off-target effects, and systemic damage (Maeda et al., 2000). The significance of PNPs in cancer therapy is further scored by their ability to circumvent multidrug resistance (MDR), which is a common obstacle in effective cancer treatment. Encapsulated drugs within the core of PNPs protect them from premature degradation and efflux pumps of cells, thus enhancing drug accumulation at the tumor site (Wang & Langer, 2012). On the other hand,

 DOI: 10.1201/9781003799351-4

surface modification of NPs with targeting ligands (e.g., antibodies and peptides) enables specific recognition of the receptors on the cancer cells, resulting in enhanced selectivity and reducing off-target effects (Peer et al., 2020). The innovative design of PNPs provides sustained and controlled release of the drug, improving the pharmacokinetics and reducing the frequency of administration, making the formulations more patent compliant (Chenthamara et al., 2019). Table 4.1 summarizes different types of PNP developed using natural and artificial polymers for anticancer applications.

TABLE 4.1
Applications, Advantages, and Disadvantages of Commonly Used Polymeric Nanoparticles

Class	Matrix Material	Applications	Advantages	Disadvantages	Ref.
Natural	Chitosan	Hemostatic, medical dressing, hydrogel, drug carrier, gene transfer	Biocompatible, antimicrobial, innocuous, easily degradable, adsorbable, film formation	Poor spinnability, poor strength, low water-solubility	Ding & Guo (2022)
	Starch	Hemostatic, tissue-engineered scaffold, drug carrier, bone repair material	Extensive availability, low price, degradation products safe and non-toxic, non-antigenic	Poor mechanical strength, hydrophobic, poor blocking performance	Pei et al. (2024)
	Alginate	Pharmaceutical excipient, Pepcid complete, medical dressings	Hypo toxicity, biocompatibility, suppresses tumor growth, enhances immunity	Less biodegradable, poor cell attachment	Abasalizadeh et al. (2020)
	Cellulose	Pharmaceutical adjuvant and drug carrier	Extensive availability, cheap	Rare adverse reactions	Islam et al. (2021)
Biosynthetic	poly—beta hydroxy-butyrate (PHB)	Drug carrier, tissue engineering	Biodegradable, safe, non-toxic, good physical and chemical properties	High crystallinity, thermally unstable	Moghaddam et al. (2016)
Synthetic co-polymers	Polylactic (PLA)	Anti-adhesion materials, patch, drug-delivery carrier, bone-fixing device, suture, tissue-engineered scaffold	Biocompatibility, good mechanical properties, safe, non-toxic	Poor toughness, degradation speed slow, hydrophobicity, lack of reactive side chain groups	Tyler et al. (2016)
	Polyurethane	Excipients, medical bandage	Cheap, rich availability, good mechanical properties	Slow degradation	Morales-González et al. (2022)
	Poly (lactic-glycolic acid) (PGLA)	Absorbable suture, drug delivery, bone screw fixation, tissue repair	Controllable biodegradability, biocompatibility	Expensive	Sampath et al. (2014)
	Polymethyl methacrylate resin (PMMA)	Bone-fixation materials, dental materials, artificial crystal	Easy operation, good biocompatibility	Monomer cytotoxicity, quick oxidation	Zhang et al. (2019)

4.2 LOADING OF ANTICANCER AGENTS INTO PNPS

The process of incorporating pharmaceutical ingredients into a carrier system like PNPs is known as "drug loading." It is necessary to load a substantial amount of drug into such systems so as to lower the amount of matrix material to be administered to the patient. In general, the drug is either incorporated at the time of PNP synthesis or the drug molecules get surface adsorbed while incubating the nanocarrier with a concentrated drug solution (Govender et al., 1999) (Panyam et al., 2004). A frequently employed technique is the solvent evaporation method, in which the drug is dissolved or distributed into a polymer solution followed by solvent extraction to create drug-loaded nanoparticles (Bilati et al., 2005). Overall, there are three approaches for loading the anticancer drugs into PNPs.

4.2.1 Physical Encapsulation

Physical encapsulation refers to the method of incorporating drugs or other bioactive agents into nanoparticles (NPs) without chemical bonding of drugs with the polymer matrix. This results in a colloidal drug carrier system made up of aqueous pockets encircled by a hydrophobic membrane (Couvreur et al., 2002) as shown in Figure 4.1. 'Emulsion technique' is commonly employed to create an oil-in-water (O/W) or water-in-oil-in-water (W/O/W) emulsion depicting adequate control over particle size and drug distribution. The drug is dissolved in an organic phase (also containing polymer) followed by evaporation of organic solvent leading to the formation of solid NPs. A relatively simple method is 'Nanoprecipitation', where polymer and drug are dissolved into a solvent followed by adding it to a non-solvent to precipitate the PNPs (Layre, 2005).

There are many other physical encapsulation methods, such as:

- **Microencapsulation**: The process of microencapsulation entails the encapsulation of medicinal molecules in tiny particles or capsules. Spray drying, coacervation, and solvent evaporation are a few techniques that can be used to accomplish microencapsulation. After

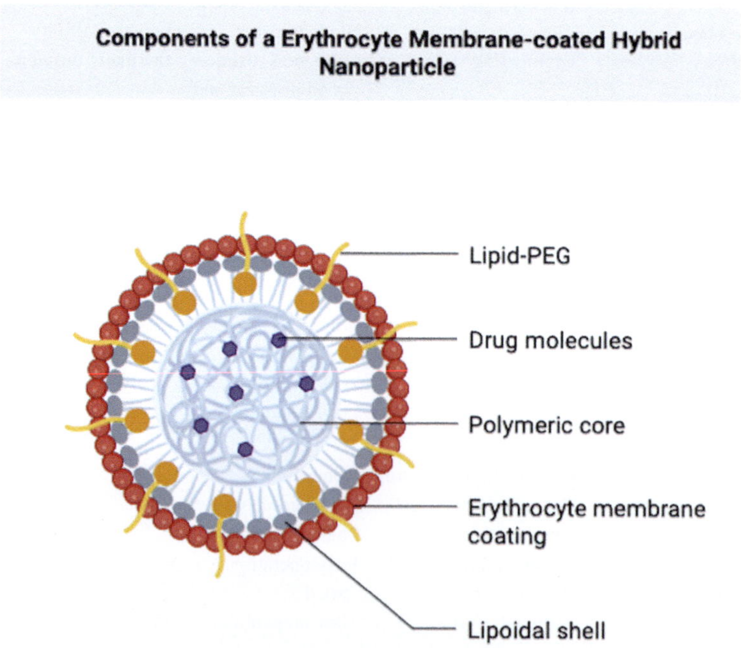

FIGURE 4.1 Physical encapsulation of anticancer drugs into PNPs

the medication has been dissolved or dispersed in a polymer solution, the solvent is withdrawn, leaving the drug-containing solid particles behind.

- **Liposome Encapsulation:** Liposomes are vesicles made of lipid bilayers that have an aqueous core and a lipid membrane that, respectively, can encapsulate hydrophilic and hydrophobic medicinal molecules. Liposome encapsulation offers a flexible drug delivery platform because of its biocompatibility and capacity to transport two different kinds of medicines at once as shown in Figure 4.2.
- **Polymer Matrix Encapsulation:** By using processes like solvent casting, hot melt extrusion, or compression molding, drug molecules can be physically confined inside a polymer matrix. The medicine is distributed throughout the polymer matrix, and the end product is a formulation that can be tablets, films, or implants. However, in view of the toxicity of organic solvents, researchers have developed 'Ionic Gelation' method and 'Supercritical Fluid Technology' to produce uniform sized NPs. The efficiency and stability of the drug within PNPs is determined by techniques like UV-Vi's spectroscopy, HPLC, and various imaging methods.

4.2.2 Chemical Encapsulation

The process of covalent attachment of anticancer drugs to the PNPs is known as chemical encapsulation or conjugation method. The drug's stability, solubility, controlled release, and targeting abilities are all intended to be improved by this method (Adhikari et al., 2017; Markovic et al., 2022). Functional groups on both the drug and polymer, such as amine, carboxyl, or thiol groups, are utilized to form chemical linkages in the presence of coupling agents like carbodiimides (e.g., EDC/NHS) (Singh et al., 2008). The number of reactive sites on the backbone determines the amount of medication loaded in the polymer systems such as polylactic acid (PLA), polyglycolic acid (PGA), and polyethylene glycol (PEG). Many times, a spacer or linker molecule is incorporated between the drug and the polymer to enhance the biophysical properties of the drug-polymer conjugate. These linkers may be cleavable under specific conditions (e.g., pH-sensitive and enzyme-responsive, etc.) to ensure drug release at the target site (Dutta et al., 2019). For instance, hydrazone bonds exhibit prolonged release of drugs in a lower pH environment and significant stability in a neutral pH environment (Tang et al., 2021). A common reduction-responsive linker is the disulfide bond (Sun et al., 2019). To accomplish tumor-targeted medication delivery, these connections can help chemotherapeutic medicines release in tumor cells more quickly and selectively.

4.3 RELEASE OF ANTICANCER AGENTS FROM PNPs

The properties of PNPs and the surrounding biological environment are critical factors for controlling the targeted release of anticancer drugs. Controlled release refers to the movement of drug molecules at a predictable and rationally programmed rate to achieve an optimal serum-drug

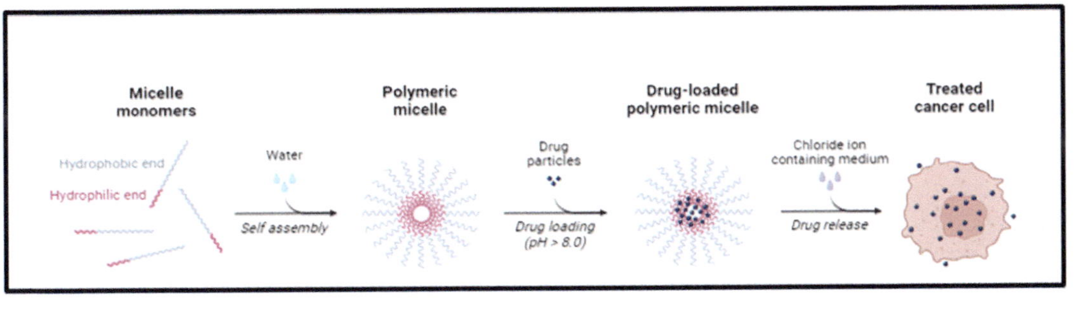

FIGURE 4.2 Micelles feature a hydrophilic shell and a hydrophobic center, the latter being able to encapsulate hydrophobic drugs based on their structure

concentration, as shown in Figure 4.3a and b. The factors influencing drug release profile include chemical composition and structural arrangement (cross-linking density, crystallinity) of the polymer system; molecular weight, solubility, and stability of the loaded drug and size, surface area, and morphology of prepared PNPs (Sokolsky-Papkov et al., 2007). Smaller particles or those with larger surface areas tend to release drugs faster due to higher surface-to-volume ratios (Singh, 2014). Such fine-tuning of the dosage form enhances the safety, efficacy, reliability, and convenience of drug therapy (Rosenbauer et al., 2010).

The simplest mechanisms of drug release from PNPs involve (i) diffusion-controlled process (drug diffusion and matrix degradation), (ii) swelling-controlled release using hydrophilic polymers (hydrogels), (iii) erosion-controlled release via surface erosion or bulk erosion of polymer matrix, and (iv) stimuli responsive release using pH sensitive polymer systems (e.g., acrylates) or temperature- or enzyme-responsive systems such as Poly(N-isopropylacrylamide) and Poly(ethylene glycol)-Poly(ε-caprolactone) (PEG-PCL) copolymer micelles, respectively as shown in Figure 4.3a.

4.4 FUNCTIONALIZATION STRATEGIES TO ENHANCE TARGETING

Functionalization techniques are essential for enhancing the targeting power of drug loading systems, providing accurate and effective delivery of therapeutic substances to targeted body locations. Through the customization of drug carrier surface chemistry, scientists can use diverse biological stimuli and interactions to accomplish targeted accumulation at specific target tissues

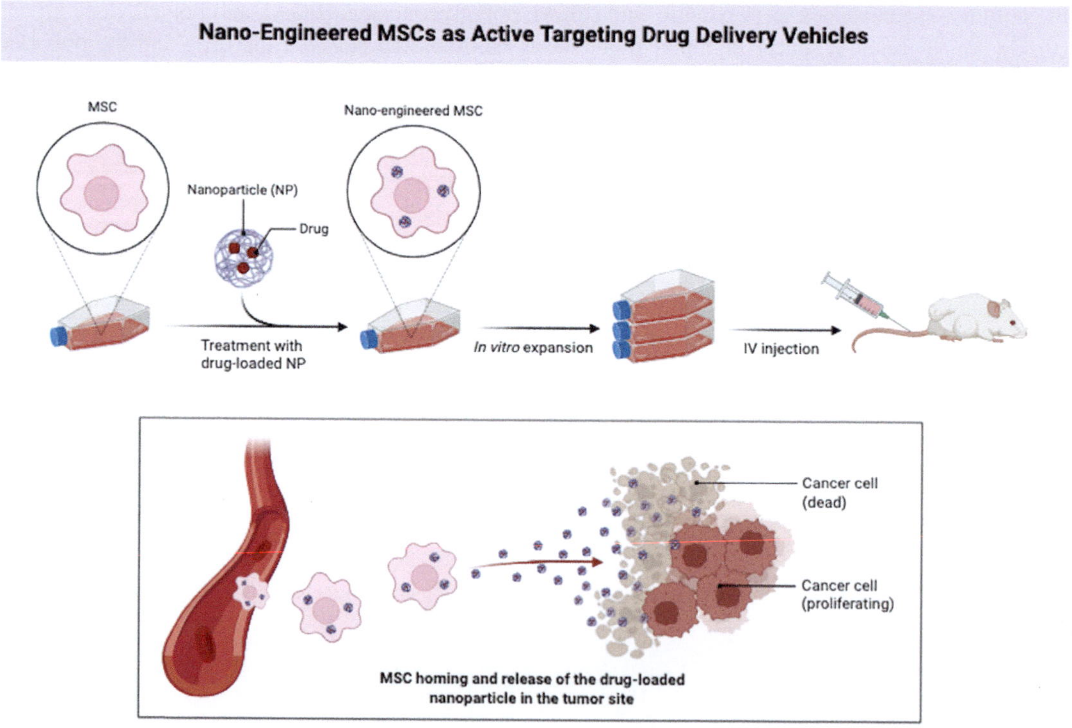

FIGURE 4.3 (a) Diffusion targeting drug delivery vehicle; (b) stimuli-responsive nanocarriers for drug delivery to the tumor site.

or cells. Targeting moieties that identify overexpressed receptors on sick cells can be attached by strategies like ligand conjugation, which makes it easier for receptor-mediated endocytosis and internalization of drug-loaded carriers. Through pH-responsive functionalization, regulated drug release is triggered at the target place by taking advantage of the acidic milieu found in intracellular compartments or tumor tissues. Stealth coatings also reduce nonspecific interactions, increasing accumulation at target areas and extending circulation time (Chenthamara et al., 2019). Researchers have discussed various functionalization strategies that enhance targeting capabilities, such as surface modification with antibodies or small molecules that specifically bind to cancer cell receptors (Park, 2017). In yet another review, various polymer and linker designs that enable precise cleavage by target enzymes have been suggested for improving the therapeutic index of anticancer drugs (Shahriari et al., 2019)

4.4.1 Mechanism of Action

Modern oncology aims at increasing the efficacy of therapeutic agents while minimizing the adverse side effects associated with traditional chemotherapy. This may be achieved via a) active or b) passive targeting of the drugs to the site using different strategies like using PNPs, taking into account the biocompatibility, safety, efficacy, and regulatory aspects of NPs manufacturing.

4.4.2 Active Targeting

Active targeting process involves the modification of PNPs with specific ligands (molecules that attach particularly to overexpressed receptors on cancer cells), such as antibodies, peptides, or small molecules, leading to selective localization of loaded drugs to the intended site of action (Varkouhi et al., 2011). For instance, overexpressed folate receptors on cancer cells can be targeted using folate- or vitamin B9-conjugated PNPs (Bellotti et al., 2009). Ligands play an important role in guiding the drugs to specific cells or tissues, enhancing the precision and efficiency of drug delivery. Once targeting ligands are selected, it becomes necessary to explore the complex mechanism controlling ligand attachment in order to maximize the effectiveness of the targeted system (Yan et al., 2024). Ligands attached to PEG-based PNPs are displayed on the particle surface leading to prolonged circulation and controlled drug release thereby creating an ideal system for targeted delivery (Yoo & Park, 2004). The longer the particles stay in blood circulation, the more would be the chances to interact with target receptors on the cancer cells, thus increasing the efficacy of targeted delivery systems.

4.4.3 Passive Targeting

Passive targeting approach is based on the unique characteristics of the tumor microenvironment without the need of ligands, primarily the enhanced permeability and retention (EPR) effect, a phenomenon observed in many types of tumor (Kim & Cho, 2022). Ignoring the use of ligands makes the design and production of nanoparticles simpler and potentially less expensive. Extremely rapid growth of the tumor cells necessitates the formation of new blood vessels, called angiogenesis. Such vessels are typically abnormal with wide fenestrations in the endothelial layer leading to enhanced permeability as shown in Figure 4.4. This property of the tumor microenvironment is exploited to allow anticancer drugs carrying PNPs (10–200 nm) to penetrate into the tumor interstitial (Bazak et al., 2014). Once nanoparticles enter the tumor site, they are less likely to be removed quickly due to poor lymphatic drainage systems. However, considering the significant variation in the extent of EPR effect in different types of tumors, between patients, and even within different areas of the same tumor, physicochemical properties of PNPs (size, shape, surface charge and hydrophobicity/hydrophilicity balance) become important in the efficacy of treatment.

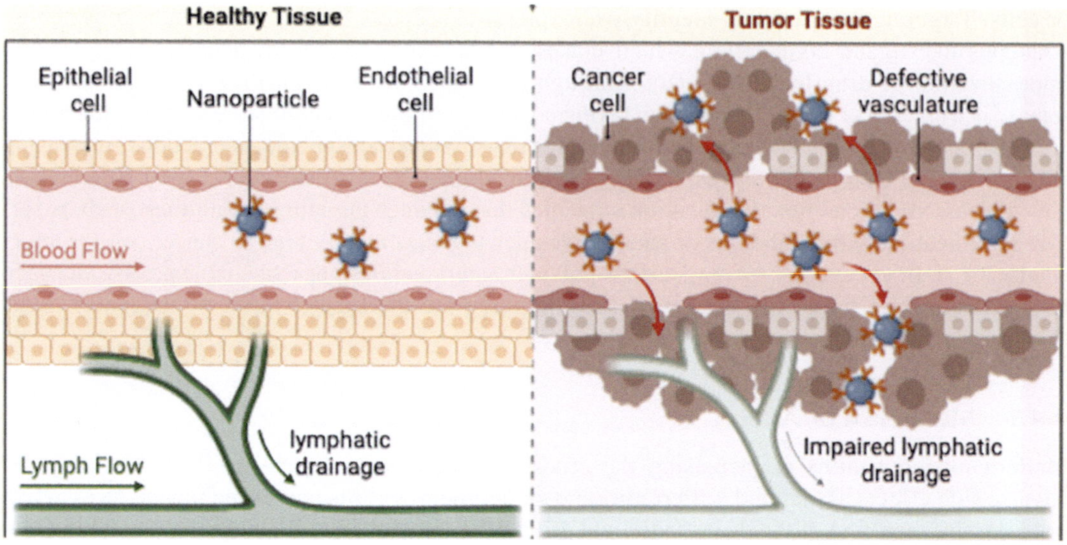

FIGURE 4.4 Enhanced permeability of blood vessels inside tumor due to abnormal wide fenestrations allow entry of drug carrying PNPs.

4.5 PRE-CLINICAL AND CLINICAL TRIALS WITH PNPs

The efficacy, safety, and pharmacokinetics of newly designed and engineered PNPs need to be tested in preclinical animal studies before human clinical trials are carried out (Kim et al., 2001). Common animal models for cancer therapy include i) transgenic and xenograft models of rodents (rats, mice) owing to their ease of handling and well-characterized genetics and physiology, and ii) larger animal models like rabbits and dogs when larger blood volumes are needed for pharmacokinetic analysis. The preclinical evaluation is done through imaging techniques (MRI, PET, CT scan), biochemical analysis of blood and tissues, histopathological examination under microscope, and Pk/Pd analysis to determine the absorption, distribution, metabolism, and excretion of the drug (Li et al., 2020). All animal studies must comply with national and international regulations on the ethical use of animals in research, such as the Guide for the Care and Use of Laboratory Animals (Yang et al., 2013). Extensive pre-clinical research is followed by human clinical trials to ensure that the new treatment is both effective and safe for human use. A list of PNPs under clinical trials for cancer treatment and the patented materials is shown in Tables 4.2 and 4.3, respectively. Researchers may use databases such as ClinicalTrials.gov to fetch detailed information on ongoing and completed clinical trials worldwide.

4.6 DIAGNOSTIC AND THERAGNOSTIC APPLICATIONS OF PNPs IN CANCER TREATMENT

The breakthrough of nanotechnology provides a novel approach for upgrading traditional treatments along with precise, accurate diagnosis and continuous monitoring of the disease (Dristant et al., 2023). PNPs can be loaded with imaging agents (e.g., gadolinium, iron oxide, or fluorescent dyes) and targeted to tumor site to enhance contrast in imaging modalities such as MRI, PET, or optical imaging as shown in Figure 4.5. This allows a real-time monitoring of tumor progression in the patient body and the assessment of treatment efficacy. The combined diagnostic and therapeutic capabilities offered by PNPs facilitate a personalized treatment approach allowing the physicians to track real-time movement of drugs and indicate any changes in treatment plans based on the tumor response.

TABLE 4.2
List of Polymeric Nanoparticles under Clinical Trials

Product	Type	Chemical structure	Phase	Application	Ref.
ABI-009	Albumin based nanoparticle	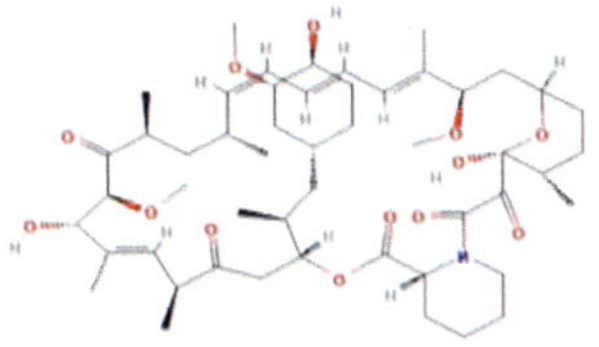	Phase I/II	Solid tumor	Wagner et al. (2021)
Nanotax	Polymer based nanoparticle	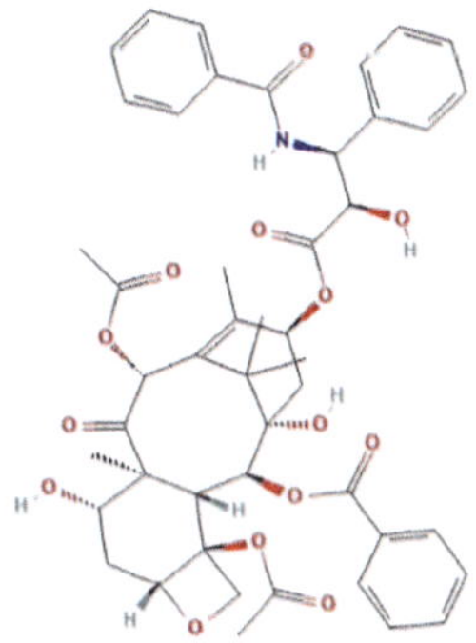	Phase I	Peritoneal neoplasms	Pandey & Dureja (2018)
BIND-014	PEG-PLGA Polymer based nanoparticle	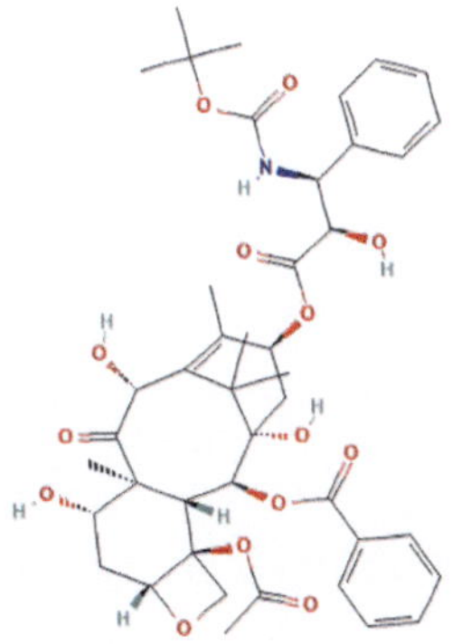	Phase I/II	NSCLC	Chen et al., 2016
Docetaxel-PNP	Polymer based nanoparticle	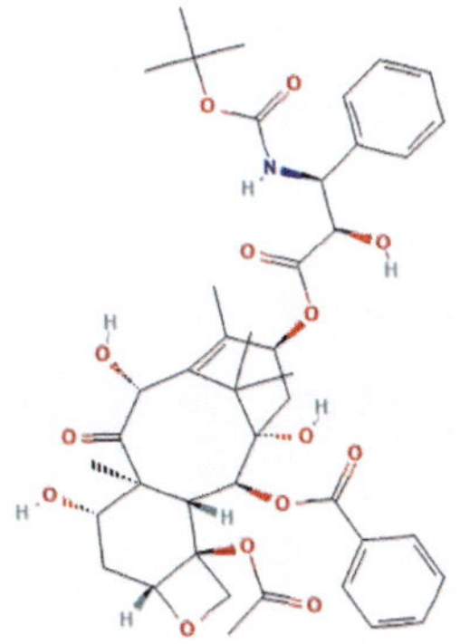	Phase I	Solid tumor	Chen et al., 2016

(Continued)

TABLE 4.2 ***(Continued)***
List of Polymeric Nanoparticles under Clinical Trials

Product	Type	Chemical structure	Phase	Application	Ref.
Cyclosert	Cyclodextrin based nanoporticle	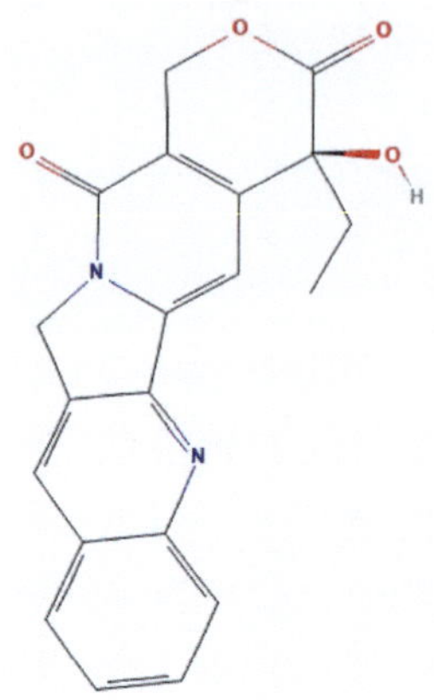	Phase I/II	Renal cell carcinoma, solid tumor, NSCLC, rectal cancer	Liu et al., 2022
Abraxane	Albumin based nanoparticle	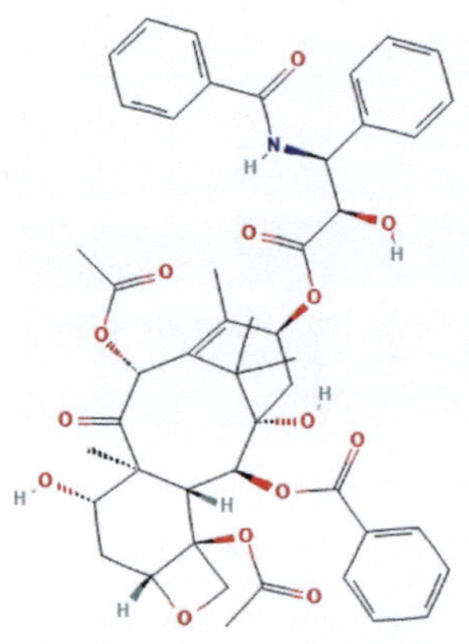	Approved	Pancreatic cancer, NSCLC, breast cancer	Liu et al., 2022
DHAD-PBCA-NPs	Polymer based nanoparticle	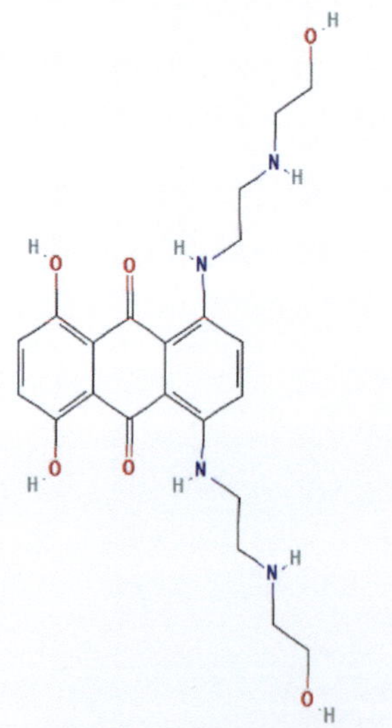	Phase II	Hepatocellular carcinoma	Liu et al., 2022

TABLE 4.2 *(Continued)*
List of Polymeric Nanoparticles under Clinical Trials

Product	Type	Chemical structure	Phase	Application	Ref.
BA-003	Polymer based nanoparticle	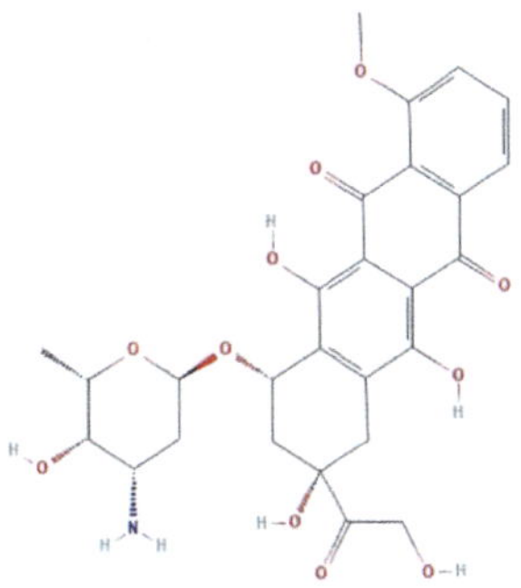	Phase III	Hepatocellular carcinoma	Pandey & Dureja, 2018
ABI-008	Albumin based nanoparticle	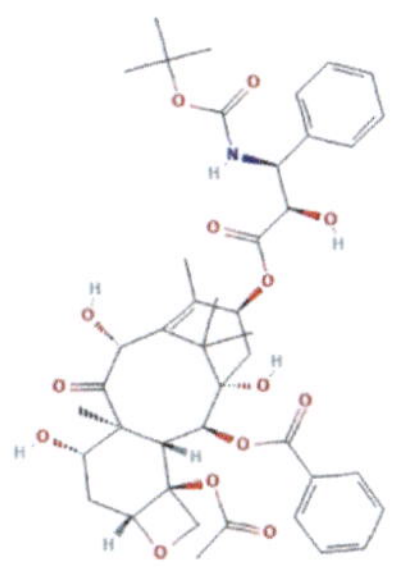	Phase I/II	Prostate cancer	Pandey & Dureja, 2018
ProLindac	HPMA-polymeric nanoparticle	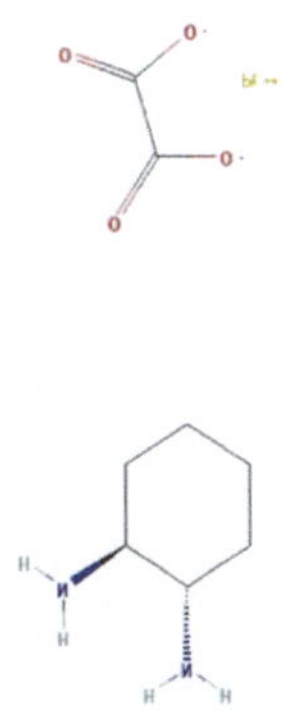	Phase II/III	Advanced ovarian cancer	Wheate & Walker, 2010

4.7 SAFETY CONCERNS

Nanomaterials offer several advantages because of their high surface/ volume ratio, high reactivity, and tunable characteristic features. However, there are concerns regarding danger to the environment and public health (Ray et al., 2009). These concerns primarily relate to the interaction of nanomaterials with biological systems and the unexpected toxicological effects (Saleh, 2021). The major safety issues associated with PNPs includes the following:

- **Matrix material safety**—Some polymers or their degradation products could potentially elicit an immune response or cause inflammation. On the other hand, non-biodegradable polymers may accumulate and result in long-term health issues.

TABLE 4.3
Recent Patents in PNPs for Cancer Therapy

Study Title	Patent no.	Original assignee	Grant year	Ref.
Treating liver cancer and inhibition of metastasis with nanoparticles targeting chemokine receptor type-4 (CXCR4).	US9415011B1	National Tsing Hua University, USA	2016	Chen et al., 2016
Method for synthesizing curcumin loaded (in a hydrophobic core) polymer-based nanoparticles with a hydrophilic shell with one or more chemotherapeutic agents.	US20130330412A1	The Johns Hopkins University, Baltimore, MD, USA	2013	Maitra & Pramanik, 2013
Therapeutic nanoparticle that includes an active agent or therapeutic agent, e.g. vinorelbine or vincristine or pharmaceutically acceptable salts thereof, and one, two, or three biocompatible polymers.	US9351933B2	Bind Therapeutics, Inc., USA	2016	Zale et al., 2016
Disclosing therapeutic nanoparticles comprising about 1 to about 20 weights% of a mechanistic target of rapamycin (mTOR, an atypical serine/threonine kinase) inhibitor and to about 70 to 99 weight% biocompatible polymers.	US9579284B2	Pfizer Inc., USA	2017	Zale et al., 2016
Discussing the nanoparticles of polyester having properties suited for encapsulating fluorescent dyes together with therapeutic drugs, resulting in theragnostic particles, useful in therapeutic treatments and diagnostic methods of cancer.	US9555008B2	University of Central Florida Research Foundation, Inc., USA	2017	Perez & Santra, 2017
Delivering a drug as nanoparticles for killing tumor cells in association with ultrasound (ranging from low to medium intensity).	US9138476B2	Academia Sinica, USA	2015	Kosheleva et al., 2015

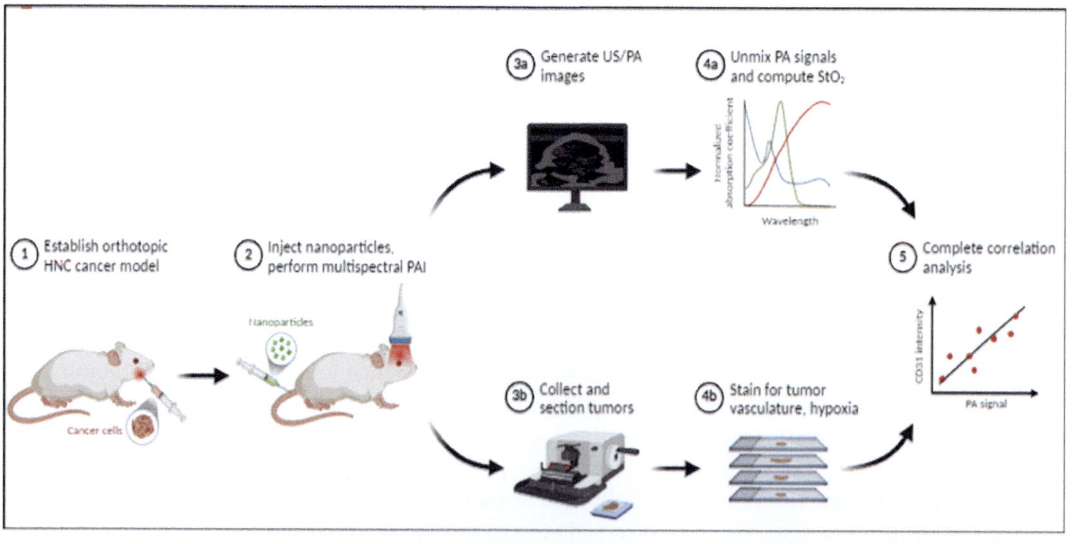

FIGURE 4.5 (a) Magnetic resonance imaging (MRI) of cancer cells, (b) CT scan with single Positron emission tomography (PET), (c) photoacoustic imaging of cancer model.

- **Genotoxicity**—Certain engineered polymeric materials may damage DNA, therefore, evaluating the genotoxic potential of PNPs is essential.
- **Protein Corona Formation**—When nanoparticles enter the bloodstream, proteins can adsorb on their surface, forming a "protein corona" that interferes with their interaction mechanism, thereby triggering an immune response or leading to rapid clearance from circulation.
- **Eco-toxicity**—The potential accumulation of PNPs in ecosystems and their effect on wildlife and plant life are important considerations.

4.8 CHALLENGES IN PNPs DRUG DELIVERY SYSTEMS

Despite several advantages offered by PNPs, there are various challenges associated with their development and clinical applications. The main challenge includes avoiding systemic toxicity and inflammation caused by the accumulation of PNPs in tissues. To address this limitation, research groups widely utilize biodegradable polymers in the development of PNPs, such as polylactic acid, poly lactic glycolic acid, and polycaprolactone that help reduce toxicity, improve drug release, and enhance biocompatibility. Additionally, natural polymers like alginate, chitosan, albumin, and gelatin have also been used in the development of PNPs (Cheng, 2021). Another challenge is to conjugate specific ligands onto the PNPs due to complexity of the surface and missed accuracy of the conjugation reaction. This poses challenges in evaluating and scaling up the formulation development process. Also, ensuring the reproducibility is a major concern to make the process cost-effective. Lack of standardized guidelines specific to nanoparticles complicates the approval process.

4.9 CONCLUSION AND FUTURE PROSPECTS

PNPs stand at the forefront of innovations in cancer treatment, presenting versatile applications in both diagnostics and therapeutics. Over the past decade, there has been a remarkable advancement in development of biodegradable and/or stimuli-responsive PNPs, resulting in the emergence of tailored properties. These advanced PNPs have been specifically designed to achieve site-specific controlled delivery, ensuring the safety of delivered agents, and prolonged circulation times. The continuous progress in this field holds great promise for improving targeted therapies and enhancing patient outcomes.

A multidisciplinary approach involving chemistry, biology, materials science, engineering, and regulatory science is necessary to overcome current challenges associated with PNPs in oncology. There is an urgent need to improve synthesis and formulation techniques to enhance reproducibility, scalability, and stability of NPs. Smart materials may be developed, which can respond to specific biological signals to improve delivery efficiency and reduce side effects. On the other hand, a better prediction and mitigation of immune responses is necessary to enhance the understanding of PNPs-biology interactions. Additionally, development of more specific guidelines and tests for nanoparticle therapies would unlock the full potential of PNPs in drug delivery systems. The use of multi-material printing and three-dimensional (3D) printing integrates the benefits of multiple functional materials with promising potential in fulfilling the need for patient-centric personalized treatment (Kapoor et al., 2025). Several inner complex structures like stromal tissues and channels of different sizes may be printed through 3D printing techniques.

REFERENCES

Abasalizadeh, F., Moghaddam, S. V., Alizadeh, E., Akbari, E., Kashani, E., Fazljou, S. M. B., & Akbarzadeh, A. (2020). Alginate-based hydrogels as drug delivery vehicles in cancer treatment and their applications in wound dressing and 3D bioprinting. Journal of Biological Engineering, 14, 1–22.

Adhikari, R., Agostini, M., Ky, N. A., Araki, T., Archidiacono, M., Bahr, M., . . . & Zuber, K. (2017). A white paper on keV sterile neutrino dark matter. Journal of Cosmology and Astroparticle Physics, 2017(01), 025.

Bazak, R., Houri, M., El Achy, S., Hussein, W., & Refaat, T. (2014). Passive targeting of nanoparticles to cancer: A comprehensive review of the literature. Molecular and Clinical Oncology, 2(6), 904–908.

Bellotti, E., Cascone, M. G., Barbani, N., Rossin, D., Rastaldo, R., Giachino, C., Cristallini, C. (2021). Targeting Cancer Cells Overexpressing Folate Receptors with New Terpolymer-Based Nanocapsules: Toward a Novel Targeted DNA Delivery System for Cancer Therapy. Biomedicines, 9(9), 1275.

Bilati, U., Allémann, E., & Doelker, E. (2005). Development of a nanoprecipitation method intended for the entrapment of hydrophilic drugs into nanoparticles. European Journal of Pharmaceutical Sciences, 24(1), 67–75.

Chen, Y. C., Liu, J. Y., & Gao, D. Y. (2016a). Method for treatment of liver cancer and inhibition of metastasis with CXC-chemokine-receptor 4-targeted nanoparticle. US Patent 9415011B1.

Chen, Y. C., Liu, J. Y., & Gao, D. Y. (2016b). U.S. Patent No. 9,415,011. Washington, DC: U.S. Patent and Trademark Office.

Cheng, Y. (2021). Design of Polymers for Intracellular Protein and Peptide Delivery. Chinese Journal of Chemistry, 39, 1443–1449.

Chenthamara, D., Subramaniam, S., Ramakrishnan, S. G., Krishnaswamy, S., Essa, M. M., Lin, F. H., & Qoronfleh, M. W. (2019). Therapeutic efficacy of nanoparticles and routes of administration. Biomaterials Research, 23(1), 20.

Couvreur, P., Barratt, G., Fattal, E., Legrand, P., & Vauthier, C. (2002). Nanocapsule technology: a review. Critical reviews in therapeutic drug carrier systems, 19(2), 99–134.

Ding, J., & Guo, Y. (2022). Recent advances in chitosan and its derivatives in cancer treatment. Frontiers in Pharmacology, 13, 888740.

Dristant, U., Mukherjee, K., Saha, S., & Maity, D. (2023). An overview of polymeric nanoparticles-based drug delivery system in cancer treatment. Technology in Cancer Research & Treatment, 22, 1533033 8231152083.

Govender, T., Stolnik, S., Garnett, M. C., Illum, L., & Davis, S. S. (1999). PLGA nanoparticles prepared by nanoprecipitation: Drug loading and release studies of a water-soluble drug. Journal of Controlled Release, 57(2), 171–185.

Islam, S. U., Ul-Islam, M., Ahsan, H., Ahmed, M. B., Shehzad, A., Fatima, A., & Lee, Y. S. (2021). Potential applications of bacterial cellulose and its composites for cancer treatment. International Journal of Biological Macromolecules, 168, 301–309.

Jin, C., Wang, K., Oppong-Gyebi, A., & Hu, J. (2020). Application of nanotechnology in cancer diagnosis and therapy-a mini-review. International Journal of Medical Sciences, 17(18), 2964.

Kedar, U., Phutane, P., Shidhaye, S., & Kadam, V. (2010). Advances in polymeric micelles for drug delivery and tumor targeting. Nanomedicine: Nanotechnology, Biology and Medicine, 6(6), 714–729.

Kim, S. K., & Cho, S. W. (2022). The Evasion Mechanisms of Cancer Immunity and Drug Intervention in the Tumor Microenvironment. Frontiers in Pharmacology, 13, 868695.

Kim, S. C., Kim, D. W., Shim, Y. H., Bang, J. S., Oh, H. S., Kim, S. W., & Seo, M. H. (2001). In vivo evaluation of polymeric micellar paclitaxel formulation: Toxicity and efficacy. Journal of Controlled Release, 72(1–3), 191–202.

Kosheleva, O. K., Lai, P., Chen, N. G., Hsiao, M., & Chen, C.-H. (2015). Nanoparti-cle-assisted ultrasound for cancer therapy. US Patent 9138476B2.

Layre, A. M., Gref, R., Richard, J., Requier, D., Chacun, H., Appel, M., Domb, A. J., & Couvreur, P. (2005). Nanoencapsulation of a crystalline drug. International journal of pharmaceutics, 298(2), 323–327.

Li, J., Li, X., de Cui, F., Du, Y. Z., Yuan, H., & Hu, F. Q. (2008). Folate-conjugated polymer micelles for active targeting to cancer cells: Preparation, in vitro evaluation of targeting ability and cytotoxicity. Nanotechnology, 19(4), 045102.

Li, Q., Li, X., & Zhao, C. (2020). Strategies to obtain encapsulation and controlled release of small hydrophilic molecules. Frontiers in Bioengineering and Biotechnology, 8, 437.

Liu, L., Dehner, C., Grandhi, N., Lyu, Y., Borcherding, D. C., Chrisinger, J. S., . . . & Hirbe, A. C. (2022). The impact of TSC-1 and-2 mutations on response to therapy in malignant PEComa: A multicenter retrospective analysis. Genes, 13(11), 1932.

Maitra, A., & Pramanik, D. (2013). Smart polymeric nanoparticles which overcome multidrug resistance to cancer therapeutics and treatment-related systemic toxicity. US Patent 20130330412A1.

Markovic, M. D., Panic, V. V., Savic, S. I., Ugrinovic, V. D., Pjanovic, R. V., Spasojevic, M. M., & Spasojevic, P. M. (2022). Biobased thermo/pH sensitive poly (N-isopropylacrylamide-co-crotonic acid) hydrogels for targeted drug delivery. Microporous and Mesoporous Materials, 335, 111817.

Moghaddam, S., Taghi Khorasani, M., Hosseinkazemi, H., Biazar, E., & Fazeli, M. (2016). Fabrication of polyhydroxy butyrate (PHB)/γ-Fe2O3 nanocomposite film and its properties study. Journal of Biomaterials Science, Polymer edition, 27(9), 793–804.

Morales-González, M., Díaz, L. E., Dominguez-Paz, C., & Valero, M. F. (2022). Insights into the design of polyurethane dressings suitable for the stages of skin wound-healing: A systematic review. Polymers, 14(15), 2990.

Nazir, S., Hussain, T., Ayub, A., Rashid, U., & MacRobert, A. J. (2014). Nanomaterials in combating cancer: Therapeutic applications and developments. Nanomedicine: Nanotechnology, Biology and Medicine, 10(1), 19–34.

Pandey, P., & Dureja, H. (2018). Recent patents on polymeric nanoparticles for cancer therapy. Recent Patents on Nanotechnology, 12(2), 155–169.

Panyam, J., Williams, D., Dash, A., Leslie-Pelecky, D., & Labhasetwar, V. (2004). Solid-state solubility influences encapsulation and release of hydrophobic drugs from PLGA/PLA nanoparticles. Journal of Pharmaceutical Sciences, 93(7), 1804–1814.

Park, K. (2017). The drug delivery field at the inflection point: Time to fight its way out of the egg. Journal of Controlled Release, 267, 2–14.

Parveen, S., & Sahoo, S. K. (2008). Polymeric Nanoparticles for Cancer Therapy. Journal of Drug Targeting, 16(2), 108–123.

Pei, J., Yan, Y., Jayaraman, S., Rajagopal, P., Natarajan, P. M., Umapathy, V. R., . . . & Mironescu, M. (2024). A review on advancements in the application of starch-based nanomaterials in biomedicine: Precision drug delivery and cancer therapy. International Journal of Biological Macromolecules, 130746.

Perez, J. M., & Santra, S. (2017). Synthesis of hyperbranched amphiphilic polyester and theranostic nanoparticles thereof. US Patent 9555008.

Prabhu, H. R., Patravale V. B., & Joshi M. D. (2015). Polymeric nanoparticles for targeted treatment in oncology: Current insights. International Journal of Nanomedicine, 10, 1001–1018.

Ray, P. C., Yu, H., & Fu, P. P. (2009). Toxicity and environmental risks of nanomaterials: challenges and future needs. Journal of environmental science and health. Part C, Environmental carcinogenesis & ecotoxicology reviews, 27(1), 1–35.

Rosenbauer, E. M., Wagner, M., Musyanovych, A., & Landfester, K. (2010). Controlled release from polyurethane nanocapsules via pH-, UV-light-or temperature-induced stimuli. Macromolecules, 43(11), 5083–5093.

Saleh, T. A. (2021). Protocols for synthesis of nanomaterials, polymers, and green materials as adsorbents for water treatment technologies. Environmental Technology & Innovation, 24, 101821.

Sampath, M., Lakra, R., Korrapati, P., & Sengottuvelan, B. (2014). Curcumin loaded poly (lactic-co-glycolic) acid nanofiber for the treatment of carcinoma. Colloids and Surfaces B: Bio Interfaces, 117, 128–134.

Shahriari, M., Zahiri, M., Abnous, K., Taghdisi, S. M., Ramezani, M., & Alibolandi, M. (2019). Enzyme responsive drug delivery systems in cancer treatment. Journal of Controlled Release, 308, 172–189.

Singh, D., McMillan, J. M., Kabanov, A. V., Sokolsky-Papkov, M., & Gendelman, H. E. (2014). Bench-to-bedside translation of magnetic nanoparticles. Nanomedicine, 9(4), 501–516.

Singh, N., Kamath, V., Narasimhamurthy, K., & Rajini, P. S. (2008). Protective effect of potato peel extract against carbon tetrachloride-induced liver injury in rats. Environmental Toxicology and Pharmacology, 26(2), 241–246.

Smith, A. B., & Jones, C. D. (2006). Polymeric nanoparticles for cancer therapy: Advantages and challenges. Journal of Nanomedicine, 10(5), 123–135

Sokolsky-Papkov, M., Agashi, K., Olaye, A., Shakesheff, K., & Domb, A. J. (2007). Polymer carriers for drug delivery in tissue engineering. Advanced drug delivery reviews, 59(4-5), 187–206.

Sun, Q., Bi, H., Wang, Z., Li, C., Wang, X., Xu, J., . . . & Yang, P. (2019). Hyaluronic acid-targeted and pH-responsive drug delivery system based on metal-organic frameworks for efficient antitumor therapy. Biomaterials, 223, 119473.

Tang, L., He, S., Yin, Y., Liu, H., Hu, J., Cheng, J., & Wang, W. (2021). Combination of nanomaterials in cell-based drug delivery systems for cancer treatment. Pharmaceutics, 13(11), 1888.

Tyler, B., Gullotti, D., Mangraviti, A., Utsuki, T., & Brem, H. (2016). Polylactic acid (PLA) controlled delivery carriers for biomedical applications. Advanced Drug Delivery Reviews, 107, 163–175.

Varkouhi, A. K., Lammers, T., Schiffelers, R. M., Van Steenbergen, M. J., Hennink, W. E., & Storm, G. (2011). Gene silencing activity of siRNA polyplexes based on biodegradable polymers. European Journal of Pharmaceutics and Biopharmaceutics, 77(3), 450–457.

Wagner, A. J., Ravi, V., Riedel, R. F., Ganjoo, K., Van Tine, B. A., Chugh, R., . . . & Dickson, M. A. (2021). nab-Sirolimus for patients with malignant perivascular epithelioid cell tumors. Journal of Clinical Oncology, 39(33), 3660.

Wang, A.Z., Langer, R., Farokhzad, O.C. (2012). Nanoparticle delivery of cancer drugs, Annual Review of Medicine. 63, 185–198.

Wheate, N. J., Walker, S., Craig, G. E., & Oun, R. (2010). The status of platinum anticancer drugs in the clinic and in clinical trials. Dalton Transactions, 39(35), 8113–8127.

Yan, Y., Ju, J., Dong, S., Wang, Y., Huang, L., Cui, L., & Cui, G. (2021). In situ polymerization permeated three-dimensional Li+-percolated porous oxide ceramic framework boosting all solid-state lithium metal battery. Advanced Science, 8(9), 2003887.

Yan, S., Na, J., Liu, X., Wu, P. (2024). Different Targeting Ligands-Mediated Drug Delivery Systems for Tumor Therapy. Pharmaceutics. 16(2), 248.

Yang, Y., Pan, D., Luo, K., Li, L., & Gu, Z. (2013). Biodegradable and amphiphilic block copolymer–doxorubicin conjugate as polymeric nanoscale drug delivery vehicle for breast cancer therapy. Biomaterials, 34(33), 8430–8443.

Yoo, H. S., & Park, T. G. (2004). Folate receptor targeted biodegradable polymeric doxorubicin micelles. Journal of Controlled Release, 96(2), 273–283.

Zale, S. E., Troiano, G., Ali, M. M., Hrkach, J., & Wright, J. (2017). Therapeutic polymeric nanoparticles with mTOR inhibitors and methods of making and using same. US Patent 9579284B2.

Zale, S. E., Troiano, G., Ali, M. M., Krkach, J., & Wright, J. (2016). Therapeutic polymeric nanoparticles comprising vinca alkaloids and methods of making and using same. US Patent 9351933B2.

Zhang, Y., Xiao, J. F., Yang, H. F., Jiao, Y., Cao, W. W., Shi, H. M., & Xiao, Y. H. (2019). N-Acetyl cysteine as a novel polymethyl methacrylate resin component: Protection against cell apoptosis and genotoxicity. Oxidative Medicine and Cellular Longevity, 2019.

5 Nanomedicines for Cancer Imaging, Diagnosis, and Therapy

Vaishali Makwana,[1] Ratul Dutta,[1] Pratik Katare,[1] Poonam Dogra,[1] Megha M. Unnimaya,[2] Vibha Choudhary,[2] Suchona Ghosh,[2] Sujith M. Subrahmanian,[2] and Jyotsnendu Giri[2]

[1]Centre for Interdisciplinary Programs, Indian Institute of Technology Hyderabad, Kandi, Telangana, India

[2]Department of Biomedical Engineering, Indian Institute of Technology Hyderabad, Kandi, Telangana, India

5.1 INTRODUCTION TO NANOMEDICINE IN ONCOLOGY

Nanomedicine has rapidly become a revolutionary area at the crossroads of nanotechnology, biology, and clinical medicine. In the specific context of oncology, precision, efficacy, and individualized methods for the diagnosis and treatment of cancers have never been more in demand. Since cancer is the world's leading cause of morbidity and mortality, mainstream models in oncologic care are being challenged in order to more effectively address nagging shortcomings in the form of late-stage diagnosis, diverse tumor biology, adverse effects at the systemic level, and resistance to therapy. Against this backdrop, nanomedicine delivers a new set of engineered tools—they can be constructed to penetrate any complex biological barrier, operate at molecular levels of precision, and integrate several clinical tasks such as imaging, therapy, and monitoring in a multifunctional platform.

This developing science holds the potential not only for better results in single patients, but also for significant progress toward equity in the provision of cancer care worldwide. The following sections provide introduction to the worldwide burden of cancer, outstanding clinical demands, as well as the size and potential of nanomedicine in fundamentally changing strategies for imaging, diagnosing, treating, and performing theranostics for cancers.

5.1.1 Global Cancer Burden and Unmet Clinical Needs

Cancer continues to be a major cause of morbidity and mortality all over the world, presenting enormous challenges to healthcare systems and society in general. Globally, there were nearly 20 million new cancers and 9.7 million deaths from cancer in 2022 as per the most recent projections from the World Health Organization (WHO) and International Agency for Research on Cancer (IARC). The estimated figure for the coming years is just as frightening: by the year 2050, the number of new cancers per year is set to increase to a figure of 33 million, while deaths from cancers are estimated to be 18.2 million. These statistics typify the necessity for transformative interventions in prevention, as well as therapy. Incidence is not equally distributed all over the world; the highest relative increase is seen in the highest HDI countries, but the highest proportional increase is in the lowest HDI countries, in which there is a predicted increase of 142% and 99% in new cancers by the year 2050, respectively ("Global Cancer Observatory" 2025).

DOI: 10.1201/9781003799351-5

Incidence in the United States follows these patterns closely. Projected in 2025 are an estimated 2,041,910 new cancer diagnoses and 618,120 deaths from cancer, representing a rate of cancer incidence at 445.8 per 100,000 people and mortality at 145.4 per 100,000 people (2019–2023 data). Mortality inequalities still exist in spite of advancements in early care and treatment: the highest rates of cancer deaths are experienced by non-Hispanic Black men (203.6 per 100,000), while the lowest occur among non-Hispanic Asian/Pacific Islander women (83.1 per 100,000). Aging populations, shifting lifestyles, increasing obesity, tobacco, alcohol, and air pollution add to the cancer load—all significant factors in the risk for cancers ("Global Cancer Observatory" 2025).

Progress in conventional surgical oncology, chemotherapy, and radiation therapy has benefited many, but many gaps remain. Late presentation, variable tumor biology, and toxicity-imposed limitations on therapy effectiveness all cause suboptimal rates of survival, especially in resource-scarce environments. Recurrence of cancer, metastasis, and resistance to drugs all limit the effectiveness of existing interventions. Therefore, there is a pressing, unserved clinical need for novel modalities that provide more specific targeting, higher efficacy, and fewer adverse effects while meeting the expanding mandate for personalized and equitable care ("Global Cancer Observatory" 2025).

5.1.2 Why Nanomedicine for Cancer? Scope and Promise

Nanomedicine, as the medical application of nanotechnology to diagnose, treat, and monitor, is born at the intersection of materials science, biology, and engineering. It is clear why nanotechnology is being used in oncology: nanoscale carriers can be engineered to interact with biological systems at the molecular level, and here is offered a distinctive prospect for the control of cancers. The nanomedicine's signature property is the capacity to encapsulate, protect, and selectively deliver cargo in the form of drugs, genes, or imaging agents directly to tumors while minimizing damage to normal tissues and maximizing therapeutic effect.

Recent reports emphasize extensive applications of nanomedicine in oncology, including target-specific drug delivery, personalized oncology, tumor imaging, and monitoring of therapy outcomes. In a prototype example, nanoparticles can be surface-modified with ligands that specifically recognize and bind to overexpressed receptors on cancer cells, leading to the effective internalization and intracellular release of anticancer drugs. Such precision targeting minimizes systemic toxicity while enabling higher local concentrations of drugs at the tumor, overcoming one of the significant drawbacks of conventional therapies. Nanomedicine, therefore, dramatically expands the treatment arsenal available to oncologists (Shi et al. 2016).

The recent leap in mRNA-based gene therapies is illustrative. The refined development of lipid nanoparticles (LNPs) for safe and effective mRNA delivery has, in the wake of the COVID-19 pandemic, catalyzed research into cancer vaccines and gene editing therapies. Optimized LNPs and polymer-based nanoparticles not only shield mRNA from degradation but also ensure precise delivery to target tissues, holding promise for cancer immunotherapies and rare disease treatments. Biodegradable nanocarriers and hybrid nano systems further diversify the toolbox, providing avenues for regenerative therapies and improved environmental sustainability in healthcare (Uchida 2022).

Cancer nanomedicines are more than drugs or pharmacology. Comprehensive applications are on the horizon for nanomaterials for imaging, including contrast agents for magnetic resonance imaging (MRI), computed tomography (CT) scans, positron emission tomography (PET) scans, and optical and ultrasound modalities. These nano-enabled contrast agents for imaging applications are designed for tumor-specific contrast, real-time in situ monitoring, and multiplexed sensing, thus boosting precision for diagnoses and early therapy intervention (Kaunitz 2018; Gholami et al. 2020a; Tatsugami et al. 2022).

Here is the Timeline of key milestones in nanomedicine development for oncology, highlighting major advancements from the discovery of liposomes (1964) to modern platforms such as lipid nanoparticle mRNA cancer vaccines (2019) and high-throughput nanoPRISM screening (2022) (Figure 5.1).

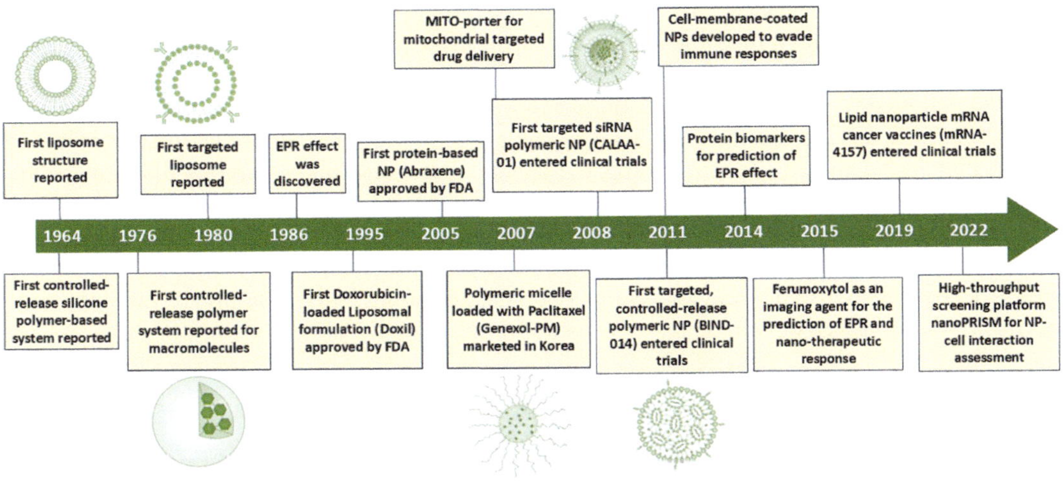

FIGURE 5.1 Timeline of key milestones in nanomedicine for oncology.

5.1.3 Defining Imaging, Diagnosis, Therapy, and Theragnostic—And How They Integrate

The multidisciplinary management of cancer hinges on four interdependent pillars: imaging, diagnosis, therapy, and the emerging field of theranostics.

Imaging is at the heart of oncology, allowing visualization of tumors for the aims of diagnosis, staging, and planning of therapy. Classical modalities (e.g., PET, MRI, ultrasound, CT) are significantly supplemented by nanotechnology nowadays. Nano-contrast agents and nanoprobes, engineered for stability and for functionalization, have higher sensitivity and specificity compared with their small-molecule counterparts, and are not only effective for the detection, but for the real-time monitoring of tumor dynamics as well (Gholami et al. 2020a; J. L. Coll 2011; Cherry 2009a).

Diagnosis involves the determination of tumor type, grade, and molecular profile correctly—a function that is increasingly dependent on advanced imaging, molecular diagnostics, and liquid biopsy platforms. Incorporation of nano sensors and nanomaterials-based multiplexed assays for signal detection and multiplexed assays, respectively, enable earlier and more specific diagnosis (Y. Zhang et al. 2019a).

Nanomedicine therapy involves treatments that treat the cancer directly, often using nanoparticles to deliver chemotherapeutic agents, nucleic acids, or proteins in a more targeted manner. These nanoparticles can potentially cross biological barriers successfully, be activated by stimuli in the tumor microenvironment (e.g., by pH or enzyme action), and release in a controlled manner the substances that are to be delivered, reducing unwanted systemic effects (Sivanand et al. 2025).

Theranostics, the integration of 'therapy' and 'diagnostics'-is a revolutionary idea in personalized medicine. Theranostic agents integrate diagnostic modalities (e.g., tumor imaging or biomarker identification) and therapeutic applications (e.g., drug delivery or radiotherapy) into a nanoscale platform, often a single entity. Radiotheranostics are exemplars, using radionuclide-labeled agents that visualize as well as treat tumors: diagnostic radionuclides allow PET/SPECT imaging to ensure target expression, whereas therapeutic radionuclides provide cytotoxic radiation to malignant cells, sometimes using agents that overlap between these two (e.g., lutetium-177). By doing so, this strategy allows for personalized selection and monitoring of therapy, precise determination of drug delivery, and real-time provider feedback. Theranostics actually completes the 'diagnosis-to-therapy' loop: a patient's tumor is initially visualized using a diagnostic component, validating the presence and size of a particular biomarker or target (e.g., PSMA or somatostatin receptor). When positive, therapy is deployed using the corresponding therapeutic nanoagent—occasionally with the same platform but with different radionuclide payload. It allows for a fundamentally more personalized approach, with tailoring of intervention to the patient's specific disease profile while still monitoring response and optimizing dosing.

With continued progress in the field, the coming together of imaging, diagnostics, therapy, and theranostics will fuel the future of precision oncology—allowing for earlier identification, patient-specific therapies, and real-time tracking of therapeutic response. This integration has the potential to manage the worldwide burden of cancer by reducing access barriers, increasing efficiency, and boosting effectiveness of care, especially as nanomedicine penetrates wider segments of the population, even those in resource-constrained environments. These combined platforms are not only about scientific breakthroughs but also about much-needed hope for overcoming the ubiquitous and increasing world burden of cancer.

5.2 NANOPARTICLE DESIGN AND TUMOR TARGETING STRATEGIES

In early detection and diagnosis of cancer, nano-oncology has developed rapidly in the last three decades. As researchers delved into the research related to cancer and nanomedicine, the attention shifted toward precise tumor targeting, followed by efficient nanomedicine delivery. Back in the year 1986, when Matsumura and Maeda first elucidated that macromolecules of a specific size range get accumulated in the solid tumors via a certain phenomenon known as Enhanced Permeability and Retention (EPR) effect. This discovery further paved the way for the delivery of drugs and nanomedicine to the targeted tumor location (Matsumura and Maeda 1986). However, the EPR effect imposes a significant challenge for the nanomedicines to be clinically translational. Certain tumors showing non-leaky vasculature remain impermeable to the EPR effect, showing limited effect for nanomedicines to target. In this regard, nanoparticle design has emerged as a crucial aspect for various tumor-targeting strategies. Strategies and designs, such as decorating the nanoparticle system with ligands, fragments of antibodies, peptides, nucleic acid aptamers, and small molecules, have gained special interest for targeting specific cancer cell receptors. Studies have shown that these ligands promote increased internalization and induce apoptosis in cancer cells. The tumor microenvironment (TME) remains an inherent physiological barrier that cannot be overlooked by researchers in establishing clinical therapy. The cellular TME is influenced by different cell types with constant cellular interactions, secretion of soluble molecules, and vesicles, thereby stimulating the ECM and tumor spread. Considering the features of TME, they possess a significantly acidic environment with hypoxic and high interstitial pressure conditions, which influence the progression of the tumor niche. The distribution and permeability of the nanomaterials are highly affected by these adverse conditions in terms of stability and functionality. Fortunately, researchers have designed various spatiotemporally controlled stimuli-responsive nanomaterials that respond to tumor-specific internal stimuli (Minh Hoang et al. 2025).

5.2.1 Targeting Approaches

Effective tumor targeting remains one of the most important goals of cancer nanomedicine, as it determines the capability of nanocarriers to selectively accumulate at tumor sites while minimizing off-target toxicity. The complicated biological barriers related to tumor vasculature, the tumor microenvironment (TME), and intracellular transport require the development of complex targeting strategies. Nanoparticle-mediated tumor targeting can be broadly categorized into passive and active approaches. Passive targeting is mainly based on unique pathophysiological features of tumors, such as increased vascular permeability and impaired lymphatic drainage, while active targeting utilizes specific ligands that can recognize and bind to overexpressed receptors or biomarkers on cancer cells and components of the TME. Collectively, these strategies can enhance drug accumulation, cellular uptake, and therapeutic efficacy, and thus increase the clinical potential of nanomedicine-based cancer therapies (Cheng et al. 2025; Rajoriya et al. 2024).

5.2.1.1 Passive Targeting

Passive targeting is defined as the encapsulation or incorporation of small molecules (cargo) in the NPs to extend their lifespan during systemic circulation and minimize side effects without target specificity to a specific tissue. The enhanced permeability and retention (EPR) effect allows nanoparticles to build up and stay in the body because tumor blood vessels are more permeable, and lymphatic drainage is not good enough. Despite the EPR effect remaining a potent phenomenon for passive targeting of nanomaterials, its naïve view remains controversial. To illustrate, one may speculate that the eruption points at the leaky vasculature of tumor cells improve NP extravasation into the interstitial tumor space. Studies have shown that the extracellular gaps (~2000 nm) in the tumor vasculature are seldom encountered, and passive extravasation is responsible for only a lesser number of NP entries into mouse solid tumors. In recent times, some NPs (ranging between 10 and 30 nm gold NPs) created micrometer-sized openings between ECs even in the absence of an EPR effect, termed as "nanoparticle-induced endothelial leakiness" (NanoEL) effect (Setyawati et al. 2017).

5.2.1.2 Active Targeting

Over the past few years, researchers have been focusing on creating new ways to fight cancer using nanomedicine. Their goal is to develop tiny systems that can seek out and target specific parts of the tumor microenvironment (TME). To do this, they attach special molecules, like peptides, antibodies, and aptamers, to the surface of these nanosystems. This process, called covalent conjugation, helps the nanosystems bind more effectively to their intended targets. Studies have shown that this approach leads to a better buildup of nanoparticles right where they are needed, including the extracellular matrix (ECM), cancer-associated fibroblasts (CAFs), and various immune cells within the TME (Thakkar et al. 2020).

NPs in the biological environment rapidly cover themselves with layers of biomolecules (mostly proteins), forming a protein corona. The strength of the corona depends on the affinity of proteins, which accordingly results in the formation of either a hard or soft corona. The composition and binding affinity of the protein corona largely determine their chemical and biological responses, including cellular functionalities and lifetime. Selective targeting-based nanomedicine designs: tumor cells, tumor microenvironment, and immune microenvironment for pH-sensitive nanomaterials are engineered to exploit the acidic tumor microenvironment (TME), thereby enabling site-specific activation and controlled drug release. This responsiveness is typically achieved through several mechanisms, including the protonation of ionizable functional groups that promote micelle assembly or disassembly, acid-cleavable linkers such as 2,3-dimethylmaleic amide (DMMA), or the incorporation of acid-labile materials like calcium carbonate and calcium phosphate, which undergo decomposition under acidic conditions. The hypoxic TME is prone to release ROS, forming a higher potential difference between intra- and extracellular spaces. Previous studies have shown that, under hypoxic conditions, black hole quencher 3 (BHQ3) modified carboxymethyl dextran has shown an increase in the rate of release of DOX. It can be attributed to the cleavage of the azo bond by the BHQ3. The extracellular matrix of solid tumors, particularly its dense collagen fibers and glycosaminoglycans, constitutes a major physical barrier to nanoparticle transport. Approaches such as surface charge modification, ligand conjugation, physicochemical tuning, and enzymatic collagen degradation have been explored to enhance intratumorally penetration. However, the structural complexity and heterogeneity of collagen remain poorly understood, underscoring the need for deeper mechanistic insights to guide the rational design of more effective nanocarriers (Minh Hoang et al. 2025).

Apart from the physiological changes of TME, immune cells remain a potent driving factor for tumor progression and nanoparticle targeting. Solid tumors have been found to recruit immune cells, which are responsible for immunosuppression, eventually favoring tumor growth. Interactions between nanoparticles and immune as well as stromal cells, often mediated through endocytosis or degradation pathways, can trigger immune activation and promote clearance from the body, thereby restricting therapeutic benefit. Recognizing this limitation, recent strategies have turned toward reprogramming the tumor microenvironment, with particular emphasis on targeting immunosuppressive cell populations, to prolong nanoparticle retention and improve treatment efficacy. In this regard, immunotherapy has become a new mainstay for cancer researchers since it can very well adjust the immune system to find and kill cancer cells. Recent nanomedicine strategies have integrated diverse immunotherapeutic modalities, including T-cell–targeted agents, cytokine delivery systems, immune checkpoint inhibitors, and cancer vaccines (Nam et al. 2019). The integration of these strategies has enabled researchers to obtain deeper insights into the TME, leading to the fabrication of better and effective nanotherapeutic approaches offering new hope for suffering cancer patients.

After achieving penetration of the complex TME barriers, it can be a major challenge for the nanomedicines to enter the tumor cells, as they only selectively accumulate in tumor tissue. To achieve target-specific treatment, nanocarriers require modifications through engineered targeting methods. Herein, antibodies and peptides have gained wide recognition for specific binding to antigens and receptors on tumor cell surfaces for targeting. Targets like epidermal growth factor receptor (EGFR), human epidermal growth factor receptor-2 (HER2) have shown promising targeting opportunities by antibody-based therapies with remarkable efficacy (Martin et al. 2023).

5.2.2 Nanostructure Designs for Organelle-Specific Targeting

In addition to internalization into target cells, nanomaterials should accumulate in key organelles and mediate apoptosis pathways, thereby decreasing off-target toxicity to healthy cells. Firstly, mitochondria can be a promising targeting organelle, as it is often referred to as a 'suicide weapon store' of eukaryotic cells, serving convergence points for lethal signal transduction cascades. The higher negative membrane potential of mitochondria in tumor cells compared to normal cells serves as a distinctive feature for designing mitochondrion-specific therapeutic nanomaterials. While designing mitochondrion-targeting nanocarriers, charge-mediated targeting can be closely looked into, as positively charged nanostructures show binding affinity to the mitochondrial membrane and increase local drug concentration. Studies have shown that delocalized lipophilic cations (DLCs) and transition metals have enhanced mitochondrial targeting abilities. These nanocomposites have been shown to induce effective death of cancerous cells by generating oxygen-based free radicals. Apart from charged molecules, researchers have also found mitochondrial-permeable peptides (MPPs) to enhance penetration efficacy. Yet, significant challenges remain, particularly in addressing the high heterogeneity of mtDNA and in finding the right balance between stimulating immune responses and avoiding immune evasion in clinical applications.

Genetic mutations and chromatin remodeling are important contributors to the generation of tumors. The cell nucleus remains another key player in both processes. In cancer, the nucleus-regulated processes of aging, apoptosis, and cell cycle are frequently suppressed, enabling cancer cells to endure and multiply. Furthermore, drug resistance is facilitated by the nucleus, which makes it possible for cancer cells to withstand chemotherapy. As such, it is a prime target for study and cancer gene therapy (Yang et al. 2022). Researchers have focused on altering nanodrugs with nuclear localization single peptides or transcription peptides to improve their ability to get into the nucleus. The nuclear pore complexes (NPCs) present within the nuclear envelope (NE) function as principal gateways for protein trafficking between the nucleus and cytoplasm. While small molecules can diffuse easily through these pores, larger macromolecules like proteins pass through active transport. In this regard, nuclear localization signal (NLS), which is an amino acid sequence, plays an important role as a molecular key for passage through nuclear pores. For example, surface modification with different NLS peptides on biodegradable silica nanocapsules (BSNPs) has increased the precise delivery of nucleus-targeting proteins. This showed tumor cell apoptosis by delivery of dNase I to the nuclear interior (Du et al. 2023).

Lastly, lysosomes have shown potential for another targeting organelle for nanomaterials. Lysosomes, also termed the 'suicidal bags' of eukaryotic cells, are very dynamic in nature for showing functionalities like degradation, clearance, and cellular waste recycling. Compared to normal cells, the lysosomes of tumor cells have relatively weak membranes, along with higher cathepsin activity. This results in the tumor cells being more prone to lysosomal membrane permeabilization (LMP), eventually leading to lysosome-dependent cellular death. After that, it has been seen that the tumor cells store redox-active iron in their lysosomes for improved metalloprotein turnover and metabolism. Therefore, when excess iron ions are released in the cytoplasm, they induce the Fenton reactions, which finally release ROS species. Based on this hypothesis, researchers have fabricated several nanostructures, like copper nanodots (CNDs), iron-based nanoparticles, which have been shown to induce ferroptosis, which is a STING1-mediated iron-catalyzed necrosis (Levine and Kroemer 2019).

Most organelle-targeting nanomedicines developed to date have been designed with a focus on single organelles. This strategy has the advantage of simplifying design and accelerating the development of nanomedicines capable of producing specific therapeutic outcomes. Nonetheless, several organelles, including the endoplasmic reticulum, Golgi apparatus, proteasomes, ribosomes, and autophagosomes, remain comparatively underexplored as therapeutic targets. By using functional regulation and precise structural targeting, extending nanomedicine design to these compartments may create new opportunities for improving efficacy. Innovative materials and unique nanostructures will probably need to be integrated for such advancements to occur. Crucially, though, this mostly "linear" design methodology emphasizes one-to-one interactions and represents a simplified understanding of cellular physiology. This oversimplification overlooks the complex crosstalk and dynamic interplay among organelles, potentially missing opportunities to exploit synergistic effects or to avoid antagonistic ones, that could substantially improve therapeutic outcomes (Tan et al. 2025).

5.2.3 Nanostructure Designs for Organelle Escape

Apart from achieving therapeutic efficacy by targeting specific organelles and delivering the encapsulated cargo, the nanocarriers face several cellular obstacles in their delivery route. As cellular organelles exhibit complex, interconnected functionalities, nanodrugs should be protected from premature degradation and deactivation mediated by lysosomes and proteosomes. Non-specific drug delivery can not only reduce the therapeutic efficiency but may also lead to genotoxicity. In this context, organelle escape plays a pivotal role. They act as a "relay station" which leads the nanoparticle system to perceive enrichment in specific compartments, such as lysosomes, before being transported to their intended targets. By minimizing cytoplasmic dispersion, this mechanism significantly enhances the precision and overall efficacy of organelle-targeted therapies. In this section, we have reviewed mainly three types of organelles that serve as escape strategies for specific tumor treatments. The most prevalent escape routes include the lysosomal escape mechanism, followed by the nuclear and proteosome escape processes (Figure 5.2) (Gao et al. 2023).

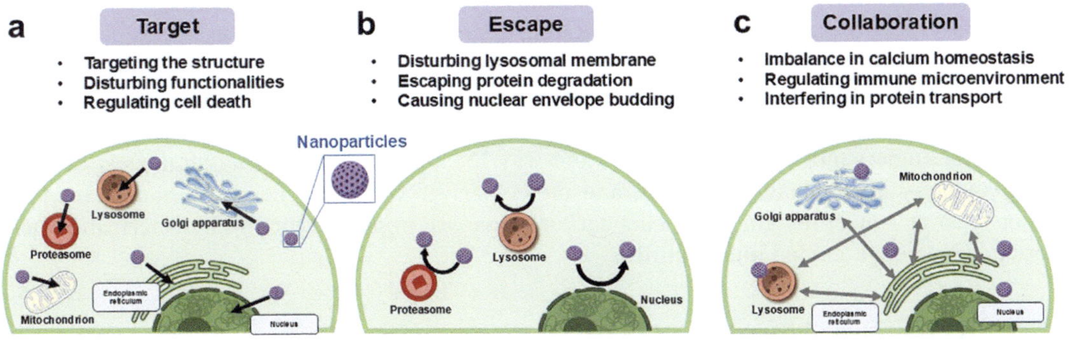

FIGURE 5.2 Schematic illustration of the organelle-involved employment of a nanoparticle showing (a) targeting, (b) escaping, and (c) collaborating strategies for specific tumor therapy

As previously stated, lysosomes function as degradation compartments. They remain responsible for the degradation of most of the biosynthetic products. They produce several degradation enzymes, like hydrolases, which undergo degradation of nanocarriers to ensure their escape. Lysosomal escape describes the process by which molecules or nanoparticles evade degradation within lysosomes after endocytosis, enabling them to reach their intended organelle targets and release their therapeutic payload. Achieving efficient lysosomal escape is therefore crucial, as it not only enhances the precision of drug delivery but also prevents unwanted cytoplasmic dispersion that could diminish therapeutic efficacy. Several mechanisms have been explored to achieve this, including the proton sponge effect, lysosomal membrane disruption, and membrane fusions (C.-G. Liu et al. 2020).

In the late 1990s, the proton sponge effect was first hypothesized. It suggests that certain cationic polymers are responsible for mediating osmotic swelling. This further worsens the lysosomal acidification, followed by lysosomal lysis and release of cellular contents. Researchers found this phenomenon fascinating to meditate on lysosomal escape by modification of nanocarriers. They found that certain chemical modifications, like the introduction of protonatable amine fractions or disulfide bonds on nanodrugs, aid in keeping the proton pump active, followed by a sequence of events, ultimately leading to the proton sponge effect. When the nanodrugs unknowingly enter the nucleus, their efficacy gets compromised. In addition, if nanodrugs build up in the nucleus inappropriately, they can trigger harmful side effects such as genetic damage, metabolic imbalances, or disruptions in the normal signaling cascade. However, there is still a limitation about nanodrugs designed to escape the nucleus. Nevertheless, several studies based on nuclear viral escape have provided insights regarding the development of nanocarriers for targeting organelles (Allen and Yokota 2024).

For constructing nanodrugs targeting different organelles, consideration should be taken for the interactions between various organelles. The nanodrugs should have the capacity to target organelles and avoid being mis-targeted by other non-specific organelles. Overall, these studies suggest that, while fabricating nanosystems, more importance should be given to their specificity to get maximum therapeutic efficacy. There are still many complex mechanisms underlying the organelle targeting that remain unaddressed. For instance, former designs have usually focused on the impact of lysosomes on targeting nanodrugs, without considering that there can be potential hurdles that lysosomes can pose to nanodrugs targeting other organelles (Wang et al. 2021).

5.3 NANOTECHNOLOGY FOR CANCER IMAGING

Accurate and early detection of cancer is essential in improving treatment outcomes, guiding therapeutic decisions, and monitoring disease progression. Conventional imaging modalities, including magnetic resonance imaging (MRI), computed tomography (CT), positron emission tomography (PET), single-photon emission computed tomography (SPECT), ultrasound, and optical imaging have revolutionized oncology; however, these modalities are often limited by sensitivity, specificity, spatial resolution, and contrast enhancement. Nanotechnology offers innovative solutions to these challenges by developing engineered nanoparticles as advanced imaging probes and contrast agents. Nanoparticles, due to their size, surface properties, and multifunctionality, can be targeted to tumor sites, increase signal intensity, provide molecular-level imaging, and enable real-time monitoring of disease. Furthermore, the integration of multi-imaging modalities into a single nanoplatform has paved the way for multimodal imaging strategies, offering complementary anatomical, functional, and molecular information. Therefore, nanotechnology is transforming cancer imaging, allowing earlier diagnosis, improved tumor characterization, and more precise image-guided interventions.

5.3.1 Nanoparticle Probes for MRI

Magnetic Resonance Imaging (MRI) developed by Paul Lauterbur in the year 1973 and also received FDA approval, approving its use in the clinical assets and so has been widely used in most of the hospitals worldwide. The detection is based upon the NMR signals which aligns along with the signals emitted by the hydrogen protons in the body after placing it in the magnetic field. Paul C. Lauterbur and Sir Peter Mansfield won Nobel Prize in the category of physiology and medicine in the year 2003 for the discovery of MRI. There are particularly three tissue parameters which are primarily responsible for the contrast in MRI and are basically classified as per their sensitivity corresponding to their tissue parameters like the proton density (ρ), the longitudinal (or spin-lattice) relaxation times T1, and the transverse (or spin-spin) relaxation times T2 or T2* (Kaunitz 2018).

5.3.1.1 Contrast Mechanisms and Relaxivity

These contrast agents have the capabilities for enhancing the image contrast in between the normal and the diseased tissue further providing a detailed information and status of the normal or the abnormal functioning of the underlying organ and the blood flow. These agents are been administered in the patient which causes an increment in the relaxation rates of the water protons in the tissue where the agent is getting accumulated and is been getting imaged. Paramagnetic, superparamagnetic, and ferromagnetic materials are widely explored as MRI contrast agents due to their magnetic properties. To be precise, MRI relies on two fundamental relaxation times: the longitudinal relaxation time (T_1) and the transverse relaxation time (T_2). These relaxation processes directly determine how tissues and fluids appear on MRI scans. Image contrast is displayed on a grayscale, where brighter regions correspond to higher signal intensity and darker regions to lower intensity. Typically, tissues with shorter relaxation times, such as those influenced by T_1 processes, appear bright (white), while tissues with longer relaxation times, associated with T_2 processes, appear dark (black). Intermediate relaxation properties produce grey tones, reflecting a balance between T_1 and T_2 contributions (Jacques et al. 2010).

Magnetic nanoparticle particularly Iron oxide nanoparticles are widely used in biomedical applications such as hyperthermia treatment, drug delivery targeting, and imaging contrast enhancement. However, when particle size is less than 20 nm, they are superparamagnetic in nature. Such behavior is highly useful in imaging techniques such as Magnetic Resonance Imaging (MRI). Because of their superparamagnetic character along with built-in biocompatibility, Superparamagnetic Iron Oxide Nanoparticles (SPIONs) have been identified as highly promising agents for medical imaging. In the biomedical applications, SPIONs should possess well-characterized physicochemical properties such as controlled size with narrow distribution, high aqueous stability, and high magnetic responsiveness (Girardet et al. 2023).

5.3.1.2 Gadolinium-Based Agents: Benefits and Safety Concerns

Gadolinium-based contrast agents (GBCAs) are designed to tightly bind the gadolinium ion through specialized chelating structures, which can be either linear or macrocyclic in nature. Because free gadolinium ions are highly toxic, the ligand framework that holds them plays a crucial role in determining the agent's safety and classification. At present, gadolinium-based contrast agents (GBCAs) are the only class of contrast agents approved for routine MRI use in clinical practice. Broadly, they are divided into two groups: linear chelates such as Gd (III)–DTPA and its derivatives, and macrocyclic chelates such as Gd (III)–DOTA. Both types can effectively enhance MRI contrast by altering the relaxation behavior of water protons, and both display strong thermodynamic stability. However, linear chelates are less kinetically stable and can undergo transmetalation with endogenous ions like Zn (II), which increases the risk of releasing free gadolinium in the body. In contrast, macrocyclic chelates form more rigid complexes, offering superior kinetic stability and minimizing gadolinium release under normal physiological conditions. For this reason, macrocyclic agents are often favored in targeted imaging applications. Gadolinium-based contrast agents (GBCAs) are widely employed in clinical MRI because their strong paramagnetic capabilities are effective for high-quality signal improvement. Long-term safety is now an issue of growing controversy. (White et al. 2006).

Alternative MRI nanoprobes:

5.3.2 Nanoplatforms for PET and SPECT

Radiation-based targeting has gained importance as a dual tool for cancer diagnosis and therapy. Although advances in oncology have improved treatment outcomes, dose-limiting toxicities such as hepatotoxicity and nephrotoxicity remain major hurdles. Nanoparticle-based carriers are being explored to address these limitations, as they can circulate longer, accumulate at tumor sites, and support multiple targeting strategies. Parallel progress in radiopharmaceutical development and imaging technologies, particularly with more sensitive radioactive tracers, has further enhanced the accuracy and reliability of nuclear medicine for cancer detection and monitoring (Julius et al. 2025).

5.3.2.1 Strategies for Radiolabeling Nanoparticles

Nanotechnology has enabled the creation of innovative materials that serve as versatile platforms in fields ranging from biosensing and bioimaging to nanomedicine, drug delivery, and theranostics. Within this space, nanoparticles (NPs) hold particular promise for multimodal imaging because of their unique characteristics of having a nanoscale dimensions (1–100 nm), adjustable imaging properties, and multifunctional potential. Among these attributes, particle size plays a pivotal role in tumor imaging. Their small size allows nanoparticles to exploit the enhanced permeability and retention (EPR) effect, leading to higher accumulation of imaging agents in tumor tissues. Radiolabeling methods are broadly grouped into four categories: (a) chelator-based radiolabeling (indirect), (b) direct particle bombardment, (c) chelator-free radiolabeling and (d) synthesis using a mixture of radioactive and nonradioactive precursors. Thus, the radiolabeled nanoparticles can be described as nanoscale materials engineered to stably incorporate a radionuclide within their structure. Unlike traditional small-molecule radiotracers, the addition of radionuclides usually causes minimal alteration to the overall design of nanoparticles. This is largely because of the inherent size difference, the nanoparticle's relatively large surface area accommodates the small amount of radionuclide required for effective SPECT or PET imaging, meaning the structural and functional characteristics of the material remain largely intact. (Pellico et al. 2021).

5.3.3 Use of Nanoparticles for CT and Photoacoustic Imaging

Computed tomography (CT) and photoacoustic imaging (PAI) are two powerful imaging modalities that can provide complementary anatomical and functional information for cancer diagnosis. While CT provides excellent spatial resolution and deep tissue imaging, its sensitivity can be limited by the performance of conventional contrast agents. Similarly, photoacoustic imaging combines the advantages of optical and ultrasound imaging, allowing high-resolution imaging of biological tissues with a deeper penetration depth than conventional optical approaches. Nanotechnology has greatly improved both modalities by developing nanoparticle-based contrast agents with enhanced imaging ability, extended circulation time and tumor-targeting ability. In particular, nanoparticles of high atomic number (high-Z) elements such as gold, bismuth, and lanthanides have shown improved X-ray attenuation for CT imaging, while plasmonic and carbon-based nanomaterials have strong optical absorption properties, resulting in strong photoacoustic signals. These engineered nanoplatforms not only improve image quality and the sensitivity of tumor detection, but also enable theranostic applications by integrating imaging, targeted drug delivery, and therapy into one system. As a result, nanoparticle-enabled CT and photoacoustic imaging are emerging as powerful tools for accurate cancer diagnosis, treatment planning, and real-time monitoring of therapy.

5.3.3.1 Conventional Iodine Agents and Their Limitations

Iodinated contrast agents remain the standard choice for enhancing X-ray and CT scans in applications such as tumor detection, coronary angiography, and perfusion imaging. In most otherwise healthy patients, these agents are considered safe, with adverse reactions usually mild and self-limiting. However, their use carries significant risks in individuals with impaired renal function, and potential interactions with concurrent medications must also be considered. Reported complications from CT contrast agents generally fall into two categories renal effects and systemic reactions with their frequency and severity closely linked to the physicochemical characteristics, particularly the osmolarity, of the formulations currently in use (Thomsen and Morcos, 2009).

Toxicity Drug Interactions and Renal Excretion: The major safety issue with iodinated contrast agents is Contrast-Induced Nephropathy (CIN), which refers to an acute decline in kidney function (Thomsen and Morcos, 2009). Patients with pre-existing moderate to severe chronic kidney disease (CKD) are particularly at risk. Older high-osmolar contrast media (HOCM) were linked with a higher frequency of CIN and other acute side effects, whereas newer low-osmolar (LOCM) and iso-osmolar (IOCM) formulations show improved safety. Other adverse reactions, though less common and usually mild, may include anaphylactoid responses. These agents can interact with certain medications. For example, their use in patients taking metformin raises the risk of lactic acidosis. Co-administration with nephrotoxic drugs such as NSAIDs or cyclosporine can worsen CIN, while concurrent use of diuretics may predispose patients to dehydration. Iodinated contrast agents are eliminated largely unchanged by the kidneys via passive glomerular filtration, with most being cleared within 24–48 hours in individuals with normal renal function. In contrast, patients with CKD show impaired clearance, leading to prolonged circulation and elevated blood concentrations (Rajpoot et al. 2022).

5.3.3.2 High-Z Nanoparticle for CT Imaging

Nanoparticles composed of elements with a high atomic number (high-Z) have emerged as promising tools to enhance the effectiveness of radiotherapy. By tailoring their surface properties, these nanoparticles can be engineered to accumulate more selectively in tumor tissue than in healthy cells. Once localized within the tumor, high-Z nanoparticles interact with radiation to amplify its therapeutic impact, thereby improving treatment outcomes without adding significant toxicity to surrounding normal tissues. Beyond their direct radio sensitizing action, these nanoparticles can also be designed to deliver drug-based sensitizers, functioning as dual-mode systems that combine physical and pharmacological mechanisms (Mostafavi et al. 2025).

5.3.3.3 Spectral and Dual-Energy CT Approaches

Spectral CT, also called as the Dual-energy CT involves scanning an object at two different energy levels, allowing for characterization of materials that conventional single-energy CT cannot distinguish. This technique works by separating materials based on how their attenuation coefficients vary with energy. Dual energy analysis can be performed in two ways: using image data or raw data. The latter approach reduces beam-hardening artifacts, making the analysis more precise. Virtual monochromatic images generated through this method show higher iodine contrast at lower energy levels, which enhances the visibility of contrast-enhanced lesions. Additionally, material decomposition techniques such as creating iodine or edema specific maps further improve the detection of lesions commonly seen in routine clinical practice (Tatsugami et al. 2022).

5.3.4 Nanomaterials in Optical and Fluorescence Imaging

Optical imaging relies on detecting light as it passes through biological tissues. Since tissues are not fully transparent, the quality of information obtained is strongly influenced by tissue thickness and optical properties. A useful "window" for such imaging lies in the near-infrared (NIR) range

(650–900 nm), where absorption and scattering are relatively low, allowing deeper penetration. In fluorescence imaging, fluorophores absorb photons and then re-emit them at longer wavelengths as they return to their ground state. This emission can be captured with sensitive detectors such as cooled CCD cameras, though depth is usually limited to around 1 cm. Time-resolved fluorescence can extend this to about 3 cm by filtering out background noise and exploiting the nanosecond-scale lifetimes of fluorophores. Beyond simple signal detection, fluorescence lifetime imaging has also been used to probe local microenvironments, including variations in pH, refractive index, ion concentration, and oxygen levels (J.-L. Coll 2011).

5.3.4.1 Nanocarriers for Fluorescent Dyes

Cross-linked micelles are self-assembled nanostructures formed from amphiphilic block copolymers and further stabilized through covalent bonds. Their tuneable sizes (~5–150 nm) allow efficient tumor accumulation, and they can encapsulate near-infrared (NIR) dyes such as cyanine and BODIPY without premature leakage. These micelles have been engineered for enhanced stability, biocompatibility, and long circulation times, making them versatile carriers for fluorescence imaging and photodynamic therapy. A variety of nanocarriers can be used, loaded with fluorescent dyes for fluorescence imaging, which are explained as follows:

Polymersomes are hollow, vesicle-like structures composed of amphiphilic block copolymers. They can encapsulate both hydrophobic and hydrophilic fluorophores, such as Nile Red or calcein, while shielding the dyes from quenching. The outer PEG corona provides "stealth" properties, prolonging circulation and enabling ligand attachment for active targeting. Modified polymersomes have been applied for deep-tissue imaging and multifunctional theranostics. Solid polymer matrices, including PMMA, PAA, and PLGA, serve as dense cores for dye entrapment. This design minimizes dye leakage and allows surface modifications for targeting ligands. Highly branched dendrimers and surface-cross-linked biodegradable nanoparticles provide multiple reactive groups for covalent dye attachment (Choudhary et al. 2024). This architecture ensures high dye loading, stability, and in some designs, controlled release, making them promising for sustained tumor imaging applications. Phospholipid vesicles such as liposomes remain classic nanocarriers for fluorophores. PEGylation extends circulation time, while surface modification with peptides or antibodies provides tumor-specific targeting. Liposomal systems have been widely applied for both imaging and drug delivery. Biodegradable poly (lactic acid) (PLA) and poly (lactic-co-glycolic acid) (PLGA) nanoparticles are FDA-approved and extensively studied for fluorescence imaging. They can encapsulate NIR dyes like ICG, Cy5, or DY-700, achieving high tumor-to-background ratios. Covalent conjugation with targeting ligands further improves specificity (Delledonne et al. 2023).

5.3.4.2 Near Infrared Fluorescence Imaging Using Nanomaterials

Near-infrared (NIR) fluorescence imaging has gained significant importance in both biomedical research and clinical practice because of its high spatial resolution and ability to penetrate tissues more deeply than visible light. Traditional NIR imaging operates in the NIR-I window (700–950 nm), which allows improved visualization compared to visible wavelengths but still faces challenges such as photon scattering, absorption by biological components, and interference from tissue autofluorescence. As a result, conventional NIR fluorescence is largely restricted to superficial lesions or requires surgical exposure of tumor-bearing regions to achieve useful imaging depth (Hong et al. 2014).

5.3.5 Multimodal Platforms (MRI/PET/Fluorescence Hybrids)

Superparamagnetic iron oxide nanoparticles (SPIONs) such as Feraheme (FH) have been explored as hybrid nanoplatforms for PET/MRI when radiolabeled with tracers like [^{89}Zr]. PET-MRI leverages the high sensitivity of PET alongside the excellent soft-tissue contrast of MRI. FH typically produces dark T2 contrast, which is sometimes difficult to interpret clinically for instance, in detecting lymph node metastases. However, when radiolabeled, FH generates bright PET signals that overcome these limitations. Studies have confirmed its suitability for chelate-free labelling and demonstrated its application in PET–MRI (Gholami et al. 2020b).

Tumor-associated macrophages (TAMs), which are linked with poor cancer prognosis, can be quantitatively monitored using SPIONs and perfluorocarbon nanoemulsions. MRI allows TAM visualization, while PET with 18F-FDG provides complementary data on tumor metabolism, together enabling a powerful prognostic tool. Dendrimers (7–12 nm) also stand out due to their deep tumor penetration and capacity for targeted drug release. G5 PAMAM dendrimers functionalized with PARACEST MRI agents have been applied for dual MRI–optical glioma imaging, successfully identifying tumors at millimeter resolution. Finally, multimodal platforms integrate with PAI, which offers high spatial resolution and deep tissue penetration through optical excitation. Mesoporous carbon nanospheres (Meso-CNS) demonstrated broad UV–vis–NIR absorption, strong photoacoustic signals, and efficient doxorubicin loading, making them potent theranostic tools. Likewise, gold nanoparticles, with their strong absorption and fluorescence properties, have been tested in dual PAI–fluorescence systems for drug delivery and real-time imaging (Desai et al. 2023).

5.3.6 Advantages versus Limitations

Nanomaterials hold significant promise in biomedicine because most biomolecules such as DNA, proteins, enzymes, and hemoglobin naturally exist at the nanometer scale. Working within this dimension provides a high surface-to-volume ratio, creating ample sites for interaction with biological systems. This leads to greater sensitivity, improved specificity, and faster reaction times. In recent years, platforms such as quantum dots, metallic nanoparticles, liposomes, dendrimers, micelles, and polymeric nanoparticles have gained attention for cancer imaging and therapy. In contrast, conventional treatment strategies face notable drawbacks, including poor solubility, uneven biodistribution, limited stability, and challenging metabolism, which together reduce therapeutic efficiency and increase toxicity. Moreover, their lack of selectivity often damages healthy cells alongside cancerous ones. Smart nanomaterials are designed to address these shortcomings, offering more targeted, stable, and effective alternatives.

Advantages:

Radiolabeled nanoparticles incorporating high-atomic-number elements offer several key advantages for cancer imaging and diagnosis. Their high-Z composition enables stronger signals compared to conventional contrast agents, enhancing attenuation in CT, relaxivity in MRI, and photon emission in PET/SPECT, which results in clearer tumor visualization even at low doses. Beyond single-modality use, these nanoparticles can be engineered as multimodal platforms, carrying multiple imaging labels such as PET/MRI or CT/fluorescence hybrids, thereby providing complementary anatomical, functional, and molecular information within a single probe. Importantly, many high-Z radiolabeled nanoparticles act not only as contrast agents but also as radiosensitizers, creating theranostic systems that combine imaging with enhanced therapeutic outcomes, particularly in radiotherapy. Their tuneable physicochemical properties including size, surface chemistry, and payload further support the development of patient tailored nanoplatforms, paving the way for highly personalized cancer imaging and therapy.

Limitations

Despite their promise, radiolabeled nanoparticles incorporating high-Z elements also face several limitations that restrict their widespread clinical translation. A key drawback is limited tissue penetration depth, especially for optical and photoacoustic imaging, which hampers the visualization of deep-seated tumors. Quantification remains another challenge, as variations in nanoparticle size, surface chemistry, and labelling efficiency can affect signal intensity and make standardization difficult across studies. Furthermore, while animal experiments often demonstrate excellent targeting and clearance, translating these results to humans is complicated by differences in pharmacokinetics, biodistribution, and tumor microenvironment. Safety concerns also persist, particularly regarding the long-term toxicity (Vasdev et al. 2022), immunogenicity, and potential accumulation of non-biodegradable nanoparticles in vital organs such as the liver, spleen, or kidneys. Manufacturing and regulatory hurdles add to the complexity, since consistent large-scale synthesis with reproducible properties is still challenging. These gaps collectively highlight the need for further optimization and rigorous evaluation before radiolabeled nanoparticles can be fully integrated into routine cancer imaging and therapy.

5.4 NANO-ENABLED CANCER DIAGNOSIS

Early detection is also instrumental in reducing the cancer effects by detecting the disease early, when treatment can be most effective. Early tumor detection significantly increases the likelihood of successful intervention. It enables increased survival rates and an improved life for patients. Quick diagnosis of cancer augments prognosis, but it also minimizes the socio-economic impact of high-end treatment and care. As a result, improving diagnostic capacity has become a major challenge for researchers. Biosensors are defined as analyzing systems consisting of a biological recognition element with a transducer, and are used to quantify specific biological or chemical compounds (Kokilavani et al. 2024). Of the numerous technologies developed to enhance cancer diagnostics, biosensors have proven to be versatile tools for fast and accurate tumor detection. Different biomarkers, like nucleic acids and proteins, generate biochemical signals which is detected by biosensors. The potential to enable biosensors to quantify biomarkers for early-stage tumor detection makes biosensors crucial in cancer medicine development. Biosensors consist of components that function as a unit to detect and quantify molecules with higher accuracy. The primary sensing device is the detector. It generally uses biological recognition components like enzymes, antibodies, or nucleic acids to identify the analyte. The transducer further converts the sensed interaction to a measurable physical signal when the analyte is detected. This signal is subsequently processed and amplified by the signal processing system, which displays the output in a user-friendly way. Because of its integrated design, biosensors may produce quick, sensitive, and specific detection, which is advantageous in a variety of fields of study and business, including environmental monitoring and medical diagnostics (Kokilavani et al. 2024).

The advancement of cancer-based biosensors has shown potential for nanoparticle-based biosensing. It enabled high-throughput cancer detection, taking advantage of nanoparticles' distinct characteristics for highly selective and sensitive detection. Nanomaterials provide a larger surface area and superior biocompatibility, which render them extremely well-suited for biomedical and biosensing purposes. Their ease of functionalization with various biomolecules increases the targeting susceptibility of tumor marker detection. This upliftment of nanoparticle-conjugated biosensors helps well in complicated biological milieus, providing fast and accurate detection essential for early diagnosis of diseases. Apart from their sensitivity, biosensors based on nanoparticles are very stable and robust, and thus enhance the overall sensing performance and lifespan of the platform. Their incorporation quenches background noise, improves signal transduction, and allows miniaturization (Foroozandeh et al. 2024).

In this regard, the emergence of liquid biopsies, including circulating tumor DNA (ctDNA), circulating tumor RNA (ctRNA), tumor-derived extracellular vesicles (EVs), and circulating tumor cells (CTC), has enhanced the shift of diagnosing cancer in a non-invasive way. These approaches enable a multifunctional diagnosis of tumor biology, treatment responses, and disease progression pathways. Clinicians can now easily elucidate molecular insights and understand the TME without invasive tissue biopsies from tumor analytes obtained from body fluids. For non-invasive genotyping from blood, to targeted or whole-genome sequencing of ctDNA, they can be used to determine the tumor-associated mutations. This greatly helps in determining the early responsiveness of therapy. Exosomal miRNA, lncRNA, proteins, and metabolites constitute complementary biomarkers of functional activity (Wan et al. 2017).

5.4.1 Emergence of Nanomaterial-Based Biosensors for Cancer Diagnosis

Recently, nanoparticle-incorporated biosensors have emerged as an emerging platform for quick recognition of diverse biomarkers and analytes. This marked great importance for cancer diagnosis applications. With the growing recognition of diverse biomarkers and analytes in non-invasive body fluids, nanomaterial-enabled biosensors are emerging as a promising platform for cancer diagnostics. Their integration with nanomaterials imparts exceptional sensitivity, allowing rapid and reliable detection.

5.4.1.1 Nanomaterial-Based Biosensors Using Liquid Biopsy for Early-Stage Tumor Detection

Progress in liquid biopsy has allowed it to be used in early tumors for treatment response monitoring and MRD assessment. As with screening and early detection, early cancer releases much smaller amounts of ctDNA, CTCs, and EVs, relative to advanced cancer, which is a challenge to detect liquid biomarkers here. However, approaches like the analysis of greater volumes of blood, the use of multiparameter assays, and the utilization of new technologies have considerably enhanced detection rates to support wonderful progress in the application of liquid biopsy in the early environment. Studies have shown that a novel dual-functional surface layer has been engineered using poly-L-lysine (PLL). This surface is further functionalized with peptide nucleic acid (PNA), which improves its binding specificity. The modification significantly enhances nanoparticle-assisted surface plasmon resonance (SPR). Using this approach, tumor-associated circulating tumor DNA (ctDNA) can be detected directly from plasma samples with high sensitivity. The wild-type (WT) and Kirsten rat viral sarcoma (KRAS) mutant genomic DNA was discriminated by the nanoparticle system in human plasma. This shows the importance of a nanosystem-based point-of-care device for colorectal cancer diagnosis (Bellassai et al. 2021).

5.4.1.2 Nanomaterial-Based Biosensors Using Exosomes or Extracellular Vesicles as Biomarkers for Cancer Detection

With the paradigm shift toward the usage of liquid biopsy for molecular analysis of TME, and adding to surgical biopsy. In this regard, exosomes have been used extensively by researchers for early cancer detection.

Extracellular vesicles (EVs) are generally small, lipid-based particles that are released by cells. They carry important biological information, such as proteins and genetic material, from their parent cells, making them valuable as markers for various diseases, including cancer.

EVs come in different sizes and are classified accordingly: small EVs, called exosomes, are 30–100 nm in diameter. They are known to transport molecules that influence cell activity and are particularly relevant in oncology. The existing interventions for detecting biomarkers were ELISA and PCR-based analyses; however, they showed high sensitivity, but require expensive and longer times. Recently, the usage of nanobiohybrid materials for fabricating biosensors has shown great potential to overcome these drawbacks (Su et al. 2020). The incorporation of conductive and porous polymers has been found to elevate the electron transport reactions. These materials have also been found to increase the electrochemical and optical properties. Apart from that, the increased surface area for sensing causes more probes to detect, which eventually enhances the sensitivity.

Several works have already been documented based on the sensing exosomes using electrochemical, electrical, colorimetric, and fluorescence sensing. Different sensors developed, using electrochemistry and electricity, enhanced the advantages of being miniaturized, label-free, and offering a quick detection time. On the other hand, metal-based nanomaterials have been widely used for creating biosensors based on electrochemical and optical properties. Wu et al. developed a biosensor using a silver nanoparticle-decorated gold nanoisland (AuNI) for glioblastoma exosome detection. This sensor, which uses an antibody against the MCT4 protein on exosome membranes, is highly durable and easy to produce. It detects exosomes by creating a light-based signal (plasmon resonance) when illuminated with visible light (L. Liu et al. 2022).

Electrochemical detection is free from the need for the use of a unique marker for recognizing exosomes. It shows cost-effectiveness by enabling the observation of the live-state cellular and exosomal activity. Nevertheless, the difficulty arises in detecting the source. Because of its low power consumption and ease of sensor downsizing, electrical exosome detection is also an efficient detection approach for on-site diagnosis and does not require a special marker. Electrical signal response based on available FETs and electrodes also becomes a disadvantage, like difficulty in signal interpretation, high signal-to-noise ratio, and difficult measurement in fluidic conditions, which must be resolved.

5.4.1.3 Nanomaterial-Based Biosensors Using Protein Biomarkers for Cancer Detection

Among other cancer biomarkers, one major category of biomarkers consists of proteins that, when found in increased or reduced levels in serum, tissue, or saliva, may reflect disease conditions. The establishment of robust, cost-effective, and effective detection and monitoring methodologies for cancer remains critical. In this regard, protein biomarkers have shown a wide range of windows for biomarker detection. This part highlighted the development of electrochemical detection methods for cancer protein biomarkers, such as prostate specific antigen (PSA), prostate specific membrane antigen (PSMA), platelet factor 4 (PF-4), interleukin 6 (IL-6), interleukin 8 (IL-8), carcinoembryonic antigen (CEA), cancer antigens (e.g., CA-125, CA-199), c-reactive protein (CRP), and alpha feto-protein (AFP) (Rusling et al. 2010).

5.4.1.3.1 Nanomaterial-Based Biosensors for Prostate Cancer

Prostate cancer is the fourth most common type of cancer worldwide and the second most common cancer diagnosed in men. In this regard, PSA has been the most precise marker studied for prostate carcinoma since its identification. In both healthy and cancerous prostate tissue, a protein called prostate-specific antigen (PSA) is produced. While a healthy prostate releases only small amounts of PSA into the blood, this amount increases significantly in people with prostate disease. Because of this, many detection methods and measures have been developed for PSA levels at different prostate cancer stages. Thanks to advances in technology, these methods have become much more accurate and efficient. Biosensors have become a great alternative to the expensive and time-consuming hospital tests. They are sensitive, selective, and can be used easily. Since the early 1990s, hundreds of different biosensors for PSA detection have been created, using various techniques like electrochemical, optical, and mass-based methods. Liu et al. presented a novel PSA recognition sensor. It is based on a resonance energy transfer (RET) phenomenon having an "on-off" switching mechanism. The idea was to synthesize nanohybrids consisting of CeO_2 nanoparticles and AuNPs incorporating graphitic carbon nitride QDs (g-CNQDs). The nano-composite exhibited strong electrochemiluminescence with $K_2S_2O_8$ as a coreactant. The reversible $Ce^{3+} \leftrightarrow Ce^{4+}$ redox process in nano-CeO_2 promoted the decomposition of coreactants, generating sulfate radicals ($SO_4^{\bullet-}$) that boosted the electrochemiluminescence signal. AuNPs facilitated electronic transfer and biomolecule anchoring sites, making significant contributions toward the efficiency of the immunosensor. The "switch-off" mechanism takes place due to silver nanoparticle-vitamin B_2 (AgNPs-VB_2) nanocomposites as quenchers. The RET property of the nanocomposites effectively affected the electrochemiluminescence intensity, allowing for highly sensitive detection of PSA (Z. Liu et al. 2023).

For the detection of prostate-specific antigen (PSA) in human serum, researchers led by Hui developed an ultrasensitive and contamination-resistant biosensor. This innovative biosensor uses a unique octabranched peptide scaffold combined with silver nanoparticle (AgNP) signal amplification. The sensor's surface is engineered with polyaniline nanowires and gold nanoparticles (AuNPs) to improve electrical signal transfer and facilitate biomolecular interactions. The key to the biosensor's function is the peptide scaffold, which has four distinct parts: an anchoring domain to attach to the surface, an anti-fouling domain (EKEKEKE) that prevents unwanted molecules from sticking to the sensor, a linking domain (PPPP), and a recognition domain (HSSKLQK) specifically designed to bind with PSA. When PSA is present, it causes the recognition domain to cleave, or break off, the peptides from the sensor's surface. This release leads to a measurable drop in the electrical signal, which is directly proportional to the amount of PSA. The biosensor was successfully tested on real clinical samples, which demonstrated its reliability for the application of early prostate cancer detection (Hui et al. 2023).

5.4.1.3.2 Nanomaterial-Based Biosensors for Ovarian Cancer

There are more than five thousand deaths due to cancer in women annually, and approximately five percent are caused by ovarian cancer (OC). OC is the seventh most frequently occurring cancer in women globally and poses a serious public health issue. The death rate due to OC is extremely high, with the figure presently standing at 63.8 %, primarily because of the lack of efficient early detection methods. OC symptoms are usually very non-specific, which makes it difficult to target. Traditionally, diagnosis of OC utilizes several well-established tests, including pelvic examinations, ultrasound, magnetic resonance imaging (MRI, biopsy, and blood tests for certain biomarkers. Although these diagnostic methods are effective in some situations, they have certain disadvantages. Recent developments in nanomaterials have further enhanced the sensitivity of biosensing techniques for the early detection of OC by overcoming intrinsic shortcomings in conventional detection techniques. Nanomaterials such as metallic NPs, MXene, and $TiO_{2,}$ have shown increased benefit for OC-based biomarker detection due to higher interaction with sensing media and recognition biomolecules (Amourizi et al. 2025). Recent advances in nanobiosensors have made it possible to measure ovarian cancer (OC) biomarkers, such as CA125, with exceptional sensitivity. One new biosensor combines Prussian blue nanoparticles (PB), MXene quantum dots (QDs), and gold nanoparticles (AuNPs). This unique combination improves stability while boosting electrical conductivity and antibody attachment. The result is an incredibly effective device that has been successfully tested on clinical serum samples, showing its potential to improve OC diagnostics (Amourizi et al. 2025).

5.4.1.3.3 Nanomaterial-Based Biosensors for Breast Cancer

Breast cancer remains the most prevalent cancer type in women globally and continues to grow in incidence. Despite improvements in early diagnosis and detection, breast cancer remains the top cause of death for women because metastatic patients are incurable and have a poor prognosis. Furthermore, mortality is extremely high. HER2 overexpression has been marked as a prominent and predictive biomarker associated with breast cancer. It is used widely for detecting the malignancy and adverse prognosis of the tumor. Even though HER2-positive breast cancers make up a significant portion of all breast cancers (15–30%), they can be difficult to treat. A major challenge is when these cancers spread (metastasize) and become resistant to the treatments designed to target them. This makes it difficult to effectively manage the disease in its advanced stages. Nonetheless, early diagnosis of breast cancer emphasizes the demand for and possible advantage of more sensitive methods. Here, recent research indicates that biosensors offer advantages with speed, cost efficiency, and specificity over approaches for biomarker detection techniques like enzyme-linked immunosorbent assay (ELISA), chemiluminescent immunoassay (CIA), molecular biology methods, and liquid biopsy. Additionally, biosensors are an excellent tool for quickly and sensitively detecting biomarkers, such as HER2, allowing for early detection (Makableh et al. 2023).

5.4.2 Limitations and Challenges

Electrochemical sensors have their benefits against conventional procedures, but they come with limitations as well. Detection approaches and device intricacies are a significant stumbling block for biosensors. Ensuring that biomolecules remain stable and active under difficult conditions is a persistent challenge, impacting how long they can be stored and remain effective. Additionally, there's a need for more research into sensitive and specific biomarkers for breast cancer, as current options often fail to predict the disease before physical symptoms appear.

Despite such challenges, the domain of biosensor technology is full of promise, though with calls for stern analysis and innovation. Most biosensors are now designed to detect a single target, but they face challenges in detecting multiple targets concurrently. Further, integration and miniaturization still lack pace.

In cancer detection, electrochemical biosensor development is hindered by complex production processes that include several steps and tagged reagents. A major challenge that arises is slow covalent bond formation in sensor fabrication. It becomes quite challenging for the current electrochemical cytosensors to identify CTCs in cancer patients' blood effectively. There is also a lack of studies on the most favorable amount of biomarker concentration for detecting breast cancer in human serum (Gajdosova et al. 2020).

Exosomes, although hopeful biomarkers, also need careful characterization at the single-vesicle level to avoid receptor heterogeneity. Apart from this, quantum dots (QDs) also face problems in handling and reception of signal difficulties relative to nanoparticles or enzymes. Scientific research has delivered improvements in electrochemical sensors by conjugation with enzyme-based and metallic nanoparticles. Despite such uprising research ideas, the translational impact remains hampered due to a lack of proper validation studies, insufficient comparisons of performance with well-established methods, and unsolved analytical challenges such as nonspecific binding and reproducibility. In addition, the high costs of nanomaterials and complicated immunosensor procedures are further obstacles (Jarahi Khameneh et al. 2024).

Despite these difficulties, electrochemical biosensors have promise for early cancer diagnosis and improved patient outcomes. The realization of this potential, however, requires great investment from the government and healthcare facilities in terms of pushing the technology toward commercialization. Overcoming these challenges will involve creating highly sensitive and stable biological sensors that have the capacity to transform cancer diagnosis and patient outcomes.

5.5 THERAPEUTIC NANOMEDICINE MODALITIES

Therapeutic nanomedicine offers a versatile platform to overcome the limitations of conventional therapies by enabling precise delivery, controlled release, and multimodal treatment strategies. Various nanocarrier systems—including liposomes, polymers, inorganic nanoparticles, and hybrid platforms—are being engineered to enhance efficacy, reduce toxicity, and tackle challenges such as multidrug resistance, poor penetration, and immune evasion. The following sections outline key nanomedicine modalities ranging from chemotherapy and immunotherapy to gene editing, phototherapies, radiosensitization, and their synergistic combinations, highlighting both their transformative potential and existing limitations.

5.5.1 Chemotherapy Delivery

Nanocarrier-enabled chemotherapy seeks to raise intratumoral drug exposure while reducing systemic toxicity, using platforms such as PEGylated/non-PEGylated liposomes, albumin nanoparticles, polymeric micelles and solid polymer nanoparticles. Multiple clinically used formulations validate this approach—for example, pegylated liposomal doxorubicin (PLD/Doxil), liposomal irinotecan (Onivyde), liposomal daunorubicin (DaunoXome), non-PEGylated liposomal doxorubicin (Myocet), albumin-bound paclitaxel (nab-paclitaxel/Abraxane), and polymeric micellar paclitaxel (Genexol-PM)—each illustrating how nanoscale carriers alter pharmacokinetics, tissue distribution and tolerability to reshape the therapeutic window. At the same time, translational analyses remind us that nanoparticle tumor delivery remains limited and heterogeneous in humans, prompting designs that leverage stimulus-responsiveness, active targeting, tumor-penetration strategies, and combination regimens to overcome barriers including multidrug resistance (MDR) (Table 5.1) (Bhatia et al. 2022).

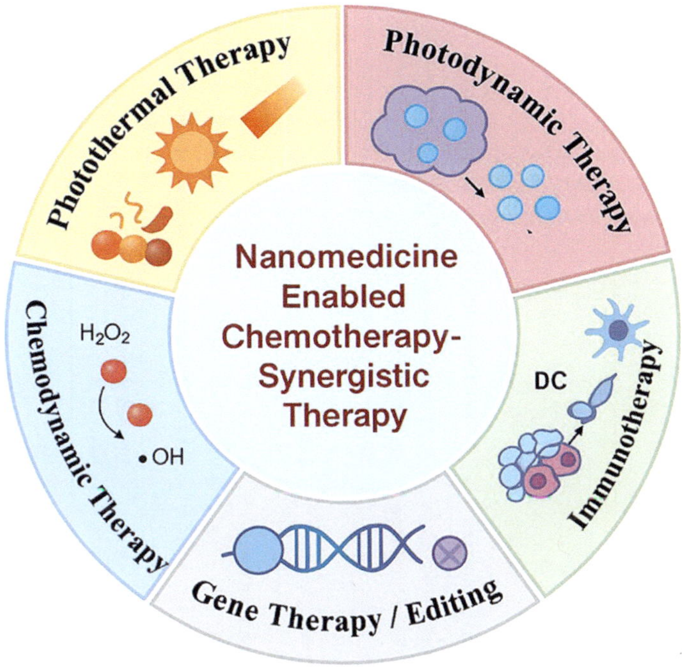

FIGURE 5.3 Nanomedicine-enabled synergistic therapies with chemotherapy.

5.5.1.1 Liposomes

Pegylated liposomal doxorubicin (Doxil/Caelyx) also invented the long-circulating liposome through the addition of a steric PEG coat, which reduces RES uptake and thus elevates tumor AUC and lowers the cardiotoxicity/alopecia profile of free doxorubicin. Early randomized studies in Kaposi's sarcoma showed clinical activity, and later investigations in breast and ovarian cancer established dosing and safety profiles. These outcomes prompted the overall clinical establishment of the liposomal anthracyclines. Mechanistically, the liposome encapsulation of doxorubicin changes its plasma/tissue kinetics, and pegylation adds further half-life prolongation and an inclination toward skin accumulation (hand-foot syndrome), which serves as an example of formulation-dependent adverse events compared to the parent drug (Gill et al. 1996).

Liposome daunorubicin (DaunoXome) and non-PEG liposome doxorubicin (Myocet) illustrate formulation variation. DaunoXome showed efficacy in AIDS-related Kaposi's sarcoma and was evaluated in other solid tumors; Myocet was tested (as monotherapy/in combination with taxanes or trastuzumab) in HER2-positive breast cancer metastatic disease, in which the non-PEG vesicles tried to reduce exposure/dermal toxicity and focus synergy with traditional agents. These products illustrate the capability of lipid formulation, surface chemistry, and state of pegylation to modulate clinical performance/toxicity. Liposomal irinotecan (nal-IRI/Onivyde) incorporated liposomal topology into a topoisomerase-I inhibitor. In NAPOLI-1, nal-IRI + 5-FU/leucovorin enhanced overall survival compared to 5-FU/leucovorin alone in gemcitabine-refractory metastatic pancreatic cancer, resulting in FDA approval in 2015. The liposome increased intratumoral conversion to the active metabolite, SN-38, and prolonged exposure, which translates into a clinically significant survival benefit and solidifies nal-IRI (Nikolova et al. 2022).

In addition to approved drugs, recent liposome engineering focuses on TME–responsive release. pH-sensitive liposomes utilize slightly acidic extracellular pH (≈6.5–6.9) to induce doxorubicin release through PE-based formulations, which contain acid-labile stabilizers, while enzyme-sensitive

TABLE 5.1
FDA-Approved and Late-Stage Nanomedicines for Chemotherapy Delivery

Formulation (Trade Name)	Carrier Type	Payload	Indication(s)	Status/Trial Phase	Key Advantages	Key Limitations	References
Doxil®/ Caelyx®	PEGylated liposome	Doxorubicin	Kaposi's sarcoma, ovarian, breast cancer	FDA approved (1995)	Reduced cardiotoxicity; prolonged circulation	Hand–foot syndrome, skin accumulation	Barenholz (2012)
Myocet®	Non-PEGy lated liposome	Doxorubicin	Metastatic breast cancer (EU)	Approved in EU	Lower cutaneous toxicity versus Doxil	Shorter half-life	Batist et al. (2006)
DaunoXome®	Liposome	Daunorubicin	Kaposi's sarcoma	FDA approved (1996)	Improved tolerability	Limited use outside KS	Northfelt et al. (1998)
Onivyde®	Liposome	Irinotecan	Pancreatic cancer (2L)	FDA approved (2015)	Enhanced SN-38 exposure; survival benefit	GI toxicity	Wang-Gillam et al. (2016)
Abraxane®	Albumin NP	Paclitaxel	Breast, NSCLC, pancreatic	FDA approved (2005)	Cremophor-free; gp60/ SPARC uptake	Peripheral neuropathy	Gradishar et al. (2005)
Genexol-PM®	Polymeric micelle	Paclitaxel	Breast cancer	Approved in Korea	Solubilization without Cremophor	Limited global adoption	Kim et al. (2004)

pegylation (e.g., MMP-cleavable PEG) bolsters regional uptake by eliminating PEG near the tumor sites. These approaches seek to balance circulation stability and in-site payload release, enhancing effectiveness in poorly perfused, heterogeneous tumors (Nikolova et al. 2022).

5.5.1.2 Albumin Nanoparticles

Nanoparticle albumin-bound paclitaxel (nab-paclitaxel/Abraxane) deletes Cremophor EL (abrogating premedication-related hypersensitivity), increases tolerated dose intensity, and employs albumin's endogenous transport system. Proposed mechanisms are gp60/caveolin-1-mediated transcytosis through endothelium and preferential tumor accumulation, which might be mediated by SPARC (secreted protein acidic and rich in cysteine), although SPARC's prognostic significance is disputed across indications. In the clinic, nab-paclitaxel has been approved in various settings (e.g., metastatic breast cancer; combination regimens in NSCLC and pancreatic cancer), and it frequently has higher response rates or convenient dosing compared to solvent-based paclitaxel. The nab platform also prompts novel albumin-hitchhiking designs (e.g., small molecule/peptide–albumin binders or 30-nm albumin NPs) to utilize the same trafficking pathways for varied payloads (taxanes, kinase inhibitors) and facilitate combination strategies (e.g., simultaneous stromal modulation in desmoplastic tumors). These derivatives seek to further optimize tumoral uptake and reduce off-target exposures (Suwannasom et al. 2023).

5.5.1.3 Polymeric Micelles and Polymeric Nanoparticles

Polymeric micelles (PEG-PLA, PCL, PLGA) solubilize hydrophobic cytotoxics and alter biodistribution. Genexol-PM (polymeric micellar paclitaxel) advanced to Phase III comparisons with solvent-based paclitaxel, while NK105 showed enhanced antitumor activity in xenografts and advanced to early clinical trials, including radiotherapy modality combination studies. Increasingly, multi-stimuli sensitive micelles and polymersomes combine pH/redox responsiveness, enzyme-cleavable coupling, and switchable size for deep penetration and intracellular release. In cancers, redox-sensitive disulfides and others use high glutathione to induce payload release, whereas matrix metalloproteinase-sensitive shells shrink and traverse highly crosslinked matrices. Such "programmed" carriers try to circumvent mass-transport bottlenecks that prevent uniform intratumoral medication distributions (Oerlemans et al. 2010).

MDR requires membrane efflux pumps (e.g., P-glycoprotein/ABCB1), intracellular trafficking/sequestration, variable apoptotic thresholds, and TME-induced difficulties. Nanocarriers can evade MDR by endocytic absorption, co-delivery of efflux modulators/ROS inducers, organelle targeting (e.g., lysosome escape), and pharmacokinetic stabilization giving cytotoxic pressure. The Pluronic micellar doxorubicin SP1049C directly modulates P-gp and cellular energetics and showed action and fair tolerability in Phase I/II clinical trials in GI malignancies above the mid-levels, as well as CSC elimination and reduced tumorigenicity, consistent with polymer-mediated MDR reversal. Other than Pluronic, pH-sensitive Pluronic micelles generating oxidative stress reverse MDR synergistically, and TME-sensitive micelles/liposomes release the medicine inside the tumor front before efflux by employing acidity or redox potential (Oerlemans et al. 2010).

5.5.2 Immunotherapy

Immunotherapy has become one of oncology's most revolutionary paradigms by delivering prolonged responses and potential cures in minority patients in whom conventional therapy is not effective. Nevertheless, the clinical benefits are still limited to minority patients due to barriers such as immune tumor evasion, lacking enough immunogenicity, systematic toxicities, and heterogeneous tumor microenvironments. The answers are given by nanomedicine by increasing the pharmacokinetics, biodistribution, and spatiotemporal control of immunomodulators. NPs can carry adjuvants to antigen-presenting cells (APCs), tumor-associated antigens or neoantigens can be entrapped by them, in situ vaccination can be permitted by them, and the tumor immune microenvironment (TIME) can be modified by them. By combining rationally designed nanocarriers with immunotherapeutic agents such as immune checkpoint inhibitors (ICIs), cytokines, and anticancer vaccines, nanomedicine has the prospect for broadening the effectiveness and safety of anticancer immunotherapy (Lee Ventola 2017).

5.5.2.1 Nano-Adjuvants: Engineering Innate Immune Activation

Modern vaccines offer evidence that adjuvant chemistry and nanoscale formulation are able to redefine immunity at its very foundation. GlaxoSmithKline's AS01 adjuvant platform (MPL + QS-21 in liposomes) in commercialized vaccines, such as Shingrix and RTS, S, is the best evidence: liposomal co-delivery of TLR4 agonist and saponin induces vigorous cellular as well as humoral responses. Cervarix, in comparison, puts MPL together with aluminum salts (AS04, not in liposomes) and demonstrates that adjuvant architecture has an effect (Jin et al. 2023).

These clinical precedents stimulate oncology-specific nano-adjuvants that encapsulate PAMPs (TLR ligands, STING activators) in polymeric vesicles, liposomes, or hybrid carriers to enhance dendritic-cell (DC) maturation and cross-priming. A prototype is STING-activating polymersomes that increase cytosolic delivery of cGAMP, reconstruct suppressive tumor microenvironments, and complement checkpoint blockade in vivo. Groundbreaking vaccine work demonstrates that properly formulated TLR agonists can "program" response size and duration—principles directly applicable to cancer vaccines. The adjuvant chemistry (e.g., MPL, QS-21), microenvironment-responsive release (pH, redox), and compartment targeting (lymph node versus tumor) are at the same level as the active itself. It is for this reason that adjuvant system choices (AS01 versus AS04) and nanopackage information often include explanations for efficacy and tolerability variations seen between vaccines and potential cancer nanovaccines (Jin et al. 2023).

5.5.2.2 APC-Targeting Nanoparticles: Precision Delivery to Dendritic Cells and Lymph Nodes

Potent antitumor T cells rely on effective cross-presentation by DCs. The nanoparticles allow for receptor-mediated uptake and lymph-node targeting:

These mannosylated carriers exploit the DCs' CD206 for increased uptake and presentation of antigens via MHC-I; different studies confirm increased cross-priming by mannosylated PLGA/polyanhydride platforms. Albumin "hitchhiking" to TDLNs: amphiphile vaccines (antigen/agonist linked to an albumin-binding lipid tail) piggy-back on endogenous albumin trafficking to lymph nodes, greatly amplifying $CD8^+$ T-cell priming in mice and informing clinical derivatives like ELI-005/ELI-002 (H. Liu et al. 2014).

5.5.2.3 Neoantigen Delivery and mRNA Nano Vaccines

Personalized mRNA vaccines delivered by lipid nanoparticles (LNPs) are now showing randomized clinical signals. In resected high-risk melanoma, the individualized vaccine mRNA-4157 (V940) plus pembrolizumab significantly improved recurrence-free survival in a Phase 2b trial. In pancreatic ductal adenocarcinoma, the autogene-cevumeran (BNT122) mRNA vaccine induced robust, vaccine-specific $CD8^+$ T-cell responses that correlated with delayed recurrence in an adjuvant Phase 1 study—an important feasibility signal in a notoriously "cold" tumor (Nguyen et al. 2025).

Behind these outcomes lies a decade of platform science showing us particle charge and composition can be tuned to target RNA-containing particles to DCs in vivo in the absence of specific ligands, and organ tropism, endosomal escape, and tolerability are strongly dictated by LNP formulation. These trials confirm an end-to-end mutation → neoantigen prediction → LNP vaccine development pipeline, paving the way to combination regimens (ICB, RT, cytotoxics) and to minimal residual disease settings in which systemic toxicity budgets are narrow (Nguyen et al. 2025).

5.5.2.4 In Situ Vaccines and Antigen-Capturing Nanoparticles (AC-NPs)

Instead of delivering exogenous antigen, in situ vaccination transforms the tumor into its own source of antigen. Protein-releasing, antigen-capture nanoparticles (functionalized to covalently bind proteins released upon local therapy) increased APC uptake and the abscopal effect when used in combination with anti-PD-1, providing cures in otherwise unresponsive melanoma models. The phototherapies and the in-situ strategies are natural complements of one another. In a benchmark experiment, PLGA-ICG-R837 nanoparticles allowed photothermal ablation by NIR while they concurrently administered a TLR7 agonist; when anti-CTLA-4 was added, this induced systemic antitumor immunity to distantly located lesions in mice (Chao et al. 2025).

Despite remarkable progress, several translational challenges remain. Anti-PEG antibodies are increasingly recognized as a translational hurdle, since they can accelerate nanoparticle clearance or trigger hypersensitivity reactions upon repeat dosing of PEGylated formulations. At the same time, delivery heterogeneity and inconsistent trial outcomes highlight the need for careful patient stratification, rational cargo selection, and robust, fit-for-purpose manufacturing analytics to ensure reproducibility and clinical impact.

5.5.3 Gene Therapy/Editing

Gene therapy and genome editing have emerged as revolutionary strategies for cancer treatment through correction of the genetic abnormalities that support tumor initiation, progression, and therapeutic resistance. In contrast to conventional therapies that mainly target cancer symptoms or fast-dividing cells, gene-based interventions aim to modify, replace, silence, or repair disease-associated genes at the molecular level. The clinical potential of these strategies has been further accelerated by advances in nanotechnology, which offers safe and efficient delivery systems for nucleic acids, such as plasmid DNA, messenger RNA (mRNA), small interfering RNA (siRNA), microRNA (miRNA), and CRISPR/Cas-based genome-editing tools. By precisely altering gene expression, these technologies hold promise for personalized cancer treatment, improved therapeutic efficacy, and reduced off-target toxicity, making gene therapy and gene editing central to next-generation oncology (Park et al. 2025).

5.5.3.1 siRNA and miRNA Delivery Systems

RNA interference (RNAi) has been identified as an effective method of controlling gene expression after transcription. Small interfering RNAs (siRNAs) silence complementary messenger RNA transcripts by their destruction, and larger gene networks responsible for oncogenesis are controlled by microRNAs (miRNAs). Naked RNAs are short-lived, quickly hydrolyzed by nucleases, and poorly internalized by cells. Nanomedicine has been used to shield the RNA molecule and facilitate its delivery.

Historic approval of the first FDA-approved therapeutic siRNA, patisiran (Onpattro), formulated in lipid nanoparticles (LNPs), confirmed the effectiveness of systemic RNAi therapy in human beings by knocking down transthyretin in hereditary amyloidosis. In the field of oncology, Atu027, a liposome-formulated siRNA against PKN3, was explored in a phase I trial and exhibited safety and signs of disease stabilization. Another therapeutic, TKM-080301, an siRNA against polo-like kinase 1 (PLK1) formulated in LNPs, was assessed in hepatocellular carcinoma; its result exhibited manageable toxicities but restricted effectiveness. Polymeric and dendrimer nanoparticles are also employed extensively. For example, poly(amidoamine) (PAMAM) dendrimers of siRNA targeted against Bcl-2 induced apoptosis and tumor regression in preclinical cancer (M. Liu et al. 2025).

5.5.3.2 Plasmid DNA and mRNA Nanomedicines

Plasmid DNA (pDNA) therapies enable long-term protein expression but require nuclear entry, which limits efficiency in non-dividing cells. The most notable example, Allovectin-7, a lipid-based pDNA encoding HLA-B7 and β2-microglobulin, advanced to phase III clinical trials in melanoma but failed to demonstrate clinical benefit. Messenger RNA (mRNA), on the other hand, requires only delivery to the cytosol, yet it was more efficient and safer by nature due to the lack of genomic integration. The effectiveness of COVID-19 mRNA vaccines revealed the scalability and clinical relevance of LNP-based mRNA delivery (Uchida 2022).

Applications in oncology have progressed immensely, where mRNA-4157 (Moderna) has exhibited drastically enhanced recurrence-free survival in combination with pembrolizumab in melanoma cases. Likewise, BNT122 (BioNTech) has revealed immunogenicity and safety in initial-phase trials.

5.5.3.3 CRISPR/Cas Genome Editing via Nanoparticles

CRISPR/Cas9 genome editing enabled targeted genome knockdown, repair, and modulation, revolutionizing oncology research. Delivery remains a constraint. Viral vectors are efficient but risk insertional mutagenesis and immunological responses. Nanoparticles provide temporary, safer delivery. LNPs containing Cas9 mRNA and sgRNAs edited Pcsk9 in hepatocytes, lowering mice cholesterol. PD-L1-targeted LNPs restored T cell immunity and tumor regression in mice models. Another improvement was tumor-specific LNPs coated with hyaluronic acid, which delivered CRISPR/Cas9 to CD44+ breast cancer cells and broke oncogenic drivers. Endosomal escape, nuclear transport, and off-target editing remain. Engineering high-fidelity Cas9 variants like eSpCas9 and SpCas9-HF1 with transitory nanoparticle delivery decreases unintentional edits and enhances safety.

Nanoparticle-mediated gene therapy translation is difficult. Due to reticuloendothelial system uptake, nanoparticles aggregate in the spleen and liver, reducing tumor delivery. Selective organ targeting (SORT) lipids reorient LNP tropism toward extrahepatic organs, improving delivery specificity. Size-switching nanoparticles and matrix-degrading proteases are being developed to overcome dense extracellular matrices and disorganized vasculature, which hinder tumor penetration. Future plans include developing theranostic nanoparticles (e.g., CRISPR carriers visible to MRI) for real-time tracking and biomarker-based patient selection to match medicines to tumor biology. Nanoparticle-enabled gene therapy and editing should remain a cornerstone of precision medicine in oncology (Rauf et al. 2025).

5.5.4 Photothermal Therapy

Photothermal therapy (PTT) is a nanomedicine approach that utilizes photosensitive nanomaterials to photo-convert near-infrared (NIR) illumination into heat to produce localized hyperthermia that kills cancer cells or makes them sensitive to other therapies. The rationale for PTT is the possibility of spatially controlled, minimally invasive tumor eradication with little damage to adjacent normal tissues. NIR wavelengths, especially within the so-called biological transparency windows (NIR-I: 650–950 nm; NIR-II: 1000–1700 nm), transmit deeper into tissues than visible light, enabling irradiation of tumors several centimeters underneath the skin surface. Nanoparticles designed to exhibit high photothermal conversion efficiency intratumorally accumulate due to the enhanced permeability and retention (EPR) effect or through active targeting ligands, where it is possible to produce enough heat under laser irradiation to trigger apoptosis, necrosis, and in most instances, immunogenic cell death (ICD). Besides direct eradication, PTT also functions as an activator trigger for the release from thermosensitive nanocarriers and as an adjunct modality to enhance chemotherapy, radiotherapy, and immunotherapy efficacy (Bian et al. 2021).

5.5.4.1 Plasmonic Nanomaterials: Gold Nanorods, Nanoshells, and Nanocages

More widely investigated among photo-thermal agents are plasmonic gold nanostructures due to their tunable optical absorption, excellent biocompatibility, and ease of surface modification. Gold nanorods (AuNRs) possess longitudinal plasmon resonance whose wavelength is accessible into the near infrared (NIR) by adjusting their aspect ratio. Upon laser irradiation, AuNRs produce rapid and intense localized heating to induce efficient tumor ablation. Gold nanoshells comprising a silica core coated by an ultrathin layer of gold mantle selectively absorbing near infrared (NIR) light have progressed most toward the clinic. Intravenously administered silica–gold nanoshells (AuroShells®) under the control of near-IR laser irradiation were safe and effective to induce focal tumor ablation of prostate tumors without damaging adjacent structures such as the nerves and the urinary sphincter. Gold nanocages comprised by hollow porous structures with large surface-to-volume ratio provide both photothermal response and drug-loading capacity to permit combination therapies (Huang and El-Sayed 2011).

Apart from gold, plasmonic and carbon-based nanomaterials were explored, such as carbon nanotubes, graphene oxide, and copper sulfide nanocrystals. Although these materials demonstrate strong photothermal conversion, their clinical application is restricted due to long-term biodegradability concerns and potential toxicity. As an alternative, gold nanomaterials tend to be biologically well tolerated and may be tailored by attaching the PEG or tumor-targeting ligands to enhance tumoral selectivity and systemic circulation. As a group, these nanoarchitectures demonstrate the possibility to delicately tune nanoscale composition and geometry to achieve clinically relevant photothermal properties (Huang and El-Sayed 2011).

5.5.4.2 NIR-I versus NIR-II Windows

Although the majority of initial PTT research used NIR-I wavelengths, increasing interest has focused on the NIR-II window (1000–1700 nm). At these wavelengths, penetration by light is greater and scattering is less intense, resulting in greater spatial resolution and more consistent distribution of heat within tumors. A range of nanomaterials has been designed to absorb in the NIR-II spectrum, such as semiconducting polymer nanoparticles, the single-walled carbon nanotube, silver sulfide quantum dots, and rare-earth doped nanoprobes. Preclinical research involving NIR-II absorbing probes has produced efficient tumor ablation even when tumors were positioned greater than 7–8 mm below the skin surface, which is the typical penetration depth limitation of NIR-I-based therapy. Additionally, NIR-II PTT causes less induction of superficial tissue non-specific heating, resulting in greater specificity therapy (Zhao et al. 2018).

Despite these advantages, the transition from NIR-I to NIR-II remains an area of ongoing research, as NIR-II lasers are less widely available in clinical settings and safety thresholds for prolonged irradiation at these wavelengths are still under investigation. Nevertheless, the development of NIR-II responsive nanomaterials represents a major frontier for deep-tissue PTT and holds promise for expanding clinical applicability to internal malignancies (Zhao et al. 2018).

Overall, Photothermal therapy demonstrates the capability of nanomedicine to produce spatiotemporally controlled, minimally invasive tumor elimination. Progresses in plasmonic nanomaterials, especially gold nanorods, nanoshells, and nanocages, paved the way toward clinical translation, and second- or even third-generation NIR-II responsive agents offer enhanced tissue penetration and greater precision. PTT is also an adaptable complement to chemotherapy, immunotherapy, PDT, and radiotherapy, offering prospects for synergistic multi-mode regimens. Hurdles exist in biodistribution, long-term safety, and manufacturability, yet preliminary clinical results already demonstrate the promise of PTT as a safe and effective add-on to standard therapies. Future advances will entail the development of biodegradable NIR-II nanomaterials, theranostic platforms integrated with imaging-guided laser control, and rationally constructed combination regimens optimized to tumor biology. With such developments, PTT will move from a niche experimental therapy toward becoming a mainstream clinical instrument for precision oncology.

5.5.5 Photodynamic Therapy

Photodynamic therapy (PDT) represents a modality that couples a photosensitizer, a light of defined wavelength, and molecular oxygen to generate cytotoxic reactive oxygen species (ROS) that trigger tumor cell death. The PDT therapy mechanism is complex: when the photosensitizer absorbs photons and converts them into surrounding oxygen molecules to produce singlet oxygen ($^\wedge 1O_2$) and free radicals that destroy biomolecules outright, it causes damage to the tumor vasculature and elicits inflammation and immune response. Moreover, PDT provides spatial and temporal selectivity since the photosensitizer is innocuous in the dark and the region may be selectively activated by light. This localized action minimizes systemic toxicity despite the inherent shortcomings due to reliance on penetration by light and the availability of oxygen. Nanotechnology has revolutionized PDT by enhancing solubility, stability, tumor uptake, and photophysics of the photosensitizer, thus overcoming most disadvantages inherent to conventional preparations (Al-Jamal et al. 2025).

5.5.5.1 Nanocarrier-Enabled Delivery of Photosensitizers

Classic photosensitizing agents—for example, porphyrins, chlorins, and phthalocyanines—suffer from low solubility in water, aggregation at physiological conditions, and long duration skin phototoxicity. Nano delivery systems obviate these disadvantages by enhancing pharmacokinetics and tumor selectivity. Porphyrin encapsulated in liposomes, for instance, improve bioavailability and tumor accumulation with reducing off-target deposition. Accordingly, hydrophobic phthalocyanines encapsulated into polymeric nanoprobes lead to monodispersed distribution and greater singlet oxygen formation efficacy. Chlorin e6 (Ce6), the most investigated second-generation PS, was encapsulated successfully into micelles, dendrimers, and semiconductor NPs to achieve deeper tumor penetration and controlled release (G. Li et al. 2024).

Some of the most recent innovations include the upconversion nanoparticles (UCNPs) that absorb the deeply penetrating NIR light and emit the shorter wavelengths employed to activate the conventional photosensitizers. This strategy efficiently sidesteps the superficial penetration employed to activate porphyrins and chlorins and extends the applicability of PDT to deeper-lying tumors. Moreover, drug delivery functionality was integrated with imaging potential by encapsulating the nanoscale coordination polymers with the photosensitizers to develop true theranostic systems (G. Li et al. 2024).

5.5.5.2 Oxygen-Independent PDT Strategies

Most significant drawback of PDT is the dependency on molecular oxygen, which is usually low in hypoxic tumor microenvironments. Toward overcoming this limitation, oxygen-independent or oxygen-augmenting strategies have been designed. Type I PDT, producing hydroxyl and superoxide radicals by virtue of an electron transfer mechanism instead of singlet oxygen, is possible under low oxygen conditions. Nanoparticles encapsulated with Type I sensitizers—for example, aza-BODIPY derivatives—were found to be effective even in hypoxic tumors.

Otherwise, oxygen-generating nanocarriers provide exogenous oxygen delivery or catalytic in situ oxygen generation. Perfluorocarbon nanoparticles, whose oxygen solubility is exceptionally high, serve as O_2 reservoirs releasing O_2 after irradiation. In the same context, catalase-encapsulated nanoparticles lyse the inherent hydrogen peroxide into oxygen, relieving hypoxia while concurrently allowing PDT. Manganese dioxide (MnO_2)-based nanomaterials constitute another family of oxygen-generating nanomaterials, lysing H_2O_2 and manipulating tumor redox balance alongside the provision of MRI contrast. These developments enhance PDT efficacy besides incorporating both therapeutic and diagnostic properties (X. Li et al. 2023).

5.5.5.3 Nanoparticle-Enabled Combination PDT Strategies

The combination of PDT with other modalities is increasingly appreciated. PDT may be used to combine with chemotherapy, where ROS induced by light increase drug uptake and cytotoxicity. Porphyrin–doxorubicin co-loaded liposomes have exhibited synergistic tumor regression when PDT-generated ROS lyse the endosomal membranes and release chemotherapeutic agents into the cytosol. PDT is also complementary to photothermal therapy (PTT), where heat enhances tumor oxygenation and consequently ROS formation, while PDT enhances PTT-triggered immunogenic cell death. The most encouraging combination seems to be the one with immunotherapy. Immunogenic cell death induced by PDT unleashes tumor-associated antigens and danger signals, attracting dendritic cells and activating cytotoxic T cell response. Combined with checkpoint inhibitors like anti-PD-1, PDT was able to induce effective systemic immunity that was responsible for regression of treated tumors as well as abscopal effects on nontreated lesions. PDT thus turned out to be an effective collaborator for the in-situ vaccination approach (Rajagopal et al. 2025).

Some photosensitizers already possess regulatory clearance within traditional formulations, such as Photofrin® (porfimer sodium), Verteporfin® (Visudyne), and Talaporfin sodium (Laserphyrin), essentially for esophageal, lung, and head and neck malignancies. Nonetheless, the development of nanoparticle-based formulations continues to move into clinical and translational pipelines. As examples, Ce6 and porphyrin derivative-based nanoparticle preparations are currently in early-phase tests for solid tumors to enhance the selectivity toward tumors and diminish systemic adverse effects. Furthermore, the Japan regulatory body approved near-infrared photoimmunotherapy (NIR-PIT) for the treatment of recurrent head and neck tumors, illuminating the clinical potential of photo-activated nanomedicine. NIR-PIT utilizes antibody–photosensitizer conjugates (e.g., anti-EGFR antibody conjugated to IR700 dye) that selectively accumulate within tumor cells and trigger abrupt necrotic cell death upon irradiation, accompanied by potent immunogenic effects. Though it is not traditional PDT per se, NIR-PIT constitutes an alternative line of photo-based nanomedicine gaining real-world traction (Rajagopal et al. 2025).

In summary, Photodynamic therapy has transformed from a specialty modality with restricted penetration depth to a cross-platform approach to tumor ablation, immune stimulation, and combinational therapies. Nanotechnology has played the key role in this transformation by offering solutions to solubility problems, biodistribution limitations, and tumor-selectivity challenges and by facilitating imaging-guided and oxygen-independent PDT approaches. By developing the field to employ upconversion systems, catalase-laden nanoclusters, MnO_2-based oxygen delivery carriers, and NIR-activated carriers, the PDT is becoming increasingly tolerant to the heterogeneities encountered within tumors. The immunogenic impact on PDT makes it an effective augmenter of immunotherapy even having the capability to turn the ‘cold’ tumors into ‘hot’ tumors amendable to checkpoint blockade. Though the problems of light penetration depth, patient-specific oxygenation of tumors, and large-scale nanocarrier fabrication remain, the future prospects of PDT nanomedicine strongly indicate increasing clinical impact especially when used as part of the multimodal regimens.

5.5.6 Radio Sensitization

Radiotherapy is a cornerstone of cancer therapy, used by an estimated 50–60% of cancer patients sometime during the course of therapy. Its treatment efficacy is based on the induction of double-strand breaks in DNA and the formation of free radicals that ultimately lead to apoptosis, mitotic catastrophe, or senescence in tumor cells. Normal tissue toxicity and inherent radio resistance due to hypoxia or repair competency in tumors, though, prevent greater success. Nanomedicine has surfaced as an effective approach to enhance radiation effects selectively within tumors through radio sensitization by exploiting nanoparticles that engage ionizing radiation to boost local energy deposition, generation of radicals, or biological response modulation. Specifically, those nanomaterials of high-atomic-number (high-Z) character, such as gold, hafnium oxide, bismuth, gadolinium, and platinum nanoparticles, strongly absorb X-rays or γ-rays to generate cascading secondary electrons that enhance local DNA damage as well as ROS formation in cancer cells. This physical dose enhancement when accompanied by tumor-selective delivery promises enhanced radiotherapy efficacy while restricting off-target damage (Gong et al. 2021).

5.5.6.1 High-Z Nanoparticles as Physical Dose Enhancers

Gold nanoparticles (AuNPs) are the most researched nanomaterial-based radiosensitizers. As a result of their large Z (Z = 79) and strong photoelectric absorption cross-section, AuNPs are efficient producers of secondary electrons when a kilovoltage spectrum is used. A number of preclinical studies have confirmed the discovery that tumor-anchored AuNPs improve DNA damage and tumor regression when administered with radiation therapy alone. Functionalization of AuNPs by PEG, antibodies, or peptides enhances their systemic circulation and tumor specificity and enhances the therapeutic indexes further (Carbone et al. 2025). Hafnium oxide nanoparticles (HfO_2 NPs), marketed under the name NBTXR3 (Hensify®), mark the pinnacle of clinical translation. NBTXR3 is administered intratumorally and is triggered by conventional radiotherapy beams to produce greater dose deposition and immunogenic tumor cell death. It was approved by Europe for the treatment of soft tissue sarcoma and is being tested in head and neck cancer, metastatic cancer to the liver, and other solid tumors (Gong et al. 2021).

Bismuth (Bi)-containing nanomaterials ($Z = 83$) are becoming increasingly popular due to their strong X-ray absorption capability and inherent imaging contrast. Examples include the development of radio sensitization-engineered bismuth sulfide and bismuth oxide nanoparticles that offer both radio sensitization capability and CT imaging guidance. Likewise, when it comes to platinum-based nanomaterials, aside from their role as the high-Z radiosensitizers, these compounds offer chemotherapeutic action through DNA crosslinking that facilitates the dual mechanism of killing tumors (Gong et al. 2021).

5.5.6.2 Hypoxia-Targeted and Oxygen-Generating Nanomedicine Radiosensitizers

Another important factor decreasing radiotherapy efficacy is tumor hypoxia, which decreases ROS formation due to radiation. To counteract this, nanocarriers have been developed to eliminate hypoxia by producing or delivering oxygen. Manganese dioxide (MnO_2) nanoparticles catalyze the degradation of the naturally occurring hydrogen peroxide into oxygen by breaking it down, thus enhancing the tissue oxygenation within tumors and radiosensitivity. Perfluorocarbon nanoemulsions function as oxygen carriers and release the oxygen near the tumor, enhancing the generation of radicals when irradiated (Debnath et al. 2024).

Alternatively, hypoxia-activated prodrugs (e.g., tirapazamine) have been co-delivered with radio sensitizing nanoparticles to exploit low-oxygen niches for selective cytotoxicity. By integrating high-Z elements with hypoxia-responsive systems, nanomedicine radiosensitizers provide a multi-pronged solution to one of radiotherapy's most entrenched challenges (Debnath et al. 2024).

5.5.6.3 Biological Pathway Modulation Through Nanocarriers

Aside from dose enhancement by physics, radio sensitization potentially can be achieved by the modulation of signal transduction pathways and DNA repair. Nanoliposomes co-delivering cytotoxins such as cisplatin or inhibitors of the response to DNA damage (e.g., ATM/ATR inhibitors, PARP inhibitors) enhance radiation therapy by overwhelming tumor repair apparatus. Liposomal preparations of cisplatin improve tumor penetration and body wide toxicity reduction while simultaneously sensitizing tumors to irradiation. Gene therapy vectors, such as siRNA- or CRISPR-containing nanoparticles, were designed to knock down important repair genes like RAD51 or DNA-PKcs and thus preclude repair of breaks induced by radiation and enhance cytotoxicity. Nanoparticle-based delivery of radio sensitizing microRNAs was investigated to reduce pro-survival signals and enhance apoptosis after irradiation. Apart for this, Nanoparticle radiosensitizers are being investigated more widely in combination regimens. As an example, radio-chemotherapy combinations with AuNPs and doxorubicin liposomes improve tumor regression over both modality arms individually. Similarly, combining radiosensitizers with photothermal or photodynamic agents generates synergistic ROS bursts and thermal stress to enhance DNA damage (Shiridokht et al. 2025).

All in all, Nanomedicine radiosensitizers constitute one of the most clinically developed interfaces between nanotechnology and oncology. By exploiting high-Z nanoparticles to achieve physical dose enhancement, oxygen-releasing systems to alleviate hypoxia, and gene-controlling carriers to achieve biological sensitization, these approaches dramatically broaden the therapeutic window of radiotherapy. With promising clinic results for hafnium oxide and gadolinium-based nanosensitizers, radiosensitization is evolving from preclinical promise toward concrete patient benefit. Future development will particularly emphasize incorporating radio sensitization into multimodality regimens combining it with immunotherapy, chemotherapy, and imaging-guided precision oncology. Despite the need to maintain careful vigilance toward toxicity, manufacturability, and regulatory paradigms, the intersection of nanomedicine and radiotherapy promises to redefine cancer care standards over the ensuing decade (Shiridokht et al. 2025).

5.5.7 Combination Strategies

The heterogeneity and complexity of tumors render monotherapies inadequate for enduring results. Cancer advances by several hallmarks' evasion of apoptosis, angiogenesis, immunological suppression, and resistance to therapy requiring multimodal intervention. Nanomedicine facilitates combination therapy through the co-delivery of several payloads, spatiotemporal release control, imaging integration, and the utilization of tumor-specific triggers (Figure 5.3). The primary advantage is synergy integrating complementary processes to improve efficacy while decreasing toxicity via lower doses.

Initial instances encompass chemo-photothermal therapy (chemo-PTT), whereby chemotherapeutics (e.g., doxorubicin, paclitaxel) are co-administered with gold nanorods or nanoshells to surmount multidrug resistance, since near-infrared (NIR) generated hyperthermia augments permeability and drug absorption. Intelligent carriers, such as polydopamine-coated mesoporous silica, enhance the synchronization of heat-activated release.

Photodynamic–immunotherapy (PDT–immuno) utilizes light-activated photosensitizers (e.g., Ce6, porphyrins) to produce reactive oxygen species (ROS), resulting in immunogenic cell death that releases tumor antigens and activates T lymphocytes when combined with PD-1/PD-L1 or CTLA-4 inhibition. These nanocarriers connect localized reactive oxygen species production to systemic immune activation, with initial trials in melanoma and head and neck malignancies currently under progress (Rajagopal et al. 2025).

The integration of PTT with gene therapy enhances the distribution of siRNA/miRNA by thermally facilitated endosomal egress. The synergy of radio–photodynamic therapy employs X-ray-responsive upconversion nanoparticles to surmount light penetration limitations, therefore extending photodynamic therapy to deep-seated cancers. The forefront exists in theranostic nanoplatforms that integrate therapy and imaging, such as iron oxide–gold core–shell nanoparticles that provide MRI/photoacoustic imaging in conjunction with photothermal therapy and drug release, facilitating real-time monitoring and precision oncology. Notwithstanding obstacles in manufacturing, CMC regulation, and toxicity management, numerous nano-combination medicines have progressed to clinical trials, demonstrating their potential for eliciting sustained, systemic cancer responses via localized interventions (Mokhtari et al. 2017).

5.5.8 Advantages versus Limitations of Therapeutic Nanomedicine Modalities for Cancer

Nanomedicine has revolutionized oncologic medication delivery and treatment. Nanocarriers' tailorable size, composition, and multiplicity of function give conventional chemotherapeutic and biologic products specificities, despite significant biological, manufacturing, and clinical barriers. This paragraph presents a balanced, extensive review of the pros and cons, laying out a clear path for nanotherapeutic development.

Modifying payload pharmacokinetics and biodistribution is a major benefit. Doxorubicin and paclitaxel have quick clearance and dose-intensity toxicity. Liposomes, polymeric micelles, and albumin nanoparticles extend systemic circulation, lower plasma levels, and aggregate better at tumor sites. For instance, PEGylated liposomal doxorubicin (Doxil) has a longer half-life and lower cardiotoxicity than traditional doxorubicin. Nab-paclitaxel (Abraxane) replaces the cytotoxic Cremophor solubilizing carrier and uses albumin transport to increase dose escalation and tolerance in different cancers. The increased permeability and retention (EPR) effect, a passive phenomenon based on leaky tumor vasculature and active targeting by ligand attachment on the nanocarrier surface are also possible with nanomedicine. Active targeting, such as folate or antibody conjugation, may increase cell-specific absorption, although efficiency depends on tumor accessibility and expression. Toxicity reduction and therapeutic index improvement are key benefits. Doxil reduced breast cancer and Kaposi's sarcoma non-hematologic toxicities. Clinical results and quality of life have improved due to these modifications. Nanocarriers release on-site payloads via pH-sensitive liposomes (initiated by acidic tumor microenvironments), temperature-sensitive liposomes (heat-triggered release), redox-sensitive polymers, and enzyme-degradable shells (Bhatia et al. 2022).

Therapy-diagnostics integration is another trademark feature. Iron oxide–gold hybrid-type nanoparticles allow contemporaneous imaging (MRI, photoacoustic) and therapy (photothermal effects) for real-time therapy result monitoring and personalized dose. Combining cytotoxic drugs with gene silencers, immunological modulators, or phototherapeutics boosts synergy. Nano vaccines with chemotherapy, photodynamic treatment, and TLR agonists enhance systemic immune response and long-term tumor control (38). Numerous nanomedicines reached the market after regulatory approval, setting translation benchmarks. Doxil (1995), Abraxane (2005), Onivyde (2015), and Genexol-PM demonstrate feasibility, commercial scalability, and clinical acceptance (Shi et al. 2016).

Despite these benefits, there are universal restrictions. Nanoparticle delivery is inconsistent due to EPR effect heterogeneity. Human tumors have variable vascularity and thick stroma, resulting in modest median tumor accumulation (≈1% of administered dose). Combine techniques like vascular normalization (with anti-VEGF medication), stroma manipulation, or physical triggers like ultrasound or heat suited to tumor microenvironments to overcome heterogeneity. MDR and limited intratumoral dispersion remain obstacles. MDR pathways and poor interstitial diffusion allow hypoxic tumor cores to survive despite nanocarrier endocytosis evading P-glycoprotein. Anti-PEG antibodies and complement activation-related pseudo allergy (CARPA) accelerate blood clearance (ABC) and challenge immunogenicity with repeated dosage. Both issues can cause infusion responses and limit multi-dose regimens (Shi et al. 2016).

Another drawback is scale-up and CMC needs. Nanomedicines require size, composition, surface chemistry, and purity consistency, which is difficult to standardize. Quality-by-design and rigorous analytics are required, but most lab-scale preparations are not GMP-ready. The translation pipe moves slowly. Preclinically verified nanomedicines number in the hundreds, yet few are approved. Failures have been linked to animal models' inability to anticipate, inefficient clinical trial designs, and suboptimal patient selection (Shi et al. 2016).

Despite these obstacles, the future seems bright. New strategies include stratifying patients by imaging modalities (e.g., PET using radiolabeled nanocarriers) to estimate EPR status, computer-aided carrier design to optimize size and ligand density, tumor-specific regimens with drugs or nanotechnology-based drugs, and smart carriers for on-demand release. Nanomedicine has transformative benefits—enhanced delivery, lower toxicity, multifunctionality, and clinical translation—but tumor heterogeneity, immunogenicity, manufacturing, safety, and regulatory complexity are major drawbacks. Design, patient selection, and translational science must be coordinated to overcome problems. Nanomedicine can transform precision oncology and patient outcomes if used wisely.

5.6 THERANOSTICS: UNIFYING IMAGING AND THERAPY

Theranostics is rapidly emerging as an essential pillar under the umbrella of precision oncology, Theranostics is a novel, patient-centric approach that couples targeted diagnosis and treatment in one single platform. It is a shift from conventional to individualized and precision medicine. Incorporating nanotechnology, theranostics enables simultaneous disease detection, targeted delivery of drugs, and monitoring the effects of treatment in real time. This approach allows for the delivery of therapeutic agents to circulate systemically, evade immune defenses, and act directly at the cellular and molecular level (Shrivastava et al. 2019) (Figure 5.4).

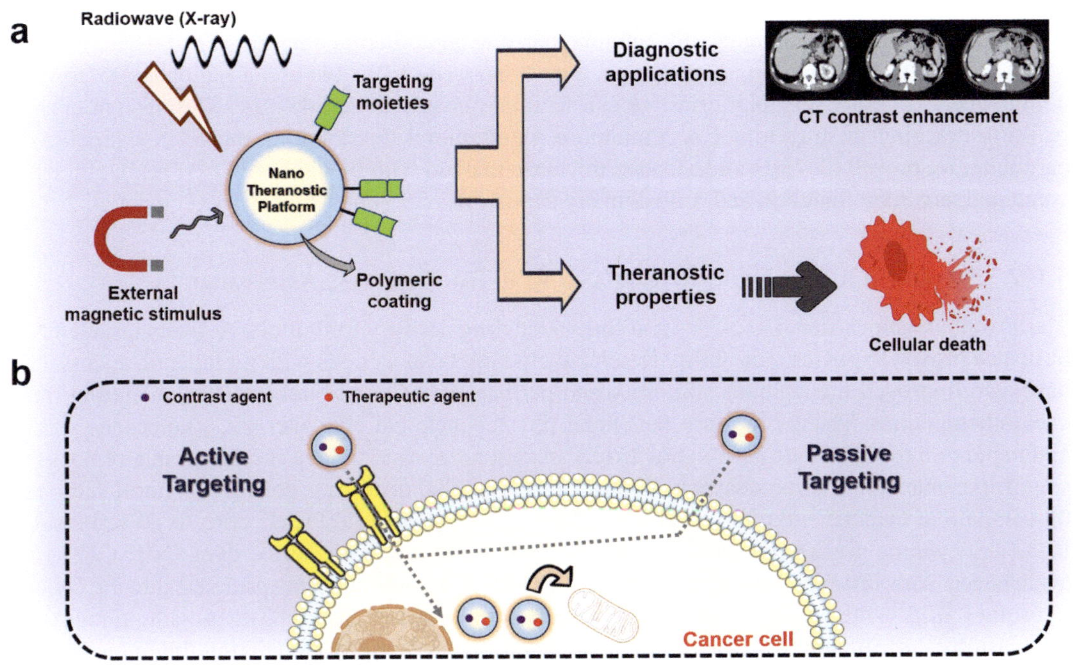

FIGURE 5.4 Nanotheranostic platform: (a) Functionalized nanoparticles enable imaging (CT contrast) and therapy under external stimuli. (b) Active and passive targeting enhance selective delivery to cancer cells.

5.6.1 Design Principles for Single-Platform Diagnosis and Treatment

Theranostics has become a leading branch of nuclear medicine, integrating diagnostic imaging with real-time, combined therapeutic interventions. A leading example is the application of ^68Ga- and ^177Lu-labeled FAP-targeting peptides, together with PET imaging, which has a major role to play in promoting cancer theranostics. and single-photon emission computed tomography (SPECT), health practitioners are able to visualize and measure specific cancer biomarkers molecules uniquely or in excess expressed by tumor cells that direct individualized treatment approaches (Shrivastava et al. 2019).

Progress in cancer diagnosis and therapy relies heavily on such key radiopharmaceuticals for theranostics. In prostate cancer, ^68Ga-PSMA PET imaging enables the detection of prostate-specific membrane antigen (PSMA), which accurately identifies tumor locations and guides targeted ^177Lu-PSMA therapy that has been shown to improve both progression-free survival (PFS) and overall survival (OS). Although originally believed to be cell-specific for prostate cancer cells, PSMA is now increasingly seen to be overexpressed in a variety of other cancers like brain metastases and high-grade gliomas, and hence it is also considered a potential agent for use in neuro-oncology. This has introduced a new mode of treatment for glioblastoma (GBM). To give one example, ^68Ga-PSMA-11 PET/CT has been very promising in the diagnosis of recurrent glioblastoma multiforme (GBM). Due to its low normal background absorption in normal brain tissue and elevated tumor-to-brain uptake ratio, this imaging agent facilitates improved demarcation of the margin of the tumor. Therefore, clinicians can more precisely target the tumor without harming surrounding normal brain tissue (Kuyumcu et al. 2021). Their success in mouse models highlights the potential of SPECT-guided imaging to maximize photodynamic therapy (PDT) and improve treatment outcomes.

It's important to first learn the fundamental principles and mechanisms of cancer imagining diagnosis and treatment. Apart from this, several theranostic nanoparticle-based strategies have been established for cancer treatment, such as photodynamic therapy (PDT), photothermal therapy (PTT), chemodynamic therapy (CDT), radiotherapy and immunotherapy. Researchers created multifunctional micelles for optical imaging, nuclear imaging, and photothermal therapy (PTT). These micelles were designed to carry two imaging agents: a near-infrared (NIR) dye and a radionuclide, forming a multivalent drug delivery platform that can facilitate image-guided therapy. This system enabled real-time tracking of drug tumor accumulation, intratumoral distribution, and release kinetics. In particular, we proved IR-780 iodide-loaded micelles, marked with rhenium-188 (^188Re), efficiently combined targeting, imaging, and drug delivery capabilities into one nanocarrier (Peng et al. 2011).

5.6.2 Imaging-Guided Drug Release and Real-Time Response Assessment

The advent of nanocarriers (NCs) has revolutionized drug delivery for tumors. Actively targeted NCs have also proved to possess the ability to selectively target cancer cells with therapeutic agents. NCs have also improved the aqueous solubility and permeation of hydrophobic drugs, including many chemotherapeutics. Thanks to these beneficial physicochemical characteristics, numerous studies and papers on the application of nanocarriers in cancer treatment have increased in a remarkable way. Liposomes are the nanocarriers that are largely utilized in drug delivery. Natural fatty acid biocompatible eutectic mixtures used as a phase change material (PCM) core to co-encapsulate ICG (indocyanine green) and DOX. Lipophilic NIR-II fluorescent cyanine dyes (NIR-C12) were synthesized with intense absorption between the NIR-II region and encapsulated into PEGylated liposomes. This is the widely accepted approach for targeting integrin αvβ3-expressing tumor cells, glioblastoma-type tumor cells, and tumor vasculature by surface functionalizing the liposome with a cyclic arginylglycylaspartic acid (cRGD) ligand. The use of polymers as carriers in the preparation of nanoformulations for (ICG) encapsulation presents significant potential within nanomedicine. Synthetic ROS-sensitive polymer with thioketal linkages (PEG-TK-ICG) that self-assembles into polymeric micelles (GA@PEG-TK-ICG PMs) with loading of indocyanine green (ICG) and glycyrrhetinic acid (GA). Such micelles show improved resistance against photobleaching, improved light-to-heat conversion efficiency, NIR-triggered drug release, excellent biocompatibility, and efficient tumor accumulation (Y. Liu et al. 2025).

In the context of chemotherapeutic drug delivery, different metallic nanomaterials, including plain metals like Au, Cu, Ag, Pt, Pd, metal oxides, metal sulfides, and metal-organic frameworks (MOFs), have been exceptionally studied as effective tumor-targeted nanocarriers. Metallic nanomaterials including gold, bismuth, lanthanides, and transition metals possess higher X-ray attenuation coefficients than iodine, making them provide improved CT image contrast at elevated tube voltages (>100 kVp). The nanomaterials made of metals like gold, bismuth, lanthanides, and transition metals are likely to resolve these challenges. The synthesis of biodegradable, TME-responsive multifunctional metal-based nanomaterials provides a potential solution with the possibility of enhanced tumor contrast with decreased doses and fewer side effects (H.-J. Yu et al. 2025).

5.6.3 Advantages (Personalization, Adaptive Therapy) versus Limitations (Complexity, Regulatory Hurdles

Theranostic nanoplatforms have embraced efficient approaches to promote the synergistic effect on cancer diagnosis and treatment. One of these efficient strategies is image-guided therapy. As aforementioned, the in vivo biodistribution and tumor-targeting function of photosensitizer-based theranostic nanoparticles can be traced with optical imaging strategies. Based on these imaging outcomes, laser irradiation can thereafter be accurately targeted to the tumor location to provide safe and effective photodynamic tumor ablation (McCarthy et al. 2005).

5.6.3.1 Combining Nanomedicines with Theranostics

Combining nanomedicine with radiation therapy (RT), such as proton and X-ray radiotherapy, not only improves outcome but also facilitates non-invasive monitoring of therapeutic efficacy.

With improving adaptive RT, nanoparticle-based diagnostic contrast agents provide in real-time assessment of tumor growth and treatment response to support personalized adjustment of therapy. Theranostic nanoparticles, which combine imaging and therapeutic functionalities, are particularly promising in this regard (Kelkar and Reineke 2011).

5.6.3.2 Improved Solubility, Bioavailability, and Reduced Toxicity

Most photosensitizers are poorly soluble in water, which restricts their therapeutic application. For overcoming this, nanoparticles like liposomes, polymeric nanoparticles, and micelles encapsulate these hydrophobic photosensitizers. This increases the solubility, stability, and bioavailability of these agents, facilitating better delivery to tumor sites. Moffitt Cancer Center's trial on adaptive abiraterone therapy for metastatic castrate-resistant prostate cancer showed significant success in patients on adaptive therapy had 46% of the time off treatment, which minimized drug-related toxicities and cost. Adaptive therapy adjusts dose intensity according to immediate patient response (e.g., tumor burden, biomarker concentration). This translates into patients being given the minimal effective dose to lower cumulative drug or radiation exposure over time. Theranostic agents (such as Lutetium-177-PSMA or DOTATATE) specifically target cancer cells by means of molecular markers (Kuyumcu et al. 2021). This minimizes off-target toxicity to healthy tissues, particularly in organs like the kidney, bone marrow, or salivary glands.

5.6.3.3 Limitations (Complexity, Regulatory Barriers)

Personalized oncology is an individualized, precision-patient approach that aims to deliver the optimal treatment to the right cancer patient at the right time. It promises significant improvement in clinical outcomes with fewer futile therapies and healthcare costs. Central to it is the use of theranostic biomarkers that are tissue, urine, or imaging-based, and guide diagnosis, therapy selection, and response monitoring. These biomarkers are subject to stringent validation for accuracy and reliability. Fast progress in genome sequencing and other omics tools has enabled the discovery of new molecular targets and greater understanding of cancer biology. This allows for earlier and more precise prediction, detection, diagnosis, and prognosis. Molecular imaging sciences also contribute by representing and measuring hallmarks of cancer in real time (Chen and Wong 2014).

There are several challenges to be addressed in moving forward with nanotheranostics. Large-scale synthesis is challenging, as complicated nanoplatforms created in the laboratory could be difficult to reproduce and produce in bulk, and maintaining sterility is a problem. Invariant packaging of imaging and therapy in a single nanoformulation is challenging due to conflicting demands in tumor targeting and pharmacokinetics that frequently fail to result in clinical synergy. There is limited regulatory control, with no established FDA guidelines for nanotheranostics. Nanotoxicity concerns, such as cytotoxicity, genotoxicity, and immunotoxicity, also remain. On an economic level, although the worth of nanomedicine is increasing, universal usage continues to face obstacles in spite of growing industry interest. There are a number of challenges that need to be overcome to fully achieve its potential. Some of these include tumor heterogeneity, the restricted commercial availability of radionuclides, and the difficulty of dosimetry, all of which complicate the efficient use of radiotheranostic therapy (Chen and Wong 2014).

5.7 CLINICAL TRANSLATION, SAFETY, AND FUTURE DIRECTIONS IN CANCER NANOMEDICINE

Cancer nanomedicine has progressed over the last several decades from an exciting research concept to a clinically relevant field with a number of nanoparticle-based formulations approved by regulatory bodies and many more in clinical trials. Despite major advances in targeted drug delivery, imaging, diagnostics, and theranostics, successful translation of nanomedicines from the laboratory to routine clinical practice remains challenging. Complex biological interactions, variability in tumor biology, manufacturing scalability, regulatory requirements, long-term safety, and pharmacokinetic behavior still impact clinical success. Meanwhile, recent advances in technologies including artificial intelligence-powered design of nanoparticles, sophisticated biomaterials, personalized medicine approaches, and multi-omics integration are providing new opportunities for the development of safer, more effective, and personalized nanotherapeutics. Here, we discuss the current clinical landscape of cancer nanomedicine, important safety and regulatory concerns, and future directions that are likely to shape the next generation of precision oncology.

5.7.1 Approved Nanomedicines, Clinical Trial Landscape, and Regulatory Challenges

In recent decades, nanomedicine has witnessed tremendous development. What was a loose network of liposome scientists, polymer chemists, chemical engineers, and experts on metal nanoparticles, mesoporous silica, and analogous materials has now become a more cohesive field of study, generating vast amounts of research and clinical evidence.

Most approved nanomedicines exploit passive targeting, whereas fewer nanocarriers employing ligand-mediated active targeting are under investigation in clinical trials. Liposomes remain the most commonly approved and clinically applied nanomedicines, predominantly due to their very good safety profile. Outside of approved products, the FDA has assigned Investigational New Drug (IND) status to some nanoformulations in recent history (Table 5.2), a majority of which consist of traditional chemotherapeutic drugs administered via established nanoparticle carriers (Tong et al. 2024).

TABLE 5.2
Nanotechnology-Based Products under Clinical Trials

Drug Candidate	Nanocarrier Type	Developer (Location)	Active Compound	Clinical Trial ID	Target Indication
Docetaxel-PNP	Polymeric nanoparticles	Samyang Biopharmaceuticals (South Korea)	Docetaxel	NCT01103791	Advanced solid tumors
ABT-888	PEGylated liposomes	AbbVie (Illinois, USA)	Temozolomide + liposomal doxorubicin	NCT01113957	Ovarian cancer
LipoVNB	Liposomes	Taiwan Liposome Company (Taiwan)	Vinorelbine tartrate	NCT02925000	Advanced malignancies
FF-10850	Liposomes	Fujifilm Pharmaceuticals (Massachusetts, USA)	Topotecan	NCT04047251	Advanced solid tumors
LY01610	Liposomes	Luye Pharma Group (China)	Irinotecan hydrochloride	NCT04381910	Small-cell lung cancer
Mitoxantrone Liposome Injection	Liposomes	CSPC ZhongQi Pharmaceutical (China)	Mitoxantrone hydrochloride	NCT04927481	Breast cancer
WGI-0301	Lipid nanoparticles	Zhejiang Haichang Biotech (China)	AKT-1 antisense oligonucleotide	NCT05267899	Advanced solid tumors
CDK-004	Exosomes	Codiak BioSciences (Massachusetts, USA)	Antisense oligonucleotide targeting STAT6	NCT05375604	Advanced hepatocellular carcinoma, gastric cancer, liver metastasis
OTX-2002	Lipid nanoparticles	Omega Therapeutics (Massachusetts, USA)	Bisictronic mRNA for c-Myc downregulation	NCT05497453	Hepatocellular carcinoma

Source: Recreated with permission from Giri et al., 2023.

5.7.1.1 Current Clinical Landscape and Regulatory Challenges

Nanotechnology has revolutionized oncology by overcoming the disadvantages of conventional cancer therapies. Nanocarrier micelles, for example, have enhanced drug solubility, facilitated targeting to cancer cells, and minimized systemic toxicity—setting the stage for clinical relevance and efficacy. Notwithstanding the progress made, the translation of such technologies from the laboratory to the clinic is both challenging and promising, requiring interdisciplinary input and extensive validation (Zhang et al. 2019).

Translational research plays a vital role in advancing nanocarriers from preclinical models to clinical application. These involve optimizing design, scalability, and consistency. Preclinical investigations examine nanocarriers in cell culture and animal models to evaluate physiological stability, and analyze potential toxic effects such as oxidative stress, inflammation, and organ accumulation. The restricted translation and small market share of nanodrugs have created doubts regarding their overall development and therapeutic efficacy. This review presents a holistic overview and discussion of the progress made in nanomedicine, as well as the major hurdles that are delaying their clinical translation (Tong et al. 2024). Effective clinical translation of nanomedicines also demands remarkable progress in large-scale production following Good Manufacturing Practices (GMP) standards. The major challenges include batch-to-batch nanoparticle quality standardization and their consistency. These concerns can be alleviated by embracing autonomous manufacturing platforms and incorporating artificial intelligence to streamline synthesis parameters, facilitate real-time monitoring of quality, and minimize production variation. In regulatory, the largest barrier is the lack of international standardization of standards and testing procedures for nanomedicines. Greater coordination and improved regulation are required to streamline the approval process and unlock the maximum benefit of nanotechnology in medicine. New approaches like photoimmunotherapy, biomarker-targeting, and exosomal miRNA inhibition hold great promise for overcoming the resistance of breast cancer. These new developments advance our knowledge of resistance mechanisms and open the door to clinical translation and personalized therapy approaches. In the future, combining computational modeling, omics platforms, and patient-derived models will be key to the development and optimization of such methods. To promote customized management of breast cancer resistance, we suggest giving top priority to translational research integrating nanotechnology and immunotherapy (Sabit et al. 2025).

5.7.2 Safety, Toxicity, and Pharmacokinetics Considerations

Cancer cell-targeting nanoparticles can carry a wide range of agents and therefore serve as useful imaging, diagnostic, and therapeutic anticancer delivery tools, all of which work to improve the efficacy and safety of treatment (Shah et al. 2025). Therapeutic activity and safety largely depend on physical parameters like particle size, morphology, surface chemistry, coating composition, and mode of delivery. They directly impact the biodistribution and accumulation of the nanoparticle in biological systems, thereby determining their clinical performance.

5.7.2.1 Delivery and Formulation

Nanocarriers or the nanoparticles with the controlled degradability and release, balance the therapeutic efficacy and safety. For more precise pre-clinical evaluation before going to human trials it's important to reduce the toxicity of these nanomaterials. Organoids and organ-on-a-chip platforms provide sophisticated 3D models for understanding nanoparticle toxicity behavior in cells and organs, gaining important insights for nanoparticle design without the use of animal models. The systems can be employed to evaluate nanoparticle toxicity in target organs, tissue penetration, cell-specific targeting, and overall therapeutic effectiveness (Gomerdinger et al. 2025).

5.7.2.2 Dose Optimization and Pharmacokinetics

In addition to the natural toxicity of the active pharmaceutical ingredients (APIs), nanodrugs and nanomaterials present other potential toxicities. These can be from the nanoparticles themselves or

FDA-approved excipients in the formulation. For example, although Doxil® lessens the cardiotoxicity that is normally found with free doxorubicin hydrochloride, it will induce other side effects, such as palmoplantar erythema syndrome and hypersensitivity reactions (Tong et al. 2024). To reduce the toxicity, it's important to do the surface modification or use the nanocarriers for the encapsulation to enhance the tissue targeting, controlled release and maintain the pharmacokinetics of the drug.

5.7.3 Emerging Materials, Supramolecular Approaches, and Omics-Based Personalized Nanomedicine

Supramolecular chemistry, an important pillar of nanotechnology, it's a promising approach because it can generate complex, multiple-function systems by means of simple and dynamic non-covalent interactions. Supramolecular materials like pillarene-based systems, virus-mimetic nanoparticles, and metal-organic frameworks (MOFs) have great promise in solving some of the long-standing challenges in cancer therapy. Through examination of their structural properties, functional operation, and therapeutic effects, we can further clarify how these next-generation nanotechnologies may be applied in clinical practice. In combination, they constitute the promise of transforming cancer diagnosis, treatment, and patient prognosis (J. Zhang et al. 2025). Amphiphilic pillarene nanostructures may also use the enhanced permeability and retention (EPR) effect to passively accumulate in tumors with maximum drug concentration in cancer cells. Example, nanosponges synthesized from amphiphilic Pillararene supramolecules that can encapsulate anticancer drugs like mitoxantrone (MTX) and doxorubicin (DOX). Metal-organic frameworks (MOFs) have unique characteristics, including structural tunability, high drug loading, and the ability to achieve combination of multiple therapeutics. For example, a ZIF-8-supported MOF co-loaded with doxorubicin (DOX) and indocyanine green (ICG) showed drastically increased tumor accumulation and enhanced induction of immunogenic cell death in 4T1 mouse models. Compared to free drugs, this MOF system induced stronger tumor inhibition, indicated by the greater expression levels of immunogenic cell death markers CRT and HMGB1, and enormously reduced volume of tumors following phototherapy (Delbianco et al. 2016).

Artificial intelligence (AI) today is more centered on developing therapeutic interventions and treatment techniques for chronic diseases like cancer, inherited diseases, and neurodegenerative disorders. Models of AI are greatly involved in both diagnostics and therapeutics, facilitating personalized medicine (PM) for a single individual or for wider populations. The ultimate objective of integrating multi-omics data is to enable fully personalized therapy. Through the association of unique omics signatures to drug response profiles, clinicians are able to stratify patients and create tailored treatment regimens. A new study integrated Quality by Design (QbD) and AI to enhance silymarin-loaded liposomes. AI was used to forecast release rate, encapsulation, and size, whereas lecithin and chitosan formulations exhibited potent cytotoxic activities (Dawoud et al. 2023). Nanocarriers may be designed with ligands that are targeted toward biomarkers found through omics studies so that therapies can be personalized to a patient's individual tumor traits and resistance patterns, thus allowing for improved treatment accuracy and efficacy.

5.7.4 Strategies to Accelerate Bench-to-Bedside Translation and Address Future Challenges

Major obstacles in bulk nanomedicine manufacture are achieving uniform particle size, uniform surface characteristics, and targeted drug loading. Regulatory requirements demand rigorous consistency of formulation, purity, and stability. New technologies like microfluidics and automated manufacturing equipment are assisting in resolving these issues. In addition, comprehensive toxicity, biodistribution, and pharmacokinetics studies must be conducted for safe and effective development. Cooperative efforts are also underway to simplify regulatory approval procedures by establishing standardized protocols and detailed guidelines. Regulatory compliance and standardization are major barriers since the regulatory agencies need strict clinical trials to ascertain toxicity, metabolism, and therapeutic effectiveness. With our ongoing insight into the biomolecular corona and its central role in defining the biological identity of nanoparticles, need next-generation analytical tools which are capable of defining these biological interactions within their native settings (R. Sivanand et al. 2025).

The rationale for the conjugation of imaging and therapeutic elements in one nanoformulation: Imaging and therapy possess different necessities with regard to tumor targeting as well as pharmacokinetics. Hence, co-delivery of both imaging and drug moieties may not lead to a significant synergistic response for clinical applications. Through simultaneous delivery of chemotherapy agents, immunotherapies, and radiotherapy agents, nanocarriers are able to target several areas of cancer biology at once, providing an edge over single-agent treatment. Nanocarriers also allow for better timing control, maximizing synergistic effects while minimizing toxicity (Gavas et al. 2021). Nanoparticles can also be used as carriers for cancer vaccines or act as adjuvants that enhance the immune response against cancer.

5.8 CONCLUSION

Nanomedicine has completely transformed the landscape of management and treatment of cancer and has led to a paradigm shift toward precision medicine-oriented, individualized patient therapy. The integration of nanotechnology in oncology offers solutions to the age-old clinical issues like late diagnoses, systemic toxicity, decreased drug bioavailability, and drug resistance during treatment. Through the logical development of nano-carriers, scientists have achieved targeted delivery of chemotherapeutic agents, nucleic acids, and immunomodulators with significant improvement of therapeutic indices and reduction of side effects.

Nanomedicine shows great promise because it allows targeted delivery to specific sites through both passive and active targeting methods. The EPR effect created a foundation for passive accumulation but researchers needed to develop ligand-functionalized nanoparticles because of the inconsistent tumor vasculature. The systems which use antibodies and peptides and aptamers and small molecules for functionalization show better binding to tumor receptors and improved penetration of the tumor microenvironment. Nanocarriers with stimulus-sensitive properties now provide improved drug delivery precision because they release therapeutic agents based on pH changes and enzymatic reactions and redox gradients and hypoxia conditions.

The development of organelle-specific targeting methods for mitochondria and nucleus and lysosomes enables researchers to activate apoptosis pathways and overcome drug resistance while controlling cellular processes from their starting points. Nanoplatforms that modify tumor-associated macrophages and enhance checkpoint inhibitor effectiveness have made nanomedicine more important for cancer immunotherapy. Nanotechnology demonstrates its broad capabilities through drug delivery systems while establishing itself as a complete therapeutic solution.

Another big change has come from using nanomaterials in diagnostic imaging and theranostics. Nanotechnology has led to better contrast agents for MRI, CT, PET, SPECT, and photoacoustic imaging. These agents improve how well images can detect problems, how accurate they are, and how well they can monitor things in real time. Instead of using traditional gadolinium-based agents, there are newer options like superparamagnetic iron oxide nanoparticles (SPIONs) and manganese-based probes. These alternatives are safer and work better, helping to reduce issues like toxicity and long-term buildup in the body. Also, nanoparticles made from high-Z elements like gold and bismuth have changed CT imaging by making dual-energy and spectral imaging possible. Photoacoustic and optical imaging agents have also made it easier to do less invasive diagnostic tests. Plus, radiolabeled nanoparticles can be used for multiple imaging methods at once, helping connect diagnosis with treatment and allowing for more personalized care plans.

Clinical translation remains a challenge. Tumor heterogeneity, variable EPR effect as well as immune clearance and protein corona formation, can all significantly affect nanoparticle behavior in vivo, efficacy, and safety. Other major hurdles include large-scale manufacturing, cost-effectiveness, long-term biocompatibility as well as regulatory approval. Standardized protocols for preclinical evaluation nanomedicine pharmacokinetics predictive models and clinical trials to validate safety and therapeutically will be welcomed by the process of overcoming these challenges.

The future of cancer nanomedicine presently lies in an approach with multi-functional hybrid systems that combine therapy and imaging/inmunomodulation within one platform. It would provide ways to accomplish accurate targeting and controlled drug release with real-time monitoring of treatment making a clinical implementation of the concept of theranostic nanomedicine possible. Furthermore, AI-driven nanoparticle design is expected to accelerate material discovery and optimization by predicting biodistribution, toxicity, and therapeutic efficacy with greater accuracy.

Personalized nanomedicine will grow out of genomic and proteomic characterization of tumors. Patient-specific tumor antigen nanovaccines, together with immune checkpoint inhibitors, promise to fulfill the great potential for effective and durable cancer immunotherapy. Similarly, gene-editing nanocarriers will soon revolutionize targeted oncogene silencing and tumor-suppressor activation approaches. Most probably they will belong to the CRISPR-Cas family of systems.

Newly evolving stimuli-responsive systems that could be triggered by more than one tumor hallmark, such as pH, hypoxia, and enzyme activity, will further broaden the dimensions of spatiotemporal control over drug release. Meanwhile, less exploited organelles and cellular pathways might open new therapeutic windows for investigation in targeted drug delivery research toward overcoming pathway-associated drawbacks found in contemporary single-organelle targeting.

Also, nanoprobes for imaging that combine MRI, PET, optical, and photoacoustic modalities are likely to provide very full pictures of diagnosis reducing the need for many different separate scans. Integration with wearable diagnostic systems and remote monitoring technologies may further advance real-time assessment of treatment response, enabling adaptive therapy strategies.

Scaling up, reproducing, and regulating things will be what brings those innovations to life. Characterization standard methods, computational models that can predict outcomes, and international guidelines to move things clinically will be what makes it possible. Material scientists working with clinicians and data scientists and even regulatory agencies are what will make sure that nanomedicine moves from being just promising research into accessible treatment that saves lives.

ACKNOWLEDGMENT

This work was supported by the Department of Biotechnology, Ministry of Science and Technology, India (BT/PR36505/NNT/28/1818/2022), Department of Science and Technology, DST-Science and Engineering Research Board (SB/S3/CE/048/2015), CRG/2020/005244 and IMPRINT (DST/IMP/2018/000687), Abdul Kalam Technology Innovation National Fellowship, Indian National Academy of Engineering, India (INAE/121/AKF/37), Higher Education Financing Agency (HEFA/CSR/IITH/01/2024-25), Ministry of Education for Prime Minister Research Fellowship (PMRF) of author Vaishali Makwana and University Grants Commission (UGC) fellowship of authors Megha M Unnimaya and Vibha Choudhary. All original figures were created with Biorender.com.

CONFLICT OF INTEREST

The authors declare that they do not have any conflicts of interest.

LIST OF ABBREVIATIONS

AFP—Alpha-Fetoprotein
AgNPs—Silver Nanoparticles
APC—Antigen-Presenting Cell
AS01—Adjuvant System 01 (liposomal MPL + QS-21)

AS04—Adjuvant System 04 (MPL + Aluminum Salt)
BHQ3—Black Hole Quencher 3
BSNPs—Biodegradable Silica Nanocapsules
CA-125—Cancer Antigen 125
CA-199—Cancer Antigen 19–9
CAF—Cancer-Associated Fibroblast
CEA—Carcinoembryonic Antigen
CKD—Chronic Kidney Disease
CNQDs—Carbon Nitride Quantum Dots
CNDs—Copper Nanodots
CRP—C-Reactive Protein
CT—Computed Tomography
CTC—Circulating Tumor Cell
ctDNA—Circulating Tumor DNA
ctRNA—Circulating Tumor RNA
DC—Dendritic Cell
DLCs—Delocalized Lipophilic Cations
DMMA—2,3-Dimethylmaleic Amide
DNA—Deoxyribonucleic Acid
DOX—Doxorubicin
EC—Endothelial Cell
ECM—Extracellular Matrix
EGFR—Epidermal Growth Factor Receptor
ELISA—Enzyme-Linked Immunosorbent Assay
EPR—Enhanced Permeability and Retention
EVs—Extracellular Vesicles
FDA—Food and Drug Administration
FH—Feraheme
GBCA—Gadolinium-Based Contrast Agent
GI—Gastrointestinal
GP60—Glycoprotein 60
HER2—Human Epidermal Growth Factor Receptor 2
HOCM—High-Osmolar Contrast Media
ICIs—Immune Checkpoint Inhibitors
ICG—Indocyanine Green
IL-6—Interleukin 6
IL-8—Interleukin 8
IOCM—Iso-Osmolar Contrast Media
KD—Kidney Disease (contextual in CIN/CKD)
KRAS—Kirsten Rat Sarcoma Viral Oncogene Homolog
LMP—Lysosomal Membrane Permeabilization
LNCs—Lipid Nanocarriers (contextual to nanomedicine)
LNP—Lipid Nanoparticle
LOCM—Low-Osmolar Contrast Media
MDR—Multidrug Resistance
MHC-I—Major Histocompatibility Complex Class I
miRNA—Micro Ribonucleic Acid
MRI—Magnetic Resonance Imaging
mtDNA—Mitochondrial DNA
MXene—Transition Metal Carbide/Nitride 2D Nanomaterial
NIR—Near-Infrared

NIR-I—Near-Infrared Window I (700–950 nm)
NK—Natural Killer (cells, contextually implied)
NLS—Nuclear Localization Signal
NP—Nanoparticle
NMR—Nuclear Magnetic Resonance
NPCs—Nuclear Pore Complexes
OC—Ovarian Cancer
PAI—Photoacoustic Imaging
PAMPs—Pathogen-Associated Molecular Patterns
PCL—Polycaprolactone
PEG—Polyethylene Glycol
PET—Positron Emission Tomography
PF-4—Platelet Factor 4
PLA—Poly(Lactic Acid)
PLGA—Poly(Lactic-co-Glycolic Acid)
PLL—Poly-L-Lysine
PMMA—Poly(Methyl Methacrylate)
PSA—Prostate-Specific Antigen
PSMA—Prostate-Specific Membrane Antigen
QDs—Quantum Dots
RES—Reticuloendothelial System
RET—Resonance Energy Transfer
RNA—Ribonucleic Acid
ROS—Reactive Oxygen Species
SPECT—Single Photon Emission Computed Tomography
SPIONs—Superparamagnetic Iron Oxide Nanoparticles
SPR—Surface Plasmon Resonance
STING—Stimulator of Interferon Genes
TAM—Tumor-Associated Macrophage
TDFLN—Tumor-Draining Lymph Node (implied in text)
TME—Tumor Microenvironment
TLR—Toll-Like Receptor
WHO—World Health Organization

REFERENCES

Al-Jamal, Ahmed N., Ali Fawzi Al-Hussainy, Bahira Abdulrazzaq Mohammed, Hadi Hussein Abbas, Issa Mohammed Kadhim, Zahraa Hassan Ward, Debarshi Kar Mahapatra, Tomy Muringayil Joseph, Ehsan kianfar, and Sabu Thomas. 2025. "Photodynamic Therapy (PDT) in Drug Delivery: Nano-Innovations Enhancing Treatment Outcomes." *Health Sciences Review* 14 (March). Elsevier: 100218. https://doi.org/10.1016/J.HSR.2025.100218.

Allen, Randall, and Toshifumi Yokota. 2024. "Endosomal Escape and Nuclear Localization: Critical Barriers for Therapeutic Nucleic Acids." *Molecules (Basel, Switzerland)* 29 (24). Molecules. https://doi.org/10.3390/MOLECULES29245997.

Amourizi, Fereshteh, Kheibar Dashtian, Rouholah Zare-Dorabei, and Shaaker Hajati. 2025. "Transformative Personalized Oxalate Biomarker Analysis through a Wrist-Worn Microneedle Device Integrated with Duplex Nanozyme Toolbox." *Sensors and Actuators B: Chemical* 423 (January): 136731. https://doi.org/10.1016/j.snb.2024.136731.

Barenholz, Yechezkel. 2012. "Doxil®—The First FDA-Approved Nano-Drug: Lessons Learned." *Journal of Controlled Release* 160 (2). J Control Release: 117–34. https://doi.org/10.1016/j.jconrel.2012.03.020.

Batist, Gerald, Lyndsay Harris, Nozar Azarnia, Lily Waiyee Lee, and Pascual Daza-Ramirez. 2006. "Improved Anti-Tumor Response Rate with Decreased Cardiotoxicity of Non-Pegylated Liposomal Doxorubicin Compared with Conventional Doxorubicin in First-Line Treatment of Metastatic Breast Cancer in

Patients Who Had Received Prior Adjuvant Doxorubicin: Results of a Retrospective Analysis." *Anti-Cancer Drugs* 17 (5): 587–95. https://doi.org/10.1097/00001813-200606000-00014.

Bellassai, Noemi, Roberta D'Agata, Almudena Marti, Andrea Rozzi, Stefano Volpi, Matteo Allegretti, Roberto Corradini, Patrizio Giacomini, Jurriaan Huskens, and Giuseppe Spoto. 2021. "Detection of Tumor DNA in Human Plasma with a Functional PLL-Based Surface Layer and Plasmonic Biosensing." *ACS Sensors* 6 (6): 2307–19. https://doi.org/10.1021/acssensors.1c00360.

Bhatia, Sangeeta N., Xiaoyuan Chen, Marina A. Dobrovolskaia, and Twan Lammers. 2022. "Cancer Nanomedicine." *Nature Reviews Cancer* 22 (10). Nature Research: 550–56. https://doi.org/10.1038/S41568-022-00496-9;SUBJMETA=1059,2321,352,631,639,67,925;KWRD=CANCER+IMAGING,CANCER+THERAPY,NANOMEDICINE.

Bian, Wangqing, Yakun Wang, Zhenxing Pan, Niping Chen, Xiaojing Li, Wing Leung Wong, Xujie Liu, Yan He, Kun Zhang, and Yu Jing Lu. 2021. "Review of Functionalized Nanomaterials for Photothermal Therapy of Cancers." *ACS Applied Nano Materials* 4 (11). American Chemical Society: 11353–85. https://doi.org/10.1021/ACSANM.1C01903.

Carbone, Giorgio Giuseppe, Stefania Mariano, Alessandra Gabriele, Sabrina Cennamo, Vitantonio Primiceri, Muhammad Rizwan Aziz, Elisa Panzarini, and Lucio Calcagnile. 2025. "Exploring the Potential of Gold Nanoparticles in Proton Therapy: Mechanisms, Advances, and Clinical Horizons." *Pharmaceutics* 17 (2). Multidisciplinary Digital Publishing Institute: 176. https://doi.org/10.3390/PHARMACEUTICS17020176.

Chao, Chih Jia, Endong Zhang, Duong N. Trinh, Edidiong Udofa, Hanchen Lin, Caylee Silvers, Jiawei Huo, et al. 2025. "Integrating Antigen Capturing Nanoparticles and Type 1 Conventional Dendritic Cell Therapy for in Situ Cancer Immunization." *Nature Communications* 16 (1). Nat Commun. https://doi.org/10.1038/S41467-025-59840-W.

Chen, Xiaoyuan, and Stephen T.C. Wong. 2014. "Cancer Theranostics." In *Cancer Theranostics*, 3–8. Elsevier. https://doi.org/10.1016/B978-0-12-407722-5.00001-3.

Cheng, H., J. Liao, Y. Ma, M. T. Sarwar, and H. Yang. 2025. "Advances in Targeted Therapy for Tumor with Nanocarriers: A Review." *Materials Today Bio* 31: 101583. https://doi.org/10.1016/J.MTBIO.2025.101583

Cherry, Simon R. 2009a. "Multimodality Imaging: Beyond PET/CT and SPECT/CT." *Seminars in Nuclear Medicine* 39 (5). Semin Nucl Med: 348–53. https://doi.org/10.1053/J.SEMNUCLMED.2009.03.001.

Choudhary, Manisha, Pratik Katare, Mrudul Deshpande, Nakshatra Chaudhari, Kuldeep Rajpoot, Aakanccha Jain, and Rakesh K. Tekade. 2024. "Dendrimers in Targeted Drug Delivery: Design, Development, and Modern Applications." In *Progress and Prospect of Nanocarriers*, 181–240. Elsevier. https://doi.org/10.1016/B978-0-12-819979-4.00004-0.

Coll, Jean-Luc. 2011. "Cancer Optical Imaging Using Fluorescent Nanoparticles." *Nanomedicine* 6 (1): 7–10. https://doi.org/10.2217/nnm.10.144.

Dawoud, Marwa H. S., Islam S. Mannaa, Amira Abdel-Daim, and Nabila M. Sweed. 2023. "Integrating Artificial Intelligence with Quality by Design in the Formulation of Lecithin/Chitosan Nanoparticles of a Poorly Water-Soluble Drug." *AAPS PharmSciTech* 24 (6): 169. https://doi.org/10.1208/s12249-023-02609-5.

Debnath, Sujit Kumar, Monalisha Debnath, Arnab Ghosh, Rohit Srivastava, and Abdelwahab Omri. 2024. "Targeting Tumor Hypoxia with Nanoparticle-Based Therapies: Challenges, Opportunities, and Clinical Implications." *Pharmaceuticals* 17 (10). Multidisciplinary Digital Publishing Institute: 1389. https://doi.org/10.3390/PH17101389.

Delbianco, Martina, Priya Bharate, Silvia Varela-Aramburu, and Peter H. Seeberger. 2016. "Carbohydrates in Supramolecular Chemistry." *Chemical Reviews* 116 (4): 1693–1752. https://doi.org/10.1021/acs.chemrev.5b00516.

Delledonne, Andrea, Elisa Guazzelli, Silvia Pescina, Annalisa Bianchera, Giancarlo Galli, Elisa Martinelli, and Cristina Sissa. 2023. "Amphiphilic Fluorinated Unimer Micelles as Nanocarriers of Fluorescent Probes for Bioimaging." *ACS Applied Nano Materials* 6 (17): 15551–62. https://doi.org/10.1021/acsanm.3c02300.

Desai, Nimeet, Pratik Katare, Vaishali Makwana, Sagar Salave, Lalitkumar K. Vora, and Jyotsnendu Giri. 2023. "Tumor-Derived Systems as Novel Biomedical Tools—Turning the Enemy into an Ally." *Biomaterials Research* 27 (1). https://doi.org/10.1186/s40824-023-00445-z.

Du, Wei, Shubo Du, Xiao Dong, Hua Bai, Jiamin Jiang, Shiping Hao, Fen Yang, et al. 2023. "Biodegradable Silica Nanocapsules Enable Efficient Nuclear-Targeted Delivery of Native Proteins for Cancer Therapy." *Biomaterials* 294 (March): 122000. https://doi.org/10.1016/j.biomaterials.2023.122000.

Foroozandeh, Amin, Mehrab Pourmadadi, Hossein SalarAmoli, and Majid Abdouss. 2024. "Aptamer-Enabled Electrochemical Bioplatform Utilizing Surface-Modified g-C3N4/MoS2/PANI Nanocomposite for Detection of CA125 Biomarker." *Sensing and Bio-Sensing Research* 45 (August): 100669. https://doi.org/10.1016/j.sbsr.2024.100669.

Gajdosova, Veronika, Lenka Lorencova, Peter Kasak, and Jan Tkac. 2020. "Electrochemical Nanobiosensors for Detection of Breast Cancer Biomarkers." *Sensors* 20 (14): 4022. https://doi.org/10.3390/s20144022.

Gao, Hongli, Jianqiao Yin, Ce Ji, Xiaopeng Yu, Jinqi Xue, Xin Guan, Shuang Zhang, Xun Liu, and Fei Xing. 2023. "Targeting Ubiquitin Specific Proteases (USPs) in Cancer Immunotherapy: From Basic Research to Preclinical Application." *Journal of Experimental & Clinical Cancer Research* 42 (1): 225. https://doi.org/10.1186/s13046-023-02805-y.

Gavas, Shreelaxmi, Sameer Quazi, and Tomasz M. Karpiński. 2021. "Nanoparticles for Cancer Therapy: Current Progress and Challenges." *Nanoscale Research Letters* 16 (1): 173. https://doi.org/10.1186/s11671-021-03628-6.

Gholami, Yaser Hadi, Hushan Yuan, Moses Q. Wilks, Richard Maschmeyer, Marc D. Normandin, Lee Josephson, Georges El Fakhri, and Zdenka Kuncic. 2020a. "A Radio-Nano-Platform for T1/T2 Dual-Mode PET-MR Imaging." *International Journal of Nanomedicine* 15. Int J Nanomedicine: 1253–66. https://doi.org/10.2147/IJN.S241971.

Gholami, Yaser Hadi, Hushan Yuan, Moses Q Wilks, Richard Maschmeyer, Marc D Normandin, Lee Josephson, Georges El Fakhri, and Zdenka Kuncic. 2020b. "A Radio-Nano-Platform for T1/T2 Dual-Mode PET-MR Imaging." *International Journal of Nanomedicine* Volume 15 (February): 1253–66. https://doi.org/10.2147/IJN.S241971.

Gill, P. S., J. Wernz, D. T. Scadden, P. Cohen, G. M. Mukwaya, J. H. von Roenn, M. Jacobs, et al. 1996. "Randomized Phase III Trial of Liposomal Daunorubicin versus Doxorubicin, Bleomycin, and Vincristine in AIDS-Related Kaposi's Sarcoma." *Journal of Clinical Oncology* 14 (8). American Society of Clinical Oncology: 2353–64. https://doi.org/10.1200/JCO.1996.14.8.2353.

Girardet, Thomas, Emilie Bianchi, Christel Henrionnet, Astrid Pinzano, Sabine Bouguet-Bonnet, Corentin Boulogne, Sébastien Leclerc, Franck Cleymand, and Solenne Fleutot. 2023. "SPIONs Magnetic Nanoparticles for MRI Applications: Microwave Synthesis and Physicochemical, Magnetic and Biological Characterizations." *Materials Today Communications* 36 (August): 106819. https://doi.org/10.1016/j.mtcomm.2023.106819.

Giri, P. M., Banerjee, A., & Layek, B. (2023). A Recent Review on Cancer Nanomedicine. Cancers, 15(8), 2256. https://doi.org/10.3390/cancers15082256

"Global Cancer Observatory." 2025. Accessed August 21. https://gco.iarc.fr/en.

Gomerdinger, Victoria F., Namita Nabar, and Paula T. Hammond. 2025. "Advancing Engineering Design Strategies for Targeted Cancer Nanomedicine." *Nature Reviews Cancer* 25 (9): 657–83. https://doi.org/10.1038/s41568-025-00847-2.

Gong, Liuyun, Yujie Zhang, Chengcheng Liu, Mingzhen Zhang, and Suxia Han. 2021. "Application of Radiosensitizers in Cancer Radiotherapy." *International Journal of Nanomedicine* 16. Dove Medical Press Ltd: 1083. https://doi.org/10.2147/IJN.S290438.

Gradishar, William J., Sergei Tjulandin, Neville Davidson, Heather Shaw, Neil Desai, Paul Bhar, Michael Hawkins, and Joyce O'Shaughnessy. 2005. "Phase III Trial of Nanoparticle Albumin-Bound Paclitaxel Compared with Polyethylated Castor Oil-Based Paclitaxel in Women with Breast Cancer." *Journal of Clinical Oncology* 23 (31). J Clin Oncol: 7794–803. https://doi.org/10.1200/JCO.2005.04.937.

Hong, Guosong, Yingping Zou, Alexander L. Antaris, Shuo Diao, Di Wu, Kai Cheng, Xiaodong Zhang, et al. 2014. "Ultrafast Fluorescence Imaging in Vivo with Conjugated Polymer Fluorophores in the Second Near-Infrared Window." *Nature Communications* 5 (1): 4206. https://doi.org/10.1038/ncomms5206.

Huang, Xiaohua, and Mostafa A. El-Sayed. 2011. "Plasmonic Photo-Thermal Therapy (PPTT)." *Alexandria Journal of Medicine* 47 (1). Taylor & Francis: 1–9. https://doi.org/10.1016/J.AJME.2011.01.001.

Hui, Ni, Ronghan Qu, Keke Xu, and Jiasheng Wang. 2023. "Prostate Specific Antigen Quantification in Human Serum Supported by the Designed Four-in-One Octabranched Peptides and AgNPs-Based Signal Amplifier." *Journal of the Taiwan Institute of Chemical Engineers* 151 (October): 105109. https://doi.org/10.1016/j.jtice.2023.105109.

Jacques, Vincent, Stéphane Dumas, Wei-Chuan Sun, Jeffrey S. Troughton, Matthew T. Greenfield, and Peter Caravan. 2010. "High-Relaxivity Magnetic Resonance Imaging Contrast Agents Part 2." *Investigative Radiology* 45 (10): 613–24. https://doi.org/10.1097/RLI.0b013e3181ee6a49.

Jarahi Khameneh, Armin, Sarvin Rahimi, Mohammed H. Abbas, Shayan Rahimi, Saeideh Mehmandoust, Abbas Rastgoo, Ashkan Heydarian, and Vahid Eskandari. 2024. "Trends in Electrochemical Biosensors for the Early Diagnosis of Breast Cancer through the Detection of Relevant Biomarkers." *Chemical Physics Impact* 8 (June): 100425. https://doi.org/10.1016/j.chphi.2023.100425.

Jin, Seung Mo, Yeon Jeong Yoo, Hong Sik Shin, Sohyun Kim, Sang Nam Lee, Chang Hoon Lee, Hyunji Kim, et al. 2023. "A Nanoadjuvant That Dynamically Coordinates Innate Immune Stimuli Activation Enhances Cancer Immunotherapy and Reduces Immune Cell Exhaustion." *Nature Nanotechnology* 18 (4). Nat Nanotechnol: 390–402. https://doi.org/10.1038/S41565-022-01296-W.

Julius, Angeline, Remya Rajan Renuka, Suresh Malakondaiah, Shenbhagaraman Ramalingam, Mukesh Kumar Dharmalingam Jothinathan, Guru Prasad Srinivasan, and Ramadurai Murugan. 2025. "Radiolabeled

Nanoparticles in Multimodal Nuclear Imaging, Diagnostics and Therapy." *Journal of Radioanalytical and Nuclear Chemistry* 334 (7): 4403–18. https://doi.org/10.1007/s10967-025-10233-9.

Kaunitz, Jonathan D. 2018. "Magnetic Resonance Imaging: The Nuclear Option." *Digestive Diseases and Sciences* 63 (5). Dig Dis Sci: 1100–01. https://doi.org/10.1007/S10620-018-4992-9.

Kelkar, Sneha S., and Theresa M. Reineke. 2011. "Theranostics: Combining Imaging and Therapy." *Bioconjugate Chemistry* 22 (10): 1879–1903. https://doi.org/10.1021/bc200151q.

Kim, Tae You, Dong Wan Kim, Jae Yong Chung, Sang Goo Shin, Sung Chul Kim, Dae Seog Heo, Noe Kyeong Kim, and Yung Jue Bang. 2004. "Phase I and Pharmacokinetic Study of Genexol-PM, a Cremophor-Free, Polymeric Micelle-Formulated Paclitaxel, in Patients with Advanced Malignancies." *Clinical Cancer Research* 10 (11). Clin Cancer Res: 3708–16. https://doi.org/10.1158/1078-0432.CCR-03-0655.

Kokilavani, R., Hiranmoy Kotal, Arunima Lala, and Saikat Kumar Jana. 2024. "Bimetallic Au-Ag Reduced Graphene Oxide Nanostructures for Enhanced Detection of Dengue Virus E Protein." *Journal of the Electrochemical Society* 171 (10): 107513. https://doi.org/10.1149/1945-7111/ad8520.

Kuyumcu, Serkan, Yasemin Sanli, and Rathan M. Subramaniam. 2021. "Fibroblast-Activated Protein Inhibitor PET/CT: Cancer Diagnosis and Management." *Frontiers in Oncology* 11 (November). https://doi.org/10.3389/fonc.2021.758958.

Lee Ventola, C. 2017. "Cancer Immunotherapy, Part 1: Current Strategies and Agents." *Pharmacy and Therapeutics* 42 (6). Medi Media USA Inc: 375. https://pmc.ncbi.nlm.nih.gov/articles/PMC5440098/.

Levine, Beth, and Guido Kroemer. 2019. "Biological Functions of Autophagy Genes: A Disease Perspective." *Cell* 176 (1–2): 11–42. https://doi.org/10.1016/j.cell.2018.09.048.

Li, Guangyao, Cong Wang, Binghui Jin, Tao Sun, Kang Sun, Shuang Wang, and Zhe Fan. 2024. "Advances in Smart Nanotechnology-Supported Photodynamic Therapy for Cancer." *Cell Death Discovery* 10 (1). Springer Nature: 1–18. https://doi.org/10.1038/S41420-024-02236-4;SUBJMETA.

Li, Xiaotong, Lei Chen, Miaoting Huang, Shaoting Zeng, Jiayi Zheng, Shuyi Peng, Yuqing Wang, Hong Cheng, and Shiying Li. 2023. "Innovative Strategies for Photodynamic Therapy against Hypoxic Tumor." *Asian Journal of Pharmaceutical Sciences* 18 (1). Elsevier: 100775. https://doi.org/10.1016/J.AJPS.2023.100775.

Liu, Chen-Guang, Ya-Hui Han, Ranjith Kumar Kankala, Shi-Bin Wang, and Ai-Zheng Chen. 2020. "Subcellular Performance of Nanoparticles in Cancer Therapy." *International Journal of Nanomedicine* Volume 15 (February): 675–704. https://doi.org/10.2147/IJN.S226186.

Liu, Haipeng, Kelly D. Moynihan, Yiran Zheng, Gregory L. Szeto, Adrienne V. Li, Bonnie Huang, Debra S. Van Egeren, Clara Park, and Darrell J. Irvine. 2014. "Structure-Based Programming of Lymph-Node Targeting in Molecular Vaccines." *Nature* 507 (7493). Nature Publishing Group: 519–22. https://doi.org/10.1038/NATURE12978.

Liu, Linlin, Abhimanyu Thakur, Wing Kar Li, Guangyu Qiu, Tian Yang, Bing He, Youngjin Lee, and Chi-Man Lawrence Wu. 2022. "Site Specific Biotinylated Antibody Functionalized Ag@AuNIs LSPR Biosensor for the Ultrasensitive Detection of Exosomal MCT4, a Glioblastoma Progression Biomarker." *Chemical Engineering Journal* 446 (October): 137383. https://doi.org/10.1016/j.cej.2022.137383.

Liu, Mohan, Yusi Wang, Yibing Zhang, Die Hu, Lin Tang, Bailing Zhou, and Li Yang. 2025. "Landscape of Small Nucleic Acid Therapeutics: Moving from the Bench to the Clinic as next-Generation Medicines." *Signal Transduction and Targeted Therapy* 10 (1). Springer Nature: 1–57. https://doi.org/10.1038/S41392-024-02112-8;SUBJMETA.

Liu, Yue, Menglong Li, Jingsi Gu, Haiyan Huang, Hui Xie, Chen Yu, Shubham Roy, et al. 2025. "Engineering of Exosome-Liposome Hybrid-Based Theranostic Nanomedicines for NIR-II Fluorescence Imaging-Guided and Targeted NIR-II Photothermal Therapy of Subcutaneous Glioblastoma." *Colloids and Surfaces B: Biointerfaces* 245 (January): 114258. https://doi.org/10.1016/j.colsurfb.2024.114258.

Liu, Zhimin, Jie Wang, Chen Cui, Limei Zheng, and Leqian Hu. 2023. "Introducing AgNPs-VB2 Composites as the Dual Signal Quenching of CeO2–AuNPs-g-CNQDs Hybrids for Ultrasensitive 'on-off' Electrochemiluminescence Immunosensing of Prostate Specific Antigen." *Talanta* 252 (January): 123886. https://doi.org/10.1016/j.talanta.2022.123886.

Makableh, Yahia, Tamara Athamneh, Manar Ajlouni, Sara Hijazi, and Aseel Alnaimi. 2023. "Enhanced Response and Selective Gold Nanoparticles/Carbon Nanotubes Biosensor for the Early Detection of HER2 Biomarker." *Sensors and Actuators Reports* 5 (June): 100158. https://doi.org/10.1016/j.snr.2023.100158.

Martin, Felicity C., Tanya B. Dorff, and Ben Tran. 2023. "The New Era of Prostate-Specific Membrane Antigen-Directed Immunotherapies and beyond in Advanced Prostate Cancer: A Review." *Therapeutic Advances in Medical Oncology* 15 (January). https://doi.org/10.1177/17588359231170474.

Matsumura, Y, and H Maeda. 1986. "A New Concept for Macromolecular Therapeutics in Cancer Chemotherapy: Mechanism of Tumoritropic Accumulation of Proteins and the Antitumor Agent Smancs." *Cancer Research* 46 (12 Pt 1): 6387–92.

McCarthy, Jason R., J. Manuel Perez, Christian Brückner, and Ralph Weissleder. 2005. "Polymeric Nanoparticle Preparation That Eradicates Tumors." *Nano Letters* 5 (12): 2552–56. https://doi.org/10.1021/nl0519229.

Minh Hoang, Chau Nguyen, Son Hai Nguyen, and Mai Thi Tran. 2025. "Nanoparticles in Cancer Therapy: Strategies to Penetrate and Modulate the Tumor Microenvironment—A Review." *Smart Materials in Medicine* 6 (2): 270–84. https://doi.org/10.1016/j.smaim.2025.07.004.

Mokhtari, Reza Bayat, Tina S. Homayouni, Narges Baluch, Evgeniya Morgatskaya, Sushil Kumar, Bikul Das, and Herman Yeger. 2017. "Combination Therapy in Combating Cancer." *Oncotarget* 8 (23). Impact Journals LLC: 38022. https://doi.org/10.18632/ONCOTARGET.16723.

Mostafavi, Mehrnaz, Farhood Ghazi, Mahboobeh Mehrabifard, Vahid Alivirdiloo, Mobasher Hajiabbasi, Fatemeh Rahimi, Ahmad Mobed, et al. 2025. "State-of-the-Art Application of Nanoparticles in Radiotherapy: A Platform for Synergistic Effects in Cancer Treatment." *Strahlentherapie Und Onkologie* 201 (6): 577–88. https://doi.org/10.1007/s00066-024-02301-y.

Nam, Jutaek, Sejin Son, Kyung Soo Park, Weiping Zou, Lonnie D. Shea, and James J. Moon. 2019. "Cancer Nanomedicine for Combination Cancer Immunotherapy." *Nature Reviews Materials* 4 (6): 398–414. https://doi.org/10.1038/s41578-019-0108-1.

Nguyen, Cao Minh, Trung T. Vu, Minh Nguyen Nguyen, Thao Suong Tran-Nguyen, Chi Thien Huynh, Quang Thanh Ha, Hoai Nghia Nguyen, and Le Son Tran. 2025. "Neoantigen-Based MRNA Vaccine Exhibits Superior Anti-Tumor Activity Compared to Synthetic Long Peptides in an in Vivo Lung Carcinoma Model." *Cancer Immunology, Immunotherapy: CII* 74 (4). Springer Science and Business Media Deutschland GmbH: 145. https://doi.org/10.1007/S00262-025-03992-7.

Nikolova, Maria P., Enamala Manoj Kumar, and Murthy S. Chavali. 2022. "Updates on Responsive Drug Delivery Based on Liposome Vehicles for Cancer Treatment." *Pharmaceutics* 14 (10). MDPI: 2195. https://doi.org/10.3390/PHARMACEUTICS14102195.

Northfelt, Donald W., Bruce J. Dezube, James A. Thommes, Becky J. Miller, Margaret A. Fischl, Alvin Friedman-Kien, Lawrence D. Kaplan, Charles Du Mond, Richard D. Mamelok, and David H. Henry. 1998. "Pegylated-Liposomal Doxorubicin versus Doxorubicin, Bleomycin, and Vincristine in the Treatment of AIDS-Related Kaposi's Sarcoma: Results of a Randomized Phase III Clinical Trial." *Journal of Clinical Oncology* 16 (7). American Society of Clinical Oncology: 2445–51. https://doi.org/10.1200/JCO.1998.16.7.2445.

Oerlemans, Chris, Wouter Bult, Mariska Bos, Gert Storm, J. Frank W. Nijsen, and Wim E. Hennink. 2010. "Polymeric Micelles in Anticancer Therapy: Targeting, Imaging and Triggered Release." *Pharmaceutical Research* 27 (12): 2569. https://doi.org/10.1007/S11095-010-0233-4.

Park, H., S. Yu, and T. Koo. 2025. "Gene Editing in Cancer Therapy: Overcoming Drug Resistance and Enhancing Precision Medicine." *Cancer Gene Therapy* 32 (12): 1293. https://doi.org/10.1038/S41417-025-00959-9

Pellico, Juan, Peter J. Gawne, and Rafael T. M. de Rosales. 2021. "Radiolabelling of Nanomaterials for Medical Imaging and Therapy." *Chemical Society Reviews* 50 (5): 3355–423. https://doi.org/10.1039/D0CS00384K.

Peng, Cheng-Liang, Ying-Hsia Shih, Pei-Chi Lee, Thomas Mon-Hsian Hsieh, Tsai-Yueh Luo, and Ming-Jium Shieh. 2011. "Multimodal Image-Guided Photothermal Therapy Mediated by 188 Re-Labeled Micelles Containing a Cyanine-Type Photosensitizer." *ACS Nano* 5 (7): 5594–607. https://doi.org/10.1021/nn201100m.

Rajagopal, Nanda, Ipshita Das, Annanya Kapur, Shruthi Nayak, Yashaswini Reddy, and Babitha Kampa Sundara. 2025. "Photodynamic Therapy Meets Nanotechnology: A Synergistic Approach for Cancer Treatment." *Translational Oncology* 62 (December). Elsevier: 102571. https://doi.org/10.1016/J.TRANON.2025.102571.

Rajoriya, V., R. Gupta, S. Vengurlekar, and U. Surendra Singh. 2024. "Nanostructured Lipid Carriers (NLCs): A Promising Candidate for Lung Cancer Targeting." *International Journal of Pharmaceutics* 655. https://doi.org/10.1016/J.IJPHARM.2024.123986

Rajpoot, Kuldeep, Pratik Katare, Muktika Tekade, Mukesh Chandra Sharma, Suryanarayana Polaka, Pinaki Sengupta, and Rakesh Kumar Tekade. 2022. "Toxicokinetic and Toxicodynamic Considerations in Drug Research." *Pharmacokinetics and Toxicokinetic Considerations—Vol II*, January. Academic Press, 751–76. https://doi.org/10.1016/B978-0-323-98367-9.00026-3.

Rauf, Mohd Ahmar, Afifa Rao, Siva Sankari Sivasoorian, and Arun K. Iyer. 2025. "Nanotechnology-Based Delivery of CRISPR/Cas9 for Cancer Treatment: A Comprehensive Review." *Cells* 14 (15). Multidisciplinary Digital Publishing Institute (MDPI): 1136. https://doi.org/10.3390/CELLS14151136.

Rusling, James F., Challa V. Kumar, J. Silvio Gutkind, and Vyomesh Patel. 2010. "Measurement of Biomarker Proteins for Point-of-Care Early Detection and Monitoring of Cancer." *The Analyst* 135 (10): 2496. https://doi.org/10.1039/c0an00204f.

Sabit, Hussein, Sanaa Rashwan, Yasser Albrahim, Al-Hassan Soliman Wadan, Faisal Radwan, Amany I. Alqosaibi, Shaimaa Abdel-Ghany, and Borros Arneth. 2025. "Targeting Resistance Pathways in Breast Cancer Through Precision Oncology: Nanotechnology and Immune Modulation Approaches." *Biomedicines* 13 (7): 1691. https://doi.org/10.3390/biomedicines13071691.

Setyawati, Magdiel I., Chor Yong Tay, Boon Huat Bay, and David T. Leong. 2017. "Gold Nanoparticles Induced Endothelial Leakiness Depends on Particle Size and Endothelial Cell Origin." *ACS Nano* 11 (5): 5020–30. https://doi.org/10.1021/acsnano.7b01744.

Shah, Kiramat Ali, Anam Razzaq, Amos Dormocara, Bengang You, Serag Eldin I. Elbehairi, Ali A. Shati, Mohammad Y. Alfaifi, Haroon Iqbal, and Jing-Hao Cui. 2025. "Current Trends in Inhaled Pharmaceuticals: Challenges and Opportunities in Respiratory Infections Treatment." *Journal of Pharmaceutical Investigation* 55 (2): 191–225. https://doi.org/10.1007/s40005-025-00729-7.

Shi, Jinjun, Philip W. Kantoff, Richard Wooster, and Omid C. Farokhzad. 2016. "Cancer Nanomedicine: Progress, Challenges and Opportunities." *Nature Reviews Cancer* 17 (1). Nature Publishing Group: 20. https://doi.org/10.1038/NRC.2016.108.

Shiridokht, Fatemeh, Parniya Kehtari, Morteza Eskandani, Alireza Farajollahi, and Somayeh Vandghanooni. 2025. "Advancing Cancer Radiotherapy: Harnessing Radiosensitizers and Nanotechnology for Enhanced Tumor Control." *International Journal of Pharmaceutics: X* 10 (December). Elsevier: 100419. https://doi.org/10.1016/J.IJPX.2025.100419.

Shrivastava, Saumya, Saloni Jain, Deepak Kumar, Shankar Lal Soni, and Mukesh Sharma. 2019. "A Review on Theranostics: An Approach to Targeted Diagnosis and Therapy." *Asian Journal of Pharmaceutical Research and Development* 7 (2): 63–9. https://doi.org/10.22270/ajprd.v7i2.463.

Sivanand, R., P. Selvakumar, and Navneet Sharma. 2025. "Nanotechnology Applications in Cancer Drug Delivery Systems: A Review." *Journal of Environmental Nanotechnology* 14 (2): 458–70. https://doi.org/10.13074/jent.2025.06.2511221.

Su, Jing, Wenhan Liu, Shixing Chen, Wangping Deng, Yanzhi Dou, Zhihan Zhao, Jianyong Li, et al. 2020. "A Carbon-Based DNA Framework Nano–Bio Interface for Biosensing with High Sensitivity and a High Signal-to-Noise Ratio." *ACS Sensors* 5 (12): 3979–87. https://doi.org/10.1021/acssensors.0c01745.

Suwannasom, Nittiya, Netsai Sriaksorn, Chutamas Thepmalee, Chonthida Thephinlap, Patcharawan Tanamatayarat, Krissana Khoothiam, Hans Bäuemler, and Nat Na-Ek. 2023. "Efficacy and Safety of Nanoparticle Albumin-Bound Paclitaxel in Advanced Non-Small Cell Lung Cancer: A Systematic Review and Meta-Analysis of Clinical Trials and Observational Studies." *Heliyon* 9 (11). Elsevier: e21903. https://doi.org/10.1016/J.HELIYON.2023.E21903.

Tan, Kexin, Haiyang Zhang, Jianyuan Yang, Hang Wang, Yongqiang Li, Guqiao Ding, Ping Gu, Siwei Yang, Jipeng Li, and Xianqun Fan. 2025. "Organelle-Oriented Nanomedicines in Tumor Therapy: Targeting, Escaping, or Collaborating?" *Bioactive Materials* 49 (July): 291–339. https://doi.org/10.1016/j.bioactmat.2025.02.040.

Tatsugami, F., T. Higaki, Y. Nakamura, Y. Honda, and K. Awa. 2022. "Dual-Energy CT: Minimal Essentials for Radiologists." *Japanese Journal of Radiology* 40 (6): 547–559. https://doi.org/10.1007/S11604-021-01233-2

Thakkar, Shreya, Dilip Sharma, Kiran Kalia, and Rakesh K. Tekade. 2020. "Tumor Microenvironment Targeted Nanotherapeutics for Cancer Therapy and Diagnosis: A Review." *Acta Biomaterialia* 101 (January): 43–68. https://doi.org/10.1016/j.actbio.2019.09.009.

Thomsen, H. S., and S. K. Morcos. 2009. "Risk of Contrast-Medium-Induced Nephropathy in High-Risk Patients Undergoing MDCT--A Pooled Analysis of Two Randomized Trials." *European Radiology* 19 (4): 891–897. https://doi.org/10.1007/S00330-008-1206-4.

Tong, Fan, Yufan Wang, and Huile Gao. 2024. "Progress and Challenges in the Translation of Cancer Nanomedicines." *Current Opinion in Biotechnology* 85 (February): 103045. https://doi.org/10.1016/j.copbio.2023.103045.

Uchida, Satoshi. 2022. "Delivery Systems of Plasmid DNA and Messenger RNA for Advanced Therapies." *Pharmaceutics* 14 (4). MDPI: 810. https://doi.org/10.3390/PHARMACEUTICS14040810.

Vasdev, Nupur, Mrudul Deshpande, Pratik Katare, Vaishali Makwana, Suryanarayana Polaka, Muktika Tekade, Pinaki Sengupta, Mukesh Chandra Sharma, Dinesh Kumar Mishra, and Rakesh Kumar Tekade. 2022. "New Emerging Technologies for Genetic Toxicity Testing." In *Pharmacokinetics and Toxicokinetic Considerations*, 175–219. Elsevier. https://doi.org/10.1016/B978-0-323-98367-9.00013-5.

Wan, Jonathan C. M., Charles Massie, Javier Garcia-Corbacho, Florent Mouliere, James D. Brenton, Carlos Caldas, Simon Pacey, Richard Baird, and Nitzan Rosenfeld. 2017. "Liquid Biopsies Come of Age: Towards Implementation of Circulating Tumour DNA." *Nature Reviews Cancer* 17 (4): 223–38. https://doi.org/10.1038/nrc.2017.7.

Wang, Ruonan, Changfeng Yin, Changren Liu, Ying Sun, Panpan Xiao, Jia Li, Shuo Yang, Wei Wu, and Xiqun Jiang. 2021. "Phenylboronic Acid Modification Augments the Lysosome Escape and Antitumor Efficacy of a Cylindrical Polymer Brush-Based Prodrug." *Journal of the American Chemical Society* 143 (49): 20927–38. https://doi.org/10.1021/jacs.1c09741.

Wang-Gillam, Andrea, Chung Pin Li, György Bodoky, Andrew Dean, Yan Shen Shan, Gayle Jameson, Teresa MacArulla, et al. 2016. "Nanoliposomal Irinotecan with Fluorouracil and Folinic Acid in Metastatic Pancreatic Cancer after Previous Gemcitabine-Based Therapy (NAPOLI-1): A Global, Randomised, Open-Label, Phase 3 Trial." *The Lancet* 387 (10018). Lancet Publishing Group: 545–57. https://doi.org/10.1016/S0140-6736(15)00986-1.

White, Gregory W., Wendell A. Gibby, and Michael F. Tweedle. 2006. "Comparison of Gd(DTPA-BMA) (Omniscan) Versus Gd(HP-DO3A) (ProHance) Relative to Gadolinium Retention in Human Bone Tissue by Inductively Coupled Plasma Mass Spectroscopy." *Investigative Radiology* 41 (3): 272–78. https://doi.org/10.1097/01.rli.0000186569.32408.95.

Yang, Jingjing, Anthony Griffin, Zhe Qiang, and Jie Ren. 2022. "Organelle-Targeted Therapies: A Comprehensive Review on System Design for Enabling Precision Oncology." *Signal Transduction and Targeted Therapy* 7 (1): 379. https://doi.org/10.1038/s41392-022-01243-0.

Yu, Hai-Jia, Jian-Hua Liu, Wei Liu, Rui Niu, Bin Zhang, Yuan Xiong, Yang Liu, Ying-Hui Wang, and Hong-Jie Zhang. 2025. "Metal-Based Nanomedicines for Cancer Theranostics." *Military Medical Research* 12 (1): 41. https://doi.org/10.1186/s40779-025-00627-x.

Zhang, Jiawei, Qingya Zhang, Xiaojia Li, Yixuan Wei, Min Qiu, Huazhe Yang, and Xiaoting Sun. 2025. "Prominent Supramolecular Systems for Cancer Therapy: From Structural Design to Tailored Applications." *European Journal of Medicinal Chemistry* 294 (September): 117754. https://doi.org/10.1016/j.ejmech.2025.117754.

Zhang, Y., M. Li, X. Gao, Y. Chen, and T. Liu. 2019. "Nanotechnology in Cancer Diagnosis: Progress, Challenges and Opportunities." *Journal of Hematology & Oncology* 12 (1). https://doi.org/10.1186/S13045-019-0833-3.

Zhao, Jingya, Dian Zhong, and Shaobing Zhou. 2018. "NIR-I-to-NIR-II Fluorescent Nanomaterials for Biomedical Imaging and Cancer Therapy." *Journal of Materials Chemistry B* 6 (3). The Royal Society of Chemistry: 349–65. https://doi.org/10.1039/C7TB02573D.

6 Inorganic Nanostructured Materials for Cancer Therapy and Diagnosis

Sarita Devi,[1] *Abhilasha Khatri*[1] *and Nirmal Prabhakar*[1]
[1]Department of Biochemistry, Panjab University, India

6.1 INTRODUCTION

Nanotechnology, operating within the nanoscale range of 1 to 100 nm, presents distinct capabilities in fabricating structures and devices tailored for cancer research and oncology. Through the integration of molecular insights with these nanostructures, advanced diagnostics, treatments, and preventive strategies for cancer can be devised. Defined by the U.S. National Nanotechnology Initiative, this domain encompasses the manipulation of materials and structures at exceptionally small scales. These nanostructures, whether utilized independently or integrated into larger systems, offer substantial potential applications in cancer research and healthcare. Despite its relatively recent exploration commencing in the 1980s, substantial progress has been achieved in implementing nano-based interventions and diagnostic tools in clinical settings, with numerous further advancements anticipated. This interdisciplinary realm brings together expertise from various fields, including physics, chemistry, engineering, computer science, and biology. Nanotechnology permeates diverse sectors such as electronics, optics, materials development, and biomedicine, catalyzing innovation across multiple domains, particularly in medical contexts.

While modern medicine has notably advanced cancer management, the disease continues to claim over six lakh lives annually in the United States alone. Despite significant progress in cancer treatments, this is imperative to enhance their specificity and mitigate systemic toxicity. Nanotechnology offers firstly enhanced early diagnosis through in vitro assays, secondly improved imaging capabilities for diagnosis and treatment monitoring, and eventually, optimized therapeutic outcomes by enhancing targeting precision, localized drug potency, and minimizing systemic toxicity. Nanoparticles (NPs), significantly smaller than human cells by factors ranging from 10^2 to 10^4, possess remarkable capabilities to engage with biomolecules both on cell surfaces and within cells themselves. The broad accessibility across various organs, biocompatibility, reduced toxicity, excellent stability, enhanced permeability and retention effect, inherent design flexibility, and adjustability of NPs can be easily adorned with diverse ligands on their surfaces, enabling insights into their interactions with live cancer cells. By facilitating swift and precise detection of cancer-related molecules, nanotechnology empowers researchers to identify molecular alterations, even within a small subset of cells. Furthermore, nanotechnology holds promise for generating entirely novel and efficacious therapeutic agents. Notably, nanomaterials demonstrate the ability to passively accumulate at tumor sites, actively target cancer cells and traverse physiological barriers such as the blood-brain barrier or the stomach epithelium.

Inorganic nanoparticles (INPs) offer significant promise for theranostics, seamlessly integrating tumor-targeted diagnosis, imaging, and therapy within a single system facilitating drug localization to kill cancer cells specifically by sparing the normal cells. Both organic and inorganic nanoparticles (Figure 6.1a) serve as imaging and therapeutic agents or as carriers for such agents. Among organic

DOI: 10.1201/9781003799351-6

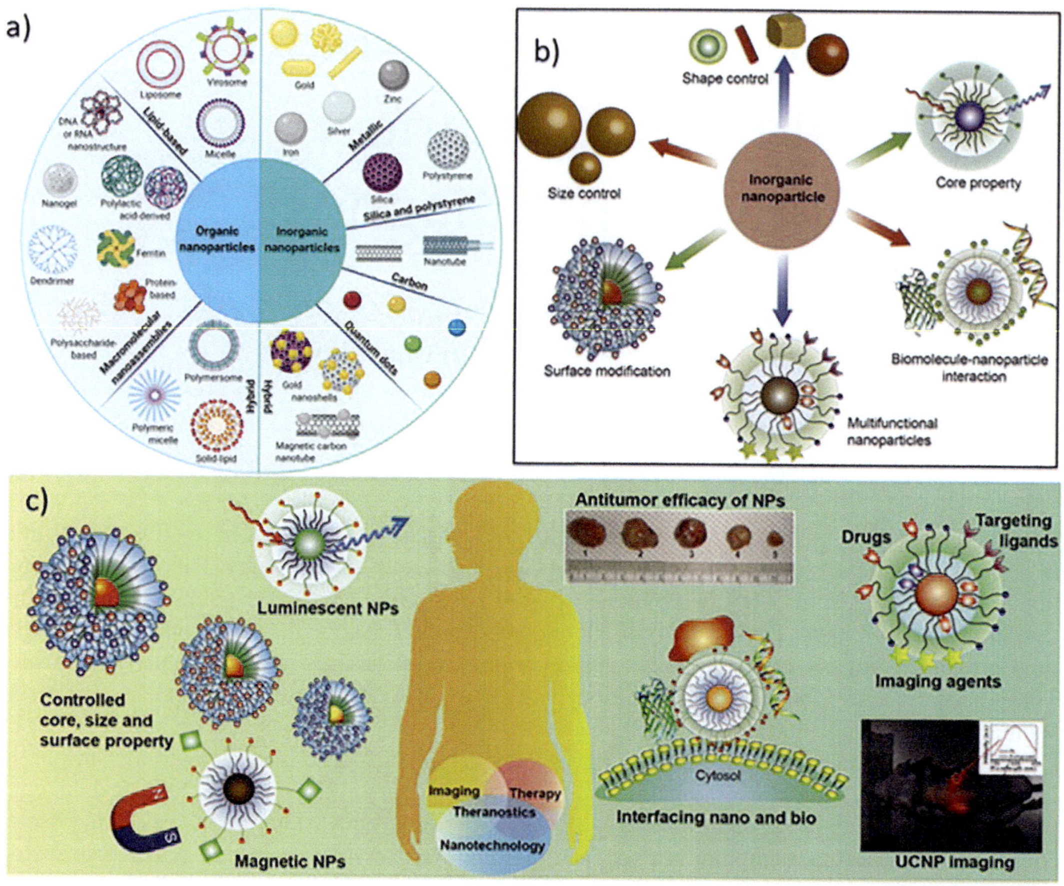

FIGURE 6.1 (a) Chemically engineered inorganic (INPs) and organic nanoparticles for cancer therapy. INPs include mainly metallic, silica, carbon, and quantum dots. Organic nanoparticles include specifically the lipid-based and macromolecular assemblies. Hybrid nanoparticles combine the advantages of both INPs and organic families to improve the biocompatibility and the stability of the nano vehicle; (b) the wide array of physical and structural properties of INPs; (c) the use of the INPs properties in biomedicine (Tonga et al. 2014).

nanoplatforms like liposomes, polymersomes, polymeric micelles, and nanoparticles, clinical translation has seen notable success (Allen and Cullis 2013; Torchilin 2007; Malam, Loizidou, and Seifalian 2009). Recently, INPs have garnered increasing attention for several reasons (Figure 6.1b): (i) their inherent optical, electronic, and magnetic characteristics often outperform those of organic counterparts, thereby enhancing both molecular imaging and therapy (Xie et al. 2011; Zrazhevskiy, Sena, and Gao 2010; Arvizo et al. 2012); (ii) their synthesis enables precise control over size, shape, charge, and composition, important for pharmacokinetics, biodistribution, and in vivo behavior (Albanese, Tang, and Chan 2012); (iii) functionalization of their surface with organic molecules allows for biocompatibility, blood circulation, and tumor targeting; and (iv) loading of a large number of therapeutic candidates without mutual interference and associated degradation such as drugs (Paul and Sharma 2020), nucleic acids (Resnier et al. 2013) and photosensitizers (Gierlich et al. 2020) aids in improvements in therapy (Figure 6.1c). Most of all, INPs have depicted intrinsic anticancer and gene-silencing performances, both of which are advantageous in cancer therapy (Debela et al. 2021).

The present chapter aims to assess the most promising recent therapeutic INP-based strategies for cancer therapy. It takes a look at the current status of INPs as imaging and therapeutic agents. The aim is both to discuss the promise of these INPs and to provide areas where questions remain and better understanding is required. Beginning The chapter with the various types of InNM including metallic nanoparticles (NPs), quantum dots (QDs), mesoporous silica nanoparticles (MSNPs), magnetic NPs (mNPs), and carbon-based nanostructures, their physicochemical properties are discussed. Following this, their imaging applications using different techniques such as magnetic resonance imaging (MRI), computed tomography (CT), positron emission tomography (PET), fluorescence imaging, and multimodal imaging approaches are presented. Furthermore, their therapeutic applications and theranostic approaches are presented. The toxicity as well as regulatory challenges and clearance mechanisms are discussed which is followed by suggesting the future direction of the material design and synthesis for cancer diagnosis and treatment.

6.2 TYPES OF INORGANIC NANOSTRUCTURED MATERIALS AND PROPERTIES

INPs lack carbon and are more stable than organic nanoparticles, hydrophilic, nontoxic, and biocompatible with living systems. INPs include metallic NPs, QDs, Si-NPs, mNPs, and carbon-based nanostructures. Their surface properties such as pore size, shapes (rod, irregular, spherical, cylindrical, tetragonal, and hexagonal), surface area to volume ratio, surface charge, structure (amorphous and crystalline), environmental factors, surface charge density, and color are distinctively beneficial in a variety of fields. The following section includes the types and properties of INPs.

6.2.1 Metallic Nanoparticles

Metal nanoparticles can be synthesized from metal precursors through either constructive or destructive mechanisms. Their unique plasma-on resonance characteristics are attributed to their distinctive optoelectrical properties (Kumar et al. 2018). Zinc (Zn), gold (Au), silver (Ag), lead (Pb), copper (Cu), cobalt (Co), cadmium (Cd), aluminum (Al), and iron (Fe) are all well-known metals to form nanoparticles of the element. The metallic NPs can be synthesized by the chemical reduction method (Turkvich/citrate reduction) (Devi et al. 2016), physical method (UV-irradiation) (Rheima et al. 2019), and biological method (plant-mediated) (Huang, Devi, et al. 2023). Noble metal nanoparticles (Au, Pt, Ag) are superior and have been applied in a diversity of biomedical applications, such as cancer treatment, diagnosis, improved radiotherapy, germicidal and fungicidal, thermal ablation, drug delivery gene transport, etc. In the field of medicine, these NPs have garnered a lot of attention due to their ability to project a range of chemical groups that help them to bind with antibodies, peptides, DNA, and RNA, as well as biocompatible polymers, such as polyethylene glycol to target a wide variety of cell types (Prasanna et al. 2019). Another unique property is the percentage of surface atoms—that is, the full-shell cluster structure, which is arranged by atom corresponding to the magic number. The magic number is either protons or neutrons that are arranged into complete shells within the atomic nucleus. A surface atom of bigger clusters is reduced as the central atoms are covered. Clusters are dispersed or aggregated clusters. The reactants having more dispersed clusters have a higher surface area so they have higher reactivity than the other (equal atoms) (Kumar et al. 2018). The advantages of metallic nanoparticles over other NPs are enhanced Rayleigh scattering, surface-enhanced Raman scattering (SERS), strong plasma absorption, biological system imaging, and their surface chemical information (Li et al. 2007). The principles of multiplexed detection using the SERS technique are shown in Figure 6.2A (Jarockyte et al. 2020). (a) Noble metal NPs having different sizes and shapes, offer unique Raman signals with narrow peaks and are used as SERS tags. (b) Schematic illustration of simultaneous detection of three tumor-associated antigens expressed in different types of cancer cells by SERS imaging (Jarockyte et al. 2020). Some of their disadvantages are (i) particle thermodynamic instability and region of high energy local minima, resulting in quality deterioration, poor corrosion resistance, and difficult structure retainment; (ii) high possibility of impurities by nitrides and oxides formation during the synthesis of these highly reactive metallic NPs; (iii) biologically toxic, carcinogenic and cause irritation due to their transparency to the cell dermis; and (iv) fine metal particles act as strong explosives leading to exothermic combustion (Granqvist and Buhrman 1976).

6.2.2 Quantum Dots

QDs are particles with a size less than 10 nm range. These are the inorganic semiconductor materials usually composed of Cd, Se, Zn, Te, Hg, and Pb (Devi, Kaur, Paul, et al. 2018; Jin et al. 2008). QDs are the most attractive luminescence label in biomedicine. The optical properties of DQs originate from interactions among electrons, holes, and their local environments (Alivisatos 1996; Chan et al. 2002). According to the semiconductor band theory, the band gap is the energy difference between the conduction band (bottom) and valence band (top). QDs absorb photons whose energy exceeds the photoluminescence (PL) excitation band gap, transferring electrons from the valence band to the conduction band. Characterized by numerous electronic states, their PL excitation spectra are wide, yet their emission bands are narrow and symmetrical. This unique trait enables different QDs to be excited by the same light source, producing various colored imaging within one biological sample. In contrast, most organic fluorescent dyes exhibit relatively narrow excitation bands and broad fluorescent bands, necessitating multiple light sources for multicolor imaging (Chan et al. 2002). By adjusting the size and composition of QDs, the emission wavelength can be fine-tuned from visible to near-infrared spectrum. Moreover, owing to their easily modifiable surfaces, QDs readily accommodate various antibodies and biomolecules, making them highly suitable for cell imaging, immunoassays (Bilan et al. 2015), and diagnostic applications. Figure 6.2B shows the multicolor capability of QD imaging in live animals. Sensitivity and spectral comparison between QD-tagged and Green Fluorescent Protein (GFP) transfected cancer cells (a), and simultaneous in vivo imaging of multicolor QD-encoded microbeads are shown (b). The right-hand images show QD-tagged cancer cells (orange, upper) and GFP-labeled cells (green, lower) (Gao et al. 2004).

QDs represent groundbreaking technological advancements with the potential application *in vitro*, particularly in detecting cancer biomarkers in molecular pathology, elucidating cancer invasion dynamics, exploring the tumor microenvironment, and offering innovative avenues for enhancing our understanding, diagnosis, classification, and treatment of cancer. Additionally, QD-based multifunctional probes are used for the anticancer drug and siRNA delivery (Medarova et al. 2007), MRI (Harisinghani et al. 2003), multiplexed molecular cancer diagnosis, (Wu et al. 2003) and *in vitro* imaging (Devi, Gupta, et al. 2018). However, despite these strides, intricate *in vivo* investigations continue to present challenges, particularly in identifying the predominant mechanisms of tumor invasion and micro-environmental compensation (Sanz-Moreno and Marshall 2010).

6.2.3 Mesoporous Silica Nanoparticles

MSNPs are presented by their porous structure, stability, inertness, and biocompatibility; therefore they are preferred for wide-ranging applications such as drug loading and delivery (Vallet-Regí et al. 2022), sensing (Devi, Kaur, Singh, et al. 2018), and catalysis (Yousefi et al. 2021). A list of approaches has been developed for their synthesis:

- Sol-gel method: a silica precursor, such as tetraethyl orthosilicate (TEOS), is hydrolyzed in the presence of a catalyst and a surfactant template, which is removed through extraction or calcination to develop the final MSNPs (Vlasenkova, Dolinina, and Parfenyuk 2019).
- Strober method: this approach involves a stabilizing substance like ammonia or ethanol during the hydrolysis and condensation of TEOS (Chen et al. 2020).
- Emulsion templating: this method is based on a water-in-oil emulsion system, where a surfactant and co-surfactant act as templates to form MSNPs (Gustafsson and Holmberg 2017).
- Reverse micelle method: In this process, surfactant is utilized to form reverse micelles in a non-polar solvent (Chen, Chen, and Shi 2014). The silica precursor is introduced into

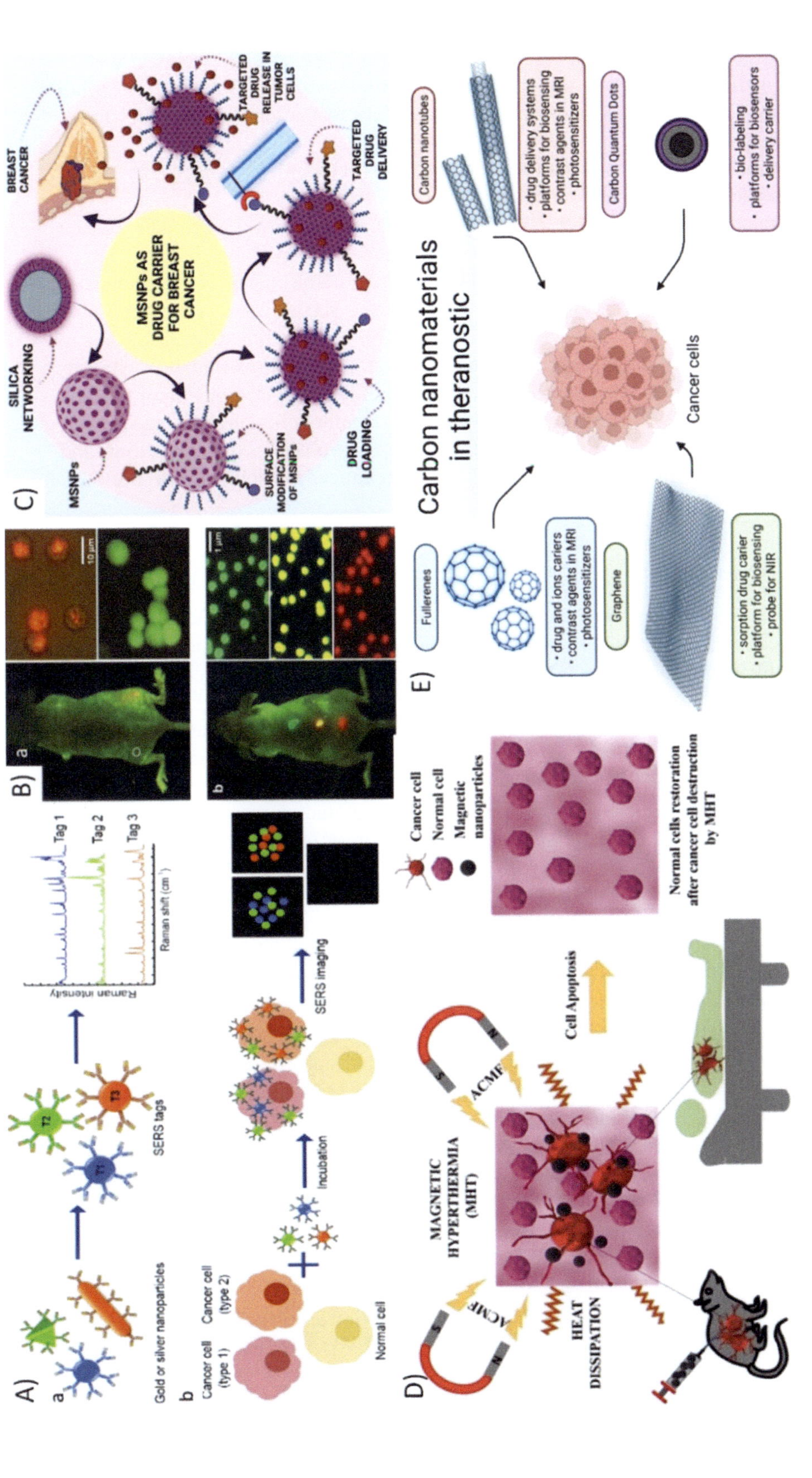

FIGURE 6.2 (A) The fundamentals of multiplexed detection utilizing the SERS technique are outlined: (a) Unique Raman signals with narrow peaks are exhibited by noble MNPs of varying size and shape, rendering them suitable as SERS tags; (b) a schematic representation demonstrates the simultaneous detection of three tumor-associated antigens expressed in different types of cancer cells through SERS imaging. [Reprinted with permission from (Jarockyte et al. 2020)]. (B) The sensitivity and multicolor imaging capabilities of QD imaging in live animals are demonstrated. [Reprinted with permission from (Gao et al. 2004)]. (C) The steps involved in the fabrication and application of MSNs as drug delivery vehicles in breast cancer [Reprinted with permission from (Thapa et al. 2023)]. (D) Role of mNPs in localized destruction of tumor cells by controlled heating of tumor specific site by external magnetic field. [Adapted from (Rajan and Sahu 2020). (E) Examples of the use of CNMs in theranostics [Taken from (Kościk, Jankowski, and Jagusiak 2021)]

the micellar solution, wherein the NPs are included. Finally, the surfactant templates are removed to obtain the MSNPs.

- Spray drying method: It involves the spraying of a silica precursor solution into a hot chamber, where the solvent evaporates, resulting in MSNPs formation, further subjected to calcination (Hong et al. 2016).
- Nano/microfluidic method: This includes managing fluids at the micro or nano size to generate desired reaction conditions. The silica precursor solutions, such as TEOS or TMOS, are produced separately and injected into a microfluidic device, forming droplets that act as confined reaction vessels. Here, the silica precursor undergoes hydrolysis and condensation to form MSNPs (Mamaeva, Sahlgren, and Lindén 2013). The characteristic properties of MSNPs that make them highly efficient drug delivery vectors are their controllable particle size and tunable porosity. Their pore size could also be tuned from 1.8 nm to 2.5 nm by using C12-C16 trimethylammonium bromide in the self-assembly of MSNPs (Botterhuis et al. 2006). Their tendency for surface modification outstands them to track the pathway of cell uptake, biodistribution *in vivo,* and targeting efficiency in cancer diagnosis and therapy (Tang, Li, and Chen 2012). The steps involved in the fabrication and application of MSNs as drug delivery vehicles in breast cancer are shown in Figure 6.2C (Thapa et al. 2023).

6.2.4 Magnetic Nanoparticles

mNPs consists of a magnetic core of maghemite (g-Fe_2O_3) or magnetite (Fe_3O_4) (Berry 2005). Other metals, such as nickel and cobalt, are also employed, although their applications are limited due to their toxicity and oxidation vulnerability (Dreaden et al. 2012). The human body has iron majorly as Ferritin, a type of protein, and its supply is restored by Iron oxide mNPs-mediated digestion of excess iron. Cationic mNPs are also present in the endosomes for a period (Salavati-Niasari, Davar, and Mir 2008). After that, during the post-cellular absorption process in the endosome and the lysosome, elemental components like iron and oxygen are stored in the body, eventually digested or destructed by hydrolytic enzymes. The adsorption, excretion, and storage of iron in the body are controlled by homeostasis. Yet being essential, the free form of iron can result in cell damage (Arosio and Levi 2002). The magnetic energy of mNPs can be converted to heat energy with the aid of an externally applied magnetic field, therefore widely applicable for hyperthermia (HT) as an efficient cancer therapeutic tool. These small mNPs easily penetrate the biological barriers to target the tumor sites specifically with a longer circulation time of NPs in the physiological environment (Chenthamara et al. 2019). The half-life circulation time is determined by MSNPs size. Smaller NPs (< 10 nm) can be entirely ejected from the renal system and larger NPs (> 200 nm) can be uptaken by phagocytosis, both eventually being unwanted for biomedical applications (Spirou et al. 2018). The injected mNPs-dosage should be low enough to avoid the possible side effects.

Localized destruction of tumor cells is achieved by controlled heating of tumor-specific sites by external magnetic field-guided mNPs, ultimately sparing the healthy cells, as shown schematically in Figure 6.2D (Rajan and Sahu 2020). It shows that the targeted mNPs are delivered to tumor cells and exposed to an alternating magnetic field (AMF). Then, the AMF energy is converted into heat by the mNP resulting in local heating (41 and 47 °C) of tumor cells (Belyanina et al. 2017).To achieve the required therapeutic temperature, the external applied magnetic field frequency should be in the low radio-frequency range (100–300 kHz) (Wu and Wang 2017). Magnetic NPs are known to dissipate the thermal energy by magnetic losses via (i) relaxation loss (Néel and Brownian relaxation loss); (ii) hysteresis heat loss; and (iii) eddy current loss (although insignificant). During clinical treatment, colloidal mNPs are injected into the tumor-specified site either actively or passively (Senapati et al. 2018). Active targeting involves the attachment of ligands on the mNP surface, which interacts with the surface receptors inside the tumor area. Passive targeting involves the attachment of mNPs to the specific sites through the leaky vasculature of the tumor and shows an enhanced permeability and retention (EPR) effect. A new approach of thermo-chemo therapy for an enhanced therapeutic effect and a greater percentage of cancer cell apoptosis is being considered by integrating the magnetic field-induced hyperthermia of nanocarriers-mNP with the controlled drug release in chemotherapy (Pradhan et al. 2010).

6.2.5 Carbon-Based Nanostructures (CNS)

Carbon is an exceptionally versatile element known for its ability to form a diverse array of structures with unique properties. These structures, known as allotropes, include "hard" diamond and "soft" graphite, with atoms arranged in hexagonal or cubic lattices (Mahor et al. 2021). Other allotropes, such as zero-dimensional (0D) fullerenes and grapheme QDs (GQDs), 1D-carbon nanotubes (CNTs), and 2D graphene sheets, have also been identified. Other CNS include nanodiamonds and Carbon nano-onions (CNOs) (Mahor et al. 2021). CNSs possess high surface area and excellent mechanical and electrical properties that promote their application also in the therapeutic and diagnostic fields. They can be used as theranostics materials specifically (Figure 6.2E) due to their unique optical characteristics and facile amalgamation with luminous substances, also due to their supramolecular π–π stacking attribute which permits a high amount of drug loading. Their excellent heat conversion capacity in the near-infrared region can be utilized for photothermal therapy. The unavoidable steps of surface functionalization include oxidation, ozonolysis, plasma treatments, and dehydrogenation which allow their usage for the controlled release of therapeutics by reducing cytotoxicity and crossing biological membranes (Li et al. 2014). Loaded CNS can be associated with the biomolecules that target the over/expressed ligands or folate receptors or tumor-associated antigens on the surface of a broad spectrum or specific type of tumor cells, accordingly (Allen 2002). For instance, CNSs have been employed in cancer phototherapy (Jiang et al. 2019), delivery of anticancer agents (Kim et al. 2017), theranostics (Wang, Bi, et al. 2018), fluorescent markers for tumor detection (Guo, Wang, and Zhao 2019), and so forth.

CNTs are large cylindrical molecules made of hexagonally arranged sp2 hybridized carbon atoms with a C–C distance of approximately 1.4 Å. They consist of single or multiple layers of graphene sheets, forming single-walled carbon nanotubes (SWCNTs) or multi-walled carbon nanotubes (MWCNTs) respectively. Both types of CNTs are capped at both ends with hemispherical carbon networks known as fullerenes. These nanotubes boast unique spectroscopic properties, with both their end and sidewalls readily amenable to covalent or non-covalent functionalization. Due to their small size, high surface area to volume ratio, and capacity to encapsulate biomolecules, they can be loaded with bioactive peptides, small-molecule drugs, proteins, or nucleic acids, by attaching via a cleavable bond (Kushwaha et al. 2013). Leveraging their ability to penetrate cells, given their diminutive size (1–100 nm) CNTs enhance the cellular uptake of therapeutic agents, safeguarding them during transit and cellular permeation. N-isopropyl acrylamide CNTs-loaded with Doxorubicin (DOX) were used for drug delivery. The smaller polymer chain length allowed the more hydrogen bonding with the drug (Maleki et al. 2020).

Graphene delivers highly interesting photoluminescence properties as well as easy surface functionalization, which leads to its biological application. The large surface area, chemical purity, large and planar sp^2 hybridization of carbon and oxygen-containing groups, physiological solubility, as well as stability of graphene oxide (GO), and free π-electrons help them for delivery of therapeutics (Pattnaik, Swain, and Lin 2016). Also, the conjugation strategies increase the biocompatibility, payload of drugs/genes via chemical conjugation or physisorption, and residence time *in vivo* (Nurunnabi et al. 2013). These materials have been explored for the delivery of chemotherapeutic agents (Zamani et al. 2018), genes (Lu et al. 2020), peptides (Ren et al. 2019), and tissue engineering (Ren et al. 2019). Vigorous oxidation of graphite was done to achieve the GO for the very first time (Hummers Jr and Offeman 1958).

Recently, the GQDs have emerged as the latest addition to the carbon nanomaterial family (Zhao et al. 2020). Comprising a few layers of graphene, GQDs exhibit a lattice distance of approximately

0.24 nm with sp2 hybridization, akin to small graphene flakes. Distinguishing them from carbon quantum dots (CQDs), which have a lattice distance of about 0.34 nm and possess an amorphous structure with sp3 hybridization, GQDs feature characteristic photoluminescence due to quantum confinement. Furthermore, GQDs share similar traits with graphene, such as a large surface area and availability of free π-electrons, making them well-suited for applications including imaging, sensing, and cancer therapy (Kumawat et al. 2017; Li et al. 2017; Zhao et al. 2020). INPs have been exploited extensively in the delivery of therapeutics, imaging, and theranostic applications.

6.3 IMAGING APPLICATIONS

To detect the specific cancer-effected cell site, different non-invasive imaging techniques are applied (Damasco et al. 2020; Aghebati-Maleki et al. 2020). The INPs with scalable sizes and strong resistance to enzyme degradation are preferred over other NMs (Damasco et al. 2020).

6.3.1 Magnetic Resonance Imaging

Cancer metastases can be successfully detected and tracked with magnetic resonance imaging (MRI) (Kumari, Ghosh, and Biswas 2016). The magnetism of H+ (proton) in body water is the basis for the MRI's working concept in humans. When the sample of interest is exposed to an external RF, the H+ proton aligns itself anti-parallel to the magnetic field. The amount of external radio frequency (RF) determines the extent of magnetization. The transverse magnetization dissipates and the aligned protons return to their initial state when the external RF is removed and the energy is released. Two separate processes can be used to identify the protons' relaxation: the longitudinal (T1 recovery) and transverse (T2-delay) relaxations. Whereas the latter creates a darker contrast, the former produces a brighter contrast. However, with the right contrast agent, either of these can be utilized to create an MRI image. Because various tissues relax at different rates and produce different pictures, this approach can differentiate between healthy and injured tissues. They may be distinguished from one another by their different rates of tissue relaxation, which also makes tumors visible (Ayrignac et al. 2019). This makes it possible to determine the size and stage of the tumor as well as diagnose the degree of tissue damage (Swayampakula, Dillis, and Abraham 2008). The reliability of MRI in identifying human early-stage cancer is improved when mNPs are conjugated to antibodies that target the proteins present in cancer cells (Neumaier et al. 2008). MRI can function on its own without the requirement for other imaging techniques.

Magnetic and Supermagnetic ferrite NPs and SPIONs were used as contrast agents for brain cancer detection (Hyder, Manjura Hoque, and Imaging 2017) (Ma et al. 2015). Pluronic F127-folate functionalized SPION was also employed as an MRI contrast agent by Quang et al. (Vu-Quang et al. 2019). Manganese ferrite nanoparticles (MFNPs) conjugated to a tumor-targeted pentapeptide (Cys-Arg-Glu-Lys-Ala) have been reported as a T1 MRI contrast agent for the detection of breast cancer (Li et al. 2020). The impact of an external magnetic field on bulk magnetite (top), Fe ions (middle), and SPIONs (bottom) is illustrated in Figure 6.3. Prior to the magnetic field's application, all magnetic moments are randomly oriented. When the external magnetic field is applied, the moments align along the z-axis of the magnetic field. Initially, the net magnetization of SPIONs surpasses that of Fe ions but falls short of bulk magnetite. After the magnetic field is removed, the moments of bulk magnetite remain fixed along the z-axis, whereas the magnetic moments of both Fe ions and SPIONs gradually relax over time until reaching equilibrium.

Apart from identifying metastates, the investigation yielded a hitherto unseen detection limit of 0.39 nm in contrast to previously documented data. The cylindrical-shaped chitosan-coated nickel-ferrite NPs were suitable for both T1 and T2 contrast agent MRI. In animal experiments, a 25% signal augmentation and a 71% signal decrease in the T1 and T2-weighted images respectively were noticed (Ahmad et al. 2015). Moreover, a prostate biomarker was targeted with the use of mouse monoclonal antibody-conjugated SPIONS as a contrast agent in T2-weighted MRI (Tietze and Alexiou 2017). The FeO core NPs effectively targeted the prostate cancer cells. Using Ultrasmall

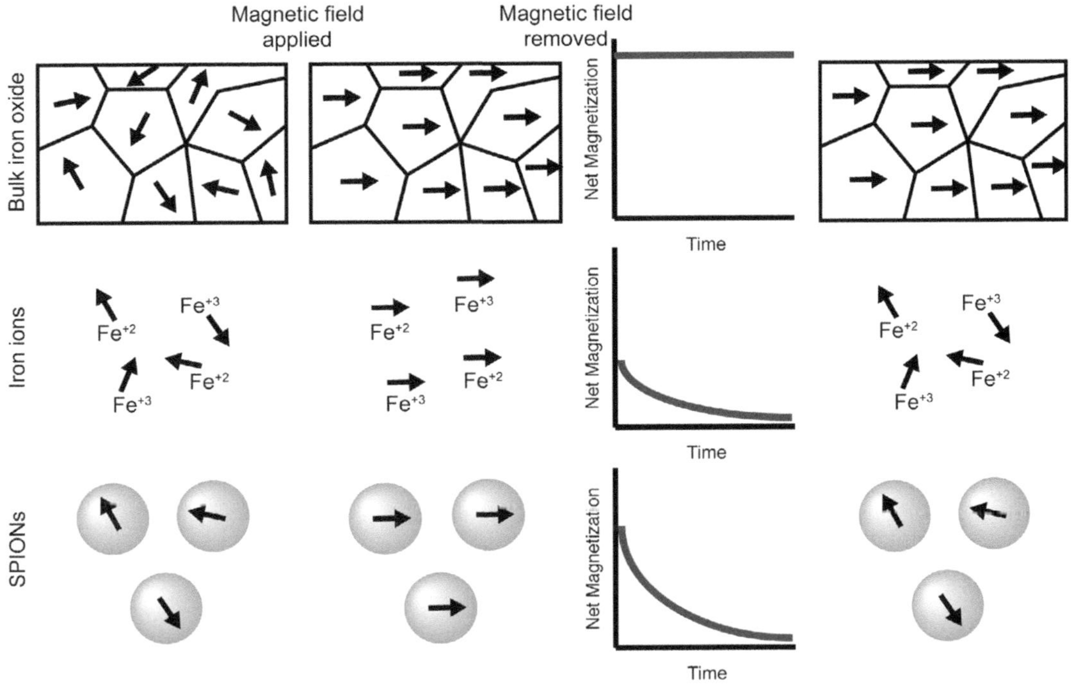

FIGURE 6.3 The impact of an external magnetic field on bulk magnetite (top), Fe ions (middle), and SPIONs (bottom) is illustrated.

Source: Reprinted with permission from (Stephen, Kievit, and Zhang 2011).

SPIONs were also tested as MRI contrasting agents for *in vivo* tumor imaging (Wang et al. 2023). When 3-amino propanol was utilized as a contrast agent instead of gadolinium butoxide, a brighter vascular image was seen, suggesting that 3-amino propanol has a role in MR tumor imaging. A dual-paclitaxel (PTX)/SPIONs-loaded Polylactic-co-glycolic acid (PLGA)-based findings of phantom MRI and relaxometry investigations demonstrated their effectiveness as T2 contrast agents (Wang et al. 2023). The NP loaded with PTX exhibited cytotoxicity and caused a delay in the *in vivo* growth of CT26 tumors. Polydopamine (PDA)-coated IONs enclosed in polyamidoamine (PAMAM) were used for theranostic activity on liver cancer cells (Jędrzak et al. 2019). The study's findings demonstrated that functionalized MNP may be effectively used in CT-PTT, or combined chemo- and photothermal treatment, to kill liver cancer cells. Additionally, the substance demonstrated competitive contrast qualities in MRI.

Therefore, it can be stated that amidst the array of mNPs, SPIONs have garnered significant attention owing to their exceptional magnetic properties, biocompatibility, and biodegradability. Concerns over toxicity often hinder the *in vivo* applications of many NPs-based contrast agents. Several formulations of SPIONs have received approval from the Food and Drug Administration as MRI contrast agents such as Lumiren® for bowel imaging, Combidex® for lymph node metastases imaging, and Feridex IV® for liver and spleen imaging.

6.3.2 Computed Tomography

Computed Tomography (CT) is one of the most effective techniques for directed diagnosis and treatment used in hospitals (Lell and Kachelrieß 2020). With the development of multidetector CT technology, the soft-tissue image's resolution is getting better (Ashraf et al. 2020). Using X-ray CT in three dimensions (3D), the structural and morphological characteristics of the sample under study can be ascertained (Aslan et al. 2020). However, to increase the sensitivity of CT scanning and enhance imaging of the tissue of interest, contrast agents with high X-ray attenuation are needed. These agents frequently include high atomic number elements like iodine, barium, and gold. The tiny iodinated molecules-based CT contrast agents have limited efficacy and rapid elimination. Only large doses can produce suitable contrast (Lusic and Grinstaff 2013). The development of NPs as next-generation CT contrast agents (Shilo et al. 2012). Multifunctional dendrimer-entrapped AuNPs loaded with gadolinium were reported to provide good dual-mode MRI/CT imaging capability *in vivo*. These complexes were expected to demonstrate excellent outcomes in early cancer diagnosis with good sensitivity and accuracy (Wen et al. 2013). Furthermore, BiNPs functionalized with antibodies showed tissue-targeted drug delivery potential (Kinsella et al. 2011). The renal route was observed to clear up the radiolabeled/tagged NPs after they were injected intravenously, increasing the contrast of the tumorous tissue. To observe the biodistribution of calcium phosphate *in vivo* through multiple administration routes, quantitative small animal positron emission tomography (PET) was used to manufacture NPs of the material. The findings showed that shortly after the intravenous injection, the NPs quickly entered the lungs and then progressively moved into the liver and spleen. Nevertheless, after being injected intramuscularly, the NPs generally stayed at the injection site, offering a fresh perspective on the treatment's long-lasting effects (Kollenda et al. 2020).

6.3.3 Positron Emission Tomography (PET)

The two main imaging modalities used in nuclear medicine are PET and Single Photon Emission Computed Tomography (SPECT) being used for imaging or diagnosing cardiovascular disorders and cancer, respectively. In both cases, the imaging signal is typically a radioisotope. PET, which requires the intravenous administration of nanomolar tracer quantities of a radioactively labeled medicine that is selective and specific for the target of interest, has emerged as the clinical method of choice for grading and restaging a variety of malignancies. By acting as signal amplifiers, NPs can increase contrast indices and improve sensitivity. One important advantage of nanoprobes over conventional biological moieties is their multimodality. Using γ rays or ß+ emitting radionuclides, SPECT or PET are used to perform radionuclide-based diagnostic imaging of cancer. The radionuclides used for SPECT-based imaging should have an energy range of 100 to 370 keV, with little particle radiation emission or higher energy γ-rays, and 100% abundance (emitting one γ-ray per decay) (Ting et al. 2010). The best radionuclides for SPECT imaging are those with half-lives that allow for imaging a few hours after injection and maintain concentration inside the target tumor throughout the imaging process. Positron (ß+) producing radionuclides are used for PET-based imaging; these radionuclides should preferably generate low-energy, short-range ß+ with 100% abundance and no higher energy cues. The instantaneous combination of these positrons with an electron leads to electron-positron annihilation, which produces two γ ray photons with identical energies of nearly 511 keV that travel in diametrically opposite directions (Velikyan and Imaging 2018; Kuntić et al. 2016; Mattoli et al. 2021; Garg et al. 2021; Chen et al. 2021). These photons are detected by a circular array of detectors positioned surrounding the patient.

To image colon cancer, dextran-coated IONPs coupled with NIR fluorochromes and PET isotopes have been employed in conjunction with a targeting vector (Nahrendorf et al. 2010). Similarly, in the case of PET/NIR-based fluorescence imaging, ferritin nanocages containing 64Cu in their cavity and the NIR fluorescent dyes Cy5.5 and RGD4C on their surface have also been created (Lin et al. 2011). Cu–In–Se QDs with a nonradioactive ZnS shell that contains 111In have recently been created for SPECT/fluorescence imaging (Sun et al. 2014).

6.3.4 Fluorescence Imaging

Fluorescent NPs hold promise as optical data storage and other technological tools in bioanalytics, medicine, gene therapy, medication delivery, and biosensing, where it is utilized to study cellular dynamics and interactions (Grunert et al. 2018). Fluorescence is a safe tool in many oncology settings as it can be used to assess invisible microscopic peritoneal metastases in advanced epithelial ovarian cancer with a strong negative predictive value (Boussedra et al. 2022); for some neuro-oncology indications for resection to the peritumoral region's functional limit with a larger resection and better results (Eatz et al. 2022; Ahrens et al. 2022); to recognize structures during robot-assisted radical prostateectomy, such as the prostate, neurovascular bundle, and lymph nodes (Rajakumar et al. 2020); to more clearly define the boundaries; for sentinel lymph node mapping in early-stage cervical and endometrial cancer (Buda et al. 2015); to support hepatic resection in liver surgery (Kan et al. 2021), and surgical resection in head and neck cancer (Voskuil et al. 2020). This surgical technique advances state-of-the-art ablation technology and has encouraging potential for the full treatment of malignant lesions in the liver and other solid organs that are more conspicuous or irregular.

Most medical and biological fluorescence imaging systems available today use dye markers, which have limits on the amount of light that each molecule can emit as well as photostability. NPs which offer robust and consistent fluorescence, present a solution to these shortcomings. It is reported the use of tailored NIR IIb fluorescence of Er-based lanthanide NPs for targeted imaging of orthotopic glioma via skull, showed better promise for imaging-guided tumor resection (Ren et al. 2020). Thermally activated delayed fluorescence (TADF) has revolutionized the field of organic light-emitting diodes by providing a long-lived delayed fluorescence component for imaging, temperature sensing, and local temperature measurement. Crucho et al. reported a simple technique for synthesizing TADF dye-doped silica NPs, which are efficiently absorbed by human cells at low incubation doses, localized in the cytoplasm, and allow for fluorescence live cell imaging (Crucho et al. 2020). It has been reported that Scheelite-like NaTb $(WO_4)^2$ NPs display particle size-dependent optical characteristics that result in green fluorescence. (Munirathnappa et al. 2020) The produced NPs demonstrated high biocompatibility in HeLa cells and are a promising contender for their role as a biomarker for cell imaging applications.

6.3.5 Multimodal Imaging Approaches

Although each imaging technique offers great spatial resolution and soft tissue contrast without causing radiation damage (Zhou et al. 2012), nevertheless, there are instances where the sensitivity is inadequate, leading to erroneous results. Multimodal imaging techniques have drawn attention as a solution since they are more effective and precise in providing information on biological and physical structures as well as their physiological functions (Lv et al. 2015).

The ability of INPs to provide simultaneous multitargeting and monitoring boosts the diagnostic and therapeutic benefits. The use of NP-based multimodal imaging probes, which are detectable by various imaging modalities, has gained immense importance in recent times (Xu et al. 2022). The development of innovative NMs with intriguing multimodal properties is made possible by the integration of magnetic and other properties into a single nanocomposite structure. Fluorescent-magnetic nanocomposites could be useful for a variety of biological applications, such as drug delivery systems, medical diagnostics, and multimodal biological imaging (Das et al. 2021). Fluorescence microscopy and MRI are two multimodal assays that could potentially employ these nanocomposites for both in *vitro* and *in vivo* bioimaging (Ganguly 2022). The promising bimodal drugs also possess both photodynamic and hyperthermic properties for the treatment of cancer (Ganguly and Margel 2020).

Upon light exposure, the FA functionalized multimodal fluorescent MNPs glow brilliantly and relax gradually. The thiol-metal bonding and surface functionalization provide a simple method for generating magneto-fluorescent Fe_3O_4-SH@QD NPs in the shape of hydrangea flowers (Chen, Zhang, et al. 2017). The effective fluorescence, superparamagnetism at RT, and fast response to an external field of magneto-fluorescent F_e3O_4-SH@QD NPs may prove advantageous for many technologies such as MRI and biolabels, targeting and photodynamic therapy, cell tracking, and separation.

Filho et al. developed a multimodal nanoprobe (BNP-Tf) that is an optically and magnetically active bimodal nanosystem made of QDs and IONPs (Cabral Filho et al. 2018). The nano platform was successful in tagging TfR at dosages that did not significantly harm HeLa cells for at least 24 hours, and it continued to function for at least two months utilizing fluorescence, flow cytometry, and MRI. Through the use of microscopy, they were able to demonstrate that HeLa cells that were selectively tagged with BNP-Tf produced a bright fluorescence as well as a high r2/rl relaxivity ratio, suggesting that this probe could be a useful tool for collecting both fluorescence and T2-weighted MR images. The multimodal imaging nanoprobes for in vivo MRI and near-INR persistent luminescence imaging were developed using near-INR luminescence NPs functionalized with Gd^{3+} complex (Abdukayum et al. 2014; Maldiney et al. 2015). In addition to these near-INR luminescence nanoprobes, metallic NPs such as fluorescent copper sulfide NPs allow for the targeting of photothermal therapy for the treatment of metastatic gastric cancer cells in lymph nodes studied in mice models, as well as non-invasive multimodality imaging (Shi et al. 2018).

MSNs coupled with gadolinium, 64Cu, and ZW800 were synthesized by Huang et al. for trimodal imaging (MRI, INR, and PET scanning). The study demonstrated that these NPs could detect micrometastases and sentinel lymph nodes with increased contrast (Huang et al. 2012). Later, it was demonstrated that radiolabeled copper (64Cu) containing porphyrosomes may be used with fluorescence imaging and PET to identify both small bone metastases of less than 2 mm and orthotopic malignancies (Liu et al. 2013). Yi et al. showed that radionuclide and CT bimodal imaging can be used to define sentinel lymph nodes in 4T1 BC mice metastatic models. The 131I-labelled CuS (copper sulfide) NPs are a good contrast agent (Yi et al. 2015). Additionally, to create multimodal NPs for MRI and fluorescence imaging to diagnose early-stage metastatic lesions, SPIONs, and gadolinium-labeled NPs were mixed with fluorescent species including QDs and UCNPs, as well as NIR dye (Qiao et al. 2017; Wang, Chen, and Zhu 2015).

6.4 THERAPEUTIC APPLICATIONS

Conventional cancer treatment techniques, including radiation, chemotherapy, and surgery, often have unfavorable side effects because they also impact healthy tissues. Since a combination of various therapy modalities is frequently employed to treat tumors, careful planning, the application of novel techniques, and the integration of diagnostic and treatment are required to customize treatments to each patient's needs and reduce side effects. The application of nanomedicine is one method to enhance care and get rid of the drawbacks of traditional cancer therapies. The application of nanotechnology to cancer diagnosis, treatment, and prevention is known as cancer nanomedicine (Damasco et al. 2020). The therapeutic applications of nanomedicine form are discussed here.

6.4.1 Targeted Drug Delivery

Modern-day research focuses on designing desirable targeted drug delivery systems for cancer therapeutics using INPs. These nanostructures used for targeted drug delivery are engineered from four main categories: metals, oxides, sulfides, and carbonaceous. Depending on their morphologies, the most common drug-delivery vehicles include nanotubes, mesoporous nanoparticles, and nanoshells. The core lies in the fact that their inner void can adsorb and retain sufficient amounts of drugs. At the same time, the open ends of pores may be capped to control the release of cargo. Since most drugs used for cancer therapies are hydrophobic, their hollow structures ace in reducing aggregation in the process of drug targeting.

Among metal NPs, the AgNPs are known to target cancer cells more efficiently. (Prabhakar et al. 2013) (Duncan et al. 2013). According to Nogueira et al., the pH stimuli play an important role in enhancing the chemotherapeutic effects of drugs on cancer cells (Nogueira et al. 2013). The substantial drug release enhancement was seen through a chitosan-based nano-formulated system with superior biodegradability, biocompatibility, pH stimuli, and reduced toxicity (Nogueira et al. 2013). The effect of prolonged exposure and ionization in an acidic environment, chitosan-NPs (CS-NPs) caused program cell death in MDA-MB-453 metastatic breast cancer cells in a pH- and time-dependent manner. Gemcitabine-loaded folic acid-capped AgNPs (CS-FA-GEM-AgNPs) were internalized in the cell organelles, such as the mitochondria, vascular area, and nucleus, as a result of the presence of FA (Karuppaiah et al. 2021). Pandey et al. developed an amygdalin-loaded AgNPs-FA nano-formulation by using chitosan microcapsule to treat breast cancer (Pandey, Ali, and Negi 2021). The encapsulation process was successfully achieved and AgNPs were seen as effective stabilizing particles owing to the presence of polar (-OH) hydroxyl groups and an amino group (-NH_2) on the polymer backbone. All such properties confirm the effective delivery of the drug to the breast cancer metastatic cell line (MDA-MB-231). The drug release rate was effectively increased at a slightly acidic pH of 6.8 rather than a pH of 7.4. At acidic pH, the hydrogen bonds were formed due to the presence of the hydroxyl group (Karuppaiah et al. 2021). Moreover, Amy/Agnp/CS treatment lowered cell viability (18–19%) more than free Amy drug treatment (cell viability, 60–62%) in the MDA-MB-231 cell line. Inference could made that maximum alteration may have occurred because of chitosan being present on the surface of the AgNPs (Karuppaiah et al. 2021). The detailed steps and application of the study are shown in Figure 6.4.

Studies regarding toxicity levels and adverse effects in the blood were conducted by bare epirubicin administration (Akter et al. 2018). HepG2 cell line-grown Ag NPs with an epirubicin cap exhibited anti-tumor efficacy at 1.92 g/ml half maximum inhibitory concentration (IC_{50}). Epirubicin-capped AgNPs with good enhanced permeability and retention (EPR) effect and in the desired size range can be utilized in medications to the targeted cancer cell without harmful side effects on healthy and normal cells. Another study carried out by Rozalen et al., illustrates that due to structural morphologies of AgNPs such as shape and size, the drug loading capabilities with various Methotrexate (MTX) concentrations were achieved as 28–40% (Rozalen et al. 2020). Moreover, the drug release capacities were enhanced to 77–80%. It was also shown that 40% of the colon cancer cells (HTC-116) were prevented from proliferating after receiving treatment with AgNPs-MTX on various cell lines. The same drug with AgNPs confirmed a low level of cytotoxicity in the zebrafish model as well (Akter et al. 2018). Through studies carried out by Ajani et al., an anti-gastric cancer therapeutic approach of tirapazamine (TPZ) conjugated with AuNPs was reported. The TPZ reduced the viability of cells in stomach cancer cells (MKN45) in low oxygen tension but underperformed in normoxic conditions. The bovine serum albumin (BSA)-conjugated AuNP enhanced the target efficiency of the TPZ. It kept the hypoxic toxin in the MKN45-induced xenograft animal model with a suitable feature of bio-distribution (Ajnai et al. 2022). Many research models these days have shown keen interest in aptamers-mediated cancer therapy. Aptamers show potential results, are easy to synthesize, non-immunogenic, and also stable. Mucin-1 and EpCAM were identified as some of the most exploited aptamers against colorectal cancer in recent research (Fu and Xiang 2020). Considering current scenarios for cancer therapy, DOX is frequently utilized in cancer research, including colorectal cancer. However, due to its detrimental impact and low response rate modifications in the drug delivery mechanism are of the utmost importance. Concerning, PrPc (aptamer)-conjugated AuNPs with DOX drug (PrPC-Apt DOA) were synthesized and loaded with DOX to check the release in a pH-dependent manner (Fu and Xiang 2020). High drug was released at pH 5.4 and consequently at pH 7.4 but unaffected by temperature. Moreover, PrPC-Apt DOA uptake was seen more in the case of PrPC-positive cells. PrPC-Apt DOA-treated cells were found in the S phase much less frequently than bare DOX-treated cells, with a higher decline in cyclin-dependent kinases including CDK-2, CDK-4, cyclin D1, and cyclin E (Go et al. 2021). Other metallic NPS, the TiO_2 (titanium dioxide) NPs is well-known to induce reactive oxygen species (ROS) production after illumination in the aqueous media with exposure to UV light (Nigam et al. 2023). In cancer treatments, TiO_2-induced ROS-mediated cell death was found as a novel application commonly referred to as PDT (photodynamic therapy). As per ongoing studies, the anticancer therapy PTX was curated to deliver these inside the liver cancer cells (HepG2) after being loaded on TiO_2 with polyethylene glycol (PEG) and FA. PEG improved the NPs' biocompatibility. FA was utilized to target the cancer

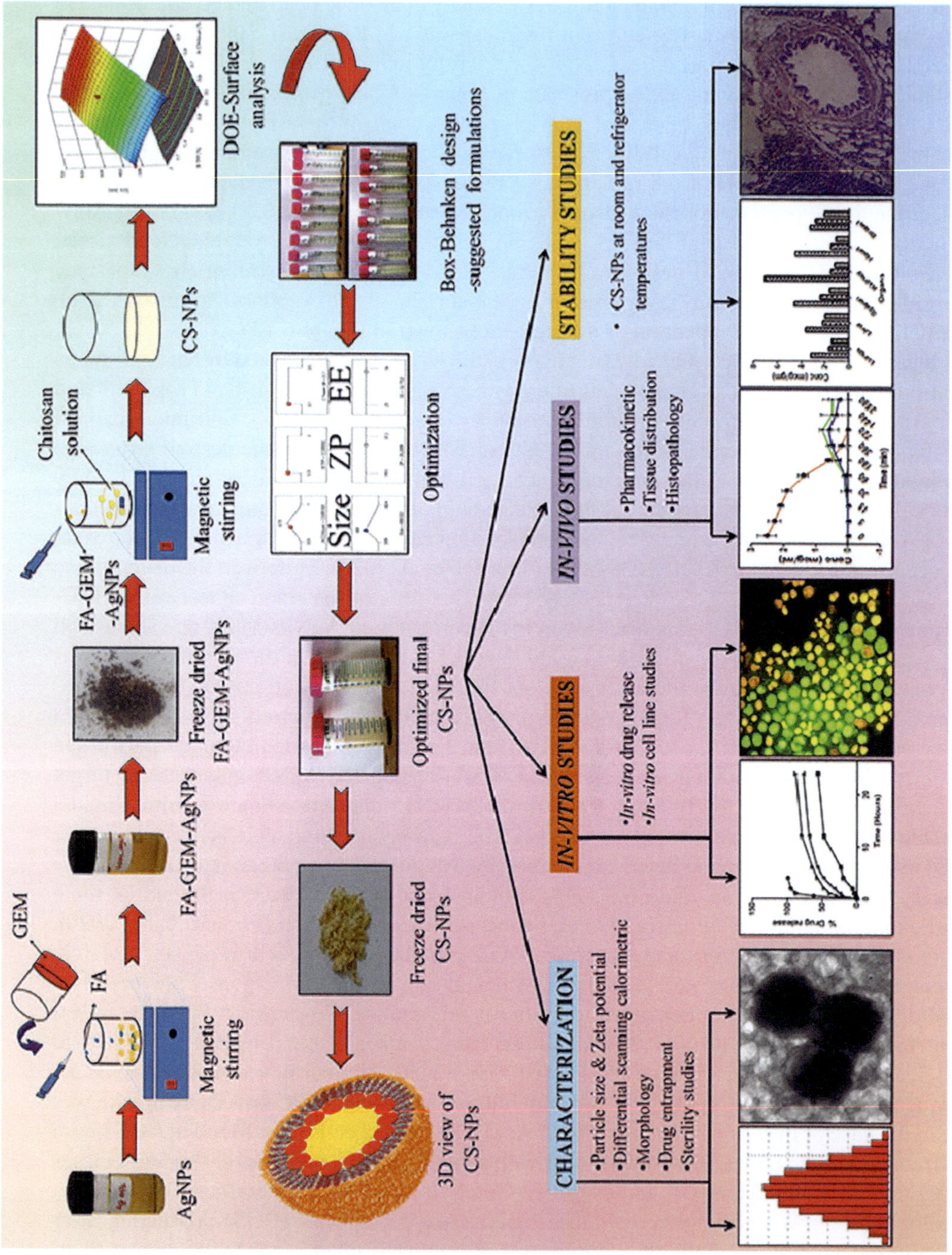

FIGURE 6.4 Synthesis and optimization of Gemcitabine-loaded chitosan-covered AgNPs/folic acid (CS-NPs). Also presented are the mitigation of the toxicity, lack of site specificity, and excretion issues associated with AgNPs and GEM; the pH-dependent cytotoxicity, apoptosis, and cellular uptake against the MDA-MB-453 metastatic breast cancer cell line; the pH-responsive release behavior both *in vitro* and *in vivo*.

Source: Reprinted with permission from Karuppaiah et al. (2021).

cell receptors. It was seen that FA–PEG–TiO_2 has high adsorption capability in case of loading and the initial release of FA–PEG–TiO_2 was fast followed by a sustained release phase. However, continuous surface modifications of the NPs, PEG, and FA functionalization reduce the ability of nanocrystals to be loaded. With an increasing concentration, TiO_2-PEG-FA treatment reduced the viability of the HepG2 cells. The cell viability employed by TiO_2-PEG-FA-PAC (Paclitaxel) was lower than that of TiO_2-PEG-FA. Lastly, TiO_2-PEG-FA had a higher IC_{50} value (59.61 mg/ml) than TiO_2-PEG-FA-PAC (22.75 mg/ml) (Venkatasubbu et al. 2013).

Other INPs, the MSNs have an exceptional ability to accept organic molecules and act as a suitable reservoir for controlled drug delivery systems (DDS) due to their stringent pore size, specific pore volume, and surface area that support a high drug payload (Vallet-Regi et al. 2001). Such NPs contain doxorubicin and L-arginine as a nitric oxide donor which were used in various research conducted *in vitro* and *in vivo* pancreatic carcinoma models (Hwang et al. 2015), (Zhang et al. 2016). The MSN/drug-treated MiaPaCa-2 human pancreatic carcinoma cells had higher cytotoxicity levels than the free drug treatment. The intervention was active to effectively deliver the drug in the SCID mouse model. The consequent study revealed that PANC-1 human pancreatic carcinoma cells treated with the silica NPs together with ultrasound-triggered release had increased levels of p53 and caspase-3 protein levels. This indicates DNA damage followed by apoptosis. Through the in vivo experiments, it was observed that there was substantial inhibition of tumor growth in nude mice. Giménez et al. loaded safranin-O and doxorubicin into PEG-capped MSNs and tested them against HeLa human cervical carcinoma cells in a glutathione (GSH)-dependent model (Gimenez et al. 2015). It was reported that the system can be retained closed at low GHS levels, allowing the drug released only at high GSH concentrations. GSH is known for its higher concentration and more reductive properties inside tumors. According to another study conducted on MSNs, it has been contemplated that the sustained delivery of drug, felodipine can be achieved by a multilayer coating of MSNs with polyelectrolytes employing the layer-by-layer (LBL) technique. The polyelectrolyte layers were crafted using natural polymers such as chitosan and acacia, which were absorbed onto the MSN surface using the LBL self-assembly technique. Felodipine was loaded using solvent deposition, with an efficacy of more than 20% entrapment. Polyelectrolyte multilayer's protective action and the felodipine's lower solubility cause minimal loss of loaded drugs after the encapsulation process. The release of felodipine from the MSNs loaded formulation was more rapid (90% of drug release within 2 hours) than the multilayered polyelectrolyte-based MSNs formulation (30% drug release in the first 2 hours). The drug sustenance effect is seen because of the blocking effect of the multilayer coating of polyelectrolytes outside felodipine-loaded MSNs. These results narrate a methodical way to sustain the release of the poorly water-soluble drug (Hu et al. 2015).

The fluorescent properties of QDs make them eligible to be used as probes with intense signal emission, making them an emerging theranostic system. QDs micelles loaded with Herceptin were used for *in vitro* and *in vivo* delivery against SK-BR3 human breast cancer and KB human nasopharyngeal epidermoid cancer cells, as well as in SKH1 mice injected with MDA-MB-231 human breast cancer cells (Nurunnabi et al. 2010) Experimental analysis stated an increased cytotoxicity dose and time-dependent effect in cell lines. Moreover, an *in vivo* antitumor effect, with shrinkage of the tumor volume and inhibition of tumor growth was seen. Another cancer study was conducted by Bagalkot et al. with QD-aptamer conjugates containing doxorubicin (Bagalkot et al. 2007). Doxorubicin is fluorescent and is capable of recognizing the extracellular domain of the prostate-specific membrane antigen to cure LNCaP human prostate adenocarcinoma cells. The research revealed that the composite was not only able to specifically detect and bind to the tumor cells but also intracellular release the drug. In a recent study, (Tian et al. 2022) visualized that diazoxide derivatives may be delivered into HeLa cells using functionalized carbon nanodiamonds (ND)-diazoxide. In contrast to the commonly available free medicines, carbon-based nanostructures exhibit persistent release. The direct measurement of the drug's local reaction at the particle and release sites can be seen. The functionalized ND-diazoxide group's reactivity to free radicals is concentration-dependent. The detection was done by functionalized NDs' capacity for quantum sensing. Hence it is feasible to monitor individual particles in individual cells during the release experiment; this unique capability provides a potent instrument to administer drugs and assess their local impact on cells.

6.4.2 Hyperthermia and Photothermal Therapy

Hyperthermia is referred to as the treatment where the tumor cells are destroyed heating them to a temperature of 40–45 °C by inducing a series of thermally induced metabolic events including apoptosis. Hyperthermic events aim to alter the extracellular microenvironment by stimulating immune responses and causing a transformation in tumor cells to an anaerobic metabolic scheme (Jose et al. 2020). Glioblastoma multiforme is an extremely aggressive brain tumor with a mean survival rate of around 4 months. Successful pre-clinical analyses were done using NP-based magnetically induced hyperthermia (NP-MIH) in glioblastoma (Gupta and Sharma 2019). It was found that MIH enhanced the potencies of commonly used chemotherapeutics by increasing the blood-brain-barrier (BBB) permeability, ultimately, increasing the drug concentrations in the tumors. Other studies have also been reported on the synergistic effect of hyperthermia and chemotherapy for cancer management (Ha et al. 2019). These studies suggest that such combinatorial treatments offer benefits over individual therapies that develop drug resistance. It is easy to understand the hyperthermic tumor destruction mechanism by considering the heat dissipation mechanisms of MNP. There are two main processes by which MNPs dissipate heat to tumor cells (Figure 6.5) (Jose et al. 2020). The first one is Néel relaxation and the second process is called Brownian relaxation. Néel relaxation occurs through the magnetic moment reorientation parallel to the applied magnetic field. On the contrary, Brownian relaxation involves the mechanical rotation of the nanomaterial as a whole toward the external magnetic field. These phenomena come into play when the material is exposed to an external alternative magnetic field (AMF) with a magnetic field reversal time shorter than the magnetic relaxation time of the material (Suto et al. 2009) (Hervault and Thanh 2014). AMF-exposed targeted MNPs can generate shear forces because of Brownian relaxation that

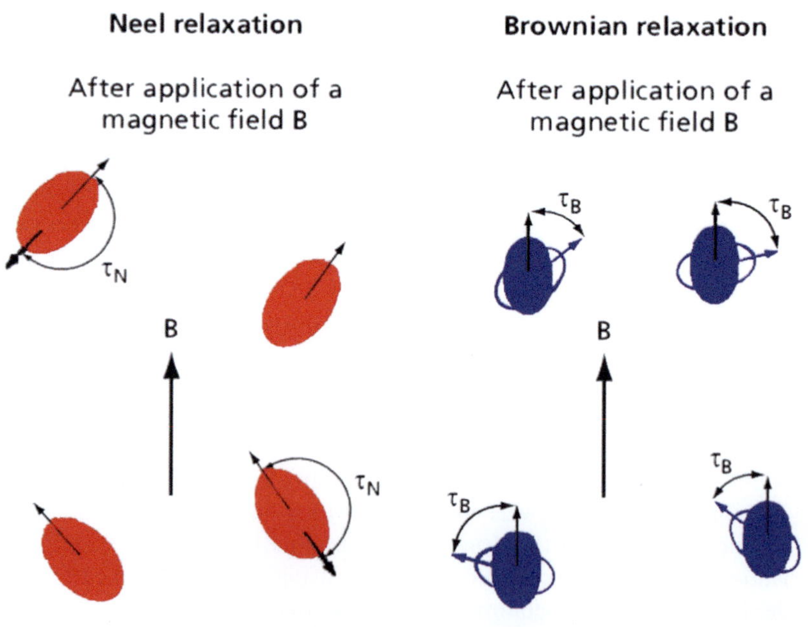

FIGURE 6.5 The schematic representation of the process of magnetic relaxation (Néel and Brownian).

Source: Adapted from Jose et al. (2020).

can directly break the cells and release lysosomal cathepsins (Chen, Chen, et al. 2017). Due to this, tumor tissues develop an impaired cooling attribute toward vascular permeability in comparison with the normal tissues resulting in lysosomal permeability and cell death (Demirci et al. 2019). Different studies state MNPs have a significant role in catalytic ROS production but an depth study of the underlying mechanism is yet to be explored (Chen, Chen, et al. 2017). Photothermal therapy (PTT) is a non-invasive therapeutic approach that uses a photothermal agent and light to produce localized heating for thermal ablation of cancer cells. By controlling the regional delivery of photothermal agents, and the direction and focus of incident light radiation, the localized heating of tumor tissues can be achieved. It greatly improves the efficiency and specificity of tumor hyperthermia with negligible side effects (Yang, Zhao, et al. 2022) (Chen et al. 2019). The selection of photothermal agents (PTAs) has a significant impact on the therapeutic efficacy of PTT. For instance, PTA must possess great thermal conductivity along with high photothermal conversion efficiency; and have strong absorption in the NIR region (700 to 1300 nm) for deep in vivo penetration. PTA should be biocompatible, less toxic, and easy to eliminate from the body

The most commonly utilized PTAs in current clinical research are indocyanine green (ICG), AuNPs, and carbon-based nanomaterials. AuNPs have shown high proficiency in cancer PTT due to their excellent biocompatibility, extensive optical properties, small size, and efficient photothermal conversion ability (Chen et al. 2016), (Asadi et al. 2021). In the growth phase of malignant tumors, there is often a large amount of neovascularization and lymphatic vessel damage around the tumor. The tumor microenvironment allows the selective accumulation of Au NPs at the tumor sites through the EPR effect, leading to enhanced therapeutic efficacy (Yang, Zhao, et al. 2022) (Maeda 2001).

For NIR light, the free electrons on the Au NPs surface undergo collective coherent oscillations guarded by the incident electric field (Kang et al. 2020) (Yang, Liang, et al. 2019). These oscillations of Au NPs enhance the surface electric field strength and, finally the light absorption and scattering capabilities (Huang and El-Sayed 2010). This oscillatory phenomenon of Au NPs in PTT is of utmost importance because Au NPs can convert light energy into heat energy via "non-radiative processes" and generate high temperatures at the site of Au NPs accumulation to induce cell death. A noteworthy feature here is that normal tissues without the accumulation of Au NPs don't fall in any damage during the entire process (Huang et al. 2008; Hirsch et al. 2003). Graphene oxide (GO) and reduced GO (rGO) are some of the most widely accepted carbon nanostructures in various applications (Gorab et al. 2023; Kargar et al. 2018). Numerous studies have been done and are under pipeline that indicate the positive effect of hyperthermia biocidal ability in wound healing (Qi et al. 2022; He et al. 2022; Lindner et al. 2021). Federico et al. initiated a study on hyaluronic acid-based (HA-EDA) electrospun membrane with GO and ciprofloxacin. Considering the photothermal activity under the NIR laser, light-triggered drug release was also seen. The combined effect of GO response to light led to laser-induced hyperthermia and antibiotic-loaded drug led to a decrease in *staphylococcus aureus* and *pseudomonas aeruginosa* pathogens viability (Federico et al. 2022). In a study conducted by Eivazzadeh-Keihan et al., a novel magnetic nanocomposite by functionalizing GO with natural polymer lignin using epichlorohydrin cross-linker was developed and then magnetized with Fe_3O_4 NPs (Eivazzadeh-Keihan et al. 2023). Under AMF, magnetic hyperthermia was achieved with a saturation magnetization value of 17.2 emu. g $^{-1}$ and a maximum specific absorption rate of 121.22 W.g^{-1}. Barra et al. used chitosan natural polymer and used magnetized rGO (rGO-$Fe_{3-x}O_4$) as a filler to develop a bionanocomposite with hyperthermia capability (Barra et al. 2023). Compared with pristine chitosan, the antioxidant activity was 9 times higher, and mechanical properties were elevated from (~ 8 MPa) for chitosan to (~ 285 MPa) for the bionanocomposite. Also, magnetic hyperthermia tests exhibited a temperature rise to 40 °C in 45 s with 50% of magnetized rGO which is relevant to the presence of rGO in the structure. It has been known through several studies that, Osteosarcoma is a drug-resistant malignant bone tumor in children which results in chemotherapy failures. Zeng et al. conjugated the mitochondria-targeting ligand (4-carboxybutyl) triphenyl phosphonium bromide (TPP) with ICG-loaded polyethyleneimine-modified PEGylated

GO sheets and prepared (TPP-PPG@ICG) for enhanced mitochondrial accumulation and PTT synergic effects under a single dose NIR irradiation (Zeng et al. 2021). This nanocomposite delivered fluorescence imaging-guided phototherapy and showed *in vivo* tumor progress inhibition capability in MG63 tumor cells.

Another common type of cancer in the world is non-melanoma skin cancer (NMSC). Cases with high-risk primary and metastasis of NMSC mostly demand multimodal therapies (Bander, Nehal, and Lee 2019; Rembielak and Ajithkumar 2019). Different light-responsive particles can be combined for synergistic effects to produce increased photothermal hyperthermia capacity in a composite. He et al. created GO@SiO_2@AuNS hybrid composite for photothermal hyperthermia application by combining the two known NIR responsive particles, spherical Au-nanoshells and GO. The composite exhibits a 30% photothermal conversion efficiency and the eradication of colorectal cancer cells (KM12C) when exposed to an 808 nm NIR laser. To create binding sites for Au NPs, GO was initially coated with a mesoporous silica layer. High photothermal conversion and biocompatibility were demonstrated by the GO@SiO_2 @AuNS hybrid (He et al. 2020). Abdi Goushbolagh et al. investigated the anticancer effects of MCNTs-COOH under NIR irradiation at various exposure times. While modified MWCNTs alone are not hazardous, 80 μg/mL MWCNTs reduced the viability of CT26 fibroblastic cells considerably after one minute of radiation (Abdi Goushbolagh et al. 2019).

To improve therapeutic results, hyperthermia can also be utilized as an adjuvant therapy in conjunction with other cancer treatment modalities. Wang et al., for example, introduced CNT@MnO_2-PEG@Ce_6 for photodynamic and PTT synergy, guided by MRI. Because of their strong cellular penetration, CNTs not only generated heat to induce hyperthermia but also transported payloads (Ce_6 and MnO_2) to cancer cells. By oxidizing H_2O_2 in the tumor microenvironment and generating ROS under NIR irradiation, photodynamic treatment (PDT) was carried out (Wang et al. 2020). Hyperthermia has been employed as a chemodynamic therapy (CDT) auxiliary technique in another study including combination therapy. A PEG-MWNTs-Fe_3O_4-GO_x nano platform was shown by Liu et al. to destroy MCF-7 malignant cells by promoting cell death. The Fenton reaction activity was enhanced by mild hyperthermia when exposed to an 808 nm laser, which in turn enhanced hydroxyl radicals (•OH) production to promote CDT (Liu et al. 2019).

Scientists are now interested in plasmonic noble metal nanoparticles, such as AgNPs, because of their exceptional capacity to use surface plasmon resonance (SPR) to transform visible and NIR light into heat. CNT/Ag NPs were created by Behnam et al. for plasmonic PTT of melanoma tumors. When utilizing CNT/Ag NPs under NIR irradiation, the histological results of the tumor tissues indicated substantial necrosis (70%), although the extent of necrosis is lesser when CNTs or Ag NPs are employed alone (Behnam, Emami, Sobhani, Koohi-Hosseinabadi, et al. 2018). Moniruzzaman et al. synthesized polyaromatic-polyphenolic CQDs. Intense multicolor imaging of cells (yellow (YCQDs), blue (B-CQDs), and green (G-CQDs)) was made possible by the synthetic substance. This was carried out in the whole visible light spectrum. The reported photothermal efficiency (PTE) was around $32.6 \pm 1\%$. Additionally, the excellent photothermal conversion led to a rise in ROS, which demonstrated strong photothermal antibacterial capabilities and damaged the *Bacillus subtilis* membrane (Moniruzzaman et al. 2022). In numerous sectors, current research has examined GQDs as PDT agents for generating ROS (Arumugasamy, Govindaraju, and Yun 2020). The bactericidal property works by breaking down the membrane and cytoplasmic exudation of drug-resistant gram-positive and gram-negative bacteria, thereby exploiting the non-invasive synergistic effect of ROS production and heat generation. A few low-sensitivity and toxicity side effects are also present. In this case, AgNPs/GQDs conjugate resulted in an efficient three-mode therapy. When 450 nm blue light is applied to nanoparticles (0.5 mg/mL), this surface connection leads to an increase in ROS generation and photothermal conversion after 10 minutes of laser treatment. Moreover, the temperature was increased by 40°C and a 14 mW/cm^2 power density. Moreover, GQD-containing compounds can be employed in drug delivery systems. These nanoparticles not only have a large specific surface area, efficient photothermal conversion, and convenience of use, but they also function as a gatekeeper during blood circulation, preventing the medicine from being released prematurely. They not only have good biocompatibility but also improve the suppression of tumor growth. A nano platform containing GQD, hyaluronic acid (HA), and mesoporous carbon nanoparticles (HMCN) has been introduced in light of these capabilities. *In vitro* and *in vivo* studies have been conducted using the HMCN for chemo-photothermal therapy, which showed the capacity to target drug delivery to cervical cancer cells that overexpress the CD44 receptor. The drug DOX (410 mg/g) into HMCN can target cancer cells precisely and offer high photothermal conversion synergistically. Therefore, the INPs are the utmost choice for anticancer thermal therapy.

6.4.3 Radiotherapy Enhancement

InNSs show great capacity for upgrading radiation treatment as they have a high ability to concentrate ionization energy inside cancer tumors (Su et al. 2014). The process that improves the vulnerability of tumors to injury by radiation is radiosensitization, which is favored by radiosensitizers. Radiosensitizers are agents that enhance the impacts of radiation on cancerous cells (Kwatra, Venugopal, and Anant 2013). Due to the EPR effect, several NPs are categorized as potential radiosensitizers to improve radiation therapy (Song et al. 2017). These INPs preferentially permeate and accumulate in tumor interstitial liquid (TIF), causing the vascular endothelium sores in strong tumors. At the same time, the retention of NPs in TIF occurs because of reduced lymphatic drainage (Klostergaard, Seeney, and Medicine 2012). Complementing nanotherapeutics works parallel with ionizing radiation that exhibits an enhanced biological response in cancer management through several approaches. The major mechanisms for this process include inhibiting DNA-repair processes and ROS production, which leads to DNA damage or other biomolecules by oxidation. Another phenomenon contributes to inhibiting tumor metastasis by controlling the tumor microenvironment (TME), and arresting the cell cycle, as shown in Figure 6.6 (Haque, Shakil, and Mahmud 2023). However, different types of NPs with radiotherapy (RT) interfere with the DNA-repair process, and ionization induces ROS generation. The combined effect of radiation together with NPs arrests the G2/M phase of the cell cycle, thus leading to cancer cell death eventually.

Ultrafine AuNPs (<5 nm), coated with multifunctional polypeptides that included a cathepsin B-responsive linker, a zwitterionic antifouling block, and a nucleus-penetrating peptide, were

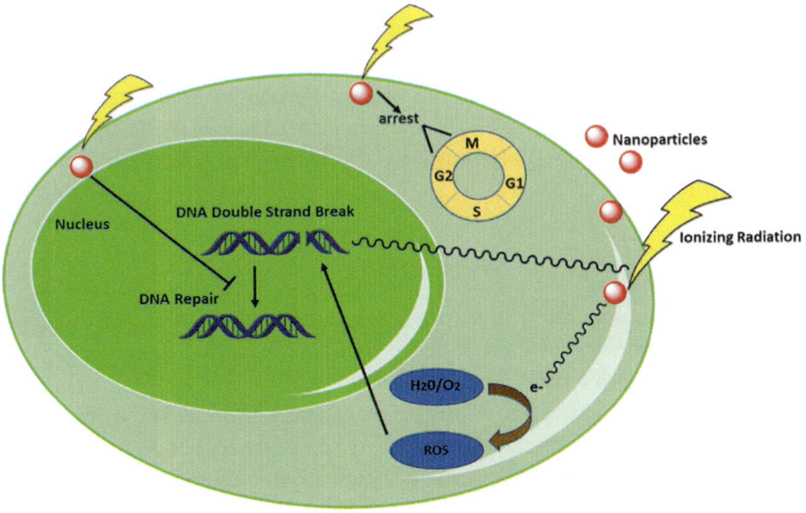

FIGURE 6.6 Biological responses of NPs aiding radiotherapy 6.

Source: Haque, Shakil, and Mahmud (2023).

selectively absorbed by tumor cells (Ding et al. 2020). These AuNPs demonstrated enhanced biocompatibility and *in vivo* targeted area enrichment. Furthermore, the ultra-small size provides the AuNPs with quick renal clearance, hence enhancing the possibility of clinical application. The ultra-small AuNPs had a positive impact on hepatocellular cancer treatment in mice when combined with X-ray irradiation. Recently, Chang et al. created CS-coated Au@Se nanocomposites (NCs) as radiosensitizers to accomplish synergistic chemo-radiotherapy based on the radiosensitization capabilities of Au NRs and the anticancer activity of Se NPs (Chang et al. 2017). Arginylglycylaspartic acid (RGD), which identifies the overexpressed $\alpha v\beta 3$ integrin receptors in a range of human cancer cells, and ACPP peptide, which is cleaved specifically by matrix metalloproteinase MMP2/9 on tumor extracellular matrix, was modified outside the CS layer to further improve the selectivity of the nanomaterials to tumor cells. According to *in vitro* tests, targeted molecular alteration led to a significant improvement in the depth of tumor infiltration of NCs. However, via altering the expression of p53 and DNA damage genes, the combination of NCs and X-ray therapy might cause intracellular ROS overproduction and induce apoptosis of A375 melanoma cells, leading to a markedly improved anticancer impact. Heterostructures based on magnetite and bismuth sulfide bimetallic NPs (BNPs) were adorned with FA and BSA and used as radiosensitizers by Nosrati and colleagues. In a 4T1 mouse model, the BNPs effectively eliminated the breast tumors without killing the mice or damaging the healthy tissues (Nosrati, Ghaffarlou, et al. 2022). A multicomponent chemoradiation agent was created based on a Bi_2S_3-Au nanosystem. The nanostructure demonstrated potential as a CT contrast agent in addition to increasing the production of free radicals. Curcumin and methotrexate were co-loaded to promote the radioprotection of healthy cells and increase damage to malignant cells, respectively. Following a single injection dose and X-ray treatment, all tumors in animal models of breast cancer were eliminated in around 20 days, with no signs of systemic damage (Nosrati, Attari, et al. 2022). Continuing with the idea of creating nano-radiosensitizers, Hu and associates created Ru-Cu nanoparticles coated in PEG that have enzyme-like characteristics and can convert H_2O_2 in cancer cells to O_2 to reduce hypoxia. In tumor-bearing mice, the effects of radiation therapy were enhanced by these incredibly sensitive nanoagents (Hu et al. 2022). Research using a Lewis Lung Carcinoma model revealed that the alloy-type Ag-Au BNPs (3:1) antitumor activity is significantly influenced by metal interactions resulting from their topological distribution (Shmarakov et al. 2017). Furthermore, it was shown that the p53/Bax/Bcl-2 and caspase apoptotic pathways cause BNP-mediated cytotoxicity (Katifelis et al. 2018). Subsequent research revealed that these BNPs decreased metastasis in SCID mice harboring 4T1 tumors. BNPs preferentially induced apoptosis via the extrinsic TRAIL-dependent mechanism, rapidly accumulating at tumor locations (Katifelis et al. 2020). PEGylated Ag-Au BNPs were also used as radiosensitizing agents on oral cancer cells (Ahmed et al. 2021). More recently, HeLa (cervical cancer) and DU 145 (prostate cancer) cells showed antiproliferative effects from Au-Ag BNPs by ROS induction (Ghosh and Singh 2021). ROS triggered the apoptotic pathway in the mitochondria, which led to the death of cancer cells (Sivamaruthi et al. 2019).

6.4.4 Combination Therapies and Synergistic Effects

Numerous studies have demonstrated that monotherapy has major difficulties in treating malignancies due to the heterogeneity of cancer cells, their proliferation, signaling pathways, microenvironments, and other factors (Barker et al. 2015; Baghban et al. 2020). Therefore, treatment plans based on combination medicines with proven efficacy are typically employed (Jadia et al. 2016; Qin et al. 2018). Combination techniques are proven to treat special drug resistance (Yardley 2013; Miyoshi et al. 2016). Combination treatments such as gene therapy, immunotherapy, PDT, and multimodal cancer chemotherapy are widely recognized (Mokhtari et al. 2017). However, the use of INPs, which provide the synergy of medication delivery and therapy, could circumvent the possibility of drug interactions when coupled, prohibiting the use of many drugs at the same time (Cascorbi 2012). Extensive research on metallic AgNPs and ceramic CeNPs indicates that these and a multitude of other INPs, including AuNPs and TiNPs possess noteworthy inherent anticancer properties (Arvizo, Bhattacharya, and Mukherjee 2010). When coupled electrostatically with the anticancer medication DOX, adjuvant AgNPs produced from bitterweed (*Andrographis paniculate* AP) showed improved cytotoxicity and synergistic efficacy against the MDA-MB-453 human breast cancer cell line (Karuppaiah et al. 2020). It was found that the order of the effectiveness of cell growth inhibition was AgNP–DOX–AP > AgNP–AP > DOX > AP. These findings imply that these intrinsic anticancer drugs perform in an effectively additive manner. When paired with DOX, CeNPs have been shown to have synergistic anticancer action (Das et al. 2017). Through electrostatic contact, the negatively charged CeNPs and positively charged DOX were conjugated. It has been shown that the synergistic effect of DOX-loaded CeNPs (CeO_2-DOX), where a gradual sustained release of DOX occurs, increases the therapeutic efficacy above DOX alone. DOX by itself showed a high cellular concentration that quickly dropped to 25% within 24 hours. CeO_2-DOX, on the other hand, similarly showed a high cellular concentration, but this one was sustained for 72 hours, tripling the repeat-dose duration. The SKOV3 ovarian cancer cells were considerably more susceptible to the *in vitro* cytotoxicity of CeO_2-DOX than to that of DOX alone. The possible additive effects of therapies are supported by these findings. Conjugation of INPs with nucleic acids has been developed as a frequent kind of biomolecule-based combination therapy since oncogenes can be suppressed utilizing one or more biomolecules (Das et al. 2017; Mansoori, Shotorbani, and Baradaran 2014). Nucleic acid distribution is exceedingly challenging because negatively charged nucleic acids with a large polyanionic surface are practically impenetrable to the cell membrane (Yang, Hinner, and Protocols 2015).

6.4.5 Overcoming Drug Resistance

Chemotherapy failure is mostly caused by multiple drug resistance (MDR) contributed by the tumor's heterogeneity, the tumor microenvironment, intracellular changes, and genetic influence. Given these hazards and unfavorable outcomes, there is a greater need than ever for the creation of novel and accurate treatment protocols. At the moment, NPs are being employed to manage the limitations of conventional treatment approaches. NMs-based drug delivery methods are precise, have good pharmacokinetics, reduce side effects, and decrease drug resistance (Dadwal et al. 2018). In the 1960s, ETH Zurich conducted the first studies on the use of nanomaterials in medicine (Li et al. 2016). Several therapeutic medications based on NMs have been produced and used for treatment since 2010, trailing closely behind the advancements in nanotechnology applications. Drug resistance has been decreased by the use of nano-based medications for TDD and as anti-neoplastics in multiple-drug combination therapy (Palazzolo et al. 2018). The MSN core and the microporous zeolite imidazolate frameworks-8 (ZIF-8) shell were integrated using polydopamine (PDA) mediated integration (PDAMSN@ZIF-8) (Wang, Guan, et al. 2018). ZIF-8 and curcumin (CUR), a P-gp efflux inhibitor, were used as plugs to stop the premature release of DOX into the cytoplasm from the mesoporous core. The drug-loaded NPs have the highest load capacity and the ability to continuously release CUR and DOX in turn under acidic circumstances. Other most prevalent nanocarriers are the iron-oxide NPs (IONPs). Once they are broken down *in vivo*, they can be integrated into the iron cycle and are biocompatible. Trimethoxysilylpropyl-ethylenediamine triacetic acid stabilized IONPs were used for magnetic targeting of particular areas (Norouzi et al. 2020). In addition, it promotes DOX aggregation in MDR glioma cells and increases the DOX circulation duration *in vivo*. Exosomes and AuNPs were utilized as medication as well as a delivery system for DOX to treat cancer cells (Zhang et al. 2019). They determined the *in vivo* biodistribution of EVdox@AuNP at a dose of 2.5 mg/kg via intravenous infusion using C57BL/6 mice and the B16F10 tumor-bearing model. This AuNP formulation accumulated more than the unconjugated AuNPs in the tumors. After the accumulation, the tumors were exposed to a laser beam for five minutes. The areas without NP accumulation saw a minor increase in temperature (to 38.1 °C), but the areas with AuNP accumulation had a fast increase in temperature (to 46.1 °C) within just one minute. These findings imply the photothermal transformation, uptake, and retention of EVdox@AuNPs in the tumor area. The DOX drug-loaded GO nanosystem as modified with two molecular beacons (MBs) was created (Yang, Song, et al. 2022). Following the uptake of the nanosystem, DOX was released into acidic endosomes. Additionally, MBs modified on the surface of GO can effectively inhibit the expression of P-gp, further prevent DOX efflux, and silence intracellular multidrug resistance 1 (MDR1) mRNA and upstream erythroblastosis virus E26 oncogene homolog 1 (ETS1) mRNA. Wang et al. used the emulsion/solvent evaporation approach to create an Au nanorod Cluster (AuCR) by combining amphibious poly (b-biotinylated poly(ethylene glycol) and curcumin-co-dithiodipropionic acid with AuNR. To release DOX at pH (pH 6.8 or 5.0), the AuCR can break down into a separate AuNR unit at an intracellular concentration of 5 mM GSH. In ADR tumor cells, the system can both increase and decrease DOX absorption and exporting to overcome the resistance (Wang, Wang, et al. 2018).

6.5 THERANOSTIC APPROACHES

Theranostics integrates the detection functionality and therapeutic characteristics into a single system for accurate cancer detection and treatment (Misra, Acharya, and Sahoo 2010). The next generation of nano theranostic anticancer candidates, radiation, light, magnetic fields, and sound waves have cemented their positions. The cross-bred NPs used in theranostics consist of an organic shell and an inorganic. The organic shell functions as a drug releaser, while the inorganic core enhances contrast. To target particular cancer cells, hybrid NPs can be coupled with targeting moieties and systematically given to patients. Numerous INPs-tailored nanocarrier systems have been employed as depots and carriers for hydrophobic compounds, which have improved pharmacokinetics, increased their bloodstream endurance and preservation, and decreased undesirable side effects by enabling tissue-specific distribution (Tian et al. 2021; Fan et al. 2019).

The impact of AuNR size was investigated on photoacoustic (PA) imaging, Pulse wave (PW) mediated-Plasmonic PTT efficacy, and SPR in a tissue-mimicking phantom at a pivotal point in the development of AuNRs for lung cancer treatment. All AuNRs showed toxicity under pulse wave illumination at a laser wavelength lower than the maximum allowable skin exposure, and the smallest AuNRs showed up to 80% cell death, proving that PW-PPTT is feasible (Knights and McLaughlan 2018). PW lasers and PA-guided PPTT can be performed using the same laser system and AuNRs to damage the tissue, and integrative theranostic applications (Sharifi et al. 2019). Similarly, by growing AgNPs atop GQDs with tannic acid (TA), Hai et al. created a multifunctional AgNP@GQDs nanocomposite (Hai et al. 2021). The nanocomposite breaks down in the presence of hydrogen peroxide (H_2O_2), releasing the oxidized TA and GQDs and oxidizing Ag0 to Ag+. By combining the H_2O_2-responsive decrease of AgNPs@GQDs with high H_2O_2 levels in cancerous cells, the nanocomposites effectively recognize and treat cancer cells. The symbiotic anticancer effect of Ag+ and oxidized TA influences the effectiveness of cell death, and the conquered GQDs are used to monitor the therapeutic efficacy through cell imaging. Zhang et al. created a biocompatible cRGD/Pt and DOX@GFNPs (RPDG) nano-formulation that improved ferroptosis and apoptosis simultaneously by upsetting the redox balance in glioblastoma cells (Zhang et al. 2021). MRI scans and *in vivo* results from tail vein injection-based pharmacological interventions indicated that the RPDGs are concentrated in the tumor sites in mice. The combination of apoptosis and ferroptosis's therapeutic advantages was enhanced and expedited with the advent of NIR. The Fenton reaction produced by Gallic acid/Fe^{2+} NPs (GFNPs) reduced Pt (IV) to Pt (III), which increased glutathione consumption (II). Comparing RPDGs to traditional treatment approaches, research shows that they immediately decrease malignancies and strengthen the immune system. Moreover, RPDGs offer superior tracer and MRI qualities. By upsetting intracellular redox equilibrium, they cause ferroptosis, which increases the effectiveness of commonly used broad-spectrum anticancer medications to treat gliomas. Thus, to treat glioma, this work opens the door for a unique strategy that targets high levels of H_2O_2 and glutathione in glioblastoma cells. In another study, a 64Cu-labeled method was created without the requirement for chelators (Duan et al. 2018). The drug-loaded MOFs were taken up by cancer cells in a size-dependent way. The *in vivo* biodistribution of drug-loaded MOF was examined using PET imaging, which was used to objectively analyze MOF in living animals. It was found that 60 nm MOF had significantly longer blood circulation and significantly greater tumor accumulation than 130 nm MOF. Several 2D-MOF nanosheets have recently been used as phototherapy agents because of their ability to produce ROS when exposed to light and their efficient absorption of NIR light. Zn-TCPP nanosheets, for example, are incredibly powerful photosensitizers for cancer PDT. These nanosheets were ideal for PDT and chemotherapy because they produced more light-triggered singlet oxygen and had a greater drug-loading capacity than their NP counterparts (Zhu et al. 2019).

The Titanium carbide (TiC)—-based magnetic MXene nanocomposite functions as an efficient PTT and imaging agent due to its colocalized SPR (Liu et al. 2018). TiO_2 NPs and biocompatible PEGylated TiO_2 NPs were also employed as PTT agents. PEGylated TiO_2 NPs shown remarkable destruction in solid tumors (Behnam, Emami, Sobhani, and Dehghanian 2018). Due to the great penetration of the NIR beam into the body and the intense photoabsorption of TiO_2-PEG at 808 nm, the *in vivo* PTT effects of TiO_2-PEG NPs in the melanoma tumor locations showed that localized NPs significantly exacerbated necrosis. The histology analysis showed that 90% of the tissue in the TiO^{2+} laser group was necrotic, proving the excellent efficacy of TiO_2-PEG NP for the PTT technique. Furthermore, Yang et al. created biodegradable MSN-ss-Gamma-aminobutyric acid (bMSN-ss-GABA), a biodegradable multifunctional drug carrier for cancer theranostics (Yang, Chen, et al. 2019). To serve as a contrast material for MRI and fluorescence imaging, the bovine serum albumin-based Gd/Au complex (BSA-Gd/Au) was enclosed on the edge of the bMSN through disulfide linkage. Next, FA was modified as a specifically focused ligand on the nanocarriers as its receptor is highly expressed in keratin-forming KB human oral epidermoid carcinoma cell lines. It was found that DOX@bMSN-ss-GABA was redox-responsive, causing rapid drug release in a tumor microenvironment where glutathione levels were elevated. Furthermore, the MRI and fluorescence imaging functions provided imaging guidance for cancer treatment. Broadly, the INP-based multifunctional nanocomposites are potent candidates to serve as a therapeutic agent for accurate nanomedicine application.

6.6 CHALLENGES AND CONSIDERATIONS

Before developing contrast agents and their nanodiagnostic counterparts for cancer diagnosis, it's crucial to consider their potential interactions within biological systems in vivo. A significant challenge in achieving effective treatment lies in overcoming the body's immune response. Upon introduction into a living organism, foreign substances are eventually cleared from the bloodstream via mechanisms such as the lymphatic and renal systems, as well as cellular uptake. Therefore, it's essential to engineer NMs capable of remaining in the body for sufficient time for imaging purposes, while ensuring cellular-level biocompatibility and eventual breakdown for removal to prevent cumulative toxicity. INPs are used to treat cancer, including brain and nervous system tumors. However, INPs can be difficult to degrade and excrete out of the body and can cause lethal effects such as inflammation and tissue cysts.

To summarize, the literature on *in vitro* and *in vivo* studies showcases the promising outcomes in treating diverse cancers using metal-based NPs with inherent anticancer properties or in combination with other therapeutic modalities. However, despite the advancements, the translation of most metal-based formulations into clinical practice remains limited primarily due to toxicity concerns. The cytotoxic nature of metallic NPs, characterized by their ability to generate ROS, induce oxidative stress, disrupt cytoskeleton integrity, and damage DNA, poses significant hurdles to their clinical approval. Therefore, future investigations must prioritize enhancing the biocompatibility of these platforms in healthy tissues, accumulating more evidence on their safety profiles and long-term effects. Another critical consideration regarding metallic NPs is their stability in biological environments, which necessitates meticulous attention through surface functionalization with various organic molecules, macromolecules, or noble metal coatings. Carbon-based NMs are less toxic than metallic NPs, as different polymers such as PEG and chitosan can be used for their functionalization with ligand-specific sites that can easily bind to the tumor cells. Using organic materials for the synthesis of CNMs has addressed the growing concern over their removal or toxicity. Also loading dual drugs in a single CNM will help in providing 100% efficiency toward tumor cells.

Although QDs, mainly from heavy metals, are potential candidates for *in vitro* cancer theranaustics, their colloidal instability hinders the advancement of *in vivo* diagnosis and therapy (Hardman 2006). Therefore, more efforts are needed to generate novel QDs to minimize toxicity and coating shell degradation and maximize detection efficiency (Smith and Nie 2009; Bottrill and Green 2011). Also, the nonspecific accumulation in organs, immune response, and genotoxic effect should be considered (Hardman 2006; Dobrovolskaia and McNeil 2007). Considering the heavy metal QDs' cytotoxicity, several low-toxicity QDs, such as by replacing Cd with Zn, have been developed (Pradhan et al. 2007). Still, extensive scrutiny of their cytotoxicity profiles is needed before QDs can be applied in any medical methods. Various research groups are attempting to prolong the circulation time of QDs by immobilizing the passivating agents, such as PEG, and optimizing their net surface charge to prevent their adsorption on the plasma proteins (Koole et al. 2008). Alternatively, clearance of INPs from the living systems is mandatory for their clinical use as contrast agents. A diameter threshold of 5–6 nm is desired, as below this, the QDs cannot escape the liver and be cleared through the kidneys (Choi et al. 2007). Moreover, the deficient data on the reproducibility, quantification, and comparability of QDs and their clinical applications are strongly limited. Different QDs have different fluorescence quantum yields according to their variable source materials and surface functionalities. Thus, the derivation and establishment of quality criteria is the essential initial step.

Magnetic NP drug delivery offers the potential for localized enhancement methods, allowing drugs to accumulate and act in predetermined areas. Iron compounds are commonly favored due to their biocompatibility and low toxicity, even being therapeutically used for iron substitution. Coating nanoparticles helps prevent agglomeration, ensures stability, and positively affects biodistribution. Various materials such as fatty acids, PEG, dextran, and chitosan can be utilized for coating. The diverse modes of action of local magnetic hyperthermia immunotherapy have been extensively explored in the past. One advantage of further developing these techniques is the ability to achieve potent immunomodulation without the use of drugs, which often leads to adverse reactions. However, hyperthermia is primarily utilized as a supplementary treatment alongside chemotherapy or radiotherapy rather than as a standalone therapy, partly due to the challenges of repeated therapy and the lack of comprehensive knowledge regarding optimal treatment parameters across different tumor types. The mNPs offer precise and uniform heating across a broader temperature range while effectively penetrating solid tumors in a non-invasive manner. Targeted heating with mNPs can induce immunogenic cell death (ICD) or other enduring anticancer immune responses through various mechanisms. Cellular stressors, such as heat, can trigger ICD, a distinctive apoptotic pathway that releases molecules called "damage-associated molecular patterns" (DAMPs) (Day, Wixson, and Shields IV 2021).

Other INPs and MSNs face several challenges, such as the control of particle size uniformity pore morphology and surface functionalization, during the synthesis and development stage, impacting their quality, scalability, stability, reproducibility, and performance. Surface modification is crucial for attaching targeting linkers, enhancing biocompatibility, and incorporating therapeutic agents. Also, reproducibility in large-scale production can be challenging due to batch-to-batch inconsistencies.

MSN-mediated cytotoxicity in cells is induced primarily by the silanol groups, disrupting the membranes through electrostatic interactions, and ROS generation, leading to cell death (Croissant et al. 2018). The glutathione depletion, membrane peroxidation, DNA damage, and mitochondrial dysfunction are the cytotoxicity factors of MSNs. Administering MSNs in multiple smaller doses shows decreased cytotoxic effects than the single large dose (Petushkov et al. 2010). The MSN surface negative charge makes stronger interactions with biological components and affects lymphocyte activity inhibition, hemolysis, immune signaling, and *in vivo* protein opsonization and causes oxidative stress, apoptosis, and tissue damage (Frickenstein et al. 2021). The formation of a protein corona due to plasma-protein interactions significantly influences MSN performance (Florek, Caillard, and Kleitz 2017). Factors such as surface functionalization, nanoparticle size, and exposure time to plasma determine protein corona formation. Poor functionalization, large size, and different shapes of MSNs may lead to improper biodegradability and retention of MSNs and lower clearance rates (Niroumand et al. 2023). As compared to the larger or smaller pore sizes, the medium pore-sized MSNs show better inhibition of cell growth and induction of tumor apoptosis and retarding tumor growth (Alberti et al. 2023). While some silica-based NMs, such as AGuIX® NPs, have received regulatory approval for clinical trials for cancer treatment (Lux et al. 2019), MSN-based drugs still require FDA approval.

6.7 FUTURE DIRECTIONS

Drawing upon the points covered in this review, it can be advocated that the development of nanoformulations with appropriate size, morphology, pore dimensions, and surface functionalization can lead to overcoming various limitations.

Controlled Radical Polymerization (CRP) techniques are revolutionizing in terms of functionalization to provide precise control over the polymerization process, enabling manipulation of the size, composition, and architecture of the polymer chains (Parkatzidis et al., 2020). In the context of MSNs, CRP techniques allow for grafting polymers, resulting in well-defined and effective functional groups on the NP surface. These polymer chains act as functional groups interacting with other molecules, thus enhancing the performance and effectiveness of functionalized MSNs by improving biocompatibility, stability, and target specificity while mitigating the ineffectiveness of functionalized moieties. Atom Transfer Radical Polymerization (ATRP) (Lorandi, Fantin, and Matyjaszewski 2022), nitroxide-mediated polymerization (NMP) (Wagner et al. 2023), and reversible addition-fragmentation chain transfer (RAFT) polymerization (Zhao et al. 2022) are few of the commonly used CRP techniques.

"Transformable" NPs, capable of modifying their shape to cross biological barriers, have gained recent attention. These NPs can be customized to respond to stimuli from their surrounding environment, facilitating morphology changes that enhance drug delivery efficiency, tumor penetration, and biocompatibility. A recent example is a gelatin/laponite/doxorubicin (GLD) comprising cross-linked gelatin-coated laponite NPs loaded with DOX (Li et al. 2023). This system undergoes size reduction in response to the matrix metallopeptidase-2 (MMP-2) enzyme, allowing easy passage through the blood-brain barrier and delivering a potent dose of anticancer medication to tumor cells.

One of the challenges in nanomedicine is to overcome biological barriers such as immune clearance (Huang et al. 2017), blood-brain barrier (BBB) (Song, Qian, and Yu 2023), endosomal entrapment (Gisbert-Garzarán, Lozano, and Vallet-Regí 2020), and lack of selective internalization and accumulation in tumor tissues (Izci et al. 2021) which impede the performance and effective delivery of therapeutic agents to target tissues or cells. A study focused on polymers evaluated the transport, uptake, and cytotoxicity of drug nanocarriers in *in vitro* BBB models. Coating with poly(ethylene glycol)–poly(ethylene imine) (PEG–PEI) copolymers initiated the uptake of rod-shaped MSNs across the BBB with insignificant damage (Baghirov et al. 2016). Thiol-modified MSNs also exhibited significantly lower neurotoxicity compared to non-functionalized MSNs, suggesting the possibility of mediating neurotoxicity by altering the surface chemistry for biomedical applications. Moreover, INPs fused with mNPs can assist in imaging and improve targeting abilities. In a recent study, mNPs subjected to dual magnetic fields demonstrated efficacy in crossing the BBB, suggesting potential application in bone metastatic prostate cancer treatment (Gupta et al. 2022).

Biomimetics is an innovative solution to overcome limitations associated with traditional cancer therapies. Coating NPs with cell membranes of biological entities enhances the precision and targeting of therapeutic agents (Zhao, Wang, and Li 2023). Biomimetic nanomedicine enhances biocompatibility by mimicking traits of natural biological materials, facilitating safe interaction with biological tissues and cells, and minimizing adverse reactions. Incorporation of INPs in biomimetic nanosystems shows promise in cancer theranostics, as demonstrated by recent studies inducing ferroptosis and ICD in gastric cancer.Mn^{2+}-doped MSNs were loaded with a cisplatin prodrug and finally coated with a cancer cell membrane (Guo et al. 2023). Its biomimetic surface allowed the NPs to enhance homologous tumor targeting, T1 signal under MRI, and immune evasion. The nano platform induced the ferroptosis-mediated ICD by depleting intracellular GSH releasing Mn^{2+} ions, and transforming cisplatin from Pt(IV) to Pt(II). It causes nuclear DNA damage, increases in lipid peroxidation content, and recruits cytotoxic T lymphocytes.

The use of "nano-regulators," nanoscale compounds that specifically modify biological processes, is another promising strategy. A recent example is a MOF-based nano-regulator targeting and delivering chemotherapeutic drugs to bone metastatic prostate cancer cells while suppressing the immune system to minimize the side effects of immunotherapy (Huang, Yuan, et al. 2023). The mitoxantrone (MTO) drug was encapsulated in a phytic acid (PA) and Fe^{3+} derived MOF nano-regulator which selectively causes the cancer cells' death through ICD while sparing the normal cells by preventing the production of TGF-β in the tumor microenvironment.

Nanomotors, incorporating INPs, represent a cutting-edge approach to achieving more target-specific deliveries with higher speed and precision. These nanoplatforms, triggered by stimuli such as enzymes or light, can autonomously self-propel toward cancer cells to deliver chemotherapeutic cargo. Additionally, advancements in nanorobotics hold potential in enhancing NPs performance, aiding in tasks such as sensing tumors, mitigating invasive surgeries, and accessing hard-to-reach tumor locations. The nanorobots-focused research is still in the early stages, due to the lack of perspective on the interactions with biological interfaces and linked complications (Kong et al. 2023). However, with the research advancement, more sophisticated nanorobots can be developed that would likely provide a significant boost to performing tasks in cancer theranostics.

Artificial Intelligence (AI) can be used to gain precise control over NPs characteristics based on abundantly available datasets and can be a game-changer in NPs design for cancer theranostics (Serov and Vinogradov 2022). AI algorithms can predict optimal NPs properties required for biocompatibility, performance, drug loading, and release, thus providing personalized cancer treatment methodologies.

Despite holding worthy promise for cancer therapies, INPs are lacking clinical translation due to their toxicity and unavailable regulatory guidelines. Overcoming these challenges requires comprehensive research, strict protocols, and collaborative efforts among academia, industry, and government agencies to ensure the safe and effective creation and usage of nanomedicines, thus advancing cancer theranostics.

6.8 CONCLUSION

In the dynamic field of cancer theranostics, the challenge of precise and targeted treatment while minimizing adverse effects remains unsolved. The constant progression of cancer often outpaces conventional treatment strategies and underscores the urgent need for innovative and effective theranostic approaches. This review has highlighted the considerable promise of INPs in addressing this challenge, thanks to their unique physicochemical properties, tunability, easy functionalization, and biocompatibility. Furthermore, the review has extensively explored the imaging and therapeutic applications of INPs in cancer, covering the metallic, silica-based, carbon-based, and magnetic NPs. The versatility of these INPs offers a transformative base for the fabrication of cancer theranostic interventions, leveraging a new era of precision medicine. The multimodal synergistic theranostics further enhance the treatment efficacy while mitigating side effects. The rationale for future research in this area is compelling. The untapped potential of INPs conjoint with emerging techniques asks description. There are countless combinations of INPs with biomolecules and other reagents still to be explored in a theranostic aspect, offering endless further possibilities and implications. Secondly, comprehensively learning the long-term effects and potential toxicity aspects linked with INPs is essential for harnessing their full potential in effective cancer theranostics. This review provides an informative overview of the current understandings in this field, emphasizing promising advancements over recent years and the imperative for further research to fully exploit the potential of INPs in cancer theranostics.

DECLARATION OF COMPETING INTEREST

The authors declare that they have no known competing financial interests or personal competing interests that could have appeared to influence the work reported.

ACKNOWLEDGMENTS

The first Author, Sarita Devi, Council of Scientific & Industrial Research (CSIR)-Pool Scientist is highly thankful to CSIR for the financial grant. The authors are grateful to the Department of Biochemistry, Panjab University.

REFERENCES

Abdi Goushbolagh, Nouraddin, Marzieh Keshavarz, Mohammad Hosein Zare, Mohammad Hossein Bahreyni-Toosi, Masoud Kargar, Bagher %J Artificial cells Farhood, nanomedicine, and biotechnology. 2019. "Photosensitizer effects of MWCNTs-COOH particles on CT26 fibroblastic cells exposed to laser irradiation." 47 (1):1326–1334.

Abdukayum, Abdukader, Cheng-Xiong Yang, Qiang Zhao, Jia-Tong Chen, Lu-Xi Dong, and Xiu-Ping Yan %J Analytical chemistry. 2014. "Gadolinium complexes functionalized persistent luminescent nanoparticles as a multimodal probe for near-infrared luminescence and magnetic resonance imaging in vivo." 86 (9): 4096–4101.

Aghebati-Maleki, Ali, Sanam Dolati, Majid Ahmadi, Amir Baghbanzhadeh, Milad Asadi, Ali Fotouhi, Mehdi Yousefi, and Leili Aghebati-Maleki %J Journal of cellular physiology. 2020. "Nanoparticles and cancer therapy: Perspectives for application of nanoparticles in the treatment of cancers." 235 (3): 1962–1972.

Ahmad, Tanveer, Hongsub Bae, Yousaf Iqbal, Ilsu Rhee, Sungwook Hong, Yongmin Chang, Jaejun Lee, Derac Sohn %J Journal of Magnetism and Magnetic Materials. 2015. "Chitosan-coated nickel-ferrite nanoparticles as contrast agents in magnetic resonance imaging." 381:151–157.

Ahmed, Shameer, Gunjan Baijal, Rudrappa Somashekar, Subramania Iyer, and Vijayashree Nayak %J International Journal of Nanomedicine. 2021. "One Pot Synthesis of PEGylated Bimetallic Gold–Silver Nanoparticles for Imaging and Radiosensitization of Oral Cancers."7103–7121.

Ahrens, Lasse Cramer, Mathias Green Krabbenhøft, Rasmus Würgler Hansen, Nikola Mikic, Christian Bonde Pedersen, Frantz Rom Poulsen, and Anders Rosendal Korshoej %J Cancers. 2022. "Effect of 5-aminolevulinic acid and sodium fluorescein on the extent of resection in high-grade gliomas and brain metastasis." 14 (3):617.

Ajnai, Giimel, Chun-Chia Cheng, Tzu-Chun Kan, Jeng-Wei Lu, Sri Rahayu, Amy Chiu, and Jungshan Chang %J Pharmaceutics. 2022. "Improving Tirapazamine (TPZ) to target and eradicate hypoxia tumors by gold nanoparticle Carriers." 14 (4):847.

Akter, Mahmuda, Md Tajuddin Sikder, Md Mostafizur Rahman, AKM Atique Ullah, Kaniz Fatima Binte Hossain, Subrata Banik, Toshiyuki Hosokawa, Takeshi Saito, and Masaaki Kurasaki %J Journal of advanced research. 2018. "A systematic review on silver nanoparticles-induced cytotoxicity: Physicochemical properties and perspectives." 9:1–16.

Albanese, Alexandre, Peter S Tang, and Warren CW Chan. 2012. "The effect of nanoparticle size, shape, and surface chemistry on biological systems." *Annual Review of Biomedical Engineering* 14:1–16.

Alberti, Sebastián, Sonja Schmidt, Simone Hageneder, Paula C Angelomé, Galo JAA Soler-lllia, Philipp Vana, Jakub Dostalek, Omar Azzaroni, and Wolfgang Knoll. 2023. "Large-pore mesoporous silica: Template design, thin film preparation and biomolecule infiltration." *Materials Chemistry Frontiers* 7 (18):4142–4151.

Alivisatos, A Paul. 1996. "Semiconductor clusters, nanocrystals, and quantum dots." *Science* 271 (5251): 933–937.

Allen, Theresa M. 2002. "Ligand-targeted therapeutics in anticancer therapy." *Nature Reviews Cancer* 2 (10): 750–763.

Allen, Theresa M, and Pieter R Cullis. 2013. "Liposomal drug delivery systems: From concept to clinical applications." *Advanced Drug Delivery Reviews* 65 (1):36–48.

Arosio, Paolo, and Sonia Levi. 2002. "Ferritin, iron homeostasis, and oxidative damage." *Free Radical Biology and Medicine* 33 (4):457–463.

Arumugasamy, Shiva Kumar, Saravanan Govindaraju, and Kyusik Yun %J Applied Surface Science. 2020. "Electrochemical sensor for detecting dopamine using graphene quantum dots incorporated with multiwall carbon nanotubes." 508:145294.

Arvizo, Rochelle R, Sanjib Bhattacharyya, Rachel A Kudgus, Karuna Giri, Resham Bhattacharya, and Priyabrata Mukherjee. 2012. "Intrinsic therapeutic applications of noble metal nanoparticles: Past, present and future." *Chemical Society Reviews* 41 (7):2943–2970.

Arvizo, Rochelle R, Resham Bhattacharya, and Priyabrata %J Expert opinion on drug delivery Mukherjee. 2010. "Gold nanoparticles: Opportunities and challenges in nanomedicine." 7 (6):753–763.

Asadi, Somayeh, Leonardo Bianchi, Martina De Landro, Sanzhar Korganbayev, Emiliano Schena, and Paola Saccomandi %J Journal of Biophotonics. 2021. "Laser-induced optothermal response of gold nanoparticles: From a physical viewpoint to cancer treatment application." 14 (2):e202000161.

Ashraf, Mohammad, Nabeel Choudhary, Syed Shahzad Hussain, Usman Ahmad Kamboh, and Naveed Ashraf %J Surgical neurology international. 2020. "Role of intraoperative computed tomography scanner in modern neurosurgery–An early experience." 11.

Aslan, Naim, Burhan Ceylan, Mümin Mehmet Koç, and Fehim Findik %J Journal of Molecular Structure. 2020. "Metallic nanoparticles as X-Ray computed tomography (CT) contrast agents: A review." 1219:128599.

Ayrignac, Xavier, Valérie Rigau, Benoit Lhermitte, Thierry Vincent, Nicolas Menjot de Champfleur, Clarisse Carra-Dalliere, Mahmoud Charif, Nicolas Collongues, Jérôme de Seze, and Sonia Hebbadj %J Journal of Neurology. 2019. "Pathologic and MRI analysis in acute atypical inflammatory demyelinating lesions." 266:1743–1755.

Bagalkot, Vaishali, Liangfang Zhang, Etgar Levy-Nissenbaum, Sangyong Jon, Philip W Kantoff, Robert Langer, and Omid C Farokhzad %J Nano letters. 2007. "Quantum dot-aptamer conjugates for synchronous cancer imaging, therapy, and sensing of drug delivery based on bi-fluorescence resonance energy transfer." 7 (10):3065–3070.

Baghban, Roghayyeh, Leila Roshangar, Rana Jahanban-Esfahlan, Khaled Seidi, Abbas Ebrahimi-Kalan, Mehdi Jaymand, Saeed Kolahian, Tahereh Javaheri, Peyman Zare %J Cell Communication and Signaling. 2020. "Tumor microenvironment complexity and therapeutic implications at a glance." 18:1–19.

Baghirov, Habib, Didem Karaman, Tapani Viitala, Alain Duchanoy, Yan-Ru Lou, Veronika Mamaeva, Evgeny Pryazhnikov, Leonard Khiroug, Catharina de Lange Davies, and Cecilia Sahlgren. 2016. "Feasibility study of the permeability and uptake of mesoporous silica nanoparticles across the blood-brain barrier." *PLoS One* 11 (8):e0160705.

Bander, Thomas S, Kishwer S Nehal, and Erica H %J Dermatologic clinics Lee. 2019. "Cutaneous squamous cell carcinoma: Updates in staging and management." 37 (3):241–251.

Barker, Holly E, James TE Paget, Aadil A Khan, and Kevin J %J Nature Reviews Cancer Harrington. 2015. "The tumour microenvironment after radiotherapy: Mechanisms of resistance and recurrence." 15 (7):409–425.

Barra, Ana, Jacek K Wychowaniec, Danielle Winning, Maria Margarida Cruz, Liliana P Ferreira, Brian J Rodriguez, Helena Oliveira, Eduardo Ruiz-Hitzky, Cláudia Nunes, and Dermot F Brougham. 2023. "Magnetic Chitosan Bionanocomposite Films as a Versatile Platform for Biomedical Hyperthermia." *Advanced Healthcare Materials*:2303861.

Behnam, Mohammad Ali, Farzin Emami, Zahra Sobhani, Omid Koohi-Hosseinabadi, Amir Reza Dehghanian, Seyed Mojtaba Zebarjad, Mohammad Hadi Moghim, and Ahmad Oryan %J Advanced pharmaceutical bulletin. 2018. "Novel combination of silver nanoparticles and carbon nanotubes for plasmonic photo thermal therapy in melanoma cancer model." 8 (1):49.

Belyanina, Irina, Olga Kolovskaya, Sergey Zamay, Ana Gargaun, Tatiana Zamay, and Anna Kichkailo. 2017. "Targeted magnetic nanotheranostics of cancer." Molecules 22 (6):975.

Berry, Catherine C. 2005. "Possible exploitation of magnetic nanoparticle–cell interaction for biomedical applications." *Journal of Materials Chemistry* 15 (5):543–547.

Bilan, Regina, Fabrice Fleury, Igor Nabiev, and Alyona Sukhanova. 2015. "Quantum dot surface chemistry and functionalization for cell targeting and imaging." *Bioconjugate Chemistry* 26 (4):609–624.

Botterhuis, Nicole E, Qianyao Sun, Pieter CMM Magusin, Rutger A Van Santen, and Nico AJM Sommerdijk. 2006. "Hollow silica spheres with an ordered pore structure and their application in controlled release studies." *Chemistry–A European Journal* 12 (5):1448–1456.

Bottrill, Melanie, and Mark Green. 2011. "Some aspects of quantum dot toxicity." *Chemical Communications* 47 (25):7039–7050.

Boussedra, Safia, Louise Benoit, Meriem Koual, Enrica Bentivegna, Huyen-Thu Nguyen-Xuan, Anne-Sophie Bats, and Henri Azaïs %J European Journal of Surgical Oncology. 2022. "Fluorescence guided surgery to improve peritoneal cytoreduction in epithelial ovarian cancer: A systematic review of available data." 48 (6):1217–1223.

Buda, Alessandro, Giampaolo Di Martino, Francesca Vecchione, Beatrice Bussi, Tiziana Dell'Anna, Sharon Palazzi, Maria Grazia Cantù, Martina Delle Marchette, and Rodolfo Milani %J International Journal of Gynecologic Cancer. 2015. "Optimizing strategies for sentinel lymph node mapping in early-stage cervical and endometrial cancer: Comparison of real-time fluorescence with indocyanine green and methylene blue." 25 (8).

Cabral Filho, Paulo E, Mariana P Cabrera, Ana LC Cardoso, Otacilio A Santana, Carlos FGC Geraldes, Beate S Santos, Maria C Pedroso de Lima, Giovannia AL Pereira, and Adriana Fontes %J Biochimica et Biophysica Acta-General Subjects. 2018. "Multimodal highly fluorescent-magnetic nanoplatform to target transferrin receptors in cancer cells." 1862 (12):2788–2796.

Cascorbi, Ingolf %J Deutsches Ärzteblatt International. 2012. "Drug interactions—principles, examples and clinical consequences." 109 (33–34):546.

Chan, Warren CW, Dustin J Maxwell, Xiaohu Gao, Robert E Bailey, Mingyong Han, and Shuming Nie. 2002. "Luminescent quantum dots for multiplexed biological detection and imaging." *Current Opinion in Biotechnology* 13 (1):40–46.

Chang, Yanzhou, Lizhen He, Zhibin Li, Lilan Zeng, Zhenhuan Song, Penghui Li, Leung Chan, Yuanyuan You, Xue-Feng Yu, and Paul K Chu %J ACS nano. 2017. "Designing core–shell gold and selenium nanocomposites for cancer radiochemotherapy." 11 (5):4848–4858.

Chen, Junqi, Chengyun Ning, Zhengnan Zhou, Peng Yu, Ye Zhu, Guoxin Tan, and Chuanbin Mao %J Progress in materials science. 2019. "Nanomaterials as photothermal therapeutic agents." 99:1–26.

Chen, Linjie, Changyou Chen, Pingping Wang, and Tao Song %J Journal of nanomaterials. 2017. "Mechanisms of cellular effects directly induced by magnetic nanoparticles under magnetic fields." 2017.

Chen, Miao, Wenjia Zhu, Jianhua Du, Chen Yang, Bing Han, Daobin Zhou, Li Huo, and Junling Zhuang %J Scientific Reports. 2021. "11C-acetate positron emission tomography is more precise than 18F-fluorodeoxyglucose positron emission tomography in evaluating tumor burden and predicting disease risk of multiple myeloma." 11 (1):22188.

Chen, Shun, Junjun Zhang, Shaokun Song, Chuanxi Xiong, and Lijie Dong %J Materials Research Express. 2017. "Hydrangea-like magneto-fluorescent nanoparticles through thiol-inducing assembly." 4 (1):015008.

Chen, Yu, Hang-Rong Chen, and Jian-Lin Shi. 2014. "Construction of homogenous/heterogeneous hollow mesoporous silica nanostructures by silica-etching chemistry: Principles, synthesis, and applications." *Accounts of Chemical Research* 47 (1):125–137.

Chen, Yu-Wei, Yu-Lin Su, Shang-Hsiu Hu, and San-Yuan Chen %J Advanced drug delivery reviews. 2016. "Functionalized graphene nanocomposites for enhancing photothermal therapy in tumor treatment." 105:190–204.

Chen, Zhe, Bo Peng, Jia-Qiong Xu, Xue-Chen Xiang, Dong-Fang Ren, Tai-Qun Yang, Shi-Yu Ma, Kun Zhang, and Qi-Ming Chen. 2020. "A non-surfactant self-templating strategy for mesoporous silica nanospheres: Beyond the Stöber method." *Nanoscale* 12 (6):3657–3662.

Chenthamara, Dhrisya, Sadhasivam Subramaniam, Sankar Ganesh Ramakrishnan, Swaminathan Krishnaswamy, Musthafa Mohamed Essa, Feng-Huei Lin, and M Walid Qoronfleh. 2019. "Therapeutic efficacy of nanoparticles and routes of administration." *Biomaterials Research* 23 (1):20.

Choi, H Soo, W Liu, P Misra, E Tanaka, JP Zimmer, and B Itty Ipe. 2007. "MG Bawendi ja JV Frangioni, Renal clearance of quantum dots." *Nature Biotechnol* 25:1165–1170.

Croissant, Jonas G, Yevhen Fatieiev, Abdulaziz Almalik, and Niveen M Khashab. 2018. "Mesoporous silica and organosilica nanoparticles: Physical chemistry, biosafety, delivery strategies, and biomedical applications." *Advanced Healthcare Materials* 7 (4):1700831.

Crucho, Carina IC, João Avó, Roberto Nobuyasu, Sandra N Pinto, Fábio Fernandes, João C Lima, Mário N Berberan-Santos, Fernando B Dias %J Materials Science and Engineering: C. 2020. "Silica nanoparticles with thermally activated delayed fluorescence for live cell imaging." 109:110528.

Dadwal, Ankita, Ashish Baldi, Raj Kumar Narang %J Artificial cells nanomedicine, and biotechnology. 2018. "Nanoparticles as carriers for drug delivery in cancer." 46 (sup2):295–305.

Damasco, Jossana A, Saisree Ravi, Joy D Perez, Daniel E Hagaman, and Marites P Melancon %J Nanomaterials. 2020. "Understanding nanoparticle toxicity to direct a safe-by-design approach in cancer nanomedicine." 10 (11):2186.

Das, Joydeep, Yun-Jung Choi, Jae Woong Han, Abu Musa Md Talimur Reza, and Jin-Hoi Kim %J Scientific reports. 2017. "Nanoceria-mediated delivery of doxorubicin enhances the anti-tumour efficiency in ovarian cancer cells via apoptosis." 7 (1):9513.

Das, Poushali, Sayan Ganguly, Shlomo Margel, and Aharon Gedanken %J Nanoscale Advances. 2021. "Tailor made magnetic nanolights: Fabrication to cancer theranostics applications." 3 (24):6762–6796.

Day, Nicole B, William C Wixson, and C Wyatt Shields IV. 2021. "Magnetic systems for cancer immunotherapy." *Acta Pharmaceutica Sinica B* 11 (8):2172–2196.

Debela, Dejene Tolossa, Seke GY Muzazu, Kidist Digamo Heraro, Maureen Tayamika Ndalama, Betelhiem Woldemedhin Mesele, Dagimawi Chilot Haile, Sophia Khalayi Kitui, and Tsegahun Manyazewal. 2021. "New approaches and procedures for cancer treatment: Current perspectives." *SAGE Open Medicine* 9:20503121211034366.

Demirci, Hakan, Naziha Slimani, Mercy Pawar, Ronald E Kumon, Prem Vaishnava, Cagri G Besirli %J Translational Vision Science and Technology. 2019. "Magnetic hyperthermia in Y79 retinoblastoma and ARPE-19 retinal epithelial cells: Tumor selective apoptotic activity of iron oxide nanoparticle." 8 (5):18–18.

Devi, Sarita, Raju K Gupta, AK Paul, Vinay Kumar, Abhay Sachdev, Packirisamy Gopinath, and S Tyagi. 2018. "Ethylenediamine mediated luminescence enhancement of pollutant derivatized carbon quantum dots for intracellular trinitrotoluene detection: Soot to shine." *RSC Advances* 8 (57):32684–32694.

Devi, Sarita, Rajwinder Kaur, Ashok K Paul, and Sachin Tyagi. 2018. "MPA-capped CdSe QD/mercaptoethylamine-capped AuNP nanocomposite-based sensor for instant detection of trinitrotoluene." *Colloid and Polymer Science* 296:427–440.

Devi, Sarita, Rajwinder Kaur, Bhupender Singh, Ashok K Paul, and Sachin Tyagi. 2018. "Fluorescent sensing assay for trinitrotoluene using fluorescein isothiocyanate conjugated mesoporous MCM-41 particles." *Journal of Nanoscience and Nanotechnology* 18 (10):6838–6849.

Devi, Sarita, Bhupinder Singh, AK Paul, and Sachin Tyagi. 2016. "Highly sensitive and selective detection of trinitrotoluene using cysteine-capped gold nanoparticles." *Analytical Methods* 8 (22):4398–4405.

Ding, Yuan, Zhongquan Sun, Zongrui Tong, Sitong Zhang, Jie Min, Qianhui Xu, Liuzhi Zhou, Zhengwei Mao, Haibing Xia, and Weilin Wang %J Theranostics. 2020. "Tumor microenvironment-responsive multifunctional peptide coated ultrasmall gold nanoparticles and their application in cancer radiotherapy." 10 (12):5195.

Dobrovolskaia, Marina A, and Scott E McNeil. 2007. "Immunological properties of engineered nanomaterials." *Nature Nanotechnology* 2 (8):469–478.

Dreaden, Erik C, Alaaldin M Alkilany, Xiaohua Huang, Catherine J Murphy, and Mostafa A El-Sayed. 2012. "The golden age: Gold nanoparticles for biomedicine." *Chemical Society Reviews* 41 (7):2740–2779.

Duan, Dongban, Hui Liu, Mengxin Xu, Mengqi Chen, Yuxiang Han, Yaxin Shi, Zhibo Liu %J ACS Applied Materials and Interfaces. 2018. "Size-controlled synthesis of drug-loaded zeolitic imidazolate framework in aqueous solution and size effect on their cancer theranostics in vivo." 10 (49):42165–42174.

Duncan, Ruth, Yee-Nee Sat-Klopsch, Angelika M Burger, Michael C Bibby, Heinz H Fiebig, Edward A Sausville %J Cancer chemotherapy and pharmacology. 2013. "Validation of tumour models for use in anticancer nanomedicine evaluation: The EPR effect and cathepsin B-mediated drug release rate." 72:417–427.

Eatz, Tiffany A, Daniel G Eichberg, Victor M Lu, Long Di, Ricardo J Komotar, and Michael E Ivan %J Journal of neuro-oncology. 2022. "Intraoperative 5-ALA fluorescence-guided resection of high-grade glioma leads to greater extent of resection with better outcomes: A systematic review." 156 (2):233–256.

Eivazzadeh-Keihan, Reza, Zeinab Pajoum, Hooman Aghamirza Moghim Aliabadi, Fatemeh Ganjali, Amir Kashtiaray, Milad Salimi Bani, Farnaz Lalebeigi, Elaheh Ziaei Ziabari, Ali Maleki, and Majid M Heravi. 2023. "Magnetic chitosan-silk fibroin hydrogel/graphene oxide nanobiocomposite for biological and hyperthermia applications." *Carbohydrate Polymers* 300:120246.

Fan, Wenpei, Wei Tang, Joseph Lau, Zheyu Shen, Jin Xie, Jianlin Shi, and Xiaoyuan Chen %J Advanced Materials. 2019. "Breaking the depth dependence by nanotechnology-enhanced X-ray-excited deep cancer theranostics." 31 (12):1806381.

Federico, Salvatore, Valentina Catania, Fabio Salvatore Palumbo, Calogero Fiorica, Domenico Schillaci, Giovanna Pitarresi, and Gaetano Giammona %J International Journal of Biological Macromolecules. 2022. "Photothermal nanofibrillar membrane based on hyaluronic acid and graphene oxide to treat Staphylococcus aureus and Pseudomonas aeruginosa infected wounds." 214:470–479.

Florek, Justyna, Romain Caillard, and Freddy Kleitz. 2017. "Evaluation of mesoporous silica nanoparticles for oral drug delivery–current status and perspective of MSNs drug carriers." *Nanoscale* 9 (40):15252–15277.

Frickenstein, Alex N, Jordan M Hagood, Collin N Britten, Brandon S Abbott, Molly W McNally, Catherine A Vopat, Eian G Patterson, William M MacCuaig, Ajay Jain, and Keisha B Walters. 2021. "Mesoporous silica nanoparticles: Properties and strategies for enhancing clinical effect." *Pharmaceutics* 13 (4):570.

Ganguly, Sayan. 2022. "Preparation/processing of polymer-graphene composites by different techniques." In *Polymer Nanocomposites Containing Graphene*, 45–74. Elsevier.

Ganguly, Sayan, and Shlomo Margel %J Biotechnology Advances. 2020. "Remotely controlled magneto-regulation of therapeutics from magnetoelastic gel matrices." 44:107611.

Gao, Xiaohu, Yuanyuan Cui, Richard M Levenson, Leland WK Chung, and Shuming Nie. 2004. "In vivo cancer targeting and imaging with semiconductor quantum dots." *Nature Biotechnology* 22 (8):969–976.

Garg, Ishan, Mark A Nathan, Ann T Packard, Eugene D Kwon, Nicholas B Larson, Val Lowe, Brian J Davis, Rimki Haloi, Mindie L Mahon, Ajit H Goenka %J Journal of Cancer Research and Therapeutics. 2021. "11C-Choline positron emission tomography/computed tomography for detection of disease relapse in patients with history of biochemically recurrent prostate cancer and prostate-specific antigen≤ 0.1 Ng/Ml." 17 (2):358–365.

Ghosh, N, and R Singh %J Rasayan J. Chem. 2021. "In vitro cytotoxicity assay of biogenically synthesized bimetallic nanoparticles." 14:486–492.

Gierlich, Piotr, Ana I Mata, Claire Donohoe, Rui MM Brito, Mathias O Senge, and Lígia C Gomes-da-Silva. 2020. "Ligand-targeted delivery of photosensitizers for cancer treatment." *Molecules* 25 (22):5317.

Gimenez, Cristina, Cristina de la Torre, Monica Gorbe, Elena Aznar, Felix Sancenon, Jose R Murguia, Ramon Martinez-Manez, M Dolores Marcos, and Pedro Amoros %J Langmuir. 2015. "Gated mesoporous silica nanoparticles for the controlled delivery of drugs in cancer cells." 31 (12):3753–3762.

Gisbert-Garzarán, Miguel, Daniel Lozano, and María Vallet-Regí. 2020. "Mesoporous silica nanoparticles for targeting subcellular organelles." *International Journal of Molecular Sciences* 21 (24):9696.

Go, Gyeongyun, Chang-Seuk Lee, Yeo Min Yoon, Ji Ho Lim, Tae Hyun Kim, and Sang Hun Lee %J International Journal of Molecular Sciences. 2021. "Prpc aptamer conjugated–gold nanoparticles for targeted delivery of doxorubicin to colorectal cancer cells." 22 (4):1976.

Gorab, Mostafa Ghafori, Hooman Aghamirza Moghim Aliabadi, Amir Kashtiaray, Mohammad Mahdavi, Milad Salimi Bani, Andisheh Etminan, Nabi Salehpour, Reza Eivazzadeh-Keihan, and Ali Maleki %J Nanoscale Advances. 2023. "Decoration of graphene oxide nanosheets with carboxymethylcellulose hydrogel, silk fibroin and magnetic nanoparticles for biomedical and hyperthermia applications." 5 (1):153–159.

Granqvist, CG, and RA Buhrman. 1976. "Ultrafine metal particles." *Journal of applied Physics* 47 (5): 2200–2219.

Grunert, Bianca, Jessica Saatz, Katrin Hoffmann, Franziska Appler, Dominik Lubjuhn, Norbert Jakubowski, Ute Resch-Genger, Franziska Emmerling, Andreas Briel %J ACS Biomaterials Science and Engineering. 2018. "Multifunctional rare-earth element nanocrystals for cell labeling and multimodal imaging." 4 (10):3578–3587.

Guo, Jingjing, Yan Wang, and Min Zhao. 2019. "Target-directed functionalized ferrous phosphate-carbon dots fluorescent nanostructures as peroxidase mimetics for cancer cell detection and ROS-mediated therapy." *Sensors and Actuators B: Chemical* 297:126739.

Guo, Weihong, Zhian Chen, Zhenhao Li, Huilin Huang, Yingxin Ren, Zhenyuan Li, Bingxia Zhao, Guoxin Li, and Yanfeng Hu. 2023. "Cancer cell membrane biomimetic mesoporous silica nanotheranostics for enhanced Ferroptosis-mediated immuogenic cell death on Gastric cancer." *Chemical Engineering Journal* 455:140868.

Gupta, Ruby, Anjali Chauhan, Tashmeen Kaur, Bijoy K Kuanr, and Deepika Sharma. 2022. "Transmigration of magnetite nanoparticles across the blood–brain barrier in a rodent model: Influence of external and alternating magnetic fields." *Nanoscale* 14 (47):17589–17606.

Gupta, Ruby, and Deepika Sharma %J ACS chemical neuroscience. 2019. "Evolution of magnetic hyperthermia for glioblastoma multiforme therapy." 10 (3):1157–1172.

Gustafsson, Hanna, and Krister Holmberg. 2017. "Emulsion-based synthesis of porous silica." *Advances in Colloid and Interface Science* 247:426–434.

Ha, Phuong Thu, Thi Thu Huong Le, Thuc Quang Bui, Hong Nam Pham, Anh Son Ho, and Linh Toan Nguyen %J New Journal of Chemistry. 2019. "Doxorubicin release by magnetic inductive heating and in vivo hyperthermia-chemotherapy combined cancer treatment of multifunctional magnetic nanoparticles." 43 (14):5404–5413.

Hai, Xin, Yuwei Li, Kaixin Yu, Shuzhen Yue, Yuanfang Li, Weiling Song, Sai Bi, and Xueji Zhang %J Chinese Chemical Letters. 2021. "Synergistic in-situ growth of silver nanoparticles with nanozyme activity for dual-mode biosensing and cancer theranostics." 32 (3):1215–1219.

Haque, Munima, Md Salman Shakil, and Kazi Mustafa Mahmud %J Cancers. 2023. "The promise of nanoparticles-based radiotherapy in cancer treatment." 15 (6):1892.

Hardman, Ron. 2006. "A toxicologic review of quantum dots: Toxicity depends on physicochemical and environmental factors." *Environmental Health Perspectives* 114 (2):165–172.

Harisinghani, Mukesh G, Jelle Barentsz, Peter F Hahn, Willem M Deserno, Shahin Tabatabaei, Christine Hulsbergen van de Kaa, Jean de la Rosette, and Ralph Weissleder. 2003. "Noninvasive detection of clinically occult lymph-node metastases in prostate cancer." *New England Journal of Medicine* 348 (25):2491–2499.

He, Shuyi, Jingyu Li, Mingjian Chen, Liehua Deng, Yuxin Yang, Zhaoyang Zeng, Wei Xiong, and Xu Wu %J International Journal of Nanomedicine. 2020. "Graphene oxide-template gold nanosheets as highly efficient near-infrared hyperthermia agents for cancer therapy."8451–8463.

He, Xiaojun, Zaian Deng, Ji-Ting Hou, Xiaoshuai Sun, Danfeng Jiang, Nahyun Kwon, Lisong Ye, Enoch Obeng, Rongdang Hu, and Yi Wang %J Advanced Materials Interfaces. 2022. "Polymetallic Hybrid Nanoplatform with Hyperthermia-Amplified Dual Enzyme-Like Activities for Efficient Speeded-Up Bacterially Infected Wound Healing." 9 (31):2201422.

Hervault, Aziliz, and Nguyễn Thị Kim Thanh %J Nanoscale. 2014. "Magnetic nanoparticle-based therapeutic agents for thermo-chemotherapy treatment of cancer." 6 (20):11553–11573.

Hirsch, Leon R, R Jason Stafford, JA Bankson, Scott R Sershen, B Rivera, RE Price, John D Hazle, Naomi J Halas, and Jennifer L West %J Proceedings of the National Academy of Sciences. 2003. "Nanoshell-mediated near-infrared thermal therapy of tumors under magnetic resonance guidance." 100 (23):13549–13554.

Hong, Shiqi, Shoucang Shen, David Cheng Thiam Tan, Wai Kiong Ng, Xueming Liu, Leonard SO Chia, Anastasia W Irwan, Reginald Tan, Steven A Nowak, and Kennan Marsh. 2016. "High drug load, stable, manufacturable and bioavailable fenofibrate formulations in mesoporous silica: A comparison of spray drying versus solvent impregnation methods." *Drug delivery* 23 (1):316–327.

Hu, Bochuan, Xiaohui Xiao, Pin Chen, Jieying Qian, Guotao Yuan, Yayi Ye, Lingli Zeng, Suqin Zhong, Xiaoli Wang, and Xiaohua Qin %J Biomaterials. 2022. "Enhancing anti-tumor effect of ultrasensitive bimetallic RuCu nanoparticles as radiosensitizers with dual enzyme-like activities." 290:121811.

Hu, Liang, Hongrui Sun, Qinfu Zhao, Ning Han, Ling Bai, Ying Wang, Tongying Jiang, and Siling Wang %J Materials Science and Engineering: C. 2015. "Multilayer encapsulated mesoporous silica nanospheres as an oral sustained drug delivery system for the poorly water-soluble drug felodipine." 47:313–324.

Huang, Ping, Xiaoqin Qian, Yu Chen, Luodan Yu, Han Lin, Liying Wang, Yufang Zhu, and Jianlin Shi. 2017. "Metalloporphyrin-encapsulated biodegradable nanosystems for highly efficient magnetic resonance imaging-guided sonodynamic cancer therapy." *Journal of the American Chemical Society* 139 (3):1275–1284.

Huang, Shu, Jun Yuan, Yong Xie, Kai Qing, Zeya Shi, Guanyu Chen, Jie Gao, Haoxiang Tan, and Wenhu Zhou. 2023. "Targeting nano-regulator based on metal–organic frameworks for enhanced immunotherapy of bone metastatic prostate cancer." *Cancer Nanotechnology* 14 (1):43.

Huang, Xiaohua, and Mostafa A El-Sayed %J Journal of advanced research. 2010. "Gold nanoparticles: Optical properties and implementations in cancer diagnosis and photothermal therapy." 1 (1):13–28.

Huang, Xiaohua, Prashant K Jain, Ivan H El-Sayed, and Mostafa A El-Sayed %J Lasers in medical science. 2008. "Plasmonic photothermal therapy (PPTT) using gold nanoparticles." 23:217–228.

Huang, Xin, Sarita Devi, Matteo Bordiga, Charles S Brennan, and Baojun Xu. 2023. "Phenolic compounds mediated biosynthesis of gold nanoparticles and evaluation of their bioactivities: A review." *International Journal of Food Science & Technology* 58 (4):1673–1694.

Huang, Xinglu, Fan Zhang, Seulki Lee, Magdalena Swierczewska, Dale O Kiesewetter, Lixin Lang, Guofeng Zhang, Lei Zhu, Haokao Gao, and Hak Soo Choi %J Biomaterials. 2012. "Long-term multimodal imaging of tumor draining sentinel lymph nodes using mesoporous silica-based nanoprobes." 33 (17):4370–4378.

Hummers Jr, William S, and Richard E Offeman. 1958. "Preparation of graphitic oxide." *Journal of the American Chemical Society* 80 (6):1339–1339.

Hwang, Angela A, Jie Lu, Fuyuhiko Tamanoi, and Jeffrey I Zink %J small. 2015. "Functional nanovalves on protein-coated nanoparticles for in vitro and in vivo controlled drug delivery." 11 (3):319–328.

Hyder, Fahmeed, S Manjura Hoque %J Contrast Media and Molecular Imaging. 2017. "Brain tumor diagnostics and therapeutics with superparamagnetic ferrite nanoparticles." 2017.

Izci, Mukaddes, Christy Maksoudian, Bella B Manshian, and Stefaan J Soenen. 2021. "The use of alternative strategies for enhanced nanoparticle delivery to solid tumors." *Chemical Reviews* 121 (3):1746–1803.

Jadia, Rahul, Cody Scandore, Prakash Rai %J International journal of nanotechnology and nanomedicine. 2016. "Nanoparticles for effective combination therapy of cancer." 1 (1).

Jarockyte, Greta, Vitalijus Karabanovas, Ricardas Rotomskis, and Ali Mobasheri. 2020. "Multiplexed nanobiosensors: Current trends in early diagnostics." *Sensors* 20 (23):6890.

Jędrzak, Artur, Bartosz F Grześkowiak, Emerson Coy, Jacek Wojnarowicz, Kosma Szutkowski, Stefan Jurga, Teofil Jesionowski, Radosław Mrówczyński %J Colloids and Surfaces B: Biointerfaces. 2019. "Dendrimer based theranostic nanostructures for combined chemo-and photothermal therapy of liver cancer cells in vitro." 173:698–708.

Jiang, Bang-Ping, Bo Zhou, Zhaoxing Lin, Hong Liang, and Xing-Can Shen. 2019. "Recent advances in carbon nanomaterials for cancer phototherapy." *Chemistry–A European Journal* 25 (16):3993–4004.

Jin, Takashi, Fumihiko Fujii, Yutaka Komai, Junji Seki, Akitoshi Seiyama, and Yoshichika Yoshioka. 2008. "Preparation and characterization of highly fluorescent, glutathione-coated near infrared quantum dots for in vivo fluorescence imaging." *International Journal of Molecular Sciences* 9 (10): 2044–2061.

Jose, Jobin, Rajesh Kumar, Seetha Harilal, Githa Elizabeth Mathew, Della Grace Thomas Parambi, Ankitha Prabhu, Md Sahab Uddin, Lotfi Aleya, Hoon Kim, and Bijo Mathew. 2020. "Magnetic nanoparticles for hyperthermia in cancer treatment: An emerging tool." *Environmental Science and Pollution Research* 27:19214–19225.

Kan, Xuefeng, Feng Zhang, Guanhui Zhou, Hongxiu Ji, Wayne Monsky, Christopher Ingraham, Chuansheng Zheng, and Xiaoming Yang %J Proceedings of the National Academy of Sciences. 2021. "Interventional real-time optical imaging guidance for complete tumor ablation." 118 (41):e2113028118.

Kang, Sung Hun, Yong Kyu Lee, Il Seok Park, In-Kyu Park, Seok Min Hong, Soon Young Kwon, Young Hee Choi, Steen J Madsen, Henry Hirschberg, and Seok Jin Hong %J BioMed Research International. 2020. "Biomimetic gold nanoshell-loaded macrophage for photothermal biomedicine." 2020.

Kargar, Samira, Samideh Khoei, Sepideh Khoee, Sakine Shirvalilou, Seied Rabi Mahdavi %J Photodiagnosis and photodynamic therapy. 2018. "Evaluation of the combined effect of NIR laser and ionizing radiation on cellular damages induced by IUdR-loaded PLGA-coated Nano-graphene oxide." 21:91–97.

Karuppaiah, Arjunan, Dinesh Babu, Divakar Selvaraj, Tamilselvan Natrajan, Ravikumar Rajan, Mrinmoy Gautam, Hariprasad Ranganathan, Karthik Siram, Jerry Nesamony, and Veintramuthu Sankar %J European Journal of Pharmaceutical Sciences. 2021. "Building and behavior of a pH-stimuli responsive chitosan nanoparticles loaded with folic acid conjugated gemcitabine silver colloids in MDA-MB-453 metastatic breast cancer cell line and pharmacokinetics in rats." 165:105938.

Karuppaiah, Arjunan, Ravikumar Rajan, Muthiah Ramanathan, and Arumugam Nagarajan %J Asian Pacific Journal of Cancer Prevention: APJCP. 2020. "Cytotoxicity and synergistic effect of biogenically synthesized ternary therapeutic nano conjugates comprising plant active principle, silver and anticancer drug on MDA-MB-453 breast cancer cell line." 21 (1):195.

Katifelis, Hector, Anna Lyberopoulou, Iuliia Mukha, Nadiia Vityuk, Gallina Grodzyuk, George E Theodoropoulos, Efstathios P Efstathopoulos, and Maria Gazouli %J Artificial cells nanomedicine, and biotechnology. 2018. "Ag/Au bimetallic nanoparticles induce apoptosis in human cancer cell lines via P53, CASPASE-3 and BAX/BCL-2 pathways." 46 (sup3):389–398.

Katifelis, Hector, Iuliia Mukha, Penelope Bouziotis, Nadiia Vityuk, Charalampos Tsoukalas, Andreas C Lazaris, Anna Lyberopoulou, George E Theodoropoulos, Efstathios P Efstathopoulos, and Maria Gazouli %J International Journal of Nanomedicine. 2020. "Ag/Au bimetallic nanoparticles inhibit tumor growth and prevent metastasis in a mouse model."6019–6032.

Kim, Sang-Woo, Yeon Kyung Lee, Jong Yeon Lee, Jeong Hee Hong, and Dongwoo Khang. 2017. "PEGylated anticancer-carbon nanotubes complex targeting mitochondria of lung cancer cells." *Nanotechnology* 28 (46):465102.

Kinsella, Joseph M, Rebecca E Jimenez, Priya P Karmali, Anthony M Rush, V Ramana Kotamraju, Nathan C Gianneschi, Erkki Ruoslahti, Dwayne Stupack, and Michael J Sailor %J Angewandte Chemie International Edition. 2011. "X-ray computed tomography imaging of breast cancer by using targeted peptide-labeled bismuth sulfide nanoparticles." 50 (51):12308–12311.

Klostergaard, Jim, Charles E Seeney %J Nanomedicine: Nanotechnology Biology, and Medicine. 2012. "Magnetic nanovectors for drug delivery." 8:S37–S50.

Knights, Oscar B, and James R McLaughlan %J International Journal of Molecular Sciences. 2018. "Gold nanorods for light-based lung cancer theranostics." 19 (11):3318.

Kollenda, Sebastian A, Jasmin Klose, Torben Knuschke, Viktoriya Sokolova, Jochen Schmitz, Magdalena Staniszewska, Pedro Fragoso Costa, Ken Herrmann, Astrid M Westendorf, and Wolfgang P Fendler %J Acta biomaterialia. 2020. "In vivo biodistribution of calcium phosphate nanoparticles after intravascular, intramuscular, intratumoral, and soft tissue administration in mice investigated by small animal PET/CT." 109:244–253.

Kong, Xiangyi, Peng Gao, Jing Wang, Yi Fang, and Kuo Chu Hwang. 2023. "Advances of medical nanorobots for future cancer treatments." *Journal of Hematology & Oncology* 16 (1):74.

Koole, Rolf, Matti M van Schooneveld, Jan Hilhorst, Karolien Castermans, David P Cormode, Gustav J Strijkers, Celso de Mello Donegá, Daniel Vanmaekelbergh, Arjan W Griffioen, and Klaas Nicolay. 2008. "Paramagnetic lipid-coated silica nanoparticles with a fluorescent quantum dot core: A new contrast agent platform for multimodality imaging." *Bioconjugate Chemistry* 19 (12):2471–2479.

Kościk, Izabela, Daniel Jankowski, and Anna Jagusiak. 2021. "Carbon nanomaterials for theranostic use." *C* 8 (1):3.

Kumar, Harish, Nagasamy Venkatesh, Himangshu Bhowmik, and Anuttam Kuila. 2018. "Metallic nanoparticle: A review." *Biomedical Journal of Scientific & Technical Research* 4 (2):3765–3775.

Kumari, Preeti, Balaram Ghosh, and Swati Biswas %J Journal of drug targeting. 2016. "Nanocarriers for cancer-targeted drug delivery." 24 (3):179–191.

Kumawat, Mukesh Kumar, Mukesh chand Thakur, Raju B Gurung, and Rohit Srivastava. 2017. "Graphene quantum dots for cell proliferation, nucleus imaging, and photoluminescent sensing applications." *Scientific Reports* 7 (1):15858.

Kuntić, Vesna, Jasmina Brborić, Zorica Vujić, and Snežana Uskoković-Marković %J Asian Journal of Chemistry. 2016. "Radioisotopes used as radiotracers for in vitro and in vivo diagnostics." 28 (2):235–241.

Kushwaha, Swatantra Kumar Singh, Saurav Ghoshal, Awani Kumar Rai, and Satyawan Singh. 2013. "Carbon nanotubes as a novel drug delivery system for anticancer therapy: A review." *Brazilian Journal of Pharmaceutical Sciences* 49:629–643.

Kwatra, Deep, Anand Venugopal, and Shrikant Anant %J Translational Cancer Research. 2013. "Nanoparticles in radiation therapy: A summary of various approaches to enhance radiosensitization in cancer." 2 (4).

Lell, Michael M, and Marc Kachelrieß %J Investigative radiology. 2020. "Recent and upcoming technological developments in computed tomography: High speed, low dose, deep learning, multienergy." 55 (1):8–19.

Li, Cuncheng, Kevin L Shuford, Q Han Park, Weiping Cai, Yue Li, Eun Je Lee, and Sung Oh Cho. 2007. "High-yield synthesis of single-crystalline gold nano-octahedra." *Angewandte Chemie-International Edition* 46 (18):3264–3268.

Li, Haiqing, Sing I Song, Ga Young Song, and Il Kim. 2014. "Non-covalently functionalized carbon nanostructures for synthesizing carbon-based hybrid nanomaterials." *Journal of Nanoscience and Nanotechnology* 14 (2):1425–1440.

Li, Shuhua, Shixin Zhou, Yunchao Li, Xiaohong Li, Jia Zhu, Louzhen Fan, and Shihe Yang. 2017. "Exceptionally high payload of the IR780 iodide on folic acid-functionalized graphene quantum dots for targeted photothermal therapy." *ACS Applied Materials & Interfaces* 9 (27):22332–22341.

Li, Wen, Han Zhang, Yehuda G Assaraf, Kun Zhao, Xiaojun Xu, Jinbing Xie, Dong-Hua Yang, and Zhe-Sheng Chen %J Drug Resistance Updates. 2016. "Overcoming ABC transporter-mediated multidrug resistance: Molecular mechanisms and novel therapeutic drug strategies." 27:14–29.

Li, Yao, Xiao Zhao, Xiaoli Liu, Keman Cheng, Xuexiang Han, Yinlong Zhang, Huan Min, Guangna Liu, Junchao Xu, and Jian Shi %J Advanced Materials. 2020. "A bioinspired nanoprobe with multilevel responsive T1-weighted MR signal-amplification illuminates ultrasmall metastases." 32 (4):1906799.

Li, Yulin, Liudi Wang, Guoqiang Zhong, Guoying Wang, Yanzhao Zhu, Jian Li, Lan Xiao, Yanhui Chu, Yan Wu, and Kaichun Li. 2023. "Size-transformable nanoparticles with sequentially triggered drug release and enhanced penetration for anticancer therapy." *Nano Research* 16 (8):11186–11196.

Lin, Xin, Jin Xie, Gang Niu, Fan Zhang, Haokao Gao, Min Yang, Qimeng Quan, Maria A Aronova, Guofeng Zhang, and Seulki Lee %J Nano letters. 2011. "Chimeric ferritin nanocages for multiple function loading and multimodal imaging." 11 (2):814–819.

Lindner, Lars H, Jean-Yves Blay, Alexander MM Eggermont, and Rolf D Issels %J European Journal of Cancer. 2021. "Perioperative chemotherapy and regional hyperthermia for high-risk adult-type soft tissue sarcomas." 147:164–169.

Liu, Tracy W, Thomas D MacDonald, Cheng S Jin, Joseph M Gold, Robert G Bristow, Brian C Wilson, and Gang Zheng %J ACS nano. 2013. "Inherently multimodal nanoparticle-driven tracking and real-time delineation of orthotopic prostate tumors and micrometastases." 7 (5):4221–4232.

Liu, Xinhe, Ying Liu, Junning Wang, Tianxiang Wei, Zhihui Dai %J ACS applied materials and interfaces. 2019. "Mild hyperthermia-enhanced enzyme-mediated tumor cell chemodynamic therapy." 11 (26): 23065–23071.

Liu, Zhuang, Menglong Zhao, Han Lin, Chen Dai, Caiyue Ren, Shengjian Zhang, Weijun Peng, and Yu Chen %J Journal of Materials Chemistry B. 2018. "2D magnetic titanium carbide MXene for cancer theranostics." 6 (21):3541–3548.

Lorandi, Francesca, Marco Fantin, and Krzysztof Matyjaszewski. 2022. "Atom transfer radical polymerization: A mechanistic perspective." *Journal of the American Chemical Society* 144 (34):15413–15430.

Lu, Yu-Jen, Yu-Hsiang Lan, Chi-Cheng Chuang, Wan-Ting Lu, Li-Yang Chan, Peng-Wei Hsu, and Jyh-Ping Chen. 2020. "Injectable thermo-sensitive chitosan hydrogel containing CPT-11-loaded EGFR-targeted graphene oxide and SLP2 shRNA for localized drug/gene delivery in glioblastoma therapy." *International Journal of Molecular Sciences* 21 (19):7111.

Lusic, Hrvoje, and Mark W Grinstaff %J Chemical reviews. 2013. "X-ray-computed tomography contrast agents." 113 (3):1641–1666.

Lux, François, Vu Long Tran, Eloise Thomas, Sandrine Dufort, Fabien Rossetti, Matteo Martini, Charles Truillet, Tristan Doussineau, Guillaume Bort, and Franck Denat. 2019. "AGuIX® from bench to bedside—Transfer of an ultrasmall theranostic gadolinium-based nanoparticle to clinical medicine." *The British Journal of Radiology* 92 (1093):20180365.

Ma, Xuehua, An Gong, Bin Chen, Jianjun Zheng, Tianxiang Chen, Zheyu Shen, Aiguo Wu %J Colloids and Surfaces B: Biointerfaces. 2015. "Exploring a new SPION-based MRI contrast agent with excellent water-dispersibility, high specificity to cancer cells and strong MR imaging efficacy." 126:44–49.

Maeda, Hiroshi %J Advances in enzyme regulation. 2001. "The enhanced permeability and retention (EPR) effect in tumor vasculature: The key role of tumor-selective macromolecular drug targeting." 41 (1): 189–207.

Mahor, Alok, Prem Prakash Singh, Peeyush Bharadwaj, Neeraj Sharma, Surabhi Yadav, Jessica M Rosenholm, and Kuldeep K Bansal. 2021. "Carbon-based nanomaterials for delivery of biologicals and therapeutics: A cutting-edge technology." *C* 7 (1):19.

Malam, Yogesh kumar, Marilena Loizidou, and Alexander M Seifalian. 2009. "Liposomes and nanoparticles: Nanosized vehicles for drug delivery in cancer." *Trends in Pharmacological Sciences* 30 (11):592–599.

Maldiney, Thomas, Bich-Thuy Doan, Damien Alloyeau, Michel Bessodes, Daniel Scherman, and Cyrille Richard %J Advanced Functional Materials. 2015. "Gadolinium-doped persistent nanophosphors as versatile tool for multimodal in vivo imaging." 25 (2):331–338.

Maleki, Reza, Hamid Hassanzadeh Afrouzi, Mirollah Hosseini, Davood Toghraie, and Sara Rostami. 2020. "Molecular dynamics simulation of Doxorubicin loading with N-isopropyl acrylamide carbon nanotube in a drug delivery system." *Computer Methods and Programs in Biomedicine* 184:105303.

Mamaeva, Veronika, Cecilia Sahlgren, and Mika Lindén. 2013. "Mesoporous silica nanoparticles in medicine—Recent advances." *Advanced Drug Delivery Reviews* 65 (5):689–702.

Mansoori, Behzad, Siamak Sandoghchian Shotorbani, and Behzad Baradaran %J Advanced pharmaceutical bulletin. 2014. "RNA interference and its role in cancer therapy." 4 (4):313.

Mattoli, Maria Vittoria, Gianluca Trevisi, Valentina Scolozzi, Amedeo Capotosti, Fabrizio Cocciolillo, Irene Marini, Valerio Mare, Luca Indovina, Massimo Caulo, and Antonella Saponiero %J Cancers. 2021. "Dynamic 11C-methionine PET-CT: Prognostic factors for disease progression and survival in patients with suspected glioma recurrence." 13 (19):4777.

Medarova, Zdravka, Wellington Pham, Christian Farrar, Victoria Petkova, and Anna Moore. 2007. "In vivo imaging of siRNA delivery and silencing in tumors." *Nature Medicine* 13 (3):372–377.

Misra, Ranjita, Sarbari Acharya, and Sanjeeb K Sahoo %J Drug discovery today. 2010. "Cancer nanotechnology: Application of nanotechnology in cancer therapy." 15 (19–20):842–850.

Miyoshi, N, SK Kundu, T Tuziuti, K Yasui, I Shimada, Y Ito %J Nanoscience and nanoengineering. 2016. "Combination of sonodynamic and photodynamic therapy against cancer would be effective through using a regulated size of nanoparticles." 4 (1):1.

Mokhtari, Reza Bayat, Tina S Homayouni, Narges Baluch, Evgeniya Morgatskaya, Sushil Kumar, Bikul Das, and Herman Yeger %J Onco target. 2017. "Combination therapy in combating cancer." 8 (23):38022.

Moniruzzaman, Md, Sayan Deb Dutta, Ki-Taek Lim, and Jongsung Kim %J Applied Surface Science. 2022. "Wet chemistry-based processing of tunable polychromatic carbon quantum dots for multicolor bioimaging and enhanced NIR-triggered photothermal bactericidal efficacy." 597:153630.

Munirathnappa, Archana K, Sachin Kumar Maurya, Kaushal Kumar, Kavitha Keshava Navada, Ananda Kulal, Nalini G Sundaram %J Materials Science and Engineering: C. 2020. "Scheelite like NaTb (WO4) 2 nanoparticles: Green fluorescence and in vitro cell imaging applications." 106:110182.

Nahrendorf, Matthias, Edmund Keliher, Brett Marinelli, Peter Waterman, Paolo Fumene Feruglio, Lioubov Fexon, Misha Pivovarov, Filip K Swirski, Mikael J Pittet, and Claudio Vinegoni %J Proceedings of the National Academy of Sciences. 2010. "Hybrid PET-optical imaging using targeted probes." 107 (17): 7910–7915.

Neumaier, Carlo Emanuele, Gabriella Baio, Silvano Ferrini, Giorgio Corte, and Antonio Daga %J Tumori. 2008. "MR and iron magnetic nanoparticles. Imaging opportunities in preclinical and translational research." 94 (2):226–233.

Nigam, Manisha, Abhay Prakash Mishra, Vishal Kumar Deb, Deen Bandhu Dimri, Vinod Tiwari, Simona Gabriela Bungau, Alexa Florina Bungau, and Andrei-Flavius Radu %J Biomedicine and Pharmacotherapy. 2023. "Evaluation of the association of chronic inflammation and cancer: Insights and implications." 164:115015.

Niroumand, Uranous, Negar Firouzabadi, Ghazal Goshtasbi, Bahareh Hassani, Parisa Ghasemiyeh, and Soliman Mohammadi-Samani. 2023. "The effect of size, morphology and surface properties of mesoporous silica nanoparticles on pharmacokinetic aspects and potential toxicity concerns." *Frontiers in Materials* 10:1189463.

Nogueira, Daniele Rubert, Lorena Tavano, Montserrat Mitjans, Lourdes Pérez, M Rosa Infante, and M Pilar Vinardell %J Biomaterials. 2013. "In vitro antitumor activity of methotrexate via pH-sensitive chitosan nanoparticles." 34 (11):2758–2772.

Norouzi, Mohammad, Vinith Yathindranath, James A Thliveris, Brian M Kopec, Teruna J Siahaan, and Donald W Miller %J Scientific reports. 2020. "Doxorubicin-loaded iron oxide nanoparticles for glioblastoma therapy: A combinational approach for enhanced delivery of nanoparticles." 10 (1):11292.

Nosrati, Hamed, Elahe Attari, Fatemeh Abhari, Murat Barsbay, Mohammadreza Ghaffarlou, Navid Mousazadeh, Rasoul Vaezi, Taras Kavetskyy, Hamed Rezaeejam, and Thomas J Webster %J Bioactive materials. 2022. "Complete ablation of tumors using synchronous chemoradiation with bimetallic theranostic nanoparticles." 7:74–84.

Nosrati, Hamed, Mohammadreza Ghaffarlou, Marziyeh Salehiabar, Navid Mousazadeh, Fatemeh Abhari, Murat Barsbay, Yavuz Nuri Ertas, Hamid Rashidzadeh, Ali Mohammadi, and Leila Nasehi %J Biomaterials advances. 2022. "Magnetite and bismuth sulfide Janus heterostructures as radiosensitizers for in vivo enhanced radiotherapy in breast cancer." 140:213090.

Nurunnabi, Md, Kwang Jae Cho, Joon Sig Choi, Kang Moo Huh, and Yong-kyu %J Biomaterials Lee. 2010. "Targeted near-IR QDs-loaded micelles for cancer therapy and imaging." 31 (20):5436–5444.

Nurunnabi, Md, Zehedina Khatun, Md Nafiujjaman, Dong-geun Lee, and Yong-kyu Lee. 2013. "Surface coating of graphene quantum dots using mussel-inspired polydopamine for biomedical optical imaging." *ACS Applied Materials & Interfaces* 5 (16):8246–8253.

Palazzolo, Stefano, Samer Bayda, Mohamad Hadla, Isabella Caligiuri, Giuseppe Corona, Giuseppe Toffoli, and Flavio Rizzolio %J Current medicinal chemistry. 2018. "The clinical translation of organic nanomaterials for cancer therapy: A focus on polymeric nanoparticles, micelles, liposomes and exosomes." 25 (34):4224–4268.

Pandey, Anushree, Asif Ali, and Yuvraj Negi %J Materials Today: Proceedings. 2021. "Synthesis of polygonal chitosan microcapsules for the delivery of amygdalin loaded silver nanoparticles in breast cancer therapy." 43:3744–3748.

Parkatzidis, Kostas, Hyun Suk Wang, Nghia P Truong, and Athina Anastasaki. 2020. "Recent developments and future challenges in controlled radical polymerization: A 2020 update." *Chem* 6 (7):1575–1588.

Pattnaik, Satyanarayan, Kalpana Swain, and Zhiqun Lin. 2016. "Graphene and graphene-based nanocomposites: Biomedical applications and biosafety." *Journal of Materials Chemistry B* 4 (48):7813–7831.

Petushkov, Anton, Nicholas Ndiege, Aliasger K Salem, and Sarah C Larsen. 2010. "Toxicity of silica nanomaterials: Zeolites, mesoporous silica, and amorphous silica nanoparticles." In *Advances in Molecular Toxicology*, 223–266. Elsevier.

Prabhakar, Uma, Hiroshi Maeda, Rakesh K Jain, Eva M Sevick-Muraca, William Zamboni, Omid C Farokhzad, Simon T Barry, Alberto Gabizon, Piotr Grodzinski, and David C Blakey. 2013. *Challenges and key considerations of the enhanced permeability and retention effect for nanomedicine drug delivery in oncology*. AACR.

Pradhan, Narayan, David M Battaglia, Yongcheng Liu, and Xiaogang Peng. 2007. "Efficient, stable, small, and water-soluble doped ZnSe nanocrystal emitters as non-cadmium biomedical labels." *Nano Letters* 7 (2):312–317.

Pradhan, Pallab, Jyotsnendu Giri, Finn Rieken, Christian Koch, Olga Mykhaylyk, Markus Döblinger, Rinti Banerjee, Dhirendra Bahadur, and Christian Plank. 2010. "Targeted temperature sensitive magnetic liposomes for thermo-chemotherapy." *Journal of Controlled Release* 142 (1):108–121.

Prasanna, SRV Siva, K Balaji, Shyam Pandey, and Sravendra Rana. 2019. "Metal oxide based nanomaterials and their polymer nanocomposites." In *Nanomaterials and polymer nanocomposites*, 123–144. Elsevier.

Qi, Xiaoliang, Xianqin Tong, Shengye You, Ruiting Mao, Erya Cai, Wenhao Pan, Chenhao Zhang, Rongdang Hu, and Jianliang Shen %J ACS macro letters. 2022. "Mild hyperthermia-assisted ROS scavenging hydrogels achieve diabetic wound healing." 11 (7):861–867.

Qiao, Han, Zhaowen Cui, Shengbing Yang, Dingkun Ji, Yugang Wang, Ying Yang, Xiuguo Han, Qiming Fan, An Qin, and Tingyu Wang %J ACS nano. 2017. "Targeting osteocytes to attenuate early breast cancer bone metastasis by theranostic upconversion nanoparticles with responsive plumbagin release." 11 (7):7259–7273.

Qin, Si-Yong, Yin-Jia Cheng, Qi Lei, Ai-Qing Zhang, and Xian-Zheng Zhang %J Biomaterials. 2018. "Combinational strategy for high-performance cancer chemotherapy." 171:178–197.

Rajakumar, Timothy, Musaab Yassin, Omar Musbahi, Eli Harris, J Francisco Lopez, Richard J Bryant, Iain DC Tullis, Borivoj Vojnovic, Freddie C Hamdy, and Alastair D Lamb %J Future Oncology. 2020. "Use of intraoperative fluorescence to enhance robot-assisted radical prostatectomy." 17 (9):1083–1095.

Rajan, Arunima, and Niroj Kumar Sahu. 2020. "Review on magnetic nanoparticle-mediated hyperthermia for cancer therapy." *Journal of Nanoparticle Research* 22:1–25.

Rembielak, Agata, and T Ajithkumar %J Clinical Oncology. 2019. "Non-melanoma skin cancer–an underestimated global health threat?" 31 (11):735–737.

Ren, Feng, Hanghang Liu, Hao Zhang, Zhilin Jiang, Bing Xia, Cécile Genevois, Tao He, Mathieu Allix, Qiao Sun, and Zhen Li %J Nano Today. 2020. "Engineering NIR-IIb fluorescence of Er-based lanthanide nanoparticles for through-skull targeted imaging and imaging-guided surgery of orthotopic glioma." 34: 100905.

Ren, Tongtong, Yufan Wang, Qilin Yu, and Mingchun Li. 2019. "Synthesis of antimicrobial peptide-grafted graphene oxide nanosheets with high antimicrobial efficacy." *Materials Letters* 235:42–45.

Resnier, Pauline, Tristan Montier, Véronique Mathieu, Jean-Pierre Benoit, and Catherine Passirani. 2013. "A review of the current status of siRNA nanomedicines in the treatment of cancer." *Biomaterials* 34 (27):6429–6443.

Rheima, Ahmed Mahdi, Mahdi A Mohammed, Shaimaa Hamed Jaber, and Shahad Abbas Hameed. 2019. "Synthesis of silver nanoparticles using the UV-irradiation technique in an antibacterial application." *Journal of Southwest Jiaotong University* 54 (5).

Rozalen, M, Manuel Sánchez-Polo, M Fernández-Perales, TJ Widmann, and José Rivera-Utrilla. 2020. "Synthesis of controlled-size silver nanoparticles for the administration of methotrexate drug and its activity in colon and lung cancer cells." *RSC Advances* 10 (18):10646–10660.

Salavati-Niasari, Masoud, Fatemeh Davar, and Noshin Mir. 2008. "Synthesis and characterization of metallic copper nanoparticles via thermal decomposition." *Polyhedron* 27 (17):3514–3518.

Sanz-Moreno, Victoria, and Christopher J Marshall. 2010. "The plasticity of cytoskeletal dynamics underlying neoplastic cell migration." *Current Opinion in Cell Biology* 22 (5):690–696.

Senapati, Sudipta, Arun Kumar Mahanta, Sunil Kumar, and Pralay Maiti. 2018. "Controlled drug delivery vehicles for cancer treatment and their performance." *Signal transduction and targeted therapy* 3 (1):7.

Serov, Nikita, and Vladimir Vinogradov. 2022. "Artificial intelligence to bring nanomedicine to life." *Advanced Drug Delivery Reviews* 184:114194.

Sharifi, Majid, Farnoosh Attar, Ali Akbar Saboury, Keivan Akhtari, Nasrin Hooshmand, Anwarul Hasan, Mostafa A El-Sayed, and Mojtaba Falahati. 2019. "Plasmonic gold nanoparticles: Optical manipulation, imaging, drug delivery and therapy." *Journal of Controlled Release* 311:170–189.

Shi, Hua, Runqi Yan, Luyan Wu, Yidan Sun, Song Liu, Zhengyang Zhou, Jian He, and Deju Ye %J Acta Biomaterialia. 2018. "Tumor-targeting CuS nanoparticles for multimodal imaging and guided photothermal therapy of lymph node metastasis." 72:256–265.

Shilo, Malka, Tobi Reuveni, Menachem Motiei, and Rachela Popovtzer %J Nanomedicine. 2012. "Nanoparticles as computed tomography contrast agents: Current status and future perspectives." 7 (2):257–269.

Shmarakov, Igor, Iuliia Mukha, Nadiia Vityuk, Vira Borschovetska, Nelya Zhyshchynska, Galyna Grodzyuk, and Anna Eremenko %J Nanoscale research letters. 2017. "Antitumor activity of alloy and core-shell-type bimetallic AgAu nanoparticles." 12:1–10.

Sivamaruthi, Bhagavathi Sundaram, Vijayan Sri Ramkumar, Govindaraju Archunan, Chaiyavat Chaiyasut, Natarajan Suganthy %J Journal of Drug Delivery Science and Technology. 2019. "Biogenic synthesis of silver palladium bimetallic nanoparticles from fruit extract of Terminalia chebula–In vitro evaluation of anticancer and antimicrobial activity." 51:139–151.

Smith, Andrew M, and Shuming Nie. 2009. "Next-generation quantum dots." *Nature biotechnology* 27 (8): 732–733.

Song, Guosheng, Liang Cheng, Yu Chao, Kai Yang, and Zhuang Liu %J Advanced materials. 2017. "Emerging nanotechnology and advanced materials for cancer radiation therapy." 29 (32):1700996.

Spirou, Spiridon V, Sofia A Costa Lima, Penelope Bouziotis, Sanja Vranješ-Djurić, Eleni K Efthimiadou, Anna Laurenzana, Ana Isabel Barbosa, Ignacio Garcia-Alonso, Carlton Jones, and Drina Jankovic. 2018. "Recommendations for in vitro and in vivo testing of magnetic nanoparticle hyperthermia combined with radiation therapy." *Nanomaterials* 8 (5):306.

Stephen, Zachary R, Forrest M Kievit, and Miqin Zhang. 2011. "Magnetite nanoparticles for medical MR imaging." *Materials Today* 14 (7–8):330–338.

Su, Xiang-Yu, Pei-Dang Liu, Hao Wu, Ning Gu %J Cancer biology and medicine. 2014. "Enhancement of radiosensitization by metal-based nanoparticles in cancer radiation therapy." 11 (2):86.

Sun, Minghao, Gobalakrishnan Sundaresan, Purnima Jose, Likun Yang, David Hoffman, Narottam Lamichhane, and Jamal Zweit %J Journal of Materials Chemistry B. 2014. "Highly stable intrinsically radiolabeled indium-111 quantum dots with multidentate zwitterionic surface coating: Dual modality tool for biological imaging." 2 (28):4456–4466.

Suto, Makoto, Yasutake Hirota, Hiroaki Mamiya, Asaya Fujita, Ryo Kasuya, Kazuyuki Tohji, Balachandran Jeyadevan %J Journal of Magnetism and Magnetic Materials. 2009. "Heat dissipation mechanism of magnetite nanoparticles in magnetic fluid hyperthermia." 321 (10):1493–1496.

Swayampakula, Anil Kumar, Charlotte Dillis, and Jame Abraham %J Expert review of anticancer therapy. 2008. "Role of MRI in screening, diagnosis and management of breast cancer." 8 (5):811–817.

Tang, Fangqiong, Linlin Li, and Dong Chen. 2012. "Mesoporous silica nanoparticles: Synthesis, biocompatibility and drug delivery." *Advanced Materials* 24 (12):1504–1534.

Thapa, Riya, Haider Ali, Obaid Afzal, Asif Ahmad Bhat, Waleed Hassan Almalki, Sami I Alzarea, Imran Kazmi, Abdulmalik Saleh Alfawaz Altamimi, Neha Jain, and Manisha Pandey. 2023. "Unlocking the potential of mesoporous silica nanoparticles in breast cancer treatment." *Journal of Nanoparticle Research* 25 (8):169.

Tian, Yuchen, Anggrek C Nusantara, Thamir Hamoh, Aldona Mzyk, Xiaobo Tian, Felipe Perona Martinez, Runrun Li, Hjalmar P Permentier, Romana Schirhagl %J ACS Applied Materials and Interfaces. 2022. "Functionalized fluorescent nanodiamonds for simultaneous drug delivery and quantum sensing in HeLa cells." 14 (34):39265–39273.

Tian, Shuyu, Rory Stevens, Bridget T McInnes, and Nastassja A Lewinski %J Micromachines. 2021. "Machine assisted experimentation of extrusion-based bioprinting systems." 12 (7):780.

Tietze, Rainer, and Christoph Alexiou %J Nanomedicine. 2017. "Improving cancer imaging with magnetic nanoparticles: Where are we now?" *Future Medicine* 12 (3):167–170.

Ting, Gann, Chih-Hsien Chang, Hsin-Ell Wang, and Te-Wei Lee %J BioMed Research International. 2010. "Nanotargeted radionuclides for cancer nuclear imaging and internal radiotherapy." 2010.

Tonga, Gulen Yesilbag, Daniel F Moyano, Chang Soo Kim, and Vincent M Rotello. 2014. "Inorganic nanoparticles for therapeutic delivery: Trials, tribulations and promise." *Current Opinion in Colloid & Interface Science* 19 (2):49–55.

Torchilin, Vladimir P. 2007. "Micellar nanocarriers: Pharmaceutical perspectives." *Pharmaceutical Research* 24:1–16.

Vallet-Regi, María, A Rámila, RP Del Real, and Pérez-Pariente %J Chemistry of Materials. 2001. "A new property of MCM-41: Drug delivery system." 13 (2):308–311.

Vallet-Regí, María, Ferdi Schüth, Daniel Lozano, Montserrat Colilla, and Miguel Manzano. 2022. "Engineering mesoporous silica nanoparticles for drug delivery: Where are we after two decades?" *Chemical Society Reviews* 51 (13):5365–5451.

Velikyan, Irina %J Contrast Media, and Molecular Imaging. 2018. "Prospective of 68 Ga radionuclide contribution to the development of imaging agents for infection and inflammation." 2018.

Venkatasubbu, G Devanand, S Ramasamy, V Ramakrishnan, and J Kumar %J Advanced Powder Technology. 2013. "Folate targeted PEGylated titanium dioxide nanoparticles as a nanocarrier for targeted paclitaxel drug delivery." 24 (6):947–954.

Vlasenkova, Mariya I, Ekaterina S Dolinina, and Elena V Parfenyuk. 2019. "Preparation of mesoporous silica microparticles by sol–gel/emulsion route for protein release." *Pharmaceutical Development and Technology* 24 (2):243–252.

Voskuil, Floris Jan, Steven Jakob de Jongh, Wouter Tjerk Rudolph Hooghiemstra, Matthijs David Linssen, Pieter Jan Steinkamp, Sebastiaan Antonius Hendrik Johannes de Visscher, Kees-Pieter Schepman, Sjoerd Geert Elias, Gert-Jan Meersma, and Pascal Klaas Christiaan Jonker %J Theranostics. 2020. "Fluorescence-guided imaging for resection margin evaluation in head and neck cancer patients using cetuximab-800CW: A quantitative dose-escalation study." 10 (9):3994.

Vu-Quang, Hieu, Mads Sloth Vinding, Thomas Nielsen, Marcus Görge Ullisch, Niels Chr Nielsen, Dinh-Truong Nguyen, and Jørgen Kjems %J Polymers. 2019. "Pluronic F127-folate coated super paramagenic iron oxide nanoparticles as contrast agent for cancer diagnosis in magnetic resonance imaging." 11 (4):743.

Wagner, Ilona, Simon Spiegel, Julian Brückel, Matthias Schwotzer, Alexander Welle, Martina H Stenzel, Stefan Bräse, Salma Begum, and Manuel Tsotsalas. 2023. "Biofunctionalization of Metal–Organic Framework Nanoparticles via Combined Nitroxide-Mediated Polymerization and Nitroxide Exchange Reaction." *Macromolecular Materials and Engineering* 308 (9):2300048.

Wang, Changyuan, Yang Wang, Wangchuan Xiao, Xiaohua Chen, Renfu Li, Zhiyong Shen, and Fengchun Lu %J BMC cancer. 2023. "Carboxylated superparamagnetic Fe3O4 nanoparticles modified with 3-amino propanol and their application in magnetic resonance tumor imaging." 23 (1):54.

Wang, Daquan, Ning Zhang, Xunan Jing, Yun Zhang, Yanzi Xu, and Lingjie Meng %J Journal of Materials Chemistry B. 2020. "Retracted Article: A tumor-microenvironment fully responsive nano-platform for MRI-guided photodynamic and photothermal synergistic therapy." 8 (36):8271–8281.

Wang, Fangfang, Zhongping Chen, and Li Zhu %J Journal of Liposome Research. 2015. "cRGD-conjugated magnetic-fluorescent liposomes for targeted dual-modality imaging of bone metastasis from prostate cancer." 25 (2):89–100.

Wang, Haitao, Jingran Bi, Bei-Wei Zhu, and Mingqian Tan. 2018. "Multicolorful carbon dots for tumor theranostics." *Current Medicinal Chemistry* 25 (25):2894–2909.

Wang, Liucan, Haidi Guan, Zhenqiang Wang, Yuxin Xing, Jixi Zhang, and Kaiyong Cai %J Molecular pharmaceutics. 2018. "Hybrid mesoporous–microporous nanocarriers for overcoming multidrug resistance by sequential drug delivery." 15 (7):2503–2512.

Wang, Yun, Feihu Wang, Ying Liu, Shaohui Xu, Yuanyuan Shen, Nianping Feng, and Shengrong Guo %J Acta Biomaterialia. 2018. "Glutathione detonated and pH responsive nano-clusters of Au nanorods with a high dose of DOX for treatment of multidrug resistant cancer." 75:334–345.

Wen, Shihui, Kangan Li, Hongdong Cai, Qian Chen, Mingwu Shen, Yunpeng Huang, Chen Peng, Wenxiu Hou, Meifang Zhu, and Guixiang Zhang %J Biomaterials. 2013. "Multifunctional dendrimer-entrapped gold nanoparticles for dual mode CT/MR imaging applications." 34 (5):1570–1580.

Wu, Kai, and Jian-Ping Wang. 2017. "Magnetic hyperthermia performance of magnetite nanoparticle assemblies under different driving fields." *AIP Advances* 7 (5).

Wu, Xingyong, Hongjian Liu, Jianquan Liu, Kari N Haley, Joseph A Treadway, J Peter Larson, Nianfeng Ge, Frank Peale, and Marcel P Bruchez. 2003. "Immunofluorescent labeling of cancer marker Her2 and other cellular targets with semiconductor quantum dots." *Nature Biotechnology* 21 (1):41–46.

Xie, Jin, Gang Liu, Henry S Eden, Hua Ai, and Xiaoyuan Chen. 2011. "Surface-engineered magnetic nanoparticle platforms for cancer imaging and therapy." *Accounts of Chemical Research* 44 (10):883–892.

Xu, Lijie, Xiaoping Jiang, Kang Liang, Meng Gao, and Biao Kong %J Aggregate. 2022. "Frontier luminous strategy of functional silica nanohybrids in sensing and bioimaging: From ACQ to AIE." 3 (1):e121.

Yang, Geng, Ting Song, Meng Wang, Mengyue Li, QingQing Su, Zhengxin Xie, Xiaoxue Xie, Hanxi Zhang, Yi Feng, and Chunhui Wu. 2022. "Recent advancements in nanosystem-based molecular beacons for RNA detection and imaging." *ACS Applied Nano Materials* 5 (3):3065–3086.

Yang, Ke, Shaojing Zhao, Baoling Li, Benhua Wang, Minhuan Lan, and Xiangzhi Song %J Coordination Chemistry Reviews. 2022. "Low temperature photothermal therapy: Advances and perspectives." 454:214330.

Yang, Nicole J, Marlon J Hinner %J Site-Specific Protein Labeling: Methods and Protocols. 2015. "Getting across the cell membrane: An overview for small molecules, peptides, and proteins."29–53.

Yang, Shuguang, Liang Chen, Xiaojun Zhou, Ping Sun, Liwen Fu, Yanling You, Man Xu, Zhengwei You, Guoyin Kai, and Chuanglong He %J Chemical Engineering Journal. 2019. "Tumor-targeted biodegradable multifunctional nanoparticles for cancer theranostics." 378:122171.

Yang, Wenjie, Huazheng Liang, Songhua Ma, Devin Wang, Jun Huang %J Sustainable Materials and Technologies. 2019. "Gold nanoparticle based photothermal therapy: Development and application for effective cancer treatment." 22:e00109.

Yardley, Denise A %J International journal of breast cancer. 2013. "Drug resistance and the role of combination chemotherapy in improving patient outcomes." 2013.

Yi, Xuan, Kai Yang, Chao Liang, Xiaoyan Zhong, Ping Ning, Guosheng Song, Dongliang Wang, Cuicui Ge, Chunying Chen, and Zhifang Chai %J Advanced Functional Materials. 2015. "Imaging-guided combined photothermal and radiotherapy to treat subcutaneous and metastatic tumors using iodine-131-doped copper sulfide nanoparticles." 25 (29):4689–4699.

Yousefi, Seyede Raheleh, Azam Sobhani, Hassan Abbas Alshamsi, and Masoud Salavati-Niasari. 2021. "Green sonochemical synthesis of BaDy 2 NiO 5/Dy 2 O 3 and BaDy 2 NiO 5/NiO nanocomposites in the presence of core almond as a capping agent and their application as photocatalysts for the removal of organic dyes in water." *RSC Advances* 11 (19):11500–11512.

Zamani, Mostafa, Mojtaba Rostami, Mozhgan Aghajanzadeh, Hamidreza Kheiri Manjili, Kobra Rostamizadeh, and Hossein Danafar. 2018. "Mesoporous titanium dioxide@ zinc oxide–graphene oxide nanocarriers for colon-specific drug delivery." *Journal of Materials Science* 53 (3):1634–1645.

Zeng, Wei-Nan, Qiu-Ping Yu, Duan Wang, Jun-Li Liu, Qing-Jun Yang, Zong-Ke Zhou, and Yi-Ping %J Journal of nanobiotechnology Zeng. 2021. "Mitochondria-targeting graphene oxide nanocomposites for fluorescence imaging-guided synergistic phototherapy of drug-resistant osteosarcoma." 19:1–19.

Zhang, Dan, Xianya Qin, Tingting Wu, Qi Qiao, Qingle Song, and Zhiping Zhang %J Biomaterials. 2019. "Extracellular vesicles based self-grown gold nanopopcorn for combinatorial chemo-photothermal therapy." 197:220–228.

Zhang, Kun, Huixiong Xu, Xiaoqing Jia, Yu Chen, Ming Ma, Liping Sun, and Hangrong Chen %J ACS nano. 2016. "Ultrasound-triggered nitric oxide release platform based on energy transformation for targeted inhibition of pancreatic tumor." 10 (12):10816–10828.

Zhang, Yulin, Kaiyan Xi, Xiao Fu, Haifeng Sun, Hong Wang, Dexin Yu, Zhiwei Li, Yuan Ma, Xinjie Liu, and Bin Huang %J Biomaterials. 2021. "Versatile metal-phenolic network nanoparticles for multitargeted combination therapy and magnetic resonance tracing in glioblastoma." 278:121163.

Zhao, Xianxian, Weiyin Gao, Hong Zhang, Xiaopei Qiu, and Yang Luo. 2020. "Graphene quantum dots in biomedical applications: Recent advances and future challenges." *Handbook of Nanomaterials in Analytical Chemistry*:493–505.

Zhao, Xiuxian, Junhua Sun, Jiachen Ma, Tongyao Liu, Zeyi Guo, Zhen Yang, Wei Yao, and Xuchuan Jiang. 2022. "Combining reversible addition-fragmentation chain transfer polymerization and thiol-ene click reaction for application of core-shell structured VO2@ polymer nanoparticles to smart window." *Sustainable Materials and Technologies* 32:e00420.

Zhao, Zhiwen, Dangge Wang, and Yaping Li. 2023. "Versatile biomimetic nanomedicine for treating cancer and inflammation disease." *Medical Review* 3 (2):123–151.

Zhou, Jing, Xingjun Zhu, Min Chen, Yun Sun, and Fuyou Li %J Biomaterials. 2012. "Water-stable NaLuF4-based upconversion nanophosphors with long-term validity for multimodal lymphatic imaging." 33 (26): 6201–6210.

Zhu, Wenjun, Yu Yang, Qiutong Jin, Yu Chao, Longlong Tian, Jingjing Liu, Ziliang Dong, and Zhuang Liu %J Nano Research. 2019. "Two-dimensional metal-organic-framework as a unique theranostic nano-platform for nuclear imaging and chemo-photodynamic cancer therapy." 12:1307–1312.

Zrazhevskiy, Pavel, Mark Sena, and Xiaohu Gao. 2010. "Designing multifunctional quantum dots for bioimaging, detection, and drug delivery." *Chemical Society Reviews* 39 (11):4326–4354.

7 Engineered Silica-Based Nanoparticles for Anticancer Drug Delivery

Angelina Gogoi,[1] Anjan Boro,[1] and Manashjit Gogoi[2]
[1]Centre for Nanoscience and Technology, Pondicherry University, Kalapet, Puducherry, India
[2]Department of Biomedical Engineering, North-Eastern Hill University, Shillong, Meghalaya, India

7.1 INTRODUCTION

Engineered nanoparticles (NPs) have enormous promise to improve illness detection and treatment in medicine, one of the technical domains in which nanotechnology has revolutionized. The surge of interest in nanotechnology has significantly increased over the past several decades, particularly in the production of NPs (Bhattacharyya et al., 2009). The applications of NPs in the medical field, especially in targeted drug delivery systems, are particularly noteworthy. These NPs increase treatment efficacy while reducing adverse effects since they target diseased cells while protecting the healthy ones, paving the way for more effective and safer treatment options in modern healthcare. (Huang et al., 2010). The advancement of cancer therapies exemplifies significant progress within this field, as there has been a notable increase in effective treatment options over recent decades. This improvement is primarily attributed to an enhanced understanding of carcinogenesis, cellular biology, and the tumor microenvironment. (Hanahan & Weinberg, 2011; Sonnenschein & Soto, 2020). SiNPs are adaptable NPs that have been extensively researched for their potential use in biomedical fields. These NPs, mainly made of SiO_2, possess biocompatibility and chemical stability and can be created with precise control over their dimensions and form. Their surface is rich in -OH/HO- groups, allowing for easy functionalization with various chemical or biological molecules (Capeletti et al., 2018). The remarkable adaptability of SiNPs positions them as up-and-coming candidates for applications in drug delivery, imaging, and therapeutic interventions. Also, their intrinsic optical and mechanical properties significantly enhance their diagnostics and tissue engineering functionality. Engineered SiNPs can be tailored using different synthetic approaches to meet specific biomedical needs. Methods such as sol-gel processing, microemulsion, and Stöber techniques allow for the creation of NPs with exact size distributions and designated surface properties. Functional modifications, such as adding targeting ligands or responsive components, can improve specificity and effectiveness (Liberman et al., 2014).

The growing interest in SiNPs for drug delivery is evident from the sharp rise in related publications over the years, as shown in Figure 7.1. This highlights the expanding research efforts and the recognition of SiNPs' potential in modern cancer therapeutic solutions.

Building on the fundamental framework of silica, MSNPs have emerged as a more advanced class of nanocarriers (NCs). MSNPs have become a focus for researchers in the field of cancer therapies. They are positioned as prospective NCs due to their benefits, which include scalable manufacture, changeable pore size (Bouchoucha et al., 2016), pore volume (Farjadian et al., 2019),

DOI: 10.1201/9781003799351-7

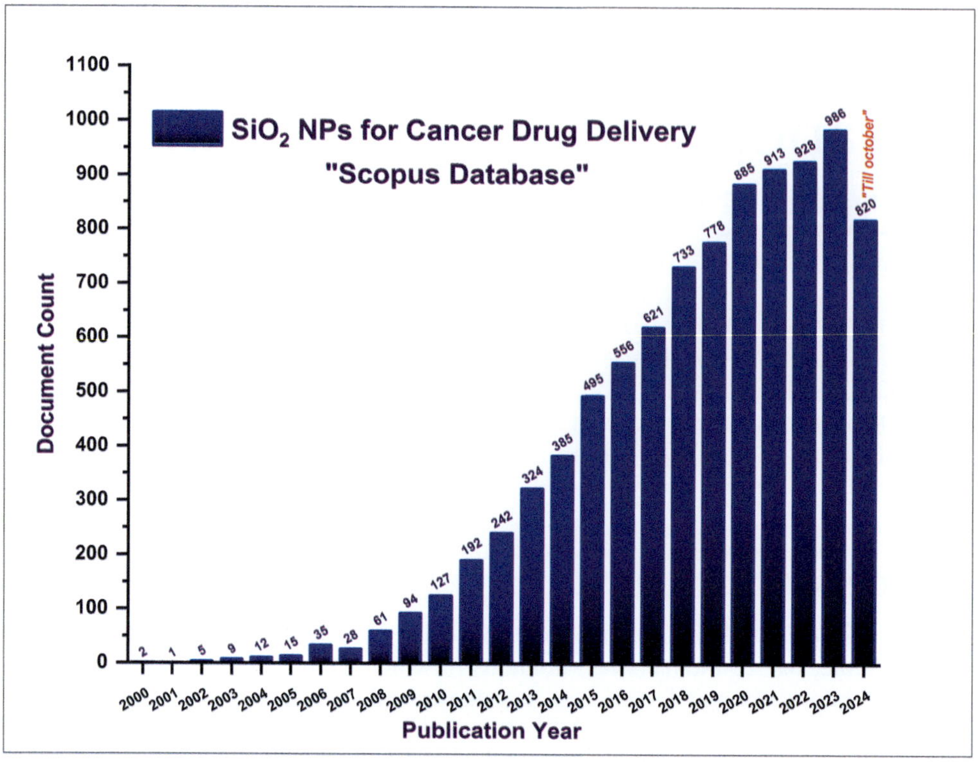

FIGURE 7.1 The number of publications contextualized within the framework of the topic of "silica nanoparticles for cancer drug delivery", indexed on the Scopus from the inception of records until October 2024.

and large surface area. For example, folate-conjugated MSNPs have a remarkable selectivity in internalizing into cancer cells while having minimal effect on normal cells. This targeting technique is largely refined by the interaction between cellular uptake kinetics and chemical functionality at the particle's surface (Silva et al., 2017). Mesoporous systems that respond to stimuli enhance the landscape even more. In these systems, the responsiveness of the probe depends on the type of responsive element and how it is attached to the surface (Albayati & Deveci, 2019). Probing further into the complex world of MSNPs, this insightful review lays out a detailed account, addressing their characteristics, various synthesis techniques, and the subtle nuances of drug administration with targeted precision. This insightful review lays out a detailed account, addressing their characteristics, various synthesis techniques, and the subtle nuances of drug administration with targeted precision. It also meticulously explores the dynamic landscape of MSNPs in treating cancer.

7.2 PROPERTIES OF SILICA-BASED NANOPARTICLES

Silica-based NPs are now widely used in nanotechnology, especially in biomedical and therapeutic fields. They are popular because they offer structural flexibility, strong stability, and can be easily adjusted for different uses. Knowing their basic properties helps improve their performance in targeted drug delivery, imaging, and diagnostics. This sections will explain the physical, chemical, and biological features that make silica NPs useful for advanced therapies.

7.2.1 Physical and Chemical Characteristics

Since SiO_2 has a large bandgap energy and is hence non-conductive, it is well known for its insulating qualities. SiO_2 has poor heat conductivity and a melting point of 1728°C, despite its brittleness and fragility (O'Hare, 1999). At higher temperatures, it also has a high refractive index and optical absorbance. In such circumstances, silica might appear as tridymite, coesite, or cristobalite, among other crystalline forms. It also has other notable physical features, including a relatively high dielectric constant (S. M. Sze, 2008). Because of its network structure, which is the result of covalent bonding between Si and O_2, it is possible to build layers on Si substrates under regulated conditions in various temperatures. The reduction in particle size facilitates the accommodation of more atoms on the surface, attributable to the corresponding increase in surface area. There is a strong correlation between the concentration of silanol groups (Si-O-H) per gram of silica and the degree of chemical modification, which includes integrating metal ions and grafting organic functional groups (Valdés et al., 2018).

7.2.2 Biocompatibility and Safety

The processes behind SiNPs biodegradation and clearance have been thoroughly studied in both in vitro and in vivo conditions. Recent studies have indicated that the biodegradation of siloxane NPs materials is primarily facilitated by the hydrolysis of siloxane bonds (Si–O–Si). This process results in the generation of silicic acid (H_4O_4Si), which is subsequently excreted from the biologi cal system (Dogra et al., 2018; Hu et al., 2021; C. Y. Lin et al., 2022). Particle size and shape, silica condensation level, pore dimension and porosity, and surface chemistry are important factors that influence how particles behave in biological systems. For example, smaller particles (<10 nm) tend rapidly through renal pathways, while larger particles are predominantly metabolized by the liver, significantly relying on hepato-biliary routes for their processing (Croissant et al., 2017; Lindén, 2018). These factors affect the body, including how they interact with proteins in the blood, cytotoxicity, degradation kinetics, and how fast the body removes them. Surface modifications, including PEGylation and the incorporation of targeted ligands, can significantly influence protein adsorption characteristics, biodistribution patterns, and the subsequent immune response (Suk et al., 2015). Amorphous SiO_2 is usually considered secure by regulatory bodies such as EMA (European Medicines Agency), FDA (United States Food and Drug Administration) etc. Amorphous SNPs are harmless, according to *in-vitro* experiments conducted on various cell lines, comprising epithelial, endothelial, fibroblast, and immune cells, including dendritic cells and macrophages (Chang et al., 2007), (Kumar et al., 2015a; Wagner et al., 2021), (Kharlamov et al., 2015; Vis et al., 2018). In these studies, viability assays such as MTT and LDH release consistently demonstrated minimal cytotoxicity across a broad range of concentrations, frequently up to 100 µg/mL. Furthermore, extensive research validates SiNPs' safety profile in biological applications (Bukara et al., 2016; Rastinehad et al., 2019; Zanoni et al., 2021).

7.2.3 Surface Modification for Enhanced Drug Loading

Improving or adding characteristics useful for medical applications is known as surface functionalization of NPs. Various types of NPs possess distinct chemical attributes that reveal unique groups that serve as functional groups on their exterior surfaces. There are two primary methods for surface modification of SiNPs: non-covalent and covalent conjugation. Non-covalent methods make use of metallic and SiO_2 NPs to facilitate weak interactions such as electrostatic, ionic, and H_2 bonding (Nell et al., 2016; Yue et al., 2019). These techniques are advantageous due to their simplicity, but they are also sensitive to other factors, including ionic concentration and pH (Lazaro et al., 2017). On the other hand, covalent bonding is more versatile (Gong et al., 2015) and enables it to be functionalized sequentially (H. Chen & He, 2015; Tian et al., 2015), which supports theranostic diagnosis (Jung et al., 2018). Covalent bonding is facilitated by linker molecules such as PEGylation (PEG) (Pagels et al., 2020), providing a variety of functionalization possibilities. PEG linkers also enhance the colloidal stability of NPs in biological environments, reducing opsonization and subsequent clearance by the immune system (Owens & Peppas, 2006). Covalent bonds are employed to target and reduce NPs toxicity, but non-covalent interactions are preferred for loading compounds such as medicines or RNA interference (RNAi) (Sanità et al., 2020). Covalent approaches, particularly click chemistry, are gaining traction due to their high efficiency, bio-orthogonality, and robust compatibility with delicate therapeutic agents (Hein et al., 2008). Furthermore, sensitive couplings such as pH-sensitivity have been investigated recently for personalized treatment techniques and adaptive drug release, especially in the acidic microenvironment of tumors (Sanità et al., 2020). For example, Schiff base linkages and hydrazone bonds have been effectively employed in pH-sensitive drug release systems, enabling targeted therapeutic activity in tumoral microenvironments while reducing systemic toxicity (Zhai et al., 2018).

7.3 SYNTHESIS METHODS

Several methods for synthesizing SiNPs have been developed, each with distinct benefits and adapted to certain purposes. Those techniques often entail the controlled hydrolysis and condensation of silicon precursors with the inclusion of stabilizing agents to modify the final characteristics of the NPs.

7.3.1 Stöber Technique

The Stöber technique is recognized as a fundamental method for synthesizing SiNPs. The process entails synthesizing porous materials through the controlled assembly of colloidal particles within a liquid medium, which results in the configuration of a gel network (Jafarzadeh et al., 2009; Singh et al., 2014). The resultant SiNPs exhibit desirable properties crucial for various applications. Researchers investigated the synthesis of porous SiNPs utilizing the Stöber method in which the silica precursor tetraethyl orthosilicate (TEOS), ammonia (NH_3) template or structure-directing agent cetyltrimethylammonium bromide (CTAB), ethanol (C_2H_5OH), and DI water were employed as chemical precursors. The process begins with the hydrolysis of TEOS, followed by a condensation reaction facilitated by NH_3. First, a solution of NH_3, H_2O, C_2H_5OH, and CTAB ($C_{19}H_{42}BrN$) was made then the mixture was vigorously agitated at elevated temperatures to ensure thorough interaction among the components. To obtain the final product, TEOS was introduced to the solution in a controlled, drop-wise manner to ensure optimal integration. The mixture was then purified to remove impurities, followed by calcination to achieve the desired physical properties (Hoffmann et al., 2006; Stöber et al., 1968). Using this technique, PNS with customized qualities fit a range of applications (Cai et al., 2001; Zhang et al., 2004).

Hydrolysis: $Si - (OR)_4 + H_2O \rightleftharpoons Si - (OR)_3(OH) + ROH$ (Singh et al., 2014)

Condensation: $(OR)_3 - Si - OH + HO - Si - (OR)_3 \rightarrow [(OR)_3Si - O - Si\,(OR)_3] + H - O - H$ (Singh et al., 2014)

In multiple studies, researchers used the multistep etching of gold cores from AuNPs@MS to create HMSNPs (Du & He, 2011). HMSNPs were formed as a result of dissolving the gold cores in thiourea solution (Y. Li et al., 2017). Meanwhile, a modified Stöber technique was used to generate MSNPs, and the surfactant template was eliminated by washing and calcination (Teng et al., 2013; Teng, Su, et al., 2014). After that, doxorubicin (DOX) was added to the collected MSNPs to create DOX@MSNPs for possible medication delivery uses (L. Chen et al., 2016; Xie et al., 2013). These investigations demonstrate the adaptability and effectiveness of sol-gel synthesis in generating a broad spectrum of SiNPs with customized structures and functions, thereby opening the possibilities for developments in several industries, including sensing, drug delivery, and catalysis.

7.3.2 Emulsion Polymerization

It involves the use of two distinct types of emulsions: *water-in-oil* (W/O) and *oil-in-water* (O/W). The micro-emulsions consist of nano colloidal that exhibit thermodynamic stability and are

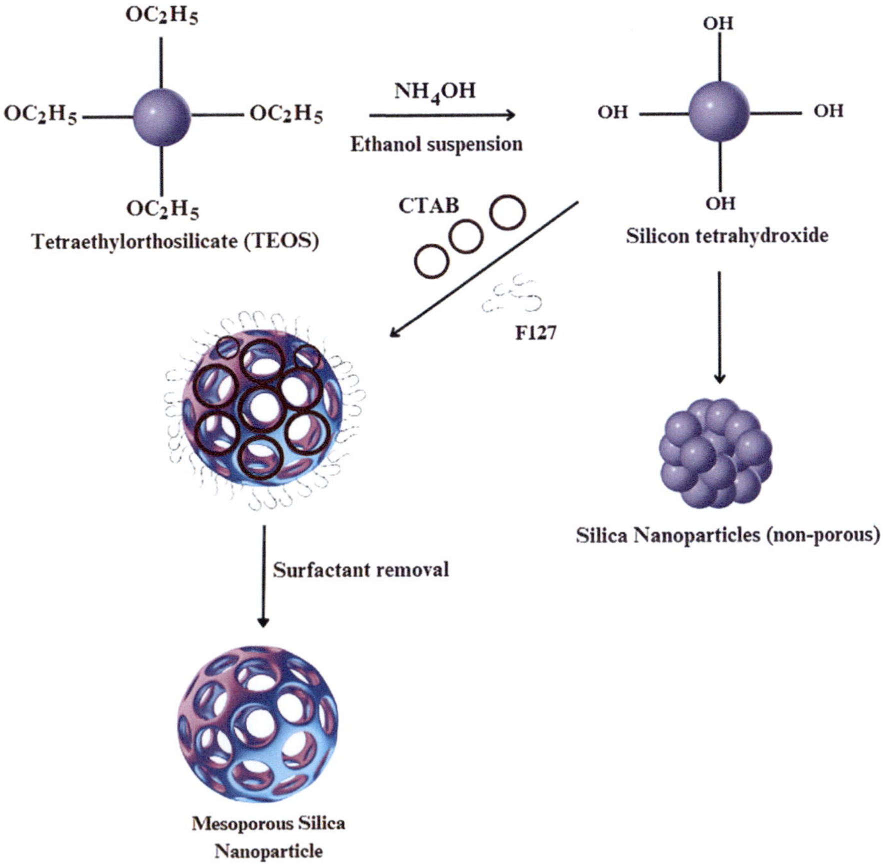

FIGURE 7.2 Stöber technique for synthesizing hollow mesoporous silica nanoparticles (HMSNPs).

stabilized by a surfactant coating. These micro-emulsions serve as nano-reactors for the synthesis of NPs. Two important variables are critical to the liquid-interface assembly strategy's success: (1) the reaction solution forms copious droplets or micelles with very stable interfaces; and (2) organosilica precursors co-assemble with SDAs on the interfaces (Ma et al., 2018). According to MSNPs prepared by Liangming Wei et al. (Wei et al., 2010), the first step involves dissolving 1gm of CTAB in a solution made of 3.5 mL of 2M NaOH and 480 mL of H_2O. After adding 7.0 mL of mesitylene, the mixture was rapidly agitated for 2 hours at 80 °C. After adding 5.0 mL of tetraethyl orthosilicate ($SiC_8H_{20}O_4$) dropwise, the reaction was allowed to proceed for an additional 2 hrs. After filtering and a methanol wash, the resultant precipitate was vacuum-dried for 24 hrs at 100 °C. Using an HCl/methanol (CH_3OH) solution, surfactant templates and mesitylene were withdrawn. Stirring 1.0g of MSNs in 100 mL CH_3OH with 0.75 mL concentrated HCL at 50 °C for 6 hrs produced the template-removed product. After filtration, the product underwent vacuum drying for 12 hours at ambient temperature. To functionalize MSNPs, 1g of MSNPs were suspended in 50 mL of dehydrated toluene. After adding 0.2 mL of room temperature water, the mixture was agitated for 3 hrs. Vinyl-trichlorosilane (1.75 mL) was then added, and the mixture was stirred for 12 hrs. Filtration was used to gather the product (V-MSNPs), which was then thoroughly cleaned with 2-propanol and vacuum-dried. For functionalization with ethyl groups (E-MSNs), the same process was followed, but 1.81 mL of ethyl-trichlorosilane ($C_2H_5Cl_3Si$) was added. It is difficult to create regulated hollow structures because, despite the introduction of the oil phase in many synthesis processes, the interfaces of oil droplets are often thermodynamically unstable (Tu et al., 2021; Y. Zhao et al., n.d.).

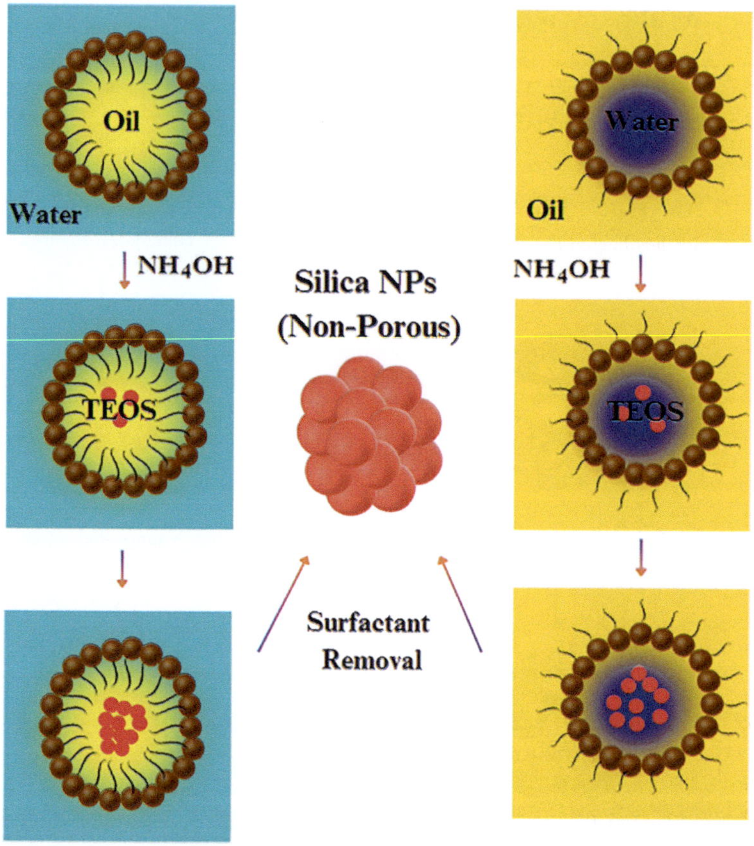

FIGURE 7.3 Emulsion polymerization for SiNPs synthesis.

Ma et al. (Ma et al., 2018) recently developed an approach to produce nano emulsion O/W interfaces with CTAB and ethanol by synthesizing steady ethane-bridged hollow periodic mesoporous organosilica (PMO) nanospheres utilizing 1,2-bis(triethoxysilyl) ethane (BTSE) as the oil-phase. Organosilica oligomers and CTAB co-assembled at stabilized BTSE O/W interfaces by a continuous reaction facilitated by NH_3, resulting in the formation of homogeneous organosilica/CTAB mesostructured shells. By adjusting the ethanol-to-water volume ratio, this one-pot approach produces hollow PMOs with a surface area of approximately 1330 m^2 g-1 and particle/cavity sizes of 100/20 nm, respectively. The synthesis of these hollow PMO nanospheres is simplified and accelerated by removing the extra oil step. Yu and colleagues (F. Lin et al., 2021) demonstrated a method to create ethane-bridged dendritic hollow PMO nanospheres using interfacial modification and composition gradient creation triggered by anion. As surfactant-directing agents (SDAs), sodium salicylate (NaSal) and CTAB were utilized. Through the formation of the Sal–/CTA^+ combination, which neutralizes CTA^+ micelles, silica core assembly, and organosilica shell co-condensation are promoted throughout the hollow structure development process. As a result, mesostructured organosilica/CTAB nanoparticles with distinct surfaces are produced. A micelle structural change is induced by sal-penetration, resulting in the formation of dendritic organosilica NPs with ≈30 nm pore size and massive radial mesostructured. The hollow cavity is obtained by selective etching of inorganic SiO_2 cores.

7.3.3 Template-Assisted Method (Soft and Hard Template)

The surfactant-templating methodology, which entails the interaction of silicate species and amphiphilic molecules through non-covalent interactions such as hydrogen bonding (H–bond) and electrostatic forces/attractions in aqueous solutions, is extensively employed in the fabrication of nanostructured materials (Fernandes et al., 2014; Manning et al., 2021). Both hydrophilic and hydrophobic regions may be found in amphiphilic surfactants. The hydrophilic-lipophilic balance (HLB) (J. G. Wang et al., 2008), which represents the proportion of polar to non-polar groups, defines the balance of these regions. Hydrophilicity is indicated by high HLB values, whereas hydrophobicity is shown by low values (Hesemann et al., 2014b; J. G. Wang et al., 2008). At the water's surface, these molecules can align so that the non-polar portion is exposed and the polar section interacts with the water. At critical micelle concentration, this disrupts surface cohesiveness, which lowers surface tension and promotes micelle production (Hesemann et al., 2014a; Kankala et al., 2022). Using a swelling agent and an extraction modified by trimethylsilylation, Hoshikawa et al. created disseminated MSNPs in an alcoholic medium that were 40–80 nm in size (Hoshikawa et al., 2010). Boonamnuayvitaya et al. studied the effects of surfactant type and concentration and used CTAB under acidic conditions to produce a high surface area (1282 m^2/g). Using an "etching-coating" method and an emulsifier-free emulsion (Boonamnuayvitaya et al., 2006), Yuan et al. created nanoscale hollow silica spheres. For distinct mesostructured SNPs, two or more templates are utilized, such as MCM-48 (J. Yuan et al., 2010). Jana et al. synthesized Si-MCM-41 materials with a rod-like shape by combining tetraalkylammonium salts with CTAB to improve ordering and stability (Jana et al., 2011). Ohkubo et al. used a combined cationic and anionic surfactant system to precisely regulate MSNPs (Ohkubo et al., 2007). Hollow SiNPs are made using hard templates such as polystyrene latex or polymeric micelles. Using polystyrene latex templates, Khanal et al. synthesized NPs with a range of shell diameters and thicknesses with smooth spherical shells and regulated dimensions using ABC triblock copolymer micelles (Khanal et al., 2007).

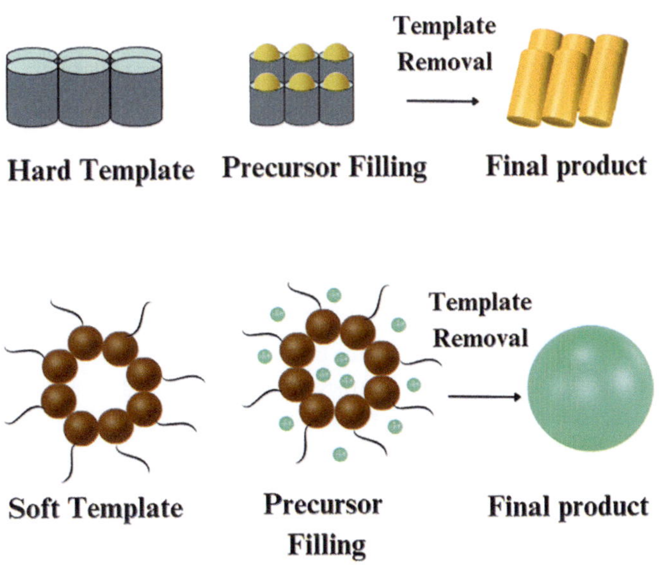

FIGURE 7.4 Template-assisted methods for SiNPs synthesis.

7.4 FUNCTIONALIZATION FOR TARGETING

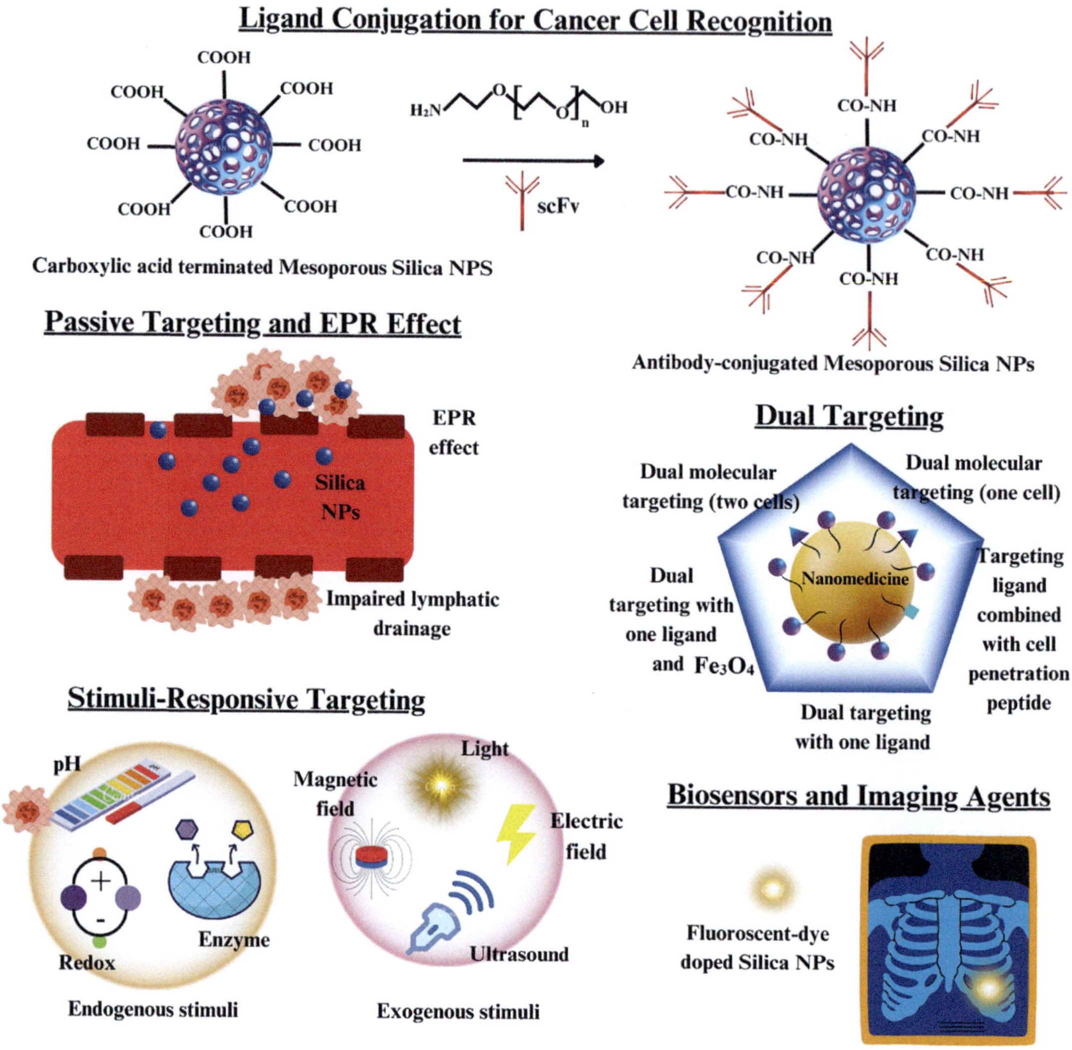

FIGURE 7.5 Functionalization of SiNPs for their various applications in cancer therapy.

7.4.1 Ligand Conjugation for Specific Cancer Cell Recognition

MSNPs are gaining recognition for their remarkable robustness, ease of functionalization, and low cytotoxicity combined with favorable hemocompatibility (Y. Zhao et al., 2024). Over the past decade, substantial research has been done toward fabricating tumor-targeted stimuli-responsive drug delivery systems. In the search for highly selective and effective tumor-targeted drug delivery platforms, numerous targeting ligands such as transferrin, particular peptides, hyaluronic acid or folic acid have been investigated in stimulus-responsive MSNPs (Carmona et al., 2015) (Xiao et al., 2014). However, achieving optimal selectivity and efficacy remains a formidable challenge in this pursuit. DOX has emerged as a prominent focus due to its widespread use in combating diverse cancers (Ganjavi et al.), including osteosarcoma bone tumors (Müller et al.). Innovative strategies have been devised to enhance the therapeutic potential of MSNPs loaded with antitumor agents. The Linlin Li group has developed a novel method for liver cancer treatment by encapsulating docetaxel within silica nanorattles, synthesized through a two-step selective-etching process and functionalized to enhance biocompatibility and systemic behavior. Nanorattles, which inherently possess amino groups on their surface, were subjected to PEGylation to enhance their dispersion stability and mitigate aggregation in biological environments. The SiO_2 nanorattles were treated with methoxypoly(ethylene glycol)-succinimidyl carbonate (mPEG-SC) to achieve this. The amino groups on the surface of the nanorattles were covalently linked to the PEG chains, resulting in stable PEGylated nanocarriers (SN-PEG) (L. Li et al., 2010a). Bertucci et al. introduced NH_2 onto the surface of MSNPs by treating them with $C_6H_{17}NOSi$. The surfactant template CTAB was eliminated through an acidic treatment with ethanol (C_2H_5OH) to facilitate unobstructed pores for drug loading. The surface NH_2 were then modified into $C_nH_{2n+1}COOH$ by reacting them with $C_4H_4O_3$, resulting in a negatively charged particle surface that enhanced the subsequent ligand conjugation process. The targeting ligand, an anti-miR221 peptide nucleic acid (PNA) modified with octaarginine (R8-PNA), was adsorbed onto the MSNPs surface via electrostatic interactions. The cationic character of the arginine-modified PNA not only promoted effective adsorption onto the negatively charged MSNPs but improved cellular uptake due to the induced positive surface charge. This ligand conjugation process provided a pore-blocking effect, facilitating the regulated release of the loaded temozolomide (TMZ), thus ensuring controlled delivery. This strategy effectively combines chemotherapy with inhibiting miRNA for glioma treatment, successfully addressing drug resistance and initiating apoptosis in resistant glioma cells (Bertucci et al., 2015). Surface modification with R8-PNA, a methacrylate nucleotide targeting miR221 miRNA, imparted enhanced pro-apoptotic effects, inducing apoptosis in T98G cells (70.9% of apoptotic cells) (Sonali et al., 2016). Moreover, Slowing et al. observed enhanced internalization of N-folate-3-aminopropyl-grafted MSNPs in HeLa cells, suggesting a folic acid (FA) receptor-mediated endocytosis mechanism (Slowing et al., 2006).

7.4.2 Passive Targeting Through Enhanced Permeability and Retention (EPR) Effect

The passive accumulation of NPs within tumors is supported by the EPR effect, which results from abnormally large open spaces of tumor vasculature and impaired lymphatic outflow. Huan Meng et al. investigated methods to augment the EPR effect and biodistribution of first-generation MSNPs to more effectively administer Dox to human squamous carcinoma xenografts in nude mice (Meng et al., 2010). Reducing the primary particle size to approximately 50 nm and surface decoration with a polyethylenimine and polyethylene glycol (PEI-PEG) copolymer for enhanced biocompatibility and circulation time while minimizing immune recognition. This allowed for the effective delivery of doxorubicin to the tumor by electrostatic attachment to phosphonate groups throughout the particle pores. This surface functionalization improved drug stability and release profiles, leveraging the EPR effect to passively accumulate NPs in tumor tissues. This design targets tumor-associated leaky vasculature, increasing drug concentration at the tumor site while minimizing off-target toxicity. (Davis et al.). Recent studies have emphasized how the shape of NPs regulates EPR-mediated tumor targeting conducted in vitro investigations into the shape-dependent cellular uptake efficiency and kinetics of SiNPs (Petros et al., 2010; Yun et al., 2009). Trewyn et al. developed MSNPs that were spherical, tube-like, hexagonal, wormhole, or helical pore structures measuring 80–150 nm in diameter and 400–1000 nm in length, which revealed endocytosis efficiency relies on cell line and shape. However, bare SiNPs characterized by exposed silanol group (≡ Si-OH) and negative charge under physiological conditions (pH ~ 7.4) exhibit inherent hemolytic activity due to interactions with red blood cell membranes, limiting their biocompatibility for tumor passive targeting (Trewyn et al., 2007a). Addressing this limitation, research has focused on incorporating organic components into the silica framework to mitigate hemolytic activity and enhance biocompatibility (Teng, Wang, et al., 2014). Organosilica NPs have thus emerged as promising candidates for drug delivery applications, with studies demonstrating significant reductions in hemolytic activity and improved biocompatibility (Y. Chen, Xu, et al., 2013; Urata et al., 2011).

7.4.3 Combination Approaches for Dual Targeting

Cancer-causing, stromal, and immune components are all in the complex assemblies comprising tumorigenic masses. Understanding the difference between pathogenic and non-pathogenic biological components is essential to enhancing the effectiveness of nanomedicine treatments. It is necessary to modify the surface of NCs using certain ligands, such as antibodies, aptamers, vitamins, peptides, or synthetic chemicals, to provide them with such selective abilities (Lorenz et al., 2020), (Zhou et al., 2017), (S. Wang et al., 2018). These ligands prefer membrane-bound receptors that are overexpressed in cancerous cells. Moreover, the technique of conjugating two ligands onto NCs increases their selectivity. Research has demonstrated the creation of synthetic peptides with specific subcellular localization, dual-ligand co-functionalized NPs, and hierarchical targeting mechanisms in NCs that interact with intracellular organelles and membrane receptors through an activatable cascade (Hoyer et al., 2012) (Guan et al., 2021). Shao et al. defined optimal configurations for targeting moieties on bifunctional NCs, highlighting the significance of Janus architectures. Their simulations revealed that Janus mesoporous silica nanoparticles (J-MSNs) with distinct surface functionalities are particularly effective for dual targeting. The asymmetric design of J-MSNs enhances specificity and efficiency in targeting applications. Magnetic J-MSNs facilitate external field-mediated targeting, improving tumor accumulation and cellular uptake of therapeutic agents such as doxorubicin while reducing systemic toxicity. Plasmonic J-MSNs utilize embedded materials such as gold or silver to enhance imaging techniques, including surface-enhanced Raman scattering (SERS) and photo-responsive drug release. These nanoparticles exhibit multi-stimuli-responsive behavior, allowing precise control of drug release triggered by pH, light, or magnetic fields. Additionally, J-MSNs functionalized with targeting ligands, such as antibodies (e.g., anti-EpCAM), effectively isolate circulating tumor cells (CTCs) and enhance drug delivery to tumor sites, capitalizing on their unique structure that enables rapid cellular internalization and addresses the challenges of physicochemical properties and inter-moiety spacing (Shao et al., 2021). Chen et al. developed a functionalization approach for MSNPs using fluorescein isothiocyanate (FITC) for hydrophobic drug loading, generation 2 PAMAM dendrimers (PAMAM-G2) for hydrophilic drug encapsulation, and HA for tumor targeting via CD44 receptor interaction. This system enables sequential drug release through stimuli-responsive mechanisms: low pH induces HA cap detachment to release doxorubicin hydrochloride (DOX.HCl), while high intracellular glutathione (GSH) levels cleave disulfide bonds to release methotrexate (MTX). The NPs got significant drug loading efficiency (MTX: ~20%, DOX.HCl: ~10%) and controlled release exceeding 90% in tumor-mimicking conditions (X. Chen & Liu, 2016). Yang et al. developed folate-conjugated fluorescent SiNPs (NPs[FITC]-PEG-Folate) which were engineered with fluorescein isothiocyanate (FITC) internally doped for high photostability and fluorescence intensity. At the same time, folate molecules were conjugated using PEG spacers to target folate receptor-positive (FR+) cancer cells specifically. With a mean size of 212 nm, these NPs exhibit sixfold higher internalization efficiency in FR+ KB cells than folate receptor-negative A549 cells, mediated by clathrin-dependent endocytosis. The presence of free folate competitively inhibited cellular uptake, confirming receptor-specific targeting (H. Yang et al., 2011). Meng et al. developed a multifunctional MSNPs platform aimed at dual-targeted delivery of Dox and P-glycoprotein (PGP) small interfering RNA (siRNA) to address multidrug resistance (MDR) in breast cancer. The MSNPs, coated with a PEI-PEG copolymer, enabled targeted delivery of therapeutics to tumor sites while reducing the uptake by the reticuloendothelial system (RES). High-throughput screening (HTS) identified Pgp siRNA as the most effective target to enhance Dox sensitivity in MDR MCF-7 xenografts. In vivo studies showed that dual-loaded MSNPs inhibited tumor growth by 80%, compared to 17% for free Dox or single-agent systems (Meng et al., 2013).

7.4.4 pH-Responsive and Stimuli-Responsive Targeting

Asymmetrical fenestrations, typically around 400 nm in diameter, characterize the abnormal vasculature of malignant tissues and serve as targets for nanoscale therapies. Rapid tumor growth and angiogenesis create leaky vessels with irregular fenestrations, allowing NPs to accumulate in the tumor microenvironment and enhancing the EPR effect. This is further influenced by molecular alterations, including the inactivation of von Hippel-Lindau (VHL) gene function and dysregulation of hypoxia-inducible factors (HIFs), which increase vascular permeability and enhance nanotherapeutic delivery to tumors (M. F. Khan et al., 2020). MSNPs are a versatile platform for stimuli-responsive drug delivery systems. Various regulatory techniques have been established, evaluating their feasibility and effectiveness. Triggers can be internal, responding to environmental cues, or external, activated by non-invasive methods such as light, pH, redox potential, ATP, or temperature (Baeza et al., 2015). Lipid or polymerized bilayers are employed as partial capping methods on the outside of MSNPs. At the site of the tumor, controlled drug release is made possible by the competitive displacement of these bilayers that occurs upon stimulation. Dynamic control over drug release can be achieved with stimuli-responsive systems, permitting accurate targeting and spatiotemporal management of therapeutic effects. The acidic microenvironment of tumor tissues (pH ~6.5–7.0), in contrast to normal physiological pH (pH ~7.4), is exploited by pH-responsive SNPs (Gao et al., 2010). pH-sensitive linkers or coatings acid-labile bonds, hydrazone, or acetal linkages (Y. Chen, Chen, et al., 2013) are utilized to conjugate drugs to the HMSNPs surface, facilitating drug release in response to acidic conditions (H. Chen et al., 2018). Moodley et al. revealed in 2020 that a polyelectrolyte-coated MSNPs exhibiting pH-sensitive drug release had organic and inorganic copolymers grafted onto the superficial surface (Moodley & Singh, 2020). Some primary gating techniques that have been studied are the attachment of SiNPs such as gold (Au) capped MSNPs for H_2O_2 responsive where the caps are linked via boronate ester bonds, sensitive to oxidative conditions and it exploits the high levels of reactive oxygen species (ROS) (L. Yang et al., 2016). Ryplida et al. developed zwitterionic carbon dots (CDs) within pH-responsive MSNPs that exploit the lower pH in tumor tissues (pH 6.5–6.9) compared to normal cells (pH 7.2–7.4). These CDs are integrated into the MSNPs core via electrostatic and hydrophobic interactions with Indocyanine Green (ICG), keeping fluorescence quenched under physiological conditions to reduce off-target effects. In acidic tumor environments, the electrostatic interactions are disrupted, releasing ICG and reactivating fluorescence to enhance imaging. Upon near-infrared (NIR) irradiation, the ICG-loaded MSNPs produce localized heat that induces apoptosis in cancer cells, with a stronger effect in acidic conditions (Ryplida et al., 2019). Kobes et al. developed MSNPs with pH-responsive coatings with protamine sulfate, glutamine, and glycine to improve cellular uptake and fluorescence detection in acidic environments. These MSNPs, loaded with Alexa Fluor 647, were integrated into decellularized liver scaffolds for monitoring cellular proliferation and scaffold colonization through longitudinal imaging (Kobes et al., 2018), Cheng et al. developed MSNPs endowed with enzyme stimuli responsive and tumor-targeting characteristics to facilitate the controlled DOX release where MSNPs functionalized with a rotaxane architecture, utilizing α-cyclodextrin as a gatekeeper, along with azido-GFLGR7RGDS peptide that incorporates tumor-targeting, cell-penetrating, and cathepsin B-cleavable sequences. This gatekeeper configuration ensured stable encapsulation of DOX under physiological conditions, thereby minimizing premature release. Once internalized by tumor cells, the overexpressed cathepsin B acted on the GFLG linker, removing the gatekeeper and initiating an "off-on" drug release mechanism. In the acidic environment of lysosomes (approximately pH 5.0), this enzymatic cleavage facilitated the release of roughly 80% of the loaded DOX within 24 hrs, subsequently inducing a significant apoptotic effect. Cellular experiments indicated that RGDS-functionalized MSNPs effectively targeted $\alpha v\beta 3$-overexpressing HeLa cells, enhancing cellular uptake and superior growth inhibition (Cheng et al., 2015). For the redox-responsive stimuli response, MSNPs utilize the high glutathione (GSH) concentration in tumor cells to trigger controlled drug release. Disulfide bonds act as gatekeepers, remaining sealed under normal conditions but breaking in the presence of GSH, allowing for targeted drug delivery and reducing side effects. Advanced designs feature multifunctional gatekeepers, such as thiolated siRNA or peptide linkers, enhancing targeting and promoting apoptosis. Structures such as cucurbituril or cyclodextrins seal the pores, releasing drugs only when exposed to reductive agents. Redox-sensitive biodegradable frameworks ensure that the NPs safely degrade after releasing their cargo, representing a promising strategy for targeted cancer therapies (Gisbert-Garzarán & Vallet-Regí, 2021; Wu et al., 2004). To alter drug release kinetics at particular temperature thresholds, thermoresponsive polymers, poly (N-isopropyl acrylamide) (PNIPAM), are grafted or doped onto the surface of mesoporous silica (Dumontel et al., 2023). The emergence of new trigger-response systems has coincided with the emergence of dual or tri-stimuli-responsive systems. These systems incorporate a dual and triple-responsive system that uses MSNPs to integrate reduction, pH, and light stimuli, etc (Martínez-Carmona et al., 2015; Moreira et al., 2016). Wen et al. developed a triple-stimuli-responsive NCs system utilizing MSNPs coated with CeO_2 and loaded with DOX and hematoporphyrin (HP). The system leverages glutathione (GSH), acidic pH, and light irradiation as triggers. In cancer cells, high intracellular GSH and low pH reduce CeO_2 to cerium ions, degrading the coating and releasing DOX. Simultaneously, light irradiation disrupts HP-DOX interactions, enhancing drug release and fluorescence signals. Furthermore, HP generates singlet oxygen ($^1O_2$) upon irradiation, enabling photodynamic therapy (PDT) (Wen et al., 2016).

7.4.5 Biosensors and Imaging Agents

SiNPs are enhancing biosensor technology by improving surface tunability and reaction kinetics, aiming for highly sensitive, specific biosensors that enable multivariate detection with reliable and repeatable performance. Their porous architecture allows for the encapsulation of signaling molecules, which can be released upon interaction with target analytes, thereby enhancing detection capabilities. For example, MSNPs functionalized with specific antibodies have been utilized for the real-time detection of cancer biomarkers, including carcinoembryonic antigen (CEA) and prostate-specific antigen (PSA) (Mladenović et al., 2024). MSNPs serve as a dual function for both recognition platforms and signal amplification mechanisms, enhancing detection sensitivity by efficiently capturing targets. They utilize techniques such as fluorescence resonance energy transfer (FRET) and electrochemical impedance spectroscopy (EIS). MSNPs-based electrochemical biosensors improve electron transfer rates, while optical biosensors immobilize and release chromogenic agents for colorimetric or fluorescence detection (Jo et al., 2015). Mathelié-Guinlet et al. demonstrated a SiNPs-assisted electrochemical biosensor capable of detecting E. coli with a limit of detection (LOD) of 10^3 CFU/mL within 30 minutes. This biosensor leverages cyclic voltammetry as the detection mechanism, where SiNPs are functionalized with polyclonal antibodies to bind to the bacteria selectively (Mathelié-Guinlet et al., 2019). The use of silica nanowires (SiNWs) functionalized with amine, biotin, or antigen moieties, leading to the development of label-free, real-time field-effect transistor (FET)-based sensors. When it came to identifying proteins (such as streptavidin and antibodies) and metal ions (such as Ca^{2+}), these sensors demonstrated remarkable sensitivity (Cui et al., 2001). Later, in 2006, Patolsky et al. expanded on this approach by combining individual axons and living mammalian neurons with SiNWs-based FETs, which allowed for a more in-depth understanding of neural activity (Patolsky et al., 2006). Kim et al. used vertically aligned SiNWs arrays as new cell culture substrates in a complementary effort that demonstrated their potential for gene transport and the clarification of biological events occurring both inside and between cells (W. Kim et al., 2007). Building on these developments, Wang et al. developed a circulating tumor cell (CTC)-capture platform by using SiNWs functionalized with cell capture agents. They showed impressive efficacy in capturing CTCs from clinical and spiked blood samples (S. Wang et al., 2011). SERS platforms based on SiNWs have enabled the ultra-sensitive detection of molecules down to single-molecule levels. The decoration of SiNWs with silver or gold nanoparticles (AgNPs) significantly enhances Raman signal amplification, enabling the detection of biological targets such as DNA and proteins with high specificity. Recent innovations, such as the development of AgNPs-coated SiNWs substrates, have allowed the detection of DNA at concentrations as low as 1 fM and provided insights into intracellular processes such as apoptosis (Peng et al.,

2014). Among imaging modalities, fluorescence technology is notable for its higher resolution and potential sensitivity in the detection of cancer cells. Herr et al. conducted a comparative analysis of fluorescence intensity between dye molecules and dye-doped SiNPs functionalized with aptamers. Their findings revealed that SiNPs modified with aptamers exhibited enhanced brightness and stability in fluorescence imaging compared to dye-aptamer conjugates alone. Flow cytometry further corroborated these results, indicating a 100-fold increase in signal intensity for SiNPs-aptamer complexes relative to single dye-labeled aptamers. As such, these dye-doped SiNPs with increased fluorescence intensity might be used to create extremely sensitive biosensors. The protective silica matrix of dye-doped SiNPs reduces photobleaching and allows for longer imaging times of tumor cells and tissues, which is another benefit over free dye molecules (Herr et al., 2006). Magnetic resonance imaging (MRI) is a vital tool for cancer diagnosis in clinical settings since it has better tissue penetrator ageing. A promising approach to improving MRI sensitivity is the incorporation of SiNPs, which can contain hundreds of MRI contrast agents, such as gadolinium chelates, in a single NP. The exceptional loading efficiency of SiNPs enhances the efficacy of MRI contrast media. The creation of a very effective MRI contrast agent based on MSNPs was developed by Taylor et al. also demonstrated the agent's effectiveness in both in vitro and in vivo MRI applications. The MSNPs-based contrast agent offers an optimal platform for MRI owing to its substantial payload of gadolinium (Gd) centers and improved water accessibility of Gd chelates (K. M. L. Taylor et al., 2008). To modify Gd chelates onto SiNPs, Lin et al. used a layer-by-layer self-assembly technique combined with fluorescence contrast agent doping during synthesis. These K7RGD-SiNPs demonstrated the capacity to identify certain tumor cells using fluorescence and magnetic resonance imaging modalities in conjunction with the inclusion of a targeting peptide (J. S. Kim et al., 2007). Lipid layering facilitated the coating of Gd chelates onto SiNPs. The resulting imaging nanocomposite demonstrated dual capability in fluorescence imaging and MRI for tumor cell identification when combined with quantum dots doping inside the same SiNPs (Koole et al., 2008).

7.5 DRUG LOADING AND RELEASE

Conventional MSNPs exhibit suboptimal targeting precision and release control alongside constrained payload capacity. Pure MSNPs fall short in efficiently transporting drugs to precise sites while ensuring controlled release, necessitating high-capacity carriers such as HMSNPs. HMSNPs leverage shell mesopores and core volume for heightened drug-loading efficiency, yet face challenges in achieving precise drug release, hindering cancer therapy. Addressing this, integrating magnetic NPs for guided targeting and polymer coatings for controlled release emerges as a promising strategy.

7.5.1 Loading Techniques and Control Loading Strategies

Numerous loading methodologies have been developed aimed at bolstering drug loading capacity and regulating release kinetics in HMSNPs drug delivery systems.

7.5.1.1 Physical Encapsulation

Drug entrapment within HMSNPs is intricately facilitated by physical encapsulation mechanisms, such as passive diffusion and adsorption, within their mesoporous structure. The solvent evaporation process entails dissolving the medicine in a volatile solvent and meticulous removal under a vacuum to ensure the drug is trapped within the nanopores. Coacervation is based on thermodynamic phase separation, which stimulates the formation of drug-loaded microdroplets in HMSNPs nanopores (Mai et al., 2013). In simple mixing, HMSNPs is incubated with drug solutions to promote the passive diffusion of drugs into the nanopores (Lu et al., n.d.; Vallet-Regí et al., 2007). When encapsulation encounters suboptimal loading efficiency and unpredictability in release kinetics, it requires further optimization and fine-tuning, such as the addition of stimuli-responsive elements to the

HMSNPs structure or the drug encapsulation process, and advanced imaging techniques to improve therapeutic outcomes (Tang et al., 2012).

7.5.1.2 Chemical Conjugation

Chemical conjugation is a delicate method that binds pharmacological agents covalently to the functional groups on the surface or confines them inside the mesoporous structure of HMSNPs (Croissant et al., 2018). Reactive compounds, containing amino or thiol functionalities, are introduced to the surface of HMSNPs to functionalize it. These groups act as anchors for drug adsorption through a variety of chemical processes, such as silanization, Amidation, Thiol-disulfide Exchange, Michael Addition Reaction, etc. (Pal et al., 2020; Rosenholm et al., 2010) or they can be pre-modified with specific functional groups depicting to react with surface moieties on HMSNs, thereby facilitating efficient conjugation (Kuthati et al., 2013).

7.5.1.3 Surface Modification

In surface modification strategies, drug loading efficiency and release kinetics are enhanced by encasing HMSNPs with polymeric, lipid, or inorganic coatings. Drug encapsulation can be enhanced via polymer coatings with PEG or PEI, which act as an inhibitor to prevent premature drug release and enhance the longevity of NPs under physiological environments. The formation of a lipid bilayer on the surface of HMSNPs emulsifies cell membranes, which facilitates cellular uptake and intracellular drug delivery (Ashley et al., 2011; Trewyn et al., 2007b). Inorganic coatings, such as silica shells or metal-organic frameworks (MOFs), can enhance drug intake even further and provide additional advantages, such as pH-responsive drug release or imaging capabilities (Horcajada et al., 2012).

7.5.2 Efficiency Evaluation

The efficiency of HMSNPs loading techniques can be evaluated through characterization techniques. UV-visible spectroscopy and fluorescence spectroscopy can be used to quantify the amount of drug loaded and drug loading efficiency by measuring absorbance or fluorescence intensity (Q. L. Li et al., 2014; Sun et al., 2018).

$$\left.\begin{aligned}\text{Drug Loading Content (wt. \%)} &= \frac{\textit{Mass of drugs in the HMSN}}{\textit{Mass of the drug loaded HMSN}}\\[2ex]\text{Drug Loading Efficiency (wt. \%)} &= \frac{\textit{Mass of drugs in the HMSN}}{\textit{Initial mass of drugs}}\end{aligned}\right\}\ \text{(Schwarzl et al., 2017)}$$

DLS can evaluate the stability and size distribution of drug-loaded NPs in solution. The release kinetics and therapeutic efficiency of drug-loaded HMSNPs can be further analyzed by *in-vitro* release studies deploying dialysis membranes or cell culture models (Yamamoto & Kuroda, 2016).

7.6 *IN VITRO* AND *IN VIVO* STUDIES

Comprehensive *in vitro* and *in vivo* analyses need to be performed for post-drug release studies to comprehend pharmacokinetics, biodistribution, and therapeutic efficacy. *In-vitro*, release kinetics, cellular uptake, and biocompatibility are scrutinized (Abu-Dief et al., 2021). In vivo, pharmacokinetic profiling and biodistribution studies are conducted, along with therapeutic efficacy assessments in relevant animal models. Toxicity evaluations, including histopathological and blood chemistry analyses, ensure systemic safety (He & Shi, 2014). The correlation coefficient R^2 value should be ~1 for the in vitro and in vivo correlation of HMSNPs (Cao et al., 2012).

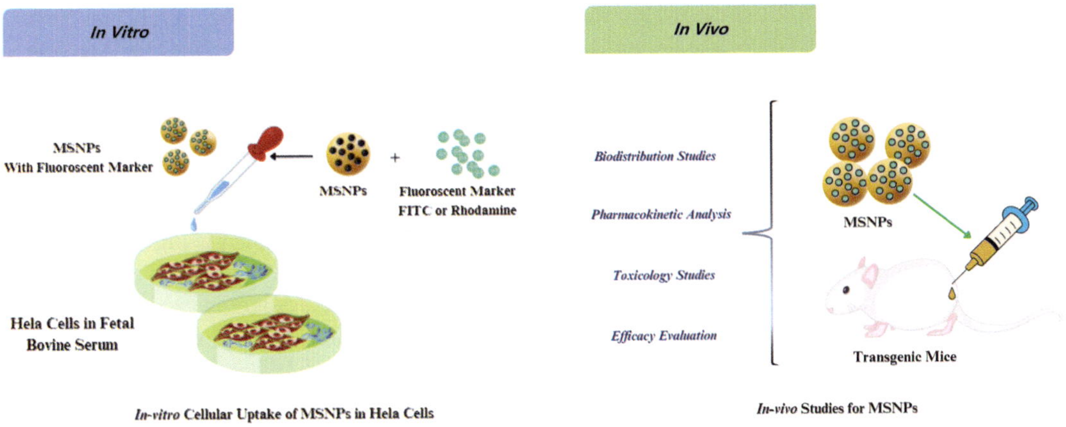

FIGURE 7.6 In vitro and in vivo studies for MSNPs.

7.6.1 *In Vitro* Studies

Investigating the cellular uptake mechanisms of HMSNPs entails meticulous experimental design and methodological execution. Primarily, an adequate cell line is selected such as TC-1 cells, HeLa cells (X. Xing et al., 2005), or A549 cells for cancer or primary macrophages for immunological studies and measured the adsorption rate and intracellular circulation of different size SiNPs (dos Santos et al., 2011; Gräslund et al., 2011), which is cultured in a complete medium supplemented such as RPMI 1640 with fetal bovine serum (FBS) and penicillin-streptomycin-glutamine, all into a humidified incubator with regulated CO_2 concentration (Shapero et al., 2011). Significant components employed in these studies encompass Cetyltrimethylammonium chloride (CTAC) aqueous solution, TEOS, disodium maleate, FITC-conjugated ovalbumin (FITC-OVA), 2′,7′-dichlorofluorescein diacetate (DCFH-DA), monochlorobimane, glutathione, sodium acetate trihydrate ($NaAc{\cdot}3H_2O$), $MnSO_4{\cdot}H_2O$, HPV16 E7 peptide (RAHYNIVTF), LysoTracker Red DND-99 and various inhibitors, as well as PE-RAHYNIVTF-MHC I dextramer and corresponding negative control PE dextramer (Andoh et al., 2006; Gräslund et al., 2011; Kumar et al., 2015b). After cell culture under standard conditions, SiNPs are functionalized with fluorescent markers such as fluorescein isothiocyanate (FITC) or rhodamine to facilitate imaging (C. Li et al., 2017). Following exposure of cells to various concentrations and duration of NPs, cellular uptake is observed in 3D visualization using fluorescent microscopy techniques, utilizing confocal microscopy. Any deviation in fluorescence escalation indicates potential NPs leakage, as it signifies the loss of self-quenching interactions among the fluorescent molecules. After excluding cell debris and doublets, the live single-cell populace is delineated through a plot of forward scatter (FSC) versus side scatter (SSC). A histogram derived from the FITC channel is then generated and scrutinized for the single-cell populace. This iterative measurement of cells not only ensures quality control but also serves as a baseline for calibrating FITC intensity in subsequent analyses (Y. Chen et al., 2009; Pack et al., 2020). Mechanistic insights into NPs internalization are elucidated via inhibition assays, where cells are pre-treated with inhibitors of specific endocytic pathways such as chlorpromazine for clathrin-mediated endocytosis or methyl-β-cyclodextrin for caveolae-mediated endocytosis (K. Chen et al., 2017).

7.6.2 *In Vivo* Studies

Various strains of mice (Transgenic E7TCR269, K14E7, C57BL/6J, CASP-1-/-, etc.) are housed under specific pathogen-free conditions at the Biological Research Facility (Lange et al., 2019). Specifically, Transgenic K14E7 mice expressing the HPV16E7 oncoprotein via the K14 promoter were employed. Female mice six to twelve weeks old are selected for the experiments (Kondoh et al., 1995). Administration of SiNPs loaded with anticancer drugs occurred via subcutaneous injection at the tail base, the required amount of PBS in microliters, with non-immunized mice serving as controls. Depletion efficacy is confirmed through blood analysis 1-day post-treatment or spleen analysis 4 days post-treatment, utilizing flow cytometry (Lu et al., 2012; Rafiq et al., 2018). Skin grafting procedures are executed, with ear skin donor mice being split into dorsal and ventral halves with forceps, E7TCR269 mice contracting double dorsal ear skins to the flank region under anesthesia (Jiang et al., 1998). Grafts are preserved and examined weekly, with graft sizes determined using imaging software. The immunization site of the skinning process for histological analysis included incubation in mild buffered formalin, paraffin insertion, and hematoxylin-eosin (H&E) staining (A. A. Khan et al., 2020). Furthermore, immunofluorescence staining is performed on skin samples encased in optimal slicing temperature substance, with slices coated with primary and secondary antibodies, followed by staining with DAPI and mounted (Haramati et al., 2007; Pakyari et al., 2016).

Important in vitro and in vivo studies carried out using SiNPs are summarized in Table 7.1.

7.6.3 Toxicity and Biocompatibility Assessments

For this assessment, the mice are seperated into treatment groups receiving different doses of SiNPs and a control group receiving saline. To assess acute toxicity, the mice are monitored meticulously for signs of distress, behavioral changes, or mortality during a specified 24- to 72-hour period while recording the acute toxicity endpoints, such as LD50 (median lethal dose) or maximum tolerated dose (MTD), based on observed adverse effects (Dieter, 1994; Shipp et al., 2006). This could involve administering doses ranging from 10 to 300 mg body weight of SiNPs via intraperitoneal injection or oral gavage (X. Chen et al., 2014). For the Hematological and Serum Biomarker Analysis, blood samples from mice are collected after the administration of NPs at designated time intervals and the RBC and WBC count, platelet count, hemoglobin levels, and hematocrit are evaluated using automated hematology analyzers (Azimipour et al., 2018; Ivanov et al., 2012). To assess systemic responses to SiNPs exposure, examine serum levels of liver enzymes (e.g., ALT, AST), renal function markers (e.g., BUN, creatinine), including inflammatory cytokines (e.g., IL-1β, TNF-α), using ELISA or multiplex assays (Mahato et al., 2021; R. Xing et al., 2016). In Subacute and Chronic Toxicity Studies, administer repeated doses of SiNPs to mice for 14–28 days (Das et al., 2021). Monitor mice daily for clinical signs, body weight changes, and behavioral abnormalities, alongside assessing organ weights and histopathological changes in major organs (e.g., liver, kidneys, lungs) to evaluate subacute and chronic toxicity (Nemmar et al., 2014). Furthermore, collect the serum samples from treated and control mice at designated time intervals for cytokine profiling to perform multiple cytokine assays or ELISA (D. P. Wang et al., 2020) and determine the levels of proinflammatory (e.g., IL-6, TNF-α) and anti-inflammatory cytokines (e.g., IL-10) in serum samples to gain insight into the immunological response induced by SiNPs (Elsabahy & Wooley, 2013; Potter et al., 2018). To completely examine toxicity profiles, correlation reports of toxicological parameters with NPs characteristics and dosing regimens are examined to aid the understanding of the relationship between NPs properties and biological reactions (Ajdary et al., 2018; Oh et al., 2010),

7.7 CHALLENGES AND FUTURE PERSPECTIVES

As nanotechnology grows, much research is being done on SiNPs, yet few of them make it to clinical trials because of the significant biological and technological obstacles. Biodistribution modulation, restricted routes of delivery, SiNPs navigating biological barriers, degradation, and toxicity are all examples of biological obstacles. The most common method of delivery, intravenous injection, has difficulties with SiNPs retention in target locations, requiring large drug concentrations with questionable therapeutic efficiency. On the other hand, combining SiNPs with magnetic NPs shows promise since it can use 3D magnetic fields to guide SiNPs against blood flow. However, issues with SiNPs quantities,

TABLE 7.1
Different Types of SiNPs for Anticancer Drug Delivery, Along with Their Respective Payloads, Treatment Models, Administration Routes, and Applications

Types of Silica Nanoparticles (SiNPs)	Payloads	Treatment Model	Administration Route	Application	Reference
Mesoporous SiNPs	Doxorubicin	In vitro and In vivo	Intravenous	Osteosarcoma, Bladder Cancer, Lobular and Ductal Carcinoma,	Y. Chen, Yang, et al. (2013)
	5-Fluorouracil	In vitro	Intravenous and Subcutaneous	Colorectal, Lobular and Squamous Cell Carcinoma	Moodley and Singh (2019)
	Methotrexate	*In-vivo*	Oral, Subcutaneous and Intramuscular	Intracranial Neoplasm, Thyroid Cancer, Lobular and Ductal Carcinoma	Shadmani et al. (2023)
Hollow Mesoporous SiNPs	Pacitaxel	*In-vitro and In-vivo*	Intravenous	Intracranial Neoplasm, Leukemia, Colorectal Carcinoma	Jia et al. (2013)
	Camptothecin	*In-vitro and In-vivo*	Oral and Transdermal	Adenocarcinoma	Babaei et al. (2020)
	Cisplatin	*In-vitro and In-vivo*	Intravenous and Intravesical	Melanoma, Ovarian Cancer, Urothelial carcinoma	Drača et al. (2021)
Core-Shell SiNPs	Docetaxel	In vivo	Intravenous and Intraperitoneal		L. Li et al. (2010b)
	Mitoxantrone	*In-vitro*	Intravenous infusion		Granja et al. (2021)
	Etoposide	*In-vivo*	Intravenous infusion	Orthotopic Lung Tumour	Z. qiang Yuan et al. (2017)
	Epirubicin	*In-vivo*	Intravenous	Murine Colorectal Carcinoma	Ansari et al. (2018)
Hybrid SiNPs	Gemcitabine	*In-vitro*	Intravenous	Pancreatic Cancer	Meng et al. (2015)
Lipid Coated SiNPs	Vinorelbine	*In-vitro*	Intravenous	Lobular and Ductal Carcinoma	Abbasfard et al. (2024)
	Irinotecan	*In-vitro*	Intravenous	Orthotopic Colon Cancer	Liu et al. (2019)
Protein Coated SiNPs	Bleomycin	*In-vitro and In-vivo*	Intramuscular, Intravenous, Subcutaneous and Intrapleural	Chronic Pulmonary Fibrosis	Bai et al. (2022)

crosstalk, and magnetic field effects continue. Scale-up synthesis, optimization, and performance prediction, all essential for clinical success, are examples of technological challenges. Large-scale manufacturing is hampered by the scaling issues with existing SiNPs formulations. Additionally, adequate research design and model representativeness create hurdles for clinical application. Particularly, models of cancer metastasis deserve consideration. Researchers are urged to hasten translation since, despite their varied and promising features, MSNPs-based cancer formulations have seen limited progress into clinical trials. Bench-to-bedside translation is critical, and advances in MSNPs synthesis and functionalization show promise for medicinal applications. MSNPs have become indispensable instruments in biomedical research during the past decade, providing a wide range of efficient treatment options. Understanding MSNPs' material characteristics and appropriateness for drug administration and other biological applications has been the subject of much research. Because of their extremely porous structure, ability to load cargo, and ability to chemically functionalize, MSNPs have proven to be remarkably versatile in delivering a wide range of therapeutic agents to target cancer cells with high efficacy. These agents include biologicals, anticancer drugs, and diagnostic agents. MSNPs have several important benefits, including increased drug solubility due to quicker rates of dissolution as well as improved systemic availability and stability in vivo. Although studies on MSNPs-based chemotherapeutic combination treatments are still in their early stages, developments in materials science and our understanding of illness will likely lead to an expansion in the potential applications of MSNPs-based drug delivery systems (DDS). Chemotherapy-based nanosystems with biocompatible MSNPs have a lot of potential for clinical application in the future. The potential uses of MSNPs-based DDS will only increase as knowledge and technology advance, opening up new avenues for flexible and adaptive developments in the field of clinical treatments.

7.8 CONCLUSION

Numerous proof-of-concept studies on the in vivo use of MSNPs in medication delivery have surfaced in recent years. Mostly focused on cancer therapy, these initiatives have sparked hope for improved diagnostic techniques and more efficient treatment plans that might reduce or eliminate side effects. Crucial to this process is the careful selection of MSNPs according to strict standards, which is a need for fruitful preclinical experiments. While most current in vivo research focuses on the delivery of cancer drugs such as DOX, Paclitaxel etc. via folate as a targeting ligand, broadening the range of possibilities to include novel cancer drugs, clinical trial candidates, or compounds pulled off the market because of severe side effects could result in significant clinical benefits. Furthermore, the investigation of novel targeting ligands and classes, in conjunction with technical developments that enable delivery to difficult anatomical locations and get beyond biological barriers such as the intestinal or blood-brain barriers, provide promising directions. Other options worth pursuing include targeting elusive cell types such as cancer stem cells, taking advantage of disease-specific microenvironments, or using disease-seeking cells as carriers. The platform's potential is further enhanced by the examination of other administration routes and the creation of externally controlled localized delivery mechanisms, such as localized photodynamic treatment and magnetic or ultrasound-guided targeting. However, comprehensive standardized biological performance testing is required to provide a solid knowledge basis for future iterations and to realize the actual therapeutic value of these developments. To advance MSNPs toward practical deployment as a potential modality for cancer theranostics shortly, current difficulties must be addressed.

REFERENCES

Abbasfard, Z., Behzad-Behbahani, A., Rastegari, B., Naeimi, S., Moghanibashi, M., & Safari, F. (2024). Overcoming breast cancer drug resistance: A novel approach using siRNA-mediated P-glycoprotein downregulation to enhance vinorelbine efficacy. *Advanced Pharmaceutical Bulletin*, *14*(2), 445–452. https://doi.org/10.34172/apb.2024.030

Abu-Dief, A. M., Alsehli, M., Al-Enizi, A., & Nafady, A. (2021). Recent advances in mesoporous silica nanoparticles for targeted drug delivery applications. *Current Drug Delivery, 19*(4), 436–450. https://doi.org/10.2174/1567201818666210708123007

Ajdary, M., Moosavi, M. A., Rahmati, M., Falahati, M., Mahboubi, M., Mandegary, A., Jangjoo, S., Mohammadinejad, R., & Varma, R. S. (2018). Health concerns of various nanoparticles: A review of their in vitro and in vivo toxicity. *Nanomaterials, 8*(9), 634. https://doi.org/10.3390/NANO8090634

Albayati, S. H. M., & Deveci, P. (2019). PH and GSH dual responsive smart silica nanocarrier for doxorubicin delivery. *Materials Research Express, 6*(6). https://doi.org/10.1088/2053-1591/AB0CDE

Andoh, Y., Mizutani, A., Ohashi, T., Kojo, S., Ishii, T., Adachi, Y., Ikehara, S., & Taketani, S. (2006). The antioxidant role of a reagent, 2′,7′-dichlorodihydrofluorescin diacetate, detecting reactive-oxygen species and blocking the induction of heme oxygenase-1 and preventing cytotoxicity. *The Journal of Biochemistry, 140*(4), 483–489. https://doi.org/10.1093/JB/MVJ187

Ansari, L., Jaafari, M. R., Bastami, T. R., & Malaekeh-Nikouei, B. (2018). Improved anticancer efficacy of epirubicin by magnetic mesoporous silica nanoparticles: In vitro and in vivo studies. *Artificial Cells, Nanomedicine, and Biotechnology, 46*(sup2), 594–606. https://doi.org/10.1080/21691401.2018.1464461

Ashley, C. E., Carnes, E. C., Phillips, G. K., Padilla, D., Durfee, P. N., Brown, P. A., Hanna, T. N., Liu, J., Phillips, B., Carter, M. B., Carroll, N. J., Jiang, X., Dunphy, D. R., Willman, C. L., Petsev, D. N., Evans, D. G., Parikh, A. N., Chackerian, B., Wharton, W.,. . . . Brinker, C. J. (2011). The targeted delivery of multicomponent cargos to cancer cells by nanoporous particle-supported lipid bilayers. *Nature Materials, 10*(5), 389–397. https://doi.org/10.1038/nmat2992

Azimipour, S., Ghaedi, S., Mehrabi, Z., Ghasemzadeh, S. A., Heshmati, M., Barikrow, N., Attar, F., & Falahati, M. (2018). Heme degradation and iron release of hemoglobin and oxidative stress of lymphocyte cells in the presence of silica nanoparticles. *International Journal of Biological Macromolecules, 118*, 800–807. https://doi.org/10.1016/J.IJBIOMAC.2018.06.128

Babaei, M., Abnous, K., Taghdisi, S. M., Taghavi, S., Sh. Saljooghi, A., Ramezani, M., & Alibolandi, M. (2020). Targeted rod-shaped mesoporous silica nanoparticles for the co-delivery of camptothecin and survivin shRNA in to colon adenocarcinoma in vitro and in vivo. *European Journal of Pharmaceutics and Biopharmaceutics, 156*, 84–96. https://doi.org/10.1016/J.EJPB.2020.08.026

Baeza, A., Colilla, M., & Vallet-Regí, M. (2015). Advances in mesoporous silica nanoparticles for targeted stimuli-responsive drug delivery. *Expert Opinion on Drug Delivery, 12*(2), 319–337. https://doi.org/10.1517/17425247.2014.953051

Bai, X., Zhao, G., Chen, Q., Li, Z., Gao, M., Ho, W., Xu, X., & Zhang, X. Q. (2022). Inhaled siRNA nanoparticles targeting IL11 inhibit lung fibrosis and improve pulmonary function post-bleomycin challenge. *Science Advances, 8*(25). https://doi.org/10.1126/SCIADV.ABN7162/SUPPL_FILE/SCIADV.ABN7162_SM.PDF

Bertucci, A., Prasetyanto, E. A., Septiadi, D., Manicardi, A., Brognara, E., Gambari, R., Corradini, R., & De Cola, L. (2015). Combined delivery of temozolomide and anti-miR221 PNA using mesoporous silica nanoparticles induces apoptosis in resistant glioma cells. *Small, 11*(42), 5687–5695. https://doi.org/10.1002/SMLL.201500540

Bhattacharyya, D., Singh, S., Satnalika, N., Khandelwal, A., & Jeon, S.-H. (2009). Nanotechnology, big things from a tiny world: A review. *Users.Encs.Concordia.Ca International Journal of u-and e-Service, Science and Technology, 2*(3). http://users.encs.concordia.ca/~mojtaba/elec6271/overview%20of%20nanotechnology.pdf

Boonamnuayvitaya, V., Tayamanon, C., Sae-Ung, S., & Tanthapanichakoon, W. (2006). Synthesis and characterization of porous media produced by a sol–gel method. *Chemical Engineering Science, 61*(5), 1686–1691. https://doi.org/10.1016/J.CES.2005.10.002

Bouchoucha, M., Cô, M.-F., Renéc, ‡, -Gaudreault, R., Andréfortin, M.-A., & Kleitz, F. (2016). Size-controlled functionalized mesoporous silica nanoparticles for tunable drug release and enhanced anti-tumoral activity. *ACS Publications Chemistry of Materials, 28*(12), 4243–4258. https://doi.org/10.1021/acs.chemmater.6b00877

Bukara, K., Schueller, L., Rosier, J., Martens, M. A., Daems, T., Verheyden, L., Eelen, S., Van Speybroeck, M., Libanati, C., Martens, J. A., Van Den Mooter, G., Frérart, F., Jolling, K., De Gieter, M., Bugarski, B., & Kiekens, F. (2016). Ordered mesoporous silica to enhance the bioavailability of poorly water-soluble drugs: Proof of concept in man. *European Journal of Pharmaceutics and Biopharmaceutics, 108*, 220–225. https://doi.org/10.1016/J.EJPB.2016.08.020

Cai, Q., Luo, Z. S., Pang, W. Q., Fan, Y. W., Chen, X. H., & Cui, F. Z. (2001). Dilute solution routes to various controllable morphologies of MCM-41 silica with a basic medium. *Chemistry of Materials, 13*(2), 258–263. https://doi.org/10.1021/cm990661z

Cao, X., Deng, W.-W., Fu, M., Wang, L., Tong, S.-S., Wei, Y.-W., Xu, Y., Su, W.-Y., Xu, X.-M., & Yu, J.-N. (2012). In vitro release and in vitro–in vivo correlation for silybin meglumine incorporated into hollow-type mesoporous silica nanoparticles. *Taylor & Francis International Journal of Nanomedicine*, *7*, 753–762. https://doi.org/10.2147/IJN.S28348

Capeletti, L. B., Loiola, L. M. D., Picco, A. S., da Silva Liberato, M., & Cardoso, M. B. (2018). Silica Nanoparticle Applications in the Biomedical Field. *Smart Nanoparticles for Biomedicine*, 115–129. https://doi.org/10.1016/B978-0-12-814156-4.00008-2

Carmona, M. M., Baeza, A., García-Castro, J., Martí Nez-Carmona, M., Rodriguez-Milla, M. A., Garcí A-Castro, J., & Vallet-Regí, M. (2015). Mesoporous silica nanoparticles grafted with a light-responsive protein shell for highly cytotoxic antitumoral therapy1. *Researchgate.Net*, *3*, 5746. https://doi.org/10.1039/C5TB00304K

Chang, J. S., Chang, K. L. B., Hwang, D. F., & Kong, Z. L. (2007). In vitro cytotoxicitiy of silica nanoparticles at high concentrations strongly depends on the metabolic activity type of the cell line. *Environmental Science and Technology*, *41*(6), 2064–2068. https://doi.org/10.1021/ES062347T/SUPPL_FILE/ES062347TSI20061226_044835.PDF

Chen, H., & He, S. (2015). PLA-PEG coated multifunctional imaging probe for targeted drug delivery. *Molecular Pharmaceutics*, *12*(6), 1885–1892. https://doi.org/10.1021/MP500512Z

Chen, H., Kuang, Y., Liu, R., Chen, Z., Jiang, B., Sun, Z., Chen, X., & Li, C. (2018). Dual-pH-sensitive mesoporous silica nanoparticle-based drug delivery system for tumor-triggered intracellular drug release. *Journal of Materials Science*, *53*(15), 10653–10665. https://doi.org/10.1007/S10853-018-2363-8

Chen, K., Li, X., Zhu, H., Gong, Q., & Luo, K. (2017). Endocytosis of nanoscale systems for cancer treatments. *Current Medicinal Chemistry*, *25*(25), 3017–3035. https://doi.org/10.2174/0929867324666170428153056

Chen, L., Zhou, X., Nie, W., Zhang, Q., Wang, W., Zhang, Y., & He, C. (2016). Multifunctional redox-responsive mesoporous silica nanoparticles for efficient targeting drug delivery and magnetic resonance imaging. *ACS Applied Materials and Interfaces*, *8*(49), 33829–33841. https://doi.org/10.1021/ACSAMI.6B11802/ASSET/IMAGES/LARGE/AM-2016-11802D_0011.JPEG

Chen, X., & Liu, Z. (2016). Dual responsive mesoporous silica nanoparticles for targeted co-delivery of hydrophobic and hydrophilic anticancer drugs to tumor cells. *Journal of Materials Chemistry B*, *4*(25), 4382–4388. https://doi.org/10.1039/C6TB00694A

Chen, X., Zhouhua, W., Jie, Z., Xinlu, F., Jinqiang, L., Yuwen, Q., & Zhiying, H. (2014). Renal interstitial fibrosis induced by high-dose mesoporous silica nanoparticles via the NF-& K;B signaling pathway. *International Journal of Nanomedicine*, *10*(1), 1–22. https://doi.org/10.2147/IJN.S73538

Chen, Y., Chen, H., research, J. S.-A. of chemical, & 2014, undefined. (2013). Construction of homogenous/heterogeneous hollow mesoporous silica nanostructures by silica-etching chemistry: Principles, synthesis, and applications. *ACS Publications Accounts of Chemical Research*, *47*(1), 125–137. https://doi.org/10.1021/ar400091e

Chen, Y., Munteanu, A. C., Huang, Y. F., Phillips, J., Zhu, Z., Mavros, M., & Tan, W. (2009). Mapping receptor density on live cells by using fluorescence correlation spectroscopy. *Chemistry—A European Journal*, *15*(21), 5327–5336. https://doi.org/10.1002/CHEM.200802305

Chen, Y., Xu, P., Chen, H., Li, Y., Bu, W., Shu, Z., Li, Y., Zhang, J., Zhang, L., Pan, L., Cui, X., Hua, Z., Wang, J., Zhang, L., & Shi, J. (2013). Colloidal HPMO nanoparticles: Silica-etching chemistry tailoring, topological transformation, and nano-biomedical applications. *Advanced Materials*, *25*(22), 3100–3105. https://doi.org/10.1002/ADMA.201204685

Chen, Y., Yang, W., Chang, B., Hu, H., Fang, X., & Sha, X. (2013). In vivo distribution and antitumor activity of doxorubicin-loaded N-isopropylacrylamide-co-methacrylic acid coated mesoporous silica nanoparticles and safety evaluation. *European Journal of Pharmaceutics and Biopharmaceutics*, *85*(3), 406–412. https://doi.org/10.1016/J.EJPB.2013.06.015

Cheng, Y. J., Luo, G. F., Zhu, J. Y., Xu, X. D., Zeng, X., Cheng, D. B., Li, Y. M., Wu, Y., Zhang, X. Z., Zhuo, R. X., & He, F. (2015). Enzyme-induced and tumor-targeted drug delivery system based on multifunctional mesoporous silica nanoparticles. *ACS Applied Materials and Interfaces*, *7*(17), 9078–9087. https://doi.org/10.1021/ACSAMI.5B00752/SUPPL_FILE/AM5B00752_SI_001.PDF

Croissant, J. G., Fatieiev, Y., Almalik, A., & Khashab, N. M. (2018). Mesoporous silica and organosilica nanoparticles: Physical chemistry, biosafety, delivery strategies, and biomedical applications. *Advanced Healthcare Materials*, *7*(4), 1700831. https://doi.org/10.1002/ADHM.201700831

Croissant, J. G., Fatieiev, Y., & Khashab, N. M. (2017). Degradability and clearance of silicon, organosilica, silsesquioxane, silica mixed oxide, and mesoporous silica nanoparticles. *Advanced Materials*, *29*(9), 1604634. https://doi.org/10.1002/ADMA.201604634

Cui, Y., Wei, Q., Park, H., & Lieber, C. M. (2001). Nanowire nanosensors for highly sensitive and selective detection of biological and chemical species. *Science*, *293*(5533), 1289–1292. https://doi.org/10.1126/SCIENCE.1062711

Das, B., Chabukdhara, M., Patra, S., & Gogoi, M. (2021). Current knowledge on toxicity of nanomaterials: Toxicity assessment and impact. *Nanotoxicology*, 339–375. https://doi.org/10.1201/9780429299742-14

Davis, M., Chen, Z., discovery, D. S.-N. reviews D., & 2008, undefined. (n.d.). Nanoparticle therapeutics: An emerging treatment modality for cancer. *Nature.Com Nature Reviews Drug Discovery*. Retrieved April 27, 2024, from https://www.nature.com/articles/nrd2614

Dieter, M. P. (1994). Toxicity and carcinogenicity studies of boric acid in male and female B6C3F1 mice. *Environmental Health Perspectives*, *102*(SUPPL. 7), 93–97. https://doi.org/10.1289/EHP.94102S793

Dogra, P., Adolphi, N. L., Wang, Z., Lin, Y. S., Butler, K. S., Durfee, P. N., Croissant, J. G., Noureddine, A., Coker, E. N., Bearer, E. L., Cristini, V., & Brinker, C. J. (2018). Establishing the effects of mesoporous silica nanoparticle properties on in vivo disposition using imaging-based pharmacokinetics. *Nature Communications*, *9*(1). https://doi.org/10.1038/S41467-018-06730-Z

dos Santos, A., Santos, dos, Varela, J., Lynch, I., Dawson, K. A., Salvati, A., dos Santos, T., & Dawson KennethADawson, K. A. (2011). Quantitative assessment of the comparative nanoparticle-uptake efficiency of a range of cell lines. *Wiley Online Library Small*, *7*(23), 3341–3349. https://doi.org/10.1002/smll.201101076

Drača, D., Edeler, D., Saoud, M., Dojčinović, B., Dunđerović, D., Đmura, G., Maksimović-Ivanić, D., Mijatović, S., & Kaluđerović, G. N. (2021). Antitumor potential of cisplatin loaded into SBA-15 mesoporous silica nanoparticles against B16F1 melanoma cells: In vitro and in vivo studies. *Journal of Inorganic Biochemistry*, *217*, 111383. https://doi.org/10.1016/J.JINORGBIO.2021.111383

Du, X., & He, J. (2011). Hierarchically mesoporous silica nanoparticles: Extraction, amino-functionalization, and their multipurpose potentials. *Langmuir*, *27*(6), 2972–2979. https://doi.org/10.1021/LA200014W/SUPPL_FILE/LA200014W_SI_001.PDF

Dumontel, B., Conejo-Rodríguez, V., Vallet-Regí, M., & Manzano, M. (2023). Natural biopolymers as smart coating materials of mesoporous silica nanoparticles for drug delivery. *Pharmaceutics*, *15*(2), 447. https://doi.org/10.3390/PHARMACEUTICS15020447

Elsabahy, M., & Wooley, K. L. (2013). Cytokines as biomarkers of nanoparticle immunotoxicity. *Chemical Society Reviews*, *42*(12), 5552–5576. https://doi.org/10.1039/C3CS60064E

Farjadian, F., Roointan, A., Mohammadi-Samani, S., & Hosseini, M. (2019). Mesoporous silica nanoparticles: Synthesis, pharmaceutical applications, biodistribution, and biosafety assessment. *Chemical Engineering Journal*, *359*, 684–705. https://doi.org/10.1016/J.CEJ.2018.11.156

Fernandes, F. M., Coradin, T., & Aimé, C. (2014). Self-assembly in biosilicification and biotemplated silica materials. *Nanomaterials*, *4*(3), 792–812. https://doi.org/10.3390/NANO4030792

Ganjavi, H., Gee, M., Narendran, A.,. . . . N. P.-C. gene, & 2006, undefined. (n.d.). Adenovirus-mediated p53 gene therapy in osteosarcoma cell lines: Sensitization to cisplatin and doxorubicin. *Nature.Com Cancer Gene Therapy*. Retrieved April 27, 2024, from https://www.nature.com/articles/7700909

Gao, W., Chan, J. M., & Farokhzad, O. C. (2010). PH-responsive nanoparticles for drug delivery. *Molecular Pharmaceutics*, *7*(6), 1913–1920. https://doi.org/10.1021/MP100253E

Gisbert-Garzarán, M., & Vallet-Regí, M. (2021). Redox-responsive mesoporous silica nanoparticles for cancer treatment: Recent updates. *Nanomaterials*, *11*(9), 2222. https://doi.org/10.3390/NANO11092222

Gong, H., Xie, Z., Liu, M., Zhu, H., & Sun, H. (2015). Redox-sensitive mesoporous silica nanoparticles functionalized with PEG through a disulfide bond linker for potential anticancer drug delivery. *RSC Advances*, *5*(73), 59576–59582. https://doi.org/10.1039/C5RA09774F

Granja, A., Lima-Sousa, R., Alves, C. G., de Melo-Diogo, D., Pinheiro, M., Sousa, C. T., Correia, I. J., & Reis, S. (2021). Mitoxantrone-loaded lipid nanoparticles for breast cancer therapy—Quality-by-design approach and efficacy assessment in 2D and 3D in vitro cancer models. *International Journal of Pharmaceutics*, *607*, 121044. https://doi.org/10.1016/J.IJPHARM.2021.121044

Gräslund, A., Madani, F., Lindberg, S., Langel, Ü., & Futaki, S. (2011). Mechanisms of cellular uptake of cell-penetrating peptides. *Journal of Biophysics*, *2011*(1), 414729. https://doi.org/10.1155/2011/414729

Guan, L., Chen, J., Tian, Z., Zhu, M., Bian, Y., & Zhu, Y. (2021). Mesoporous organosilica nanoparticles: Degradation strategies and application in tumor therapy. *View*, *2*(5), 20200117. https://doi.org/10.1002/VIW.20200117

Hanahan, D., & Weinberg, R. A. (2011). Hallmarks of cancer: The next generation. *Cell*, *144*(5), 646–674. https://doi.org/10.1016/J.CELL.2011.02.013

Haramati, J., Soppe, C., & Zúñiga, M. C. (2007). A rapid method for skin grafting in mice that greatly enhances graft and recipient survival. *Transplantation*, *84*(10), 1364–1367. https://doi.org/10.1097/01.TP.0000289994.13139.F4

He, Q., & Shi, J. (2014). MSN anti-cancer nanomedicines: Chemotherapy enhancement, overcoming of drug resistance, and metastasis inhibition. *Advanced Materials*, *26*(3), 391–411. https://doi.org/10.1002/ADMA.201303123

Hein, C. D., Liu, X. M., & Wang, D. (2008). Click chemistry, a powerful tool for pharmaceutical sciences. *Pharmaceutical Research*, *25*(10), 2216–2230. https://doi.org/10.1007/S11095-008-9616-1

Herr, J. K., Smith, J. E., Medley, C. D., Shangguan, D., & Tan, W. (2006). Aptamer-conjugated nanoparticles for selective collection and detection of cancer cells. *Analytical Chemistry*, *78*(9), 2918–2924. https://doi.org/10.1021/AC052015R

Hesemann, P., Nguyen, T. P., & El Hankari, S. (2014a). Precursor mediated synthesis of nanostructured silicas: From precursor-surfactant ion Pairs to structured materials. *Materials*, *7*(4), 2978–3001. https://doi.org/10.3390/MA7042978

Hesemann, P., Nguyen, T. P., & El Hankari, S. (2014b). Precursor mediated synthesis of nanostructured silicas: From precursor-surfactant ion Pairs to structured materials. *Materials*, *7*(4), 2978–3001. https://doi.org/10.3390/MA7042978

Hoffmann, F., Cornelius, M., Morell, J., & Fröba, M. (2006). Silica-based mesoporous organic–inorganic hybrid materials. *Angewandte Chemie International Edition*, *45*(20), 3216–3251. https://doi.org/10.1002/ANIE.200503075

Horcajada, P., Gref, R., Baati, T., Allan, P. K., Maurin, G., Couvreur, P., Férey, G., Morris, R. E., & Serre, C. (2012). Metal-organic frameworks in biomedicine. *Chemical Reviews*, *112*(2), 1232–1268. https://doi.org/10.1021/CR200256V

Hoshikawa, Y., Yabe, H., Nomura, A., Yamaki, T., Shimojima, A., & Okubo, T. (2010). Mesoporous silica nanoparticles with remarkable stability and dispersibility for antireflective coatings. *Chemistry of Materials*, *22*(1), 12–14. https://doi.org/10.1021/CM902239A/SUPPL_FILE/CM902239A_SI_001.PDF

Hoyer, J., research, I. N.-A. of chemical, & 2012, undefined. (2012). Peptide vectors for the nonviral delivery of nucleic acids. *ACS Publications Accounts of Chemical Research*, *45*(7), 1048–1056. https://doi.org/10.1021/ar2002304

Hu, Y., Bai, S., Wu, X., Tan, S., & He, Y. (2021). Biodegradability of mesoporous silica nanoparticles. *Ceramics International*, *47*(22), 31031–31041. https://doi.org/10.1016/J.CERAMINT.2021.08.129

Huang, Q., Yu, H., & Ru, Q. (2010). Bioavailability and delivery of nutraceuticals using nanotechnology. *Journal of Food Science*, *75*(1), R50–R57. https://doi.org/10.1111/J.1750-3841.2009.01457.X

Ivanov, S., Zhuravsky, S., Yukina, G., Tomson, V., Korolev, D., & Galagudza, M. (2012). In vivo toxicity of intravenously administered silica and silicon nanoparticles. *Materials*, *5*(10), 1873–1889. https://doi.org/10.3390/MA5101873

Jafarzadeh, M., Rahman, I. A., & Sipaut, C. S. (2009). Synthesis of silica nanoparticles by modified sol-gel process: The effect of mixing modes of the reactants and drying techniques. *Journal of Sol-Gel Science and Technology*, *50*(3), 328–336. https://doi.org/10.1007/S10971-009-1958-6/TABLES/5

Jana, S., Dutta, B., Honda, H., & Koner, S. (2011). Mesoporous silica MCM-41 with rod-shaped morphology: Synthesis and characterization. *Applied Clay Science*, *54*(2), 138–143. https://doi.org/10.1016/J.CLAY.2011.07.018

Jia, L., Shen, J., Li, Z., Zhang, D., Zhang, Q., Liu, G., Zheng, D., & Tian, X. (2013). In vitro and in vivo evaluation of paclitaxel-loaded mesoporous silica nanoparticles with three pore sizes. *International Journal of Pharmaceutics*, *445*(1–2), 12–19. https://doi.org/10.1016/J.IJPHARM.2013.01.058

Jiang, J., Humar, A., Gracia, B., & Zhong, R. (1998). Surgical technique for vascularized ear transplantation in mice. *Microsurgery*. https://doi.org/10.1002/(SICI)1098-2752(1998)18:1

Jo, H., Her, J., & Ban, C. (2015). Dual aptamer-functionalized silica nanoparticles for the highly sensitive detection of breast cancer. *Biosensors and Bioelectronics*, *71*, 129–136. https://doi.org/10.1016/J.BIOS.2015.04.030

Jung, E., Kang, C., Lee, J., Yoo, D., Hwang, D. W., Kim, D., Park, S. C., Lim, S. K., Song, C., & Lee, D. (2018). Molecularly engineered theranostic nanoparticles for thrombosed vessels: H2O2-activatable contrast-enhanced photoacoustic imaging and antithrombotic therapy. *ACS Nano*, *12*(1), 392–401. https://doi.org/10.1021/ACSNANO.7B06560

Kankala, R. K., Han, Y. H., Xia, H. Y., Wang, S. Bin, & Chen, A. Z. (2022). Nanoarchitectured prototypes of mesoporous silica nanoparticles for innovative biomedical applications. *Journal of Nanobiotechnology*, *20*(1), 1–67. https://doi.org/10.1186/S12951-022-01315-X/FIGURES/14

Khan, A. A., Khan, I. M., Nguyen, P. P., Lo, E., Chahadeh, H., Cerniglia, M., & Noriega, J. A. (2020). Skin graft techniques. *Clinics in Podiatric Medicine and Surgery*, *37*(4), 821–835. https://doi.org/10.1016/j.cpm.2020.07.007

Khan, M. F., Kundu, D., Gogoi, M., Shrestha, A. K., Karanth, N. G., & Patra, S. (2020). *Enzyme-Responsive and Enzyme Immobilized Nanoplatforms for Therapeutic Delivery: An Overview of Research Innovations and Biomedical Applications*, 165–200. https://doi.org/10.1007/978-3-030-47120-0_6

Khanal, A., Inoue, Y., Yada, M., & Nakashima, K. (2007). Synthesis of silica hollow nanoparticles templated by polymeric micelle with core-shell-corona structure. *Journal of the American Chemical Society*, *129*(6), 1534–1535. https://doi.org/10.1021/JA0684904/SUPPL_FILE/JA0684904SI20061127_094139.PDF

Kharlamov, A. N., Tyurnina, A. E., Veselova, V. S., Kovtun, O. P., Shur, V. Y., & Gabinsky, J. L. (2015). Silica-gold nanoparticles for atheroprotective management of plaques: Results of the NANOM-FIM trial. *Nanoscale*, *7*(17), 8003–8015. https://doi.org/10.1039/C5NR01050K

Kim, J. S., Rieter, W. J., Taylor, K. M. L., An, H., Lin, W., & Lin, W. (2007). Self-assembled hybrid nanoparticles for cancer-specific multimodal imaging. *Journal of the American Chemical Society*, *129*(29), 8962–8963. https://doi.org/10.1021/JA073062Z

Kim, W., Ng, J. K., Kunitake, M. E., Conklin, B. R., & Yang, P. (2007). Interfacing silicon nanowires with mammalian cells. *Journal of the American Chemical Society*, *129*(23), 7228–7229. https://doi.org/10.1021/JA071456K

Kobes, J. E., Georgiev, G. I., Louis, A. V., Calderon, I. A., Yoshimaru, E. S., Klemm, L. M., Cromey, D. W., Khalpey, Z., & Pagel, M. D. (2018). A comparison of iron oxide particles and silica particles for tracking organ recellularization. *Molecular Imaging*, *17*. https://doi.org/10.1177/1536012118787322

Kondoh, G., Li, Q., Paii, J., & Hakura, A. (1995). Transgenic models for papillomavirus-associated multistep carcinogenesis. *Intervirology*, *38*(3–4), 181–186. https://doi.org/10.1159/000150430

Koole, R., Van Schooneveld, M. M., Hilhorst, J., Castermans, K., Cormode, D. P., Strijkers, G. J., Donegá, C. D. M., Vanmaekelbergh, D., Griffioen, A. W., Nicolay, K., Fayad, Z. A., Meijerink, A., & Mulder, W. J. M. (2008). Paramagnetic lipid-coated silica nanoparticles with a fluorescent quantum dot core: A new contrast agent platform for multimodality imaging. *Bioconjugate Chemistry*, *19*(12), 2471–2479. https://doi.org/10.1021/BC800368X

Kumar, D., Mutreja, I., Keshvan, P. C., Bhat, M., Dinda, A. K., & Mitra, S. (2015a). Organically modified silica nanoparticles interaction with macrophage cells: Assessment of cell viability on the basis of physicochemical properties. *Journal of Pharmaceutical Sciences*, *104*(11), 3943–3951. https://doi.org/10.1002/JPS.24614

Kumar, D., Mutreja, I., Keshvan, P. C., Bhat, M., Dinda, A. K., & Mitra, S. (2015b). Organically modified silica nanoparticles interaction with macrophage cells: Assessment of cell viability on the basis of physicochemical properties. *Journal of Pharmaceutical Sciences*, *104*(11), 3943–3951. https://doi.org/10.1002/JPS.24614/ASSET/E86F8B03-58E7-4A4F-8C5F-069D59F95E11/MAIN.ASSETS/GR7.SML

Kuthati, Y., Sung, P. J., Weng, C. F., Mou, C. Y., & Lee, C. H. (2013). Functionalization of mesoporous silica nanoparticles for targeting, biocompatibility, combined cancer therapies and theragnosis. *Journal of Nanoscience and Nanotechnology*, *13*(4), 2399–2430. https://doi.org/10.1166/JNN.2013.7363

Lange, M. E., Uwiera, R. R. E., & Inglis, G. D. (2019). Housing gnotobiotic mice in conventional animal facilities. *Current Protocols in Mouse Biology*, *9*(1), e59. https://doi.org/10.1002/CPMO.59

Lazaro, I., Haddad, S., Sacca, S., Chem, C. O.-T.-, & 2017, undefined. (2017). Selective surface PEGylation of UiO-66 nanoparticles for enhanced stability, cell uptake, and pH-responsive drug delivery. *Cell.Com Chem*, *2*(4), 561–578. https://doi.org/10.1016/j.chempr.2017.02.005

Li, C., Tebo, A. G., & Gautier, A. (2017). Fluorogenic labeling strategies for biological imaging. *International Journal of Molecular Sciences*, *18*(7), 1473. https://doi.org/10.3390/IJMS18071473

Li, L., Tang, F., Liu, H., Liu, T., Hao, N., Chen, D., Teng, X., & He, J. (2010a). In vivo delivery of silica nanorattle encapsulated docetaxel for liver cancer therapy with low toxicity and high efficacy. *ACS Nano*, *4*(11), 6874–6882. https://doi.org/10.1021/NN100918A

Li, L., Tang, F., Liu, H., Liu, T., Hao, N., Chen, D., Teng, X., & He, J. (2010b). In vivo delivery of silica nanorattle encapsulated docetaxel for liver cancer therapy with low toxicity and high efficacy. *ACS Nano*, *4*(11), 6874–6882. https://doi.org/10.1021/NN100918A/SUPPL_FILE/NN100918A_SI_001.PDF

Li, Q. L., Sun, Y., Sun, Y. L., Wen, J., Zhou, Y., Bing, Q. M., Isaacs, L. D., Jin, Y., Gao, H., & Yang, Y. W. (2014). Mesoporous silica nanoparticles coated by layer-by-layer self-assembly using cucurbit[7]uril for in vitro and in vivo anticancer drug release. *Chemistry of Materials*, *26*(22), 6418–6431. https://doi.org/10.1021/CM503304P/SUPPL_FILE/CM503304P_SI_001.PDF

Li, Y., Li, N., Pan, W., Yu, Z., Yang, L., & Tang, B. (2017). Hollow mesoporous silica nanoparticles with tunable structures for controlled drug delivery. *ACS Applied Materials and Interfaces*, *9*(3), 2123–2129. https://doi.org/10.1021/ACSAMI.6B13876/ASSET/IMAGES/LARGE/AM-2016-13876Z_0004.JPEG

Liberman, A., Mendez, N., Trogler, W. C., & Kummel, A. C. (2014). Synthesis and surface functionalization of silica nanoparticles for nanomedicine. *Surface Science Reports*, *69*(2–3), 132–158. https://doi.org/10.1016/J.SURFREP.2014.07.001

Lin, C. Y., Yang, C. M., & Lindén, M. (2022). Dissolution and morphology evolution of mesoporous silica nanoparticles under biologically relevant conditions. *Journal of Colloid and Interface Science*, *608*, 995–1004. https://doi.org/10.1016/J.JCIS.2021.09.164

Lin, F., Meng, X., Tang, K., Wu, L., Yuan, R., & Liao, L. (2021). Structure modulation of periodic mesoporous organosilicas with organic salts. *Journal of Materials Science*, *56*(24), 13590–13603. https://doi.org/10.1007/S10853-021-06191-8

Lindén, M. (2018). Biodistribution and excretion of intravenously injected mesoporous silica nanoparticles: Implications for drug delivery efficiency and safety. *Enzymes*, *43*, 155–180. https://doi.org/10.1016/BS.ENZ.2018.07.007

Liu, X., Jiang, J., Chan, R., Ji, Y., Lu, J., Liao, Y. P., Okene, M., Lin, J., Lin, P., Chang, C. H., Wang, X., Tang, I., Zheng, E., Qiu, W., Wainberg, Z. A., Nel, A. E., & Meng, H. (2019). Improved efficacy and reduced toxicity using a custom-designed irinotecan-delivering silicasome for orthotopic colon cancer. *ACS Nano*, *13*(1), 38–53. https://doi.org/10.1021/ACSNANO.8B06164/SUPPL_FILE/NN8B06164_SI_001.PDF

Lorenz, B., Ali, N., Bocklitz, T., Rösch, P., & Popp, J. (2020). Discrimination between pathogenic and non-pathogenic E. coli strains by means of Raman microspectroscopy. *Analytical and Bioanalytical Chemistry*, *412*(30), 8241–8247. https://doi.org/10.1007/S00216-020-02957-2/FIGURES/3

Lu, J., Li, Z., Zink, J. I., Nanotechnology, F. T.-N., Biology, undefined, & 2012, undefined. (n.d.). In vivo tumor suppression efficacy of mesoporous silica nanoparticles-based drug-delivery system: Enhanced efficacy by folate modification. *Elsevier Biology and Medicine*. Retrieved April 27, 2024, from https://www.sciencedirect.com/science/article/pii/S1549963411002553?casa_token=IUNi38xliCAAAAAA:s_tPO11719i1SwXmrlWkIXd5s71HOD45Lx00DzfGkXBilp7YQmljf8ZGpMGIJdJHoesi3ilqaPE

Lu, J., Li, Z., Zink, J. I., & Tamanoi, F. (2012). In vivo tumor suppression efficacy of mesoporous silica nanoparticles-based drug-delivery system: Enhanced efficacy by folate modification. *Nanomedicine: Nanotechnology, Biology and Medicine*, *8*(2), 212–220. https://doi.org/10.1016/J.NANO.2011.06.002

Ma, X., Su, X., Zhang, J., Dang, M., Tao, J., Xu, P., Li, Y., Lv, P., Wei, W., & Teng, Z. (2018). Uniform and ordered periodic mesoporous organosilica thin films by a facile solution growth approach. *Journal of Porous Materials*, *25*(2), 489–494. https://doi.org/10.1007/S10934-017-0460-8

Mahato, M., Patra, S., & Gogoi, M. (2021). *Herbal Nanocarriers for Cancer Therapy*, 41–75. https://doi.org/10.1007/978-3-030-44921-6_2

Mai, W., Biology, H. M.-I., & 2013, undefined. (2013). Mesoporous silica nanoparticles: A multifunctional nano therapeutic system. *Academic.Oup.Com Integrative Biology*, *5*, 19. https://doi.org/10.1039/c2ib20137b

Manning, J. R. H., Brambila, C., & Patwardhan, S. V. (2021). Unified mechanistic interpretation of amine-assisted silica synthesis methods to enable design of more complex materials. *Molecular Systems Design & Engineering*, *6*(3), 170–196. https://doi.org/10.1039/D0ME00131G

Martínez-Carmona, M., Baeza, A., Rodriguez-Milla, M. A., García-Castro, J., & Vallet-Regí, M. (2015). Mesoporous silica nanoparticles grafted with a light-responsive protein shell for highly cytotoxic antitumoral therapy. *Journal of Materials Chemistry B*, *3*(28), 5746–5752. https://doi.org/10.1039/C5TB00304K

Mathelié-Guinlet, M., Cohen-Bouhacina, T., Gammoudi, I., Martin, A., Béven, L., Delville, M. H., & Grauby-Heywang, C. (2019). Silica nanoparticles-assisted electrochemical biosensor for the rapid, sensitive and specific detection of Escherichia coli. *Sensors and Actuators B: Chemical*, *292*, 314–320. https://doi.org/10.1016/J.SNB.2019.03.144

Meng, H., Liong, M., Xia, T., Li, Z., Ji, Z., Zink, J. I., & Nel, A. E. (2010). Engineered design of mesoporous silica nanoparticles to deliver doxorubicin and p-glycoprotein siRNA to overcome drug resistance in a cancer cell line. *ACS Nano*, *4*(8), 4539–4550. https://doi.org/10.1021/NN100690M

Meng, H., Mai, W. X., Zhang, H., Xue, M., Xia, T., Lin, S., Wang, X., Zhao, Y., Ji, Z., Zink, J. I., & Nel, A. E. (2013). Codelivery of an optimal drug/siRNA combination using mesoporous silica nanoparticles to overcome drug resistance in breast cancer in vitro and in vivo. *ACS Nano*, *7*(2), 994–1005. https://doi.org/10.1021/NN3044066/SUPPL_FILE/NN3044066_SI_001.PDF

Meng, H., Wang, M., Liu, H., Liu, X., Situ, A., Wu, B., Ji, Z., Chang, C. H., & Nel, A. E. (2015). Use of a lipid-coated mesoporous silica nanoparticle platform for synergistic gmcitabine and pclitaxel delivery to human pancreatic cancer in mice. *ACS Nano*, *9*(4), 3540–3557. https://doi.org/10.1021/ACSNANO.5B00510/SUPPL_FILE/NN5B00510_SI_001.PDF

Mladenović, M., Jarić, S., Mundžić, M., Pavlović, A., Bobrinetskiy, I., & Knežević, N. (2024). Biosensors for cancer biomarkers based on mesoporous silica nanoparticles. *Biosensors*, *14*(7), 326. https://doi.org/10.3390/BIOS14070326

Moodley, T., & Singh, M. (2019). Polymeric mesoporous silica nanoparticles for enhanced delivery of 5-fluorouracil in vitro. *Pharmaceutics*, *11*(6), 288. https://doi.org/10.3390/PHARMACEUTICS11060288

Moodley, T., & Singh, M. (2020). Sterically stabilised polymeric mesoporous silica nanoparticles improve doxorubicin efficiency: Tailored cancer therapy. *Molecules*, *25*(3), 742. https://doi.org/10.3390/MOLECULES25030742

Moreira, A. F., Dias, D. R., & Correia, I. J. (2016). Stimuli-responsive mesoporous silica nanoparticles for cancer therapy: A review. *Microporous and Mesoporous Materials*, *236*, 141–157. https://doi.org/10.1016/J.MICROMESO.2016.08.038

Müller, I., Jenner, A., Bruchelt, G.,. . . . D. N.-B. and, & 1997, undefined. (n.d.). Effect of concentration on the cytotoxic mechanism of doxorubicin—apoptosis and oxidative DNA damage. *Elsevier Biochemical and Biophysical Research Communications*. Retrieved April 27, 2024, from https://www.sciencedirect.com/science/article/pii/S0006291X96958982

Nell, K. M., Fontenot, S. A., Carter, T. G., Warner, M. G., Warner, C. L., Addleman, R. S., & Johnson, D. W. (2016). Non-covalent functionalization of high-surface area nanomaterials: A new class of sorbent materials. *Environmental Science: Nano*, *3*(1), 138–145. https://doi.org/10.1039/C5EN00170F

Nemmar, A., Albarwani, S., Beegam, S., Yuvaraju, P., Yasin, J., Attoub, S., & Ali, B. H. (2014). Amorphous silica nanoparticles impair vascular homeostasis and induce systemic inflammation. *International Journal of Nanomedicine*, *9*(1), 2279–2789. https://doi.org/10.2147/IJN.S52818

Oh, W. K., Kim, S., Choi, M., Kim, C., Jeong, Y. S., Cho, B. R., Hahn, J. S., & Jang, J. (2010). Cellular uptake, cytotoxicity, and innate immune response of silica-Titania hollow nanoparticles based on size and surface functionality. *ACS Nano*, *4*(9), 5301–5313. https://doi.org/10.1021/NN100561E/SUPPL_FILE/NN100561E_SI_001.PDF

O'Hare, P. A. G. (1999). Thermochemistry of silicon-containing materials. *Pure and Applied Chemistry*, *71*(7), 1243–1248. https://doi.org/10.1351/PAC199971071243

Ohkubo, T., Ogura, T., Sakai, H., & Abe, M. (2007). Synthesis of highly-ordered mesoporous silica particles using mixed cationic and anionic surfactants as templates. *Journal of Colloid and Interface Science*, *312*(1), 42–46. https://doi.org/10.1016/J.JCIS.2007.02.043

Owens, D. E., & Peppas, N. A. (2006). Opsonization, biodistribution, and pharmacokinetics of polymeric nanoparticles. *International Journal of Pharmaceutics*, *307*(1), 93–102. https://doi.org/10.1016/J.IJPHARM.2005.10.010

Pack, C. G., Paulson, B., Shin, Y., Jung, M. K., Kim, J. S., & Kim, J. K. (2020). Variably sized and multi-colored silica-nanoparticles characterized by fluorescence correlation methods for cellular dynamics. *Materials*, *14*(1), 19. https://doi.org/10.3390/MA14010019

Pagels, R. F., Pinkerton, N. M., York, A. W., & Prud'homme, R. K. (2020). Synthesis of heterobifunctional thiol-poly(lactic acid)-b-poly(ethylene glycol)-hydroxyl for nanoparticle drug delivery applications. *Macromolecular Chemistry and Physics*, *221*(2). https://doi.org/10.1002/MACP.201900396

Pakyari, M., Farokhi, A., Khosravi-Maharlooei, M., Kilani, R. T., Ghahary, A., & Brown, E. (2016). A new method for skin grafting in murine model. *Wound Repair and Regeneration*, *24*(4), 695–704. https://doi.org/10.1111/WRR.12445

Pal, N., Lee, J. H., & Cho, E. B. (2020). Recent trends in morphology-controlled synthesis and application of mesoporous silica nanoparticles. *Nanomaterials*, *10*(11), 2122. https://doi.org/10.3390/NANO10112122

Patolsky, F., Timko, B. P., Yu, G., Fang, Y., Greytak, A. B., Zheng, G., & Lieber, C. M. (2006). Detection, stimulation, and inhibition of neuronal signals with high-density nanowire transistor arrays. *Science*, *313*(5790), 1100–1104. https://doi.org/10.1126/SCIENCE.1128640

Peng, F., Su, Y., Zhong, Y., Fan, C., Lee, S. T., & He, Y. (2014). Silicon nanomaterials platform for bioimaging, biosensing, and cancer therapy. *Accounts of Chemical Research*, *47*(2), 612–623. https://doi.org/10.1021/AR400221G/ASSET/IMAGES/MEDIUM/AR-2013-00221G_0011.GIF

Petros, R., discovery, J. D.-N. reviews D., & 2010, undefined. (2010). Strategies in the design of nanoparticles for therapeutic applications. *Nature.Com Nature Reviews Drug Discovery*. https://doi.org/10.1038/nrd2591

Potter, T. M., Neun, B. W., Rodriguez, J. C., Ilinskaya, A. N., & Dobrovolskaia, M. A. (2018). Analysis of pro-inflammatory cytokine and type II interferon induction by nanoparticles. *Methods in Molecular Biology*, *1682*, 173–187. https://doi.org/10.1007/978-1-4939-7352-1_15

Rafiq, S., Yeku, O. O., Jackson, H. J., Purdon, T. J., van Leeuwen, D. G., Drakes, D. J., Song, M., Miele, M. M., Li, Z., Wang, P., Yan, S., Xiang, J., Ma, X., Seshan, V. E., Hendrickson, R. C., Liu, C., & Brentjens, R. J. (2018). Targeted delivery of a PD-1-blocking scFv by CAR-T cells enhances anti-tumor efficacy in vivo. *Nature Biotechnology*, *36*(9), 847–856. https://doi.org/10.1038/nbt.4195

Rastinehad, A. R., Anastos, H., Wajswol, E., Winoker, J. S., Sfakianos, J. P., Doppalapudi, S. K., Carrick, M. R., Knauer, C. J., Taouli, B., Lewis, S. C., Tewari, A. K., Schwartz, J. A., Canfield, S. E., George, A. K., West, J. L., & Halas, N. J. (2019). Gold nanoshell-localized photothermal ablation of prostate tumors in a clinical pilot device study. *Proceedings of the National Academy of Sciences of the United States of America*, *116*(37), 18590–18596. https://doi.org/10.1073/PNAS.1906929116

Rosenholm, J., Sahlgren, C., Lindén, M., Rosenholm, J. M., & Lind, M. (2010). Towards multifunctional, targeted drug delivery systems using mesoporous silica nanoparticles–opportunities & challenges. *Pubs. Rsc.Org Nanoscale*. https://doi.org/10.1039/c0nr00156b

Ryplida, B., Lee, G., In, I., & Park, S. Y. (2019). Zwitterionic carbon dot-encapsulating pH-responsive mesoporous silica nanoparticles for NIR light-triggered photothermal therapy through pH-controllable release. *Biomaterials Science*, *7*(6), 2600–2610. https://doi.org/10.1039/C9BM00160C

Sanità, G., Carrese, B., & Lamberti, A. (2020). Nanoparticle surface functionalization: How to improve biocompatibility and cellular internalization. *Frontiers in Molecular Biosciences*, *7*. https://doi.org/10.3389/FMOLB.2020.587012/FULL

Schwarzl, R., Du, F., Haag, R., & Netz, R. R. (2017). General method for the quantification of drug loading and release kinetics of nanocarriers. *European Journal of Pharmaceutics and Biopharmaceutics*, *116*, 131–137. https://doi.org/10.1016/J.EJPB.2016.12.015

Shadmani, N., Makvandi, P., Parsa, M., Azadi, A., Nedaei, K., Mozafari, N., Poursina, N., Mattoli, V., Tay, F. R., Maleki, A., & Hamidi, M. (2023). Enhancing methotrexate delivery in the brain by mesoporous silica nanoparticles functionalized with cell-penetrating peptide using in vivo and ex vivo monitoring. *Molecular Pharmaceutics*, *20*(3), 1531–1548. https://doi.org/10.1021/ACS.MOLPHARMACEUT.2C00755/SUPPL_FILE/MP2C00755_SI_001.PDF

Shao, D., Wang, Z., Chang, Z., Chen, L., Dong, W. F., & Leong, K. W. (2021). Janus metallic mesoporous silica nanoparticles: Unique structures for cancer theranostics. *Current Opinion in Biomedical Engineering*, *19*, 100294. https://doi.org/10.1016/J.COBME.2021.100294

Shapero, K., Fenaroli, F., Lynch, I., Cottell, D. C., Salvati, A., & Dawson, K. A. (2011). Time and space resolved uptake study of silica nanoparticles by human cells. *Molecular BioSystems*, *7*(2), 371–378. https://doi.org/10.1039/C0MB00109K

Shipp, A., Lawrence, G., Gentry, R., McDonald, T., Bartow, H., Bounds, J., Macdonald, N., Clewell, H., Allen, B., & Van Landingham, C. (2006). Acrylamide: Review of toxicity data and dose-response analyses for cancer and noncancer effects. *Critical Reviews in Toxicology*, *36*(6), 481–608. https://doi.org/10.1080/10408440600851377

Silva, C. R. P., Da Rocha Ferreira, F., Webler, G. D., Da Silva, A. O. S., De Abreu, F. C., & Fonseca, E. J. S. (2017). Encapsulation of mangiferin in ordered mesoporous silica type SBA-15: Synthesis and characterization. *Materials Research Express*, *4*(6), 065402. https://doi.org/10.1088/2053-1591/AA71E6

Singh, L. P., Bhattacharyya, S. K., Kumar, R., Mishra, G., Sharma, U., Singh, G., & Ahalawat, S. (2014). Sol-Gel processing of silica nanoparticles and their applications. *Advances in Colloid and Interface Science*, *214*, 17–37. https://doi.org/10.1016/J.CIS.2014.10.007

Slowing, I., Trewyn, B. G., & Lin, V. S. Y. (2006). Effect of surface functionalization of MCM-41-type mesoporous silica nanoparticles on the endocytosis by human cancer cells. *Journal of the American Chemical Society*, *128*(46), 14792–14793. https://doi.org/10.1021/JA0645943

Sze, S. M. (2008). *Semiconductor Devices: Physics and Technology*, 2nd ed. 28–33. https://books.google.com/books/about/SEMICONDUCTOR_DEVICES_PHYSICS_AND_TECHNO.html?id=d_J0ZnHjUvIC

Sonali, Agrawal, P., Singh, R. P., Rajesh, C. V., Singh, S., Vijayakumar, M. R., Pandey, B. L., & Muthu, M. S. (2016). Transferrin receptor-targeted vitamin E TPGS micelles for brain cancer therapy: Preparation, characterization and brain distribution in rats. *Drug Delivery*, *23*(5), 1788–1798. https://doi.org/10.3109/10717544.2015.1094681

Sonnenschein, C., & Soto, A. M. (2020). Over a century of cancer research: Inconvenient truths and promising leads. *PLoS Biology*, *18*(4), e3000670. https://doi.org/10.1371/JOURNAL.PBIO.3000670

Stöber, W., Fink, A., & Bohn, E. (1968). Controlled growth of monodisperse silica spheres in the micron size range. *Journal of Colloid and Interface Science*, *26*(1), 62–69. https://doi.org/10.1016/0021-9797(68)90272-5

Suk, J. S., Xu, Q., Kim, N., Hanes, J., & Ensign, L. M. (2015). PEGylation as a strategy for improving nanoparticle-based drug and gene delivery. *Advanced Drug Delivery Reviews*, *99*(Pt A), 28. https://doi.org/10.1016/J.ADDR.2015.09.012

Sun, W., Fan, J., Wang, S., Kang, Y., Du, J., & Peng, X. (2018). Biodegradable drug-loaded hydroxyapatite nanotherapeutic agent for targeted drug release in tumors. *ACS Applied Materials and Interfaces*, *10*(9), 7832–7840. https://doi.org/10.1021/ACSAMI.7B19281/ASSET/IMAGES/LARGE/AM-2017-19281R_0008.JPEG

Tang, F., Li, L., & Chen, D. (2012). Mesoporous silica nanoparticles: Synthesis, biocompatibility and drug delivery. *Advanced Materials*, *24*(12), 1504–1534. https://doi.org/10.1002/ADMA.201104763

Taylor, K. M. L., Kim, J. S., Rieter, W. J., An, H., Lin, W., & Lin, W. (2008). Mesoporous silica nanospheres as highly efficient MRI contrast agents. *Journal of the American Chemical Society*, *130*(7), 2154–2155. https://doi.org/10.1021/JA710193C

Teng, Z., Su, X., Lee, B., Huang, C., Liu, Y., Wang, S., Wu, J., Xu, P., Sun, J., Shen, D., Li, W., & Lu, G. (2014). Yolk-shell structured mesoporous nanoparticles with thioether-bridged organosilica frameworks. *Chemistry of Materials*, *26*(20), 5980–5987. https://doi.org/10.1021/CM502777E/SUPPL_FILE/CM502777E_SI_001.PDF

Teng, Z., Su, X., Zheng, Y., Sun, J., Chen, G., Tian, C., Wang, J., Li, H., Zhao, Y., & Lu, G. (2013). Mesoporous silica hollow spheres with ordered radial mesochannels by a spontaneous self-transformation approach. *Chemistry of Materials*, *25*(1), 98–105. https://doi.org/10.1021/CM303338V/SUPPL_FILE/CM303338V_SI_001.PDF

Teng, Z., Wang, S., Su, X., Chen, G., Liu, Y., Luo, Z., Luo, W., Tang, Y., Ju, H., Zhao, D., & Lu, G. (2014). Facile synthesis of yolk–shell structured inorganic–organic hybrid spheres with ordered radial mesochannels. *Advanced Materials*, *26*(22), 3741–3747. https://doi.org/10.1002/ADMA.201400136

Tian, J., Zhang, H., Liu, M., Deng, F., Huang, H., Wan, Q., Li, Z., Wang, K., He, X., Zhang, X., & Wei, Y. (2015). A bioinspired strategy for surface modification of silica nanoparticles. *Applied Surface Science*, *357*, 1996–2003. https://doi.org/10.1016/J.APSUSC.2015.09.171

Trewyn, B. G., Giri, S., Slowing, I. I., & Lin, V. S. Y. (2007a). Mesoporous silica nanoparticle based controlled release, drug delivery, and biosensor systems. *Chemical Communications*, *31*, 3236–3245. https://doi.org/10.1039/B701744H

Trewyn, B. G., Giri, S., Slowing, I. I., & Lin, V. S. Y. (2007b). Mesoporous silica nanoparticle based controlled release, drug delivery, and biosensor systems. *Chemical Communications*, *31*, 3236–3245. https://doi.org/10.1039/B701744H

Tu, D. Y., Pan, Q. M., Zhou, J. H., Tong, B., Zhang, G. T., & Wang, W. (2021). Morphological evolution and spreading flow of hollow oil droplet impact on a heated wall. *Theoretical and Computational Fluid Dynamics*, *35*(2), 209–227. https://doi.org/10.1007/S00162-020-00557-5/FIGURES/11

Urata, C., Yamada, H., Wakabayashi, R., Aoyama, Y., Hirosawa, S., Arai, S., Takeoka, S., Yamauchi, Y., & Kuroda, K. (2011). Aqueous colloidal mesoporous nanoparticles with ethenylene-bridged silsesquioxane frameworks. *Journal of the American Chemical Society*, *133*(21), 8102–8105. https://doi.org/10.1021/JA201779D

Valdés, O., Marican, A., Mirabal-Gallardo, Y., & Santos, L. S. (2018). Selective and efficient arsenic recovery from water through quaternary amino-functionalized silica. *Polymers*, *10*(6). https://doi.org/10.3390/POLYM10060626

Vallet-Regí, M., Balas, F., & Arcos, D. (2007). Mesoporous materials for drug delivery. *Angewandte Chemie—International Edition*, *46*(40), 7548–7558. https://doi.org/10.1002/ANIE.200604488

Vis, B., Hewitt, R. E., Faria, N., Bastos, C., Chappell, H., Pele, L., Jugdaohsingh, R., Kinrade, S. D., & Powell, J. J. (2018). Non-functionalized ultrasmall silica nanoparticles directly and size-selectively activate T cells. *ACS Nano*, *12*(11), 10843–10854. https://doi.org/10.1021/ACSNANO.8B03363

Wagner, J., Gößl, D., Ustyanovska, N., Xiong, M., Hauser, D., Zhuzhgova, O., Hočevar, S., Taskoparan, B., Poller, L., Datz, S., Engelke, H., Daali, Y., Bein, T., & Bourquin, C. (2021). Mesoporous silica nanoparticles as pH-responsive carrier for the immune-activating drug resiquimod enhance the local immune response in mice. *ACS Publications ACS Nano*, *15*(3), 4450–4466. https://doi.org/10.1021/acsnano.0c08384

Wang, D. P., Wang, Z. J., Zhao, R., Lin, C. X., Sun, Q. Y., Yan, C. P., Zhou, X., & Cao, J. M. (2020). Silica nanomaterials induce organ injuries by Ca2+-ROS-initiated disruption of the endothelial barrier and triggering intravascular coagulation. *Particle and Fibre Toxicology*, *17*(1), 1–21. https://doi.org/10.1186/S12989-020-00340-8/FIGURES/12

Wang, J. G., Xiao, Q., Zhou, H. J., Sun, P. C., Ding, D. T., & Chen, T. H. (2008). Anionic surfactant-templated mesoporous silica (AMS) nano-spheres with radially oriented mesopores. *Journal of Colloid and Interface Science*, *323*(2), 332–337. https://doi.org/10.1016/J.JCIS.2008.04.044

Wang, S., Li, F., Hu, X., Lv, M., Fan, C., & Ling, D. (2018). Tuning the intrinsic nanotoxicity in advanced therapeutics. *Advanced Therapeutics*, *1*(5). https://doi.org/10.1002/ADTP.201800059

Wang, S., Liu, K., Liu, J., Yu, Z. T. -F., Xu, X., Zhao, L., Lee, T., Lee, E. K., Reiss, J., Lee, Y., Chung, L. W. K., Huang, J., Rettig, M., Seligson, D., Duraiswamy, K. N., Shen, C. K.-., & Tseng, H. (2011). Highly efficient capture of circulating tumor cells by using nanostructured silicon substrates with integrated chaotic micromixers. *Angewandte Chemie*, *123*(13), 3140–3144. https://doi.org/10.1002/ANGE.201005853

Wei, L., Hu, N., & Zhang, Y. (2010). Synthesis of polymer—mesoporous silica nanocomposites. *Materials*, *3*(7), 4066–4079. https://doi.org/10.3390/MA3074066

Wen, J., Yang, K., Xu, Y., Li, H., Liu, F., & Sun, S. (2016). Construction of a triple-stimuli-responsive system based on cerium oxide coated mesoporous silica nanoparticles. *Scientific Reports*, *6*(1), 1–10. https://doi.org/10.1038/srep38931

Wu, G., Fang, Y. Z., Yang, S., Lupton, J. R., & Turner, N. D. (2004). Glutathione metabolism and its implications for health. *The Journal of Nutrition*, *134*(3), 489–492. https://doi.org/10.1093/JN/134.3.489

Xiao, D., Jia, H. Z., Zhang, J., Liu, C. W., Zhuo, R. X., & Zhang, X. Z. (2014). A dual-responsive mesoporous silica nanoparticle for tumor-triggered targeting drug delivery. *Small*, *10*(3), 591–598. https://doi.org/10.1002/SMLL.201301926

Xie, M., Shi, H., Li, Z., Shen, H., Ma, K., Li, B., Shen, S., & Jin, Y. (2013). A multifunctional mesoporous silica nanocomposite for targeted delivery, controlled release of doxorubicin and bioimaging. *Colloids and Surfaces B: Biointerfaces*, *110*, 138–147. https://doi.org/10.1016/J.COLSURFB.2013.04.009

Xing, R., Li, K. Le, Zhou, Y. F., Su, Y. Y., Yan, S. Q., Zhang, K. L., Wu, S. C., Sima, Y. H., Zhang, K. Q., He, Y., & Xu, S. Q. (2016). Impact of fluorescent silicon nanoparticles on circulating hemolymph and hematopoiesis in an invertebrate model organism. *Chemosphere*, *159*, 628–637. https://doi.org/10.1016/J.CHEMOSPHERE.2016.06.057

Xing, X., He, X., Peng, J., Wang, K., & Tan, W. (2005). Uptake of silica-coated nanoparticles by HeLa cells. *Journal of Nanoscience and Nanotechnology*, *5*(10), 1688–1693. https://doi.org/10.1166/JNN.2005.199

Yamamoto, E., & Kuroda, K. (2016). Colloidal mesoporous silica Nanoparticles. *Bulletin of the Chemical Society of Japan*, *89*(5), 501–539. https://doi.org/10.1246/BCSJ.20150420

Yang, H., Lou, C., Xu, M., Wu, C., Miyoshi, H., & Liu, Y. (2011). Investigation of folate-conjugated fluorescent silica nanoparticles for targeting delivery to folate receptor-positive tumors and their internalization mechanism. *International Journal of Nanomedicine*, *6*, 2023–2032. https://doi.org/10.2147/IJN.S24792

Yang, L., Yin, T., Liu, Y., Sun, J., Zhou, Y., & Liu, J. (2016). Gold nanoparticle-capped mesoporous silica-based H2O2-responsive controlled release system for Alzheimer's disease treatment. *Acta Biomaterialia*, *46*, 177–190. https://doi.org/10.1016/J.ACTBIO.2016.09.010

Yuan, J., Zhou, T., & Pu, H. (2010). Nano-sized silica hollow spheres: Preparation, mechanism analysis and its water retention property. *Journal of Physics and Chemistry of Solids*, *71*(7), 1013–1019. https://doi.org/10.1016/J.JPCS.2010.04.004

Yuan, Z. Q., Chen, W. L., You, B. G., Liu, Y., Yang, S. D., Li, J. Z., Zhu, W. J., Zhou, X. F., Liu, C., & Zhang, X. N. (2017). Multifunctional nanoparticles co-delivering EZH2 siRNA and etoposide for synergistic therapy of orthotopic non-small-cell lung tumor. *Journal of Controlled Release*, *268*, 198–211. https://doi.org/10.1016/J.JCONREL.2017.10.025

Yue, L., Sun, C., Cheng, Q., Ding, Y., Wei, J., & Wang, R. (2019). Gold nanorods with a noncovalently tailorable surface for multi-modality image-guided chemo-photothermal cancer therapy. *Chemical Communications*, *55*(90), 13506–13509. https://doi.org/10.1039/C9CC07131H

Yun, H., Kim, K., Gu, W., Sharma, S., Pham, V. H., Boscoboinik, J. A., Lee, S.-Y., Ferrari, M., & Decuzzi, P. (2009). Shaping nano-/micro-particles for enhanced vascular interaction in laminar flows. *Iopscience.Iop.OrgNanotechnology*, *20*, 11. https://doi.org/10.1088/0957-4484/20/49/495101

Zanoni, D. K., Stambuk, H. E., Madajewski, B., Montero, P. H., Matsuura, D., Busam, K. J., Ma, K., Turker, M. Z., Sequeira, S., Gonen, M., Zanzonico, P., Wiesner, U., Bradbury, M. S., & Patel, S. G. (2021). Use of ultrasmall core-shell fluorescent silica nanoparticles for image-guided sentinel lymph node biopsy in head and neck melanoma: A nonrandomized clinical trial. *JAMA Network Open*, *4*(3). https://doi.org/10.1001/JAMANETWORKOPEN.2021.1936

Zhai, Y., Zhou, X., Zhang, Z., Zhang, L., Wang, D., Wang, X., & Sun, W. (2018). Design, synthesis, and characterization of Schiff base bond-linked pH-responsive doxorubicin prodrug based on functionalized mPEG-PCL for targeted cancer therapy. *Polymers*, *10*(10), 1127. https://doi.org/10.3390/POLYM10101127

Zhang, Y. B., Qian, X. F., Li, Z. K., Yin, J., & Zhu, Z. K. (2004). Synthesis of novel mesoporous silica spheres with starburst pore canal structure. *Journal of Solid State Chemistry*, *177*(3), 844–848. https://doi.org/10.1016/J.JSSC.2003.09.018

Zhao, Y., Peng, F., advances, Y. K.-R., & 2021, undefined. (n.d.). Design and characterization of oil-in-water nanoemulsion for enhanced oil recovery stabilized by amphiphilic copolymer, nonionic surfactant, and LAPONITE. *Pubs.Rsc.Org RSC Advances*. Retrieved April 27, 2024, from https://pubs.rsc.org/en/content/articlehtml/2021/ra/d0ra06080a

Zhao, Y., Sun, X., Zhang, G., Trewyn, B. G., Slowing, I. I., & S-Y Lin, V. (2024). Interaction of mesoporous silica nanoparticles with human red blood cell membranes: Size and surface effects. *ACS Publications ACS Nano*, *20*(2), 51. https://doi.org/10.1021/nn103077k

Zhou, Q., Zhang, L., & Wu, H. (2017). Nanomaterials for cancer therapies. *Nanotechnology Reviews*, *6*(5), 473–496. https://doi.org/10.1515/NTREV-2016-0102/HTML

8 Gold (Au) Nanostructures Decorated Graphene Nanosheets for Photothermal Cancer Therapy

Prosenjit Mridha,[1,4] *Esha Roy,*[1,4]
Jyoti Lakshmi Hati Boruah,[2,4] *Deep Jyoti Das,*[1,4]
Rituraj Konwar,[1,4] *Manash Ranjan Das,*[3,4] *and Rinku Baishya*[1,4]
[1]Centre for Pre-clinical Studies, CSIR-North East Institute of Science and Technology, Jorhat, India
[2]Biological Sciences and Technology Division, CSIR-North East Institute of Science and Technology, Jorhat, India
[3]Materials Sciences and Technology Division, CSIR-North East Institute of Science and Technology, Jorhat, India
[4]AcSIR-Academy of Scientific and Innovative Research, Ghaziabad, Uttar Pradesh, India

8.1 INTRODUCTION

Photothermal therapy (PTT), employing light-absorbing nanoparticles, stands out as one of the most effective techniques for cancer treatment (Huang *et al.*, 2006, 2008). During PTT, near-infrared (NIR) light is absorbed by photosensitive nanoparticles, converting it into heat within tumor tissues (Gharatape *et al.*, 2016). As the temperature of malignant tumor tissues reaches 42–47 °C, apoptosis is induced in cancer cells, which are more susceptible to heat compared to normal cells, leading to rapid cell death through necrosis at higher temperatures (Nguyen *et al.*, 2017). In recent years PTT has gained great attention in curing cancer because it is highly effective against cancer as well as causes negligible damage to the nearby healthy tissues (Spyratou *et al.*, 2017; Yang *et al.*, 2010). However, appropriate light intensity and nanoparticle dose are required for the best performance of the PTT. High-intensity light as well as high doses of nanoparticles can also provoke chronic inflammation and necrosis of the normal cells (Nguyen *et al.*, 2017). Those nanoparticles exhibit effective light-to-heat conversion within the biological windows (700–1400 nm), are considered as potent photothermal agents (Jaque *et al.*, 2014). Light within this range can easily penetrate tissues due to low light absorption and scattering, allowing highly potent photothermal agents to efficiently convert light to heat even under low-power laser sources. Moreover, nanoparticles used in PTT should possess minimal toxicity and excellent solubility in biocompatible media to reduce adverse effects and ensure easy accessibility to cancerous tumors, even with low blood circulation (Farokhnezhad *et al.*, 2019). In recent years, various types of nanoparticles have been employed in PTT for cancer treatment both *in vitro* and *in vivo*, including carbon-based nanoparticles, metal-based nanoparticles, copper-based nanoparticles, black phosphorous-based nanoparticles, and others (Doughty *et al.*, 2019).

DOI: 10.1201/9781003799351-8

Among these, gold nanoparticles exhibit exceptional optical properties and efficient light-to-heat conversion, making them highly efficient candidates in biomedical applications such as photothermal therapy (Vines *et al.*, 2019), bioimaging (Wu *et al.*, 2019), diagnostics (Singh *et al.*, 2018), and biomolecule sensing (Saha *et al.*, 2012). Gold nanoparticles display intriguing shape-dependent surface plasmon resonance (SPR) characteristics. Consequently, gold nanoparticles of various shapes, including stars (Wang *et al.*, 2013; Li *et al.*, 2015), cages (Skrabalak *et al.*, 2008), rods (Murphy *et al.*, 2005), and shells (Bardhan *et al.*, 2011), have found applications in biomedical fields.

The carbon-based nanomaterials encompasses various types, among them, graphene emerged as one of the most pivotal materials. Graphene has been discovered in 2004 (Novoselov *et al.*, 2004). However, its application in biomedicine commenced around 2008 (Liu *et al.*, 2008). Graphene-based nanoparticles demonstrate the ability to absorb near-infrared (NIR) light and efficiently convert it into heat. Moreover, due to their high tumor tissue penetrance, lower toxicity, and large surface-to-volume ratio, these nanomaterials are considered superior agents compared to carbon nanotubes (CNTs) in photothermal therapy applications (Markovic *et al.*, 2011). Graphene-based nanomaterials—that is, reduced graphene oxide (rGO), graphene oxide (GO), and GO-nanocomposites—have shown excellent potential in the photothermal treatment of cancer, because of their high specific surface area, NIR light absorbance, and abundance of functional groups that can be used for effective biomolecular loading or bioconjugation (Chen *et al.*, 2016). Orecchioni *et al.* conducted a comparative study on graphene for cancer treatment, revealing that photothermal therapy (PTT) ranks as the second-largest component of cancer therapy. Their findings suggest that PTT holds promise as an effective technique for cancer treatment with minimal invasiveness (Orecchioni *et al.*, 2015). In 2010, Yang *et al.* first time used the graphene oxide (GO) in conjunction with photothermal therapy (PTT) for the successful suppression of tumors via intravenous injection (Yang *et al.*, 2010). Additionally, studies have observed that conjugating graphene-derived nanoparticles with polyethylene glycol (PEG) significantly enhances their biocompatibility and water solubility (Robinson *et al.*, 2011)

In contrast to carbon-based nanoparticles, such as graphene and other carbon nanostructures, gold nanostructures have been noted to exhibit low thermal stability when subjected to prolonged laser irradiation (Bian *et al.*, 2014). Additionally, the practical applications of gold nanoparticles are constrained by their insufficient surface functionalization (Zhang *et al.*, 2013). Typically, cetyltrimethylammonium bromide (CTAB) is utilized for the surface modification of gold nanostructures, but its toxicity to human cells poses a significant challenge. Consequently, employing gold nanoparticles alone in biomedical applications proves challenging due to these drawbacks. To mitigate toxic adverse effects, gold nanostructure materials are often combined with less toxic biocompatible materials (Zhang *et al.*, 2012). As, the graphene-based nanomaterials demonstrate excellent biocompatibility, they can serve as a protective layer for gold-based nanostructures, addressing the aforementioned issue. Moreover, the presence of a graphene shell enhances the thermal stability of gold nanostructures under continuous laser irradiation. Thus, graphene-conjugated gold nanostructures emerge as highly promising materials for photothermal therapy. Conjugating graphene with gold nanostructures also augments the surface area and the number of active sites for loading anticancer drugs, thereby increasing the potential for simultaneous photothermal therapy and chemotherapy (Farokhnezhad *et al.*, 2019). In addition to photothermal therapy (PTT), gold nanoparticle-decorated graphene emerged as an exceptional candidate for combined therapy. Cheng Xu *et al.* demonstrated that gold nanorods (AuNRs) encapsulated in nanographene oxide (NGO) shells represent an ultra-efficient candidate for chemo-photothermal cancer therapy (Xu *et al.*, 2013a). Graphene-gold hybrid nanostructures also exhibit promise for cancer-specific multimodal imaging and combined therapeutics (Yang *et al.*, 2021). Throughout this book chapter, various synthesis procedures of graphene-decorated gold nanostructures (GGNMs) and their applications in PTT, cellular uptake, biodistribution, biocompatibility, tumor tissue accumulation, and other combined photothermal therapies (such as PTT-Photodynamic therapy (PDT), Chemo-PTT, PTT-Imaging) will be briefly discussed.

8.2 GOLD NANOSTRUCTURES DECORATED GRAPHENE NANOSHEETS

In this section, we have discussed different types of gold nanostructure materials and their properties, different functionalization approaches of graphene nanosheets by gold nanostructure materials, and their characterization as well as properties.

8.2.1 Types of Gold Nanostructures (AuNPs) and Their Properties

Various types of gold nanostructures and their unique physical, chemical and optical properties are very much important for the application in different aspect.

8.2.1.1 Types

Different types of gold nanoparticles are commonly used such as gold nanospheres, gold nanostars, gold nanoshells, gold nanorods, gold nanoflowers, gold nanocubes, gold nanobipyramids, and many more. These gold-based nanoparticles exhibit unique physical, chemical, and optical properties, which made them special for application in different aspects. Because of their highly biocompatible nature, these nanoparticles are also used in biomedical applications (Vines *et al.*, 2019). Figure 8.1 represents gold nanoparticles of different sizes and shapes.

8.2.1.2 Properties

While bulk material displays some features, AuNPs display different ones. AuNPs' size and shape determine these characteristics. Gold nanoparticles show various colors, the color of gold nanoparticles can vary greatly depending on their size and can be brown, purple, blue, orange, or red when they are in solution. The surface plasmon resonance (SPR) band is visible in the 500–550 nm range for gold nanoparticles depending on their size. The incident photon's collective oscillations of conduction electrons give rise to the SPR band. This kind of band is not present in bulk materials or very small AuNPs, especially those with a diameter of less than 2 nm. In addition to particle size, other factors that affect AuNP SPR include ligands, nanoparticle form, temperature, and charge. By triggering the deactivation pathway, AuNPs turn off the nearby fluorophores and this happens because the emission spectra of fluorophores strongly align with the surface plasmon band of AuNPs, quenching the fluorescence effectively. Fluorescence

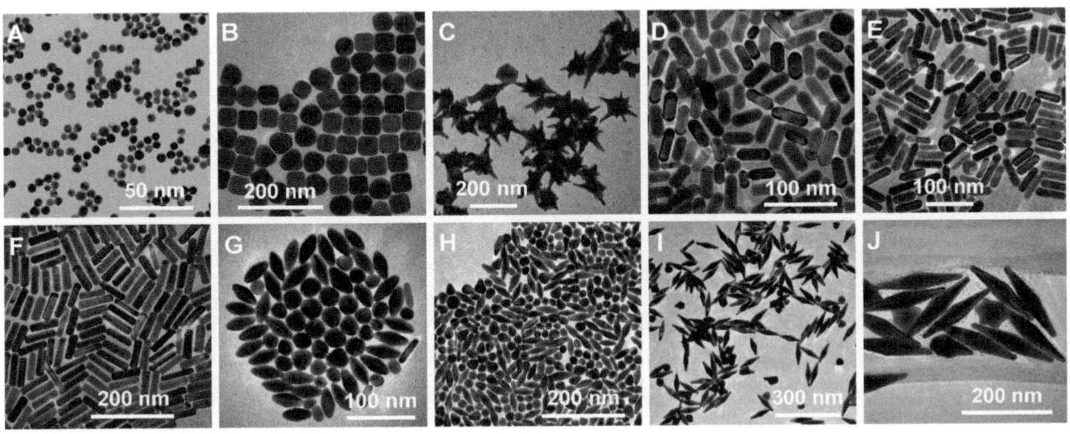

FIGURE 8.1 Typical TEM images of Au nanoparticles of various sizes and shapes. (A) Nanospheres, (B) nanocubes, (C) nanobranches, (D), (E), (F) represent nanorods of different aspect ratios. (G), (H), (I), (J) show nanobipyramids of various aspect ratios.

Source: Chen et al. (2008).

resonance energy transfer or FRET, is the term for this phenomenon, which has been seen in AuNPs as small as 1 nm. AuNPs can also quench fluorescence by a different method known as photo-induced electron transfer (PET), in which AuNPs absorb the photon and do the quenching work (Amina *et al.*, 2020; Yeh *et al.*, 2012).

8.2.2 Synthesis and Functionalization of Graphene by Gold Nanostructure Particles

The terms "in situ" and "ex-situ" are typically used to describe the two basic techniques for the conjugation of gold nanoparticles (AuNPs) with graphene sheets—that is, graphene oxide GO) and reduced graphene oxide (rGO). AuNPs grow directly on the surface of graphene in an in situ process; in contrast, in an ex-situ technique, graphene and AuNPs are synthesized separately and then merged. A direct electrostatic interaction between graphene and AuNPs can accomplish the ex-situ technique. Many different synthesis procedures come under these two broad synthesis approaches (Khalil *et al.*, 2016; Lebepe *et al.*, 2020). Table 8.1 summarizes different synthesis procedures of graphene-gold nanocomposites.

8.2.2.1 In Situ Synthesis

The following graphene-gold nanoparticle synthesis methods such as "reduction in mixed solution", "physical vapor deposition method", "hydrothermal reduction method", and "electrochemical method", come under the in situ technique. The "Reduction in mixed solution" technique is also of different types such as "simultaneous reduction", "microwave-aided deposition", "sonication-aided deposition", "photo-assisted deposition", and "radio wave-aided deposition", etc. (Khalil *et al.*, 2016).

8.2.2.1.1 Reduction in Mixed Solution

In this method, Au precursor and graphene are reduced in a mixture of solutions to synthesize Au-graphene nanostructures. Different methods under "Reduction in mixed solution" have been discussed briefly in the following section.

8.2.2.1.1.1 Simultaneous Reduction The simultaneous reduction of Au metal precursors and graphene in a mixed solution is the usual pathway for the creation of graphene–AuNPs. Using this simple and cost-effective method Byung-Seon *et al.* synthesized layer-by-layer films composed of graphene and gold nanoparticles alternatively (Kong *et al.*, 2009). Another group synthesized gold nanoparticle-graphene nanosheets through the above method utilizing sodium dodecyl sulfate (SDS) solution as a protector and disperser (Xu *et al.*, 2013b).

8.2.2.1.1.2 Microwave-Aided Deposition Huating *et al.* has developed a quick, one-step process for the successful synthesis of graphene nanosheets–gold (GNS–Au) nanocomposites using microwave radiation in aqueous conditions. Where microwaves trigger the reduction process (Hu *et al.*, 2012). Kabeer et al. also used this method to synthesize Bare-Surfaced Gold Nanostructures (BSGNs) and GO Sheets conjugate (GO-BSGN) (Jasuja *et al.*, 2010).

8.2.2.1.1.3 Sonication-Aided Deposition In this method, high-frequency ultrasound is used to reduce simultaneously graphene oxide (GO) and a gold precursor. Many scientists used this method to synthesize graphene-gold nanostructure materials (Vinodgopal *et al.*, 2010; Park *et al.*, 2011).

8.2.2.1.1.4 Photo-Assisted Deposition The photo-assisted deposition is another excellent method of graphene-gold synthesis, where light is used to enhance the reduction of gold and graphene. Caires *et al.* synthesized gold nanorods (GNRs) and graphene oxide (GO) nanocomposite materials by an easy, one-pot method, where GNRs are attached directly to the GO flakes by UV light irradiation (Caires *et al.*, 2015).

8.2.2.1.1.5 Radio Wave-Aided Deposition Stela *et al.* used the radio frequency in chemical vapor deposition (CVD) method to synthesize graphene–AuNPs composite by using a gold-magnesium oxide (Au/MgO) catalyst (Pruneanu *et al.*, 2011).

8.2.2.1.2 Physical Vapor Deposition Method

Several materials can be easily deposited onto surfaces as thin films or nanoparticles using physical vapor deposition (PVD). It uses highly controllable vacuum techniques such as thermal evaporation and sputter deposition to accomplish the condensation of a vaporized substance onto a substrate. Priyanka *et al.* used this method for the deposition of Au on GO, where the minimum thickness of Au-GO composite was 0.75 nm. The deposited Au has fragmented into a variety of sized nanoparticles, usually a few nanometers in diameter, instead of forming a homogenous thin coating (Pandey *et al.*, 2011). Zhengtang *et al.* also deposited gold atoms on few-layer graphene by physical vapor deposition method (Luo *et al.*, 2010).

8.2.2.1.3 Hydrothermal Reduction Method

Recently, the hydrothermal synthesis method gained great attention for the synthesis of nanoparticles. This synthesis process is often carried out in steel pressure vessels known as autoclaves in high-temperature and high vapor pressure (Bai *et al.*, 2012). The synthesis of graphene-AuNP composites was reported by Liu *et al.* using a microwave-assisted hydrothermal system in a Teflon-lined autoclave at 150 °C for 1 hour without the use of reducing agents (Liu *et al.*, 2014).

8.2.2.1.4 Electrochemical Method

The electrochemical method does not cause contamination of the produced materials and is straightforward, quick, and environmental friendly. Graphene-AuNP nanocomposites can now be created by electrochemical deposition techniques, which usually involve three steps: depositing graphene sheets onto an electrode, dipping the graphene-coated electrode into an electrolytic solution containing metallic precursors, and then applying an electrochemical potential (Khalil *et al.*, 2016). By electrochemically reducing GO and Au precursors in a single step, Maduraiveeran *et al.* produced a new nanocomposite of reduced GO (rGO) and Au nanocomposites that were deposited on a glassy carbon electrode (GCE) (Govindhan *et al.*, 2015).

8.2.2.2 Ex-Situ Synthesis

The ex-situ method involves two steps, first synthesis of nanoparticles and then decorating them on the graphene sheet surface. Covalent and non-covalent interactions, such as hydrogen bonds, pie-pie stacking, van der Waals contacts, or electrostatic interactions, promote this attachment. Although coating of AuNPs with the ex-situ approach is common, still AuNPs aggregate on the GO sheet as a result of this direct procedure. To stop these aggregations, some researchers have recently used stabilizers, linkers, or functionalization materials such as gum arabica (GA), polyethylene glycol, polystyrene sulfonate (PSS), cysteine (Cys), polyethyleneimine (PEI), and polyvinyl pyrrolidone (PVP) (Khalil *et al.*, 2016; Lebepe *et al.*, 2020).

8.2.2.3 Characterization of AuNPs-GO Nanostructure Materials

For the characterization of AuNPs–graphene, numerous technique is used such as Fourier-transform infrared spectroscopy (FT-IR), X-ray diffraction (XRD), UV-VIS spectroscopy, Transmission Electron Microscopy (TEM), etc., and many more. With these techniques, the conjugation of AuNPs and graphene can be confirmed. With FT-IR, different functional groups of the AuNP-graphene nanocomposites, AuNPs, and graphene can be identified. X-ray diffraction (XRD) is a useful technique for examining the interlayer variations of materials linked to graphite. The nanocomposites also exhibit specific UV-VIS peaks. TEM is used to determine the morphological difference between individual nanomaterials and nanocomposites. Figures 8.2, 8.3, 8.4 and 8.5 represent

TABLE 8.1
Summary of Different Synthesis Processes of Au-Graphene Nanocomposites

Synthesis process	Product name	Graphene derivatives	Gold precursor	Driving force of the reaction	References
Simultaneous reduction	Layer by layer RGO-AuNP	GO	$HAuCl_4.3H_2O$	Spontaneous	**Kong *et al.* (2009)**
	GNPs-GR	GO	$HAuCl_4$	High temperature	**Xu *et al.* (2013b)**
Microwave-aided deposition	GNS–Au	GO	$HAuCl_4$	Microwave	**Hu *et al.* (2012)**
	GO-BSGN	GO	$HAuCl_4.3H_2O$	Microwave	**Jasuja *et al.* (2010)**
Sonication-aided deposition	Au-RGO	GO	$HAuCl_4$	Ultrasound	**Vinodgopal *et al.* (2010)**
	RGO-Au NP	GO	$HAuCl_4.3H_2O$	Ultrasound	**Park *et al.* (2011)**
Photo-assisted deposition	GNR-GO	GO	$HAuCl_4.3H_2O$	UV-light	**Caires *et al.* (2015)**
	AuNPs-graphene	Graphene sheets	$HAuCl_4$	633 nm laser	**Cheng *et al.* (2013)**
Physical vapor deposition method	AuNP-GO	GO	Gold	Pressure	**Pandey *et al.* (2011)**
	AuNP-graphene	Graphene	Gold	Temperature and pressure	**Luo *et al.* (2010)**
Hydrothermal reduction method	Graphene-AuNP	GO sheets	$HAuCl_4$	High temperature	**Liu *et al.* (2014)**
Electrochemical method	Au-rGO	GO	Au chloride	Electrochemical potential	**Govindhan *et al.* (2015)**
Ex situ method	GO–AuNR	GO	HAuCl4	Electrostatic potential	**Hu *et al.* (2013)**
	AuNR-PEG-GO	GO	$HAuCl_4.3H_2O$	Electrostatic interaction	**Dembereldorj *et al.* (2014)**

FT-IR spectra, XRD, UV-VIS spectra, and TEM images of AuNP-graphene nanostructures. (Pham *et al.*, 2011; Huang *et al.*, 2010)

8.3 BIOCOMPATIBILITY, CELLULAR UPTAKE, AND BIODISTRIBUTION

Biocompatibiliy, cellular uptake and biodistribution are critical parameters for for their safety and efficacy.

8.3.1 Biocompatibility

The biocompatibility of nanomaterials is a critical parameter for their effective application in biological systems. Numerous studies have highlighted that factor such as size, surface charge, and capping agents play pivotal roles in influencing the cytotoxicity of nanomaterials. These characteristics can affect cellular uptake, biodistribution, and interaction with biomolecules, ultimately determining their safety and efficacy in biomedical applications (Fard *et al.*, 2015). Functionalization and property optimization of graphene-based materials have facilitated the advancement of effective and safe nanotherapeutics for cancer treatment. For instance, reduced graphene oxide (rGO) nanosheets functionalized with polyethylene glycol (PEG) chains and embedded with gold-palladium (AuPd) nanoparticles exhibit improved solubility and stability in biological media. This functionalization strategy enhances their biocompatibility, as demonstrated in studies involving HeLa cells, underscoring their potential for biomedical applications (Darabdhara *et al.*, 2015). Another study demonstrated that polydopamine (PDA)-functionalized reduced graphene oxide (rGO) embedded with gold-palladium (AuPd) nanoparticles exhibited exceptional biocompatibility. These nanostructures showed high survival rates in zebrafish embryos and excellent compatibility with L929 cell lines, highlighting their potential for applications in cancer theranostics (Das *et al.*, 2020).

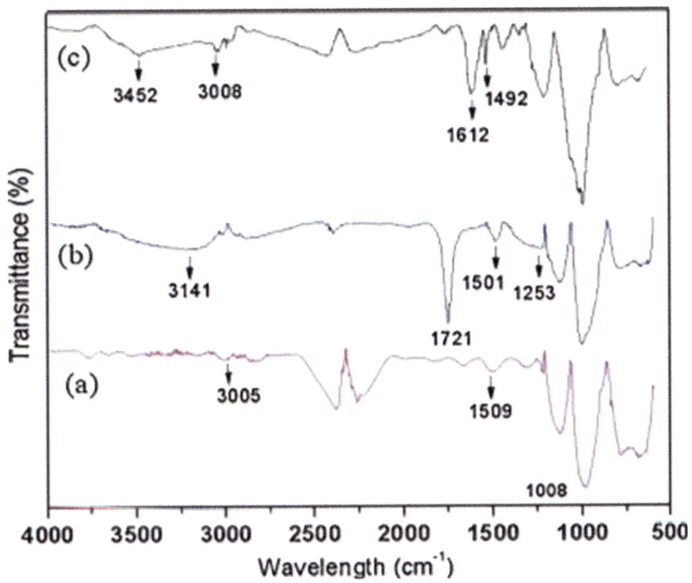

FIGURE 8.2 Representing FT-IR spectra of (a) pristine graphite, (b) graphene oxide, and (c) immobilized AuNPs on the surface of GOS, which is determined as AuNPs-i-GOS.

Source: Pham et al. (2011).

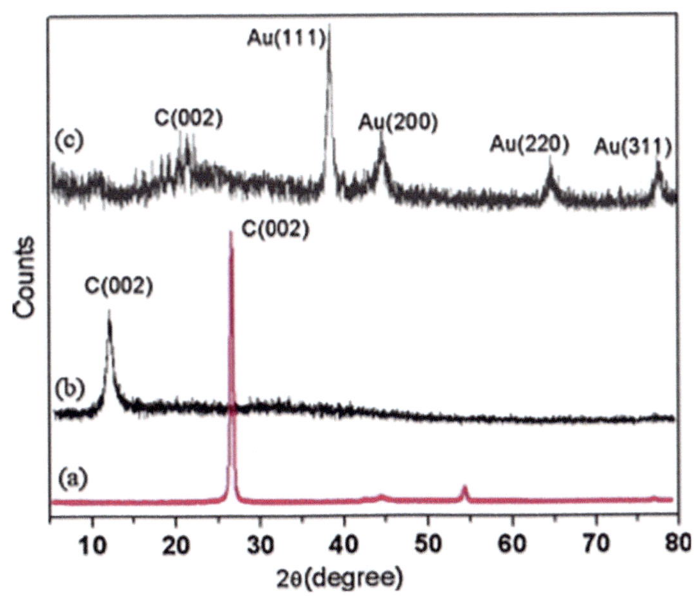

FIGURE 8.3 Showing the XRD patterns of (a) pristine graphite, (b) GO, and (c) AuNPs-i-GOS.

Source: Pham et al. (2011).

5,10,15,20-Tetrakis (3-methylpyridyl) porphyrin (TMePyP) is a highly effective photosensitizer with a remarkable ability to generate reactive oxygen species (ROS) upon light activation. These ROS can specifically interact with G-quadruplex DNA structures commonly found in cancer cells, disrupting their cell cycle and inducing cellular responses such as apoptosis or senescence, thereby

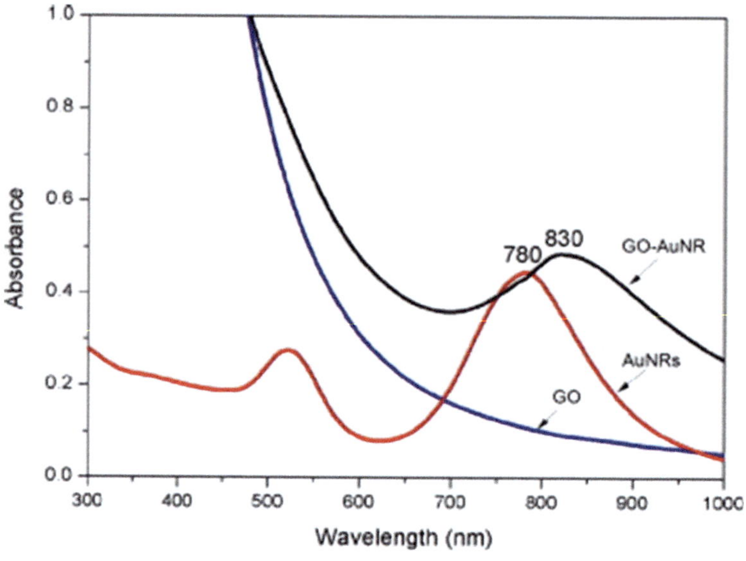

FIGURE 8.4 Representing UV–VIS spectra of GO, AuNRs, and GO–AuNR.

Source: Hu et al., (2013).

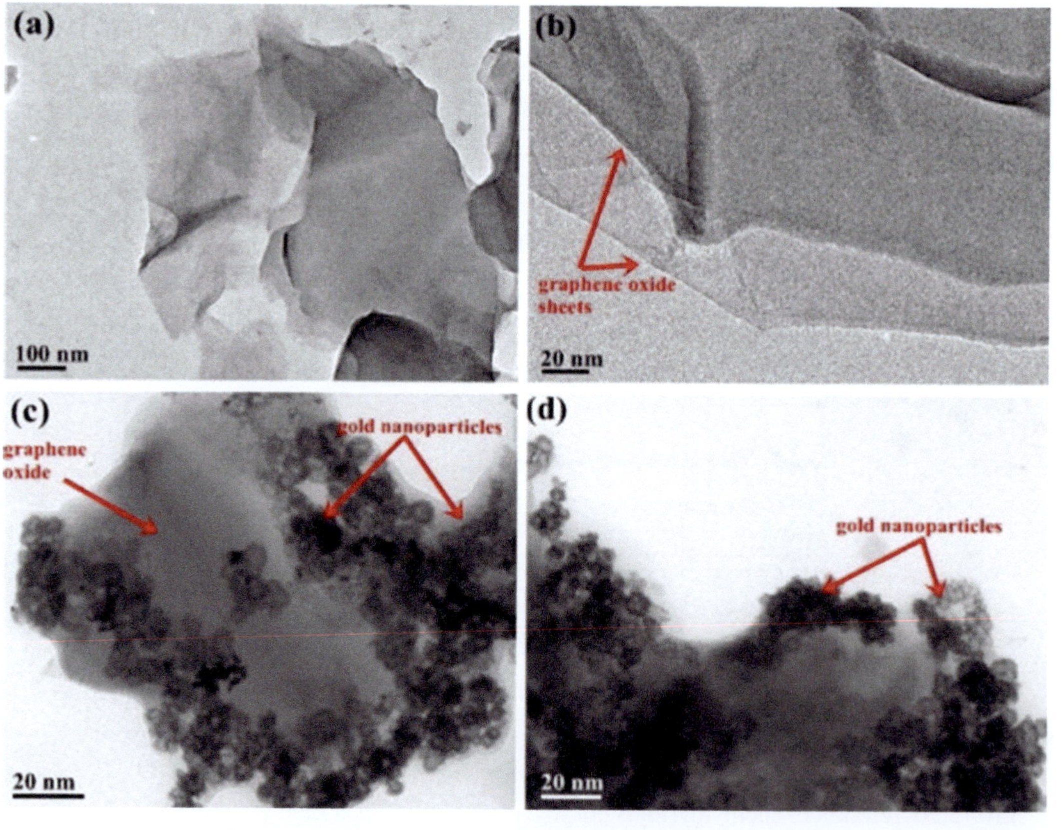

FIGURE 8.5 TEM images of graphene oxide sheets (GOS) (a and b) and immobilized AuNPs on the surface of GOS, which is determined as AuNPs-i-GOS (c and d).

Source: Pham et al. (2011).

demonstrating significant potential in photodynamic cancer therapy (Huang *et al.*, 2020). The conjugation of graphene oxide (GO)-modified gold nanorods (AuNRs) with the photosensitizer TMePyP (forming GO@AuNRs-TMePyP) resulted in a photo-synergistic therapeutic agent. This conjugate enhanced cell survivability by approximately 25%, attributed to the suppression of TMePyP activity by GO@AuNRs, thereby reducing excessive cytotoxicity. The improved cell survival highlights the biocompatibility of GO@AuNRs-TMePyP, suggesting its significant potential for biomedical applications. (Lebepe *et al.*, 2020).

8.3.2 Cellular Uptake

Effective cellular uptake of nanoparticles is governed by various physicochemical and biological parameters. The distribution and uptake of nanoparticles (NPs) at both cellular and organ levels are influenced by factors such as primary particle size and agglomeration state, which are further modulated by environmental conditions such as pH levels and dispersant composition. Additionally, the shape of nanoparticles plays a crucial role in determining their biodistribution, intracellular fate, and cellular assimilation efficiency. The elemental composition and surface characteristics also significantly affect nanoparticle behavior and localization within biological systems. In a study involving human colon cancer HT-29 cells, the endocytosis and tumor localization potential of gold nanorod-conjugated reduced graphene oxide-doxorubicin (GNRs-ICG@rGO-DOX) loaded with indocyanine green (ICG) were investigated. Following six hours of incubation, confocal laser scanning microscopy (CLSM) revealed the red fluorescence of doxorubicin (DOX) localized inside the cells. This was in contrast to the control groups, which included a blank condition (Figure 8.6 g–i) and cells treated with GNRs-ICG@rGO without DOX (Figure 8.6 j–l), confirming the efficient intracellular uptake and localization of GNRs-ICG@rGO-DOX (Maji *et al.*, 2022). Reduced graphene oxide (rGO) and doxorubicin (DOX) were functionalized with PEGylated Fe_2O_3@Au core/shell nanoparticles (Fe_2O_3@Au NPs) and incubated with HeLa cells for intervals of 1, 2, 4, and 12 hours. Cellular uptake of rGO-Fe_2O_3@Au NPs was evident due to the strong surface plasmon resonance (SPR) band at 542 nm, which was quantified by measuring the absorption of stained cells. The cellular uptake of both rGO-Fe_2O_3@Au NPs and DOX-rGO-Fe_2O_3@Au NPs increased significantly within the initial 4 hours of incubation. Furthermore, HeLa cells stained with rGO-Fe_2O_3@Au NPs exhibited decreased viability, as observed through MRI imaging, indicating the potential of these nanocomposites for theranostic applications (Chen *et al.*, 2015).

8.3.3 Biodistribution

The therapeutic efficacy and toxicity of nanoparticles are primarily influenced by their tissue distribution and pharmacokinetics parameters which are predominantly governed by their physical and chemical characteristics, including their size, surface charge, and surface chemistry. These properties play a crucial role in determining how nanoparticles are absorbed, distributed, metabolized, and eliminated within the body, ultimately impacting their safety and effectiveness in therapeutic applications (Li *et al.*, 2008). The biodistribution and tumor accumulation of hybrid graphene oxide (GO)/gold (Au) activatable probe, referred to as cationic polymer–Gold nanoparticle–Graphene Oxide activatable probe (CPGA), were evaluated using optical and photoacoustic (PA) imaging techniques. The probe was administered intravenously to mice bearing SCC7 tumors, and PA signals at the tumor site were monitored at various time points. The results demonstrated that PA signals reached a peak at 6 hours post-injection, which was consistent with the fluorescence imaging data. CPGA was observed to accumulate in tumor blood vessels over time, suggesting its potential for targeted tumor delivery. The normalized PA signals of CPGA in tumor tissues were measured at different time points, showing progressive accumulation: 1.42 ± 0.32 at 1 hour, 1.95 ± 0.25 at 4 hours, 2.5 ± 0.27 at 6 hours, and 1.71 ± 0.31 at 12 hours post-injection. These values were

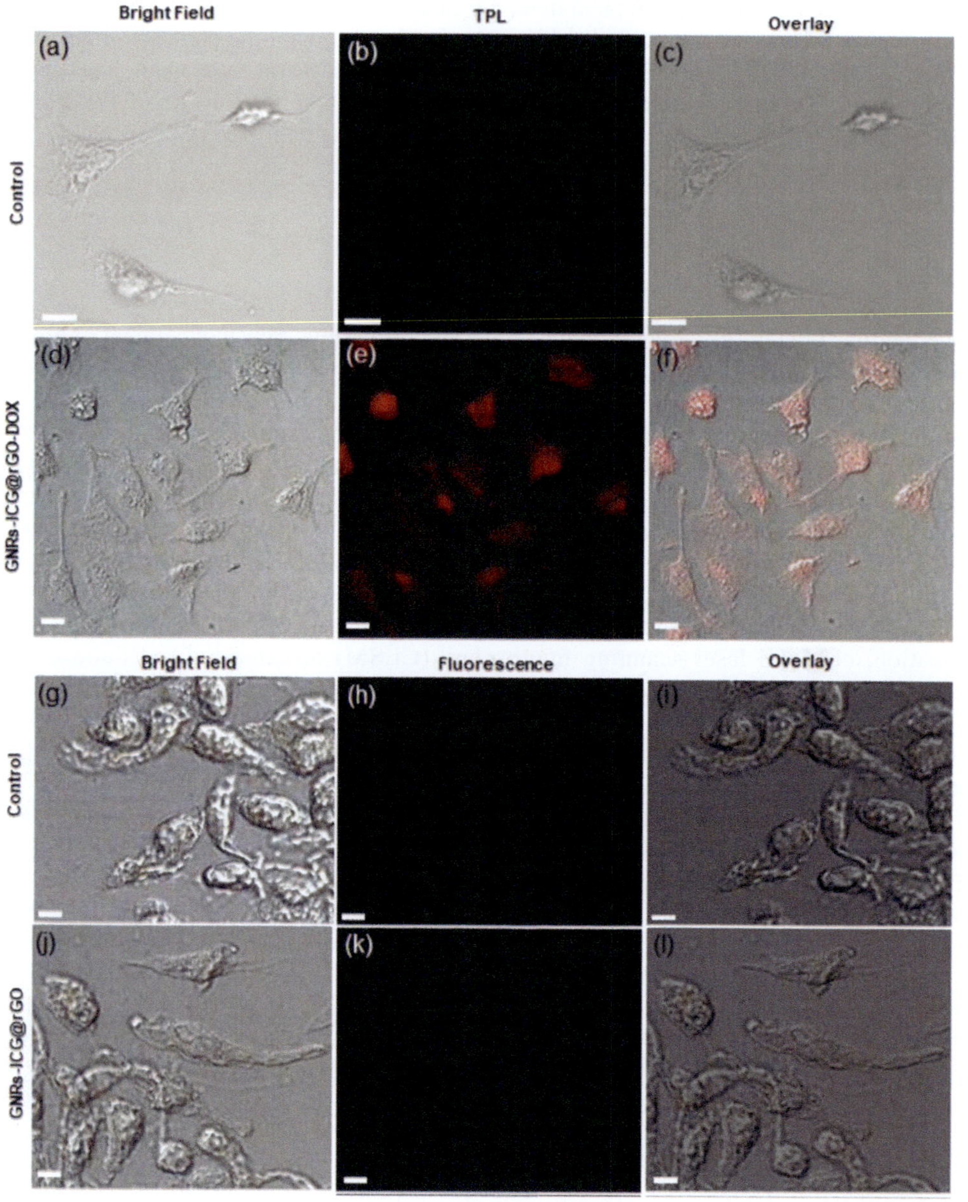

FIGURE 8.6 *In vitro* cellular uptake. TPL microscopy pictures of HT-29 cells treated with GNRs-ICG@rGO-DOX (100µg/mL) for six hours (d–f) and (a–c) as controls. CLSM picture of HT-29 cells treated with (j-l) and as a control (g-i) (scale bar = 10µm).

Source: Maji et al. (2022) (https://creativecommons.org/licenses/by-nc-nd/4.0/).

significantly higher than those observed in the control groups (CPG or Au), indicating the enhanced absorbance of the GO and Au components in CPGA, which could make it a promising candidate for photothermal therapy (PTT) in tumor ablation. Additionally, the concentration of Au in the tumor and normal organs was quantified using inductively coupled plasma mass spectrometry (ICP-MS), revealing an Au concentration of 7.06 ± 0.49% ID/g within the tumor tissue, in agreement with the ex vivo biodistribution fluorescence imaging data (Gao *et al.*, 2016).

8.4 TIMOR TISSUE ACCUMULATION

The rGO-AuNP theranostic platform, based on reduced graphene oxide (rGO)-loaded plasmonic gold nanoparticles (AuNPs), was investigated for its tumor tissue accumulation properties. This platform exhibited a sandwich nanostructure, which demonstrated enhanced photothermal and photoacoustic (PA) properties, making it suitable for PA imaging and photothermal therapy (PTT). Following intravenous administration in SKOV-3 tumor-bearing mice, the rGO-AuNPs showed significant tumor accumulation, resulting in a strong PA signal at multiple time points post-injection (Figure 8.7a). PA imaging of the tumor tissue revealed rapid accumulation of the rGO-AuNPs, with the strongest PA signal observed 24 hours after administration (Figure 8.7b), confirming the platform's potential for tumor-targeted imaging and therapy. The photoacoustic (PA) signal was

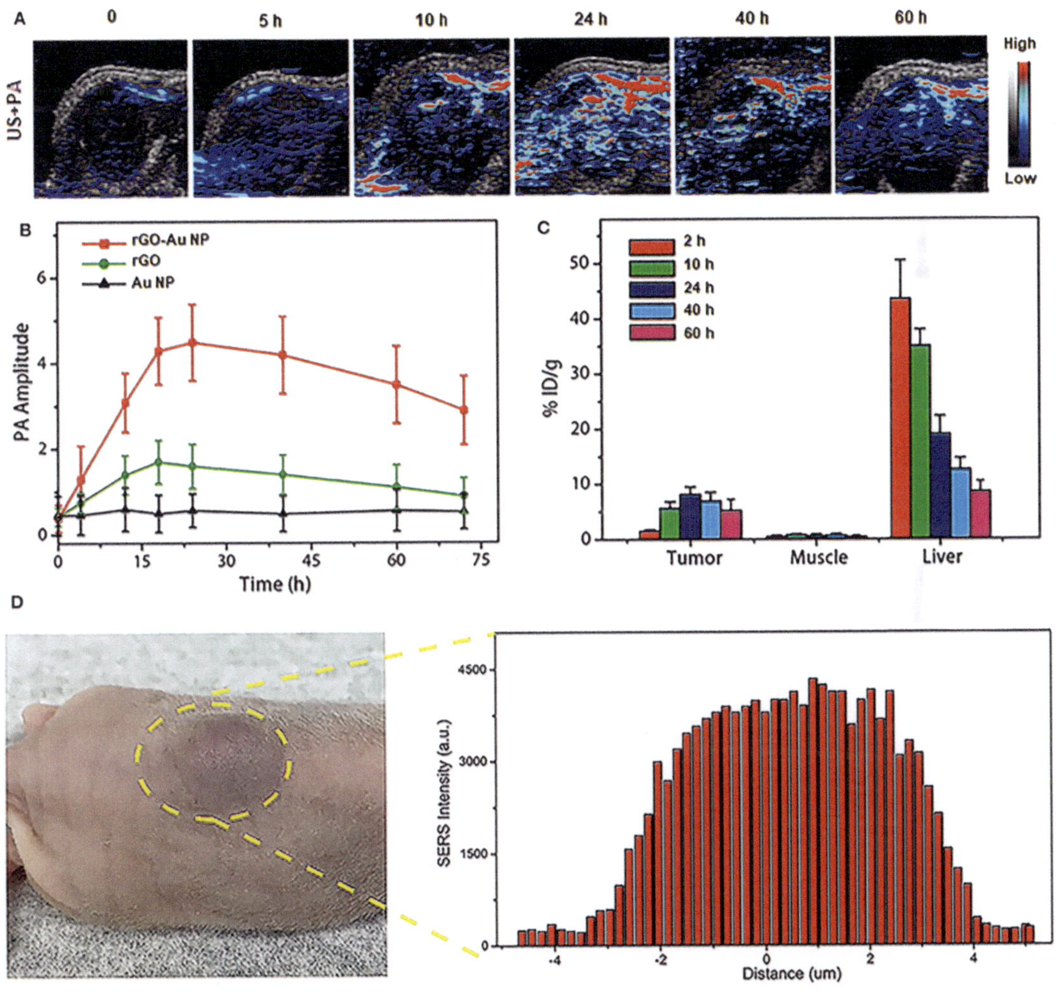

FIGURE 8.7 *In vivo* PA imaging using NIR-II. (A) Two-dimensional ultra US and PA pictures of tumor tissues in SKOV-3 tumor-bearing mice administered rGO-AuNP at different intervals after injection (B) PA signal amplitude variations in the tumor area treated with PBS, rGO, and rGO-AuNPs (C) The biodistribution of rGO-AuNP in liver, muscle, and tumor at various times (D) The *in vivo* surface-enhanced Raman scattering (SERS) signal of the tumor and the surrounding tissue is used to identify the tumor's boundary with the normal tissue.

Source: Wang et al. (2020).

predominantly observed in the tumor tissue, with negligible background signal in the skin, suggesting that NIR-II PA imaging of rGO-AuNPs offers superior contrast ratio and resolution compared to traditional NIR-I PA imaging. In vivo biodistribution studies (Figure 8.7c) revealed significant accumulation of rGO-AuNPs in the liver. However, over time, the concentration of rGO-AuNPs in the liver decreased, indicating a gradual clearance, suggesting that the nanoparticles exhibit a slow clearance rate from the liver (Wang *et al.*, 2020).

8.4.1 Active Targeting

The active targeting strategy involves the attachment of ligands or targeting moieties to the surface of nanoparticles, enabling them to specifically recognize and bind to receptors or antigens that are overexpressed on tumor cells. This approach aims to optimize therapeutic efficacy by enhancing the internalization of therapeutic payloads into cancer cells and promoting tumor-specific accumulation of nanoparticles, thereby minimizing off-target effects. Despite the challenges inherent in active targeting, ongoing research seeks to identify innovative methods to further improve the efficiency and specificity of nanoparticle-based drug delivery for cancer treatment. Future advancements in this area may lead to the development of more refined and effective anticancer therapies (Rosenblum *et al.*, 2018). To enhance targeting efficiency and retention, active targeting was introduced as an additional strategy to complement passively targeted treatments. The EPR effect forms the basis of passive targeting, wherein nanoparticles preferentially accumulate in tumor tissues due to the leaky blood vessels and compromised lymphatic drainage characteristic of tumors. To enable specific targeting, gold nanorods (Au NRs) conjugated with reduced graphene oxide (rGO) were functionalized with tumor-targeting HIV-1 Tat protein and H2N-PEG-NH2. The Tat peptide, known for its ability to target human glioblastoma astrocytoma cells (U87MG), it utilizes a terminal arginine residue that carries a positive charge, facilitating cell entry. This approach aims to assess and enhance the tumor-targeted photothermal therapeutic effect of the nanomaterials on U87MG cells (Lim *et al.*, 2000). After incubation with Au NRs@rGO-PEG and subsequent laser irradiation (808 nm, 1 W/cm², 10 minutes), nearly 97% of cells were destroyed, with an EC_{50} value of 32 µg/mL. The decline in cell viability was concentration-dependent. A significantly lower EC_{50} value of 11 µg/mL was observed with Tat-functionalized Au NRs@rGO-PEG, highlighting the beneficial effect of integrated Tat vectors. To visualize the uptake of fluorescently labeled nanoparticles, confocal microscopic images were obtained under identical conditions following incubation with 50 µg/mL Au NRs@rGO-PEG-Tat/FITC for 1, 4, and 24 hours. From 1 to 4 hours, the fluorescence intensity increased significantly, reaching its peak at 4 hours. At 24 hours, a slight decrease in fluorescence intensity was observed. The highest distribution of Au NRs@rGO-PEG-Tat/FITC was localized within the cytoplasm at the 4-hour mark. In contrast, non-vectorized nanomaterials exhibited significantly weaker signals at the same time point. The physicochemical properties of Au NRs@rGO-PEG-Tat/FITC had a pronounced impact on nanoparticle uptake by U87MG cells. Detailed analysis revealed the strongest fluorescence signal in the perinuclear region, likely corresponding to the cisternae of the Golgi complex. This finding suggests an endosomal pathway involving the engulfment of nanoparticles into the Golgi apparatus (fluorescence intensity ~10,000 a.u.) followed by endosomal recycling. Effective photothermal therapy requires significant accumulation of photothermal agents within tumor cells to ensure selective and efficient heating (Turcheniuk *et al.*, 2016).

8.4.2 Passive Targeting

Passive targeting utilizes the enhanced permeability and retention (EPR) effect, where nanoparticles accumulate in tumor tissues due to the abnormal structure of tumors. The leaky vasculature in tumors allows nanoparticles to penetrate, while impaired lymphatic drainage prevents their removal, resulting in prolonged retention. This approach improves the specificity and efficacy of drug delivery systems, making it a key strategy in cancer therapy (Maeda *et al.*, 1989). As tumor vasculature are highly chaotic and complex in nature with high porosity (100–780 nm), which is higher than normal tissue junction (6nm), nanocarriers circulating in the blood selectively enter into the interstitial spaces of tumor tissues and get accumulated there due to impaired lymphatic drainage system. Still, macrophages present in the liver and spleen can remove nanocarriers from blood circulation which can be avoided by coating with PEG which will increase the blood circulation time and selective accumulation on the tumor site (Andresen *et al.*, 2005). GO, covalently functionalized with polyethylene glycol (PEG) for improved water dispersibility and activity of anticancer drugs such as camptothecin derivative SN38 (hydrophobic anticancer drug), doxorubicin (DOX) and camptothecin (CPT), paclitaxel and improving their therapeutic efficacy in drug-resistant cancer cells (Mahato *et al.*, 2021; Liu *et al.*, 2008; Yang *et al.*, 2008; Zhang *et al.*, 2010).

8.5 PHENOMENON OF PHOTOTHERMAL THERAPY

Photothermal therapy (PTT) leverages light, typically in the near-infrared (NIR) spectrum, to elevate tissue temperature, leading to localized photocoagulation. By utilizing high-intensity light sources, PTT generates heat to achieve sub-coagulative temperatures (43–55 °C) or coagulative temperatures (55–100 °C). These temperature ranges induce rapid protein denaturation and disrupt cell membranes, effectively causing localized damage to targeted tissues. This precise thermal effect makes PTT a promising approach for minimally invasive therapeutic applications (Pattani *et al.*, 2015, Tong *et al.*, 2007). Graphene has been extensively employed in photothermal therapy (PTT) when conjugated with established photothermal materials. For instance, the hybrid nanomaterial GO@SiO_2@AuNS, comprising graphene oxide (GO), silica (SiO_2), and gold nanoshells (AuNS), demonstrates notable photothermal properties along with excellent biocompatibility. This hybrid material has been investigated for its potential to effectively destroy cancer cells. Treatment with a high concentration of GO@SiO_2@AuNS hybrid (100 $\mu g.mL^{-1}$) or near-infrared (NIR) laser irradiation (0.3 W/cm² for 20 minutes) alone does not induce significant cytotoxicity in cells. However, the combination of the GO@SiO_2@AuNS hybrid and NIR laser irradiation leads to a substantial reduction in cell viability. Specifically, with increasing concentrations of the GO@SiO_2@AuNS hybrid (10, 50, and 100 $\mu g.mL^{-1}$) under NIR laser exposure, cell viability decreases significantly, reaching

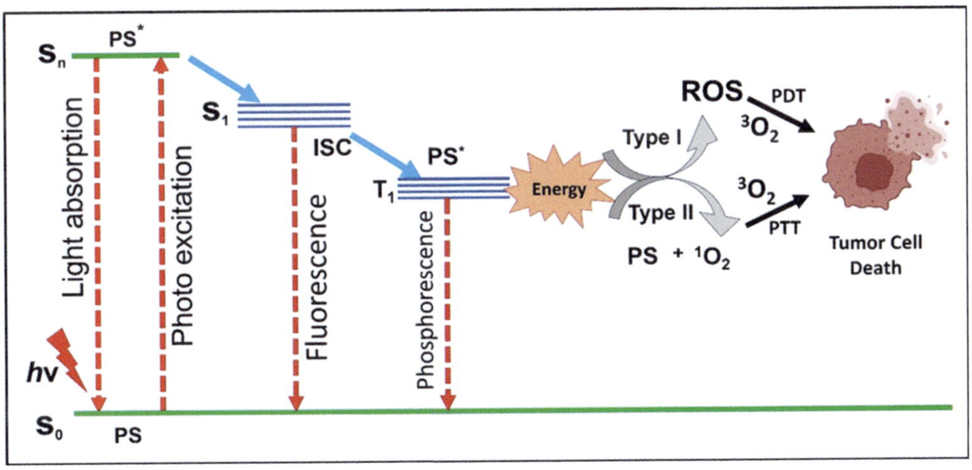

FIGURE 8.8 A simplified Jablonski diagram explaining the photophysical and photochemical basis of PDT and PTT. S_0—ground state, S_1—excited singlet state, T_1—excited triplet state, ISC—intersystem crossing, PS—Photosensitizer. Updated from the previously published work.

Source: Roy et al. (2023).

approximately 61%, 35%, and 10%, respectively. These results highlight the synergistic effect of the hybrid material and NIR irradiation in inducing photothermal cytotoxicity, demonstrating its potential for targeted cancer therapy (He *et al.*, 2020). rGO nanosheets functionalized with PEG chains and embedded with AuPd nanoparticles (NPs) were successfully photothermally ablated *in vitro* in HeLa cells when the nanocomposites were used at concentrations as low as 20 mg/mL, HeLa cells' relative cell viabilities after laser irradiation (808 nm, 10 min) showed considerable photoablation, achieving near-total (97%) cell ablation with an LC_{50} of 7 mg/mL (Darabdhara *et al.*, 2015).

For instance, when exposed to a NIR laser at a low dose of 25 $\mu g.mL^{-1}$, AuPd-rGO/PDA nanocomposites showed excellent photothermal properties, increasing temperature by almost 51 ± 3 °C in just three minutes causing cell death in MDA-MB-231 cells (Das *et al.*, 2020).

8.6 COMBINED THERAPY TECHNIQUE

Gold nanostructures have gained considerable attention as multifunctional platforms for combination therapy due to their unique optical properties, high surface-to-volume ratio, excellent biocompatibility, and ease of surface functionalization.

8.6.1 PTT and PDT

The potential of photodynamic therapy (PDT) in cancer therapy has attracted a lot of attention. It involves selectively activating photosensitizers within specific lesions by means of light as an external trigger.

Lebepe *et al.*, reported a GO-coated AuNRs nanocomposite conjugated with water soluble cationic porphyrin (TMePyP) as a photo synergistic therapeutic agent. The nanocomposite had a superior photothermal and photodynamic properties compared to individual components. The nanocomposite showed promise as a dual-function agent for cancer therapy, offering potential benefits over conventional treatments (Lebepe *et al.*, 2021). In another study, AuNRs coated with GO and conjugated with meso-tetra-(4-sulfonatophenyl) porphyrin (TPPS4) emerged as a promising dual photodynamic and photothermal agent for biomedical applications. The phototherapeutic qualities and dispersibility of GO@AuNRs are improved upon conjugation with TPPS4. It is also exhibited that GO@AuNRs-TPPS4 can tolerate freeze-drying pressure without applying cryoprotectant materials, which indicates that the material is highly stable. Due to the above characteristics, GO@AuNRs-TPPS4 can be used as a potent PTT-PDT agent (Lebepe *et al.*, 2023).

8.6.2 Chemotherapy and Photothermal Therapy (Chemo-PTT)

In recent years, PTT has become an alternative method for cancer treatment, which has gained much attention from researchers. Though PTT has highly selective and noninvasive characteristics, still it is very much site-specific—that is, it shows its effect only where the photo-absorber nanoparticles are present and NIR light is irradiated. For these reasons, researchers are finding more effective methods for cancer treatment. So, combined chemotherapy and PTT can be a more effective method for cancer treatment (Wang *et al.*, 2016). Xinhuan *et al.* successfully synthesized DNA aptamer (Apt)–modified graphene oxide–gold nanoparticle (GO–AuNP) composites. Further doxorubicin (DOX) was loaded on the GO–AuNP–Apt system which exhibits heat-stimulative and sustained release characteristics. This investigation revealed that combined therapy (Chemo-PTT) is more effective than that of single chemotherapy or PTT (Wang *et al.*, 2015). Another group synthesized Gum Arabic (GA) functionalized GO (fGO). GA functionalization increases NIR absorption and solubility of GO. Then they conjugated gold nanorods (GNRs) with fGO which forms GO@GNRs nanocomposites. Further, they attached Doxorubicin (DOX) with the above nanocomposites to enhance the Chemo-PTT efficacy. This fGO@GNRs-DOX system increases the NIR-induced drug release and the photothermal property, which makes it an ideal candidate for Chemo-PTT (Khan *et al.*, 2017). DOX-loaded core-shell gold nanorods and mesoporous silica nanoparticles capped with PEGylated graphene oxide (GNRs/SiO2/GO-PEG) are also excellent systems for Chemo-PTT. These nanocomposites (GNRs/SiO2/GO-PEG-DOX) show excellent photothermal integrity both in acidic media and in physiological conditions because of the presence of biocompatible GO-PEG. GO-PEG enhances the specific surface area of the nanocomposites which subsequently increases light-to-heat conversion efficacy between GNRs and GO-PEG. GNRs/SiO2/GO-PEG also show outstanding DOX loading efficiency and excellent light-to-heat conversion effect. GNRs/SiO2/GO-PEG-DOX nanocomposite system significantly released drugs in a pH-/NIR-dual responsive manner, which ultimately effectively enhances the Chemo-PTT effect. (Qi *et al.*, 2019). Chen *et al.* synthesized a novel bevacizumab (anticancer drug)-loaded folic acid (FA) and GO-conjugated gold nanorods (Be-FA-GO-AuN) for synergistic chemo-PTT. These nanocomposites passively target tumor tissues, where the folic acid receptors are expressed selectively. These Be-FA-GO-AuN show pH and NIR light-dependent drug release characteristics, which exhibit less cytotoxicity because of the minimum non-specific spread of the drug in the other healthy tissues (Chen *et al.*, 2021). In another study, GNRs were attached to the surface of PEGylated graphene oxide (GO-PEG) through polydopamine (PDA) to fabricate GNRs-GO-PDA nanosheets. The GNRs-GO-PDA hybrid nanosheets exhibit excellent DOX-loading capacity, photostability, and light-to-heat conversion efficiency (Qi *et al.*, 2020). Fengyang *et al.* developed a novel nanocomposite of PDA-decorated nano reduced-graphene oxide (NRGO), gold nanostars (GNS), and DOX (NRGO-GNS@DOX) for combined chemo-PTT treatment of breast cancer. Upon irradiation of NIR laser, the NRGO-GNS@DOX nanocomposites elicited chemo-PTT significantly in 4T1 breast cancer cells due to the synergistic effect of NRGO-GNS-depended PTT and DOX-induced chemotherapy (Wang *et al.*, 2016). Cheng *et al.* developed a novel nanomaterials comprising AuNR enclosed within NGO shells, which is highly effective chemo-PTT cancer therapeutic agent. Hyaluronic acid (HA) conjugation with these nanostructures (NGOHA-AuNRs) enhances its PTT efficacy than AuNRs. DOX loading on NGOHA-AuNR show highly pH-responsive and NIR light dependent drug release characteristics. Xu *et al.* reported that combined approach of Chemo-PTT using NGOHA-AuNRs-DOX resulted in four times higher cell death in compared to only PTT and 1.5 times higher cell death compared to only chemotherapy (Xu *et al.*, 2013a). Figure 8.9 presents the chemo-PTT effect on A549 (lung cancer) cell line.

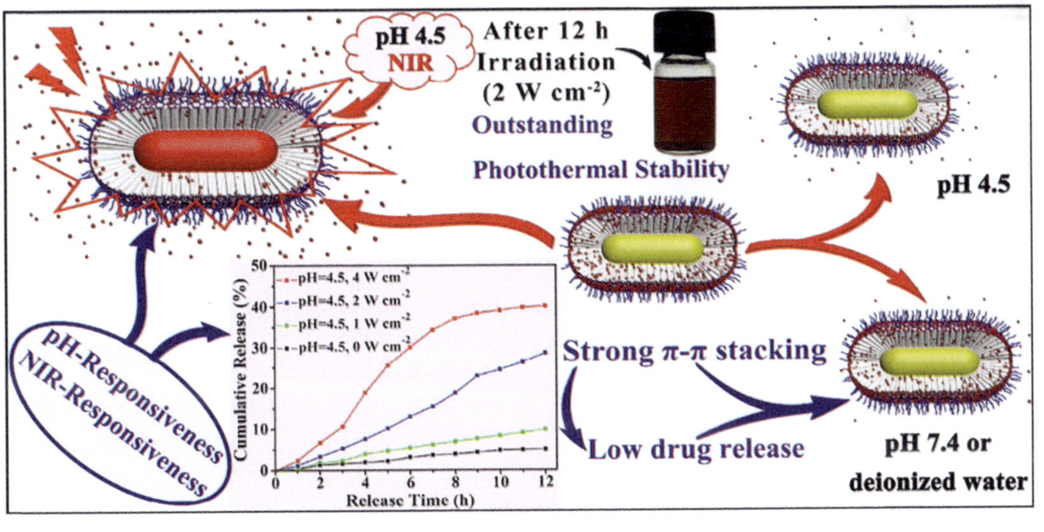

FIGURE 8.9 Diagram showing the pH- and NIR-dependent drug release mechanism of GO-PEG/SiO2-GNR nanocomposite.

Source: Qi et al. (2019).

8.6.3 PTT-Imaging

Combined PTT imaging can be one of the best options for cancer theranostics. PTT and imaging can be used for tumor ablation and diagnosis respectively. The exact location and the size of tumors along with the presence of photo absorber agents must be identified before therapy. During therapy, the treatment process must be continuously observed, and its efficacy must be evaluated after therapy. The combination of photothermal therapy and contrast-enhanced diagnostic imaging capability may be the best method to use for these purposes. A non-invasive approach to tumor detection and real-time particle localization monitoring is made possible by contrast-agent imaging techniques such as magnetic resonance imaging (MRI), computed tomography (CT), and ultrasound imaging (US). Every imaging method has benefits and drawbacks of its own. Though US imaging is very much effective still many cancers cannot be diagnosed via US imaging. Because of less sensitivity, CT imaging causes low soft tissue contrast. Combining different modalities has become more and more popular in recent years. In addition, the excitement surrounding these multimodal imaging devices has sparked a great deal of interest in the creation of multimodal contrast agents, which will increase their therapeutic effects. When numerous agents are administered, the body's blood clearance mechanisms may be under additional stress. However, this can be avoided when multimodal detectability is combined with a single agent (Jin *et al.*, 2013).

Gold nanoparticle-decorated graphene sheets have become an interesting agent for combined PTT-imaging. Gold nanoparticle conjugated reduced graphene oxide (rGO-AuNP) functionalized with PEG (rGO-AuNPs-PEG) shows excellent PTT-imaging efficacy against ovarian cancer (Wang *et al.*, 2020). α-synuclein protein was used to conjugate GO-Au and attached it on the surface of the tumor-tropic mesenchymal stem cell (MSC) to enhance its efficacy and subsequently reduce the cytotoxicity. AuNP-GO-MSCscan effectively diagnosed the tumor tissue by NIR imaging as well as effectively reduced the tumor via photothermal therapy (Kang *et al.*, 2017). The GO-GNRs nanohybrids exhibit a remarkable photothermal effect and CT imaging. At the dose of 50 μg/mL and NIR irradiation at 808 nm laser (power 0.4 W/cm^2) for 6 minutes remarkably increased the temperature. Even after several cycles of NIR irradiation, these nanoparticles exhibited very good photothermal, morphological, and optical characteristics. Excellent CT imaging properties and a photothermal impact were observed upon administration of the GO-GNRs into xenograft tumors. The combination of GO-GNRs and the preclinical CT agent iohexol improved CT imaging even more. Hence, the GO-GNR nanocomposites have considerable potential for accurate CT-image-guided photothermal tumor treatment (Sun *et al.*, 2017). A fluorescent and photoacoustic (PA) imaging-guided GO-Au composites (GA) were coated with a NIR-sensitive dye (Cy5.5) labeled-matrix metalloproteinase-14 (MMP-14) substrate (CP) to create a tumor-targeted theranostic agent (CPGA). Surface Plasmon Resonance (SPR) from both GO and Au quenches the Cy5.5 fluorescent signal, still, it can boost strong fluorescence signals after breakdown by MMP-14. When comparing the GA hybrid to Au or GO alone, it was discovered that the photothermal impact was much higher. Mice having SCC7 tumors were given CPGA intravenously, and the tumor area showed strong PA and fluorescent signals. After applying a laser to the tumors, considerable tumor inhibition was seen (Gao *et al.*, 2016). **Figure 8.10** shows near-infrared fluorescence and photoacoustic imaging-guided photothermal therapy.

Au-GO nanoparticle decorated cancer-specific nucleic acid conjugates (Au@GO NP-NACs) for combined PTT and multimodal imaging. These nanoparticles also exhibit excellent performance in cancer theranostics (Yang *et al.*, 2021).

8.7 CONCLUSION AND FUTURE PERSPECTIVES

In this book chapter, we have tried to provide a summary of the various synthesis procedures of graphene-decorated gold nanostructured materials and their applications in PTT, their biocompatibility, cellular uptake, biodistribution, tumor tissue accumulation, and other combined photothermal

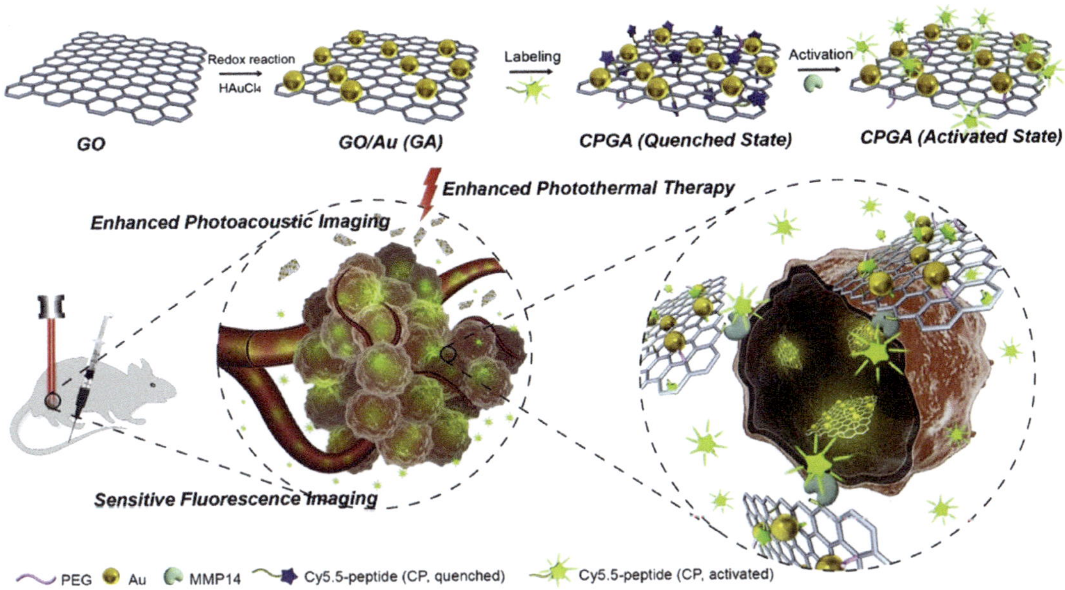

FIGURE 8.10 Schematic representation of near-infrared fluorescence and photoacoustic imaging-guided photothermal therapy of gold nanoparticle decorated graphene oxide.

Source: Gao et al. (2016).

therapy modalities such as PTT-PDT, Chemo-PTT, and PTT-Imaging. The rapid progress of nanotechnology has greatly advanced the utilization of PTT in both diagnosis and treatment of cancer. PTT involves minimally invasive procedures and maximum therapeutic outcomes. PTT and its adjuvant therapies are one of the most promising therapeutic options for cancer treatment, in which the thermal sensitivity of the target cells, the type of photothermal conversion agent, and the intensity and time span of laser light affect the cancer cells and their treatment. The photothermal agents and light wavelengths should be such that there is the least amount of damage to healthy tissues, the light should penetrate deeply into tumor tissues, killing the tumor tissues and removing the cancer cells. PTT is considered to be safe with fewer side effects because it enables targeted heating of tumor cells, minimizing harm to surrounding healthy tissues. PTT using nanomaterials has only been tested on tumor models in preclinical studies (*in vitro* and *in vivo*) necessitating further research before its clinical adoption.

In the combinatorial therapy with PTT discussed, each therapy producing synergistic effect is unique. Although this book chapter presents some encouraging features of the combined PTT therapy of gold nanostructures decorated graphene nanosheets with PDT, Chemotherapy, and Imaging, further extensive research is needed to enter clinical trials. PTT and PDT combined therapy has been shown to overcome multidrug resistance and reduce the dose-limiting toxicity linked to chemotherapeutic drugs. Chemo-PTT also reduce the dose related toxicity and enhance the efficacy in a synergistic way. Specific targeting of tumors, and faster clearance from the system are important steps in the development of functionalized gold nanostructures decorated graphene nanosheets for PTT. Passive targeting of these nanoparticles during drug delivery causes accumulation in the tissues. The functionalization of nanoparticles with active targeting molecules overcomes this barrier. Future studies on multifunctional (e.g., PTT-PDT-imaging; Chemo-PTT-imaging; Chemo-PTT-PDT-imaging etc.) Au nanostructured decorated graphene nanocomposite will improve the application of nanomaterials in PTT application in terms of diagnosis, increasing cancer treatment efficiency, and reduction in toxicity.

ACKNOWLEDGEMENT

PM and ER acknowledges Council of Scientific and Industrial Research (CSIR), India for the fellowship. The authors are grateful to the Director, CSIR-NEIST for approval with institute publication number: CSIR-NEIST/PUB/2024/113.

LIST OF ABBREVIATIONS

A.U.—Arbitrary units
Apt—Aptamer
Au/MgO—Gold-magnesium oxide Au-Gold
AuNPs—Gold nanoparticles
AuNRs—Gold nanorods
AuNs—Gold nano shells
AuPd—Gold-Palladium
Be-FA-GO-AuN—Bevacizumab-loaded folic acid (FA) and GO-conjugated gold nanorods (Be-FA-GO-AuN)
BSGNs—Bare-Surfaced Gold Nanostructures
Chemo-PTT—Chemotherapy and Photothermal therapy
CNTs—Carbon nanotubes
CLSM—Confocal laser scanning microscopy
CPGA—Cationic Polymer–Gold Nanoparticle–Graphene Oxide Activatable Probe
CPT—Camptothecin
CT—Computed tomography
CTAB—Cetyltrimethylammonium bromide
CVD—Chemical vapor deposition
Cy.5.5—Cyanine 5.5
Cys—Cysteine
DOX—Doxorubicin
EPR—Enhanced permeability and retention
FA—Folic acid
fGO—Functionalized GO
FITC—Fluorescein isothiocyanate,
FRET—Fluorescence resonance energy transfer
FT-IR—Fourier-transform infrared spectroscopy
GA—Gum arabica
GCE—Glassy carbon electrode
GGNMs—Graphene-decorated gold nanostructured materials
GNMs—Gold nanostructured materials,
GNRs/SiO2/GO-PEG—Gold nanorods and mesoporous silica nanoparticles capped with PEGylated graphene oxide
GNS—Gold nanostars
GNS-Au—Graphene nanosheets–gold
GNSs—Graphene nanosheets,
GO—Graphene oxide
GO–AuNP—Graphene oxide–gold nanoparticle
HA—Hyaluronic acid
HIV—Human Immunodeficiency Virus
ICG—Indocyanine green
ICP-MS—Inductively coupled plasma mass spectrometry
LC50—Lethal concentration 50%

MMP-14—Matrix metalloproteinase-14
MRI—Magnetic resonance imaging
MSC—Mesenchymal stem cell
NACs—Nucleic acid conjugates
NIR—Near-infrared
NRGO—Nano reduced-graphene oxide
PA—Photoacoustic
PBS—Phosphate buffered saline
PDA—Polydopamine
Pd—Palladium
PDT—Photodynamic therapy
PEG—polyethylene glycol
PEG—Poly ethylene glycol
PEI—Polyethyleneimine
PET—Photo-induced electron transfer
PSS—Polystyrene sulfonate
PTT—Photothermal therapy
PTT—Imaging: Photothermal therapy-Imaging
PVP—Polyvinyl pyrrolidone
r-GO—Reduced graphene oxide
SERS—Surface-Enhanced Raman Scattering
SiO2—Silicon dioxide
SPR—Surface plasmon resonance
TAT—Trans-Activator of Transcription
TEM—Transmission Electron Microscopy
TMePyP—Porphyrin, 5, 10, 15, 20-tetrakis (3-methyl pyridyl) porphyrin
TPPS4—Meso-tetra-(4-sulfonatophenyl) porphyrin
U87MG—Human glioblastoma astrocytoma
US—Ultrasound
UV-VIS—Ultraviolet-Visible
XRD—X-ray diffraction

REFERENCES

Amina, Sundus Jabeen, and Bin Guo. "A review on the synthesis and functionalization of gold nanoparticles as a drug delivery vehicle." *International Journal of Nanomedicine* (2020): 9823–9857.

Andresen, Thomas L., Simon S. Jensen, and Kent Jørgensen. "Advanced strategies in liposomal cancer therapy: Problems and prospects of active and tumor specific drug release." *Progress in Lipid Research* 44, no. 1 (2005): 68–97.

Bai, Song, and Xiaoping Shen. "Graphene–inorganic nanocomposites." *Rsc Advances* 2, no. 1 (2012): 64–98.

Bardhan, Rizia, Surbhi Lal, Amit Joshi, and Naomi J. Halas. "Theranostic nanoshells: From probe design to imaging and treatment of cancer." *Accounts of Chemical Research* 44, no. 10 (2011): 936–946.

Bian, Xia, Zhi-Ling Song, Yu Qian, Wei Gao, Zhen-Qian Cheng, Long Chen, Hao Liang et al. "Fabrication of graphene-isolated-Au-nanocrystal nanostructures for multimodal cell imaging and photothermal-enhanced chemotherapy." *Scientific Reports* 4, no. 1 (2014): 6093.

Caires, A. J., D. C. B. Alves, C. Fantini, A. S. Ferlauto, and L. O. Ladeira. "One-pot in situ photochemical synthesis of graphene oxide/gold nanorod nanocomposites for surface-enhanced Raman spectroscopy." *RSC Advances* 5, no. 58 (2015): 46552–46557.

Chen, Hongda, Fuyao Liu, Zhen Lei, Lina Ma, and Zhenxin Wang. "Fe 2 O 3@ Au core@ shell nanoparticle–graphene nanocomposites as theranostic agents for bioimaging and chemo-photothermal synergistic therapy." *Rsc Advances* 5, no. 103 (2015): 84980–84987.

Chen, Huanjun, Xiaoshan Kou, Zhi Yang, Weihai Ni, and Jianfang Wang. "Shape-and size-dependent refractive index sensitivity of gold nanoparticles." *Langmuir* 24, no. 10 (2008): 5233–5237.

Chen, Yu, Zhiguo Luo, Chunli Chen, Ming Luo, and Li Yuan. "Enhanced therapeutic efficacy of drug encapsulated folic acid conjugated graphene oxide-gold nanorods for chemo-photothermal therapeutics of cervical cancer." *Biotechnology & Biotechnological Equipment* 35, no. 1 (2021): 1492–1504.

Chen, Yu-Wei, Yu-Lin Su, Shang-Hsiu Hu, and San-Yuan Chen. "Functionalized graphene nanocomposites for enhancing photothermal therapy in tumor treatment." *Advanced Drug Delivery Reviews* 105 (2016): 190–204.

Cheng, Cheng-En, Chi-Yuan Lin, Hao-Yu Chang, Chen-Han Huang, Hsing-Ying Lin, Chia-Hao Chen, Chia-Chen Hsu, Chen-Shiung Chang, and Forest Shih Sen Chien. "Surface-enhanced Raman scattering of graphene with photo-assisted-synthesized gold nanoparticles." *Optics Express* 21, no. 5 (2013): 6547–6554.

Darabdhara, Gitashree, Manash R. Das, Volodymyr Turcheniuk, Kostiantyn Turcheniuk, Vladimir Zaitsev, Rabah Boukherroub, and Sabine Szunerits. "Reduced graphene oxide nanosheets decorated with AuPd bimetallic nanoparticles: A multifunctional material for photothermal therapy of cancer cells." *Journal of Materials Chemistry B* 3, no. 42 (2015): 8366–8374.

Das, Punamshree, Sushma V. Mudigunda, Gitashree Darabdhara, Purna K. Boruah, Sachin Ghar, Aravind K. Rengan, and Manash R. Das. "Biocompatible functionalized AuPd bimetallic nanoparticles decorated on reduced graphene oxide sheets for photothermal therapy of targeted cancer cells." *Journal of Photochemistry and Photobiology B: Biology* 212 (2020): 112028.

Dembereldorj, Uuriintuya, Seon Young Choi, Erdene-Ochir Ganbold, Nam Woong Song, Doseok Kim, Jaebum Choo, So Yeong Lee, Sehun Kim, and Sang-Woo Joo. "Gold nanorod-assembled PEGylated graphene-oxide nanocomposites for photothermal cancer therapy." *Photochemistry and Photobiology* 90, no. 3 (2014): 659–666.

Doughty, Austin C. V., Ashley R. Hoover, Elivia Layton, Cynthia K. Murray, Eric W. Howard, and Wei R. Chen. "Nanomaterial applications in photothermal therapy for cancer." *Materials* 12, no. 5 (2019): 779.

Fard, Javad Khalili, Samira Jafari, and Mohammad Ali Eghbal. "A review of molecular mechanisms involved in toxicity of nanoparticles." *Advanced Pharmaceutical Bulletin* 5, no. 4 (2015): 447.

Farokhnezhad, Mohsen, and Mahdi Esmaeilzadeh. "Graphene coated gold nanoparticles: An emerging class of nanoagents for photothermal therapy applications." *Physical Chemistry Chemical Physics* 21, no. 33 (2019): 18352–18362.

Gao, Shi, Liwen Zhang, Guohao Wang, Kai Yang, Minglong Chen, Rui Tian, Qingjie Ma, and Lei Zhu. "Hybrid graphene/Au activatable theranostic agent for multimodalities imaging guided enhanced photothermal therapy." *Biomaterials* 79 (2016): 36–45.

Novoselov, Kostya S., Andre K. Geim, Sergei V. Morozov, De-eng Jiang, Yanshui Zhang, Sergey V. Dubonos, Irina V. Grigorieva, and Alexandr A. Firsov. "Electric field effect in atomically thin carbon films." *science* 306, no. 5696 (2004): 666–669.

Gharatape, Alireza, Soodabeh Davaran, Roya Salehi, and Hamed Hamishehkar. "Engineered gold nanoparticles for photothermal cancer therapy and bacteria killing." *RSC Advances* 6, no. 112 (2016): 111482–111516.

Govindhan, Maduraiveeran, Mona Amiri, and Aicheng Chen. "Au nanoparticle/graphene nanocomposite as a platform for the sensitive detection of NADH in human urine." *Biosensors and Bioelectronics* 66 (2015): 474–480.

He, Shuyi, Jingyu Li, Mingjian Chen, Liehua Deng, Yuxin Yang, Zhaoyang Zeng, Wei Xiong, and Xu Wu. "Graphene oxide-template gold nanosheets as highly efficient near-infrared hyperthermia agents for cancer therapy." *International Journal of Nanomedicine* (2020): 8451–8463.

Hu, Chaofan, Jianhua Rong, Jianghu Cui, Yunhua Yang, Lufeng Yang, Yaling Wang, and Yingliang Liu. "Fabrication of a graphene oxide–gold nanorod hybrid material by electrostatic self-assembly for surface-enhanced Raman scattering." *Carbon* 51 (2013): 255–264.

Hu, Huating, Xianbao Wang, Chunhui Xu, Jinzhao Wang, Li Wan, Min Zhang, and Xiaopeng Shang. "Microwave-assisted synthesis of graphene nanosheets–gold nanocomposites with enhancing electrochemical response." *Fullerenes, Nanotubes and Carbon Nanostructures* 20, no. 1 (2012): 31–40.

Huang, Jie, Liming Zhang, Biao Chen, Nan Ji, Fenghua Chen, Yi Zhang, and Zhijun Zhang. "Nanocomposites of size-controlled gold nanoparticles and graphene oxide: Formation and applications in SERS and catalysis." *Nanoscale* 2, no. 12 (2010): 2733–2738.

Huang, Qian, Yang Chen, Liying Hao, Ronghui Zhou, Yanjing Li, Qirong Li, Bofeng Zhu, and Xiaoxiao Cai. "Pegylated carbon nitride nanosheets for enhanced reactive oxygen species generation and photodynamic therapy under hypoxic conditions." *Nanomedicine: Nanotechnology, Biology and Medicine* 25 (2020): 102167.

Huang, Xiaohua, Ivan H. El-Sayed, Wei Qian, and Mostafa A. El-Sayed. "Cancer cell imaging and photothermal therapy in the near-infrared region by using gold nanorods." *Journal of the American Chemical Society* 128, no. 6 (2006): 2115–2120.

Huang, Xiaohua, Prashant K. Jain, Ivan H. El-Sayed, and Mostafa A. El-Sayed. "Plasmonic photothermal therapy (PPTT) using gold nanoparticles." *Lasers in Medical Science* 23 (2008): 217–228.

Jaque, Daniel, L. Martínez Maestro, Blanca del Rosal, P. Haro-Gonzalez, Antonio Benayas, J. L. Plaza, E. Martín Rodríguez, and J. García Solé. "Nanoparticles for photothermal therapies." *Nanoscale* 6, no. 16 (2014): 9494–9530.

Jasuja, Kabeer, Josh Linn, Steven Melton, and Vikas Berry. "Microwave-reduced uncapped metal nanoparticles on graphene: Tuning catalytic, electrical, and Raman properties." *The Journal of Physical Chemistry Letters* 1, no. 12 (2010): 1853–1860.

Jin, Yushen, Jinrui Wang, Hengte Ke, Shumin Wang, and Zhifei Dai. "Graphene oxide modified PLA microcapsules containing gold nanoparticles for ultrasonic/CT bimodal imaging guided photothermal tumor therapy." *Biomaterials* 34, no. 20 (2013): 4794–4802.

Kang, Seokyung, Junghee Lee, Seungmi Ryu, Yeji Kwon, Kyung-Hun Kim, Dae Hong Jeong, Seung R. Paik, and Byung-Soo Kim. "Gold nanoparticle/graphene oxide hybrid sheets attached on mesenchymal stem cells for effective photothermal cancer therapy." *Chemistry of Materials* 29, no. 8 (2017): 3461–3476.

Khalil, Ibrahim, Nurhidayatullaili Muhd Julkapli, Wageeh A. Yehye, Wan Jefrey Basirun, and Suresh K. Bhargava. "Graphene–gold nanoparticles hybrid—synthesis, functionalization, and application in a electrochemical and surface-enhanced raman scattering biosensor." *Materials* 9, no. 6 (2016): 406.

Khan, M. Shahnawaz, Sunil Pandey, Mukesh L. Bhaisare, Gangaraju Gedda, Abou Talib, and Hui-Fen Wu. "Graphene oxide@ gold nanorods for chemo-photothermal treatment and controlled release of doxorubicin in mice Tumor." *Colloids and Surfaces B: Biointerfaces* 160 (2017): 543–552.

Kong, Byung-Seon, Jianxin Geng, and Hee-Tae Jung. "Layer-by-layer assembly of graphene and gold nanoparticles by vacuum filtration and spontaneous reduction of gold ions." *Chemical Communications* 16 (2009): 2174–2176.

Lebepe, Thabang Calvin, Rodney Maluleke, Nande Mgedle, and Oluwatobi Samuel Oluwafemi. "Porphyrin as a cryoprotectant for graphene oxide-coated gold nanorods to produce conjugated product with improved stability and opto-phototherapeutic properties." *Pharmaceutics* 15, no. 11 (2023): 2538.

Lebepe, Thabang Calvin, Sundararajan Parani, Vuyelwa Ncapayi, Rodney Maluleke, Grace It Mwad Mbaz, Olufunto Tolulope Fanoro, Jose Rajendran Varghese, Atsuki Komiya, Tetsuya Kodama, and Oluwatobi Samuel Oluwafemi. "Graphene oxide-gold nanorods nanocomposite-porphyrin conjugate as promising tool for cancer phototherapy performance." *Pharmaceuticals* 14, no. 12 (2021): 1295.

Lebepe, Thabang Calvin, Sundararajan Parani, and Oluwatobi S. Oluwafemi. "Graphene oxide-coated gold nanorods: Synthesis and applications." *Nanomaterials* 10, no. 11 (2020): 2149.

Li, Jingchao, Rong Cai, Naoki Kawazoe, and Guoping Chen. "Facile preparation of albumin-stabilized gold nanostars for the targeted photothermal ablation of cancer cells." *Journal of Materials Chemistry B* 3, no. 28 (2015): 5806–5814.

Li, Shyh-Dar, and Leaf Huang. "Pharmacokinetics and biodistribution of nanoparticles." *Molecular Pharmaceutics* 5, no. 4 (2008): 496–504.

Lim, Siew Pheng, and Alfredo Garzino-Demo. "The human immunodeficiency virus type 1 Tat protein upregulates the promoter activity of the beta-chemokine monocyte chemoattractant protein 1 in the human astrocytoma cell line U-87 MG: Role of SP-1, AP-1, and NF-κB consensus sites." *Journal of Virology* 74, no. 4 (2000): 1632–1640.

Liu, Hui, Xing Su, Congyue Duan, Xiaonan Dong, Shili Zhou, and Zhenfeng Zhu. "Microwave-assisted hydrothermal synthesis of Au NPs–graphene composites for H2O2 detection." *Journal of Electroanalytical Chemistry* 731 (2014): 36–42.

Liu, Zhuang, Joshua T. Robinson, Xiaoming Sun, and Hongjie Dai. "PEGylated nanographene oxide for delivery of water-insoluble cancer drugs." *Journal of the American Chemical Society* 130, no. 33 (2008): 10876–10877.

Luo, Zhengtang, Luke A. Somers, Yaping Dan, Thomas Ly, Nicholas J. Kybert, E. J. Mele, and AT Charlie Johnson. "Size-selective nanoparticle growth on few-layer graphene films." *Nano Letters* 10, no. 3 (2010): 777–781.

Maeda, H. A. Y. M., and Y. Matsumura. "Tumoritropic and lymphotropic principles of macromolecular drugs." *Critical Reviews in Therapeutic Drug Carrier Systems* 6, no. 3 (1989): 193–210.

Mahato, Mrityunjoy, Sanjukta Patra, and Manashjit Gogoi. "Herbal Nanocarriers for cancer therapy." *Nanopharmaceuticals: Principles and Applications* 2 (2021): 41–75.

Maji, Swarup Kumar, Subin Yu, Eunshil Choi, Ju Won Lim, Dohyub Jang, Ga-young Kim, Sehoon Kim, Hyukjin Lee, and Dong Ha Kim. "Anisotropic plasmonic gold nanorod–indocyanine green@ reduced graphene oxide–doxorubicin nanohybrids for image-guided enhanced tumor theranostics." *ACS Omega* 7, no. 17 (2022): 15186–15199.

Markovic, Zoran M., Ljubica M. Harhaji-Trajkovic, Biljana M. Todorovic-Markovic, Dejan P. Kepić, Katarina M. Arsikin, Svetlana P. Jovanović, Aleksandar C. Pantovic, Miroslav D. Dramićanin, and Vladimir S. Trajkovic. "In vitro comparison of the photothermal anticancer activity of graphene nanoparticles and carbon nanotubes." *Biomaterials* 32, no. 4 (2011): 1121–1129.

Murphy, Catherine J., Tapan K. Sau, Anand M. Gole, Christopher J. Orendorff, Jinxin Gao, Linfeng Gou, Simona E. Hunyadi, and Tan Li. "Anisotropic metal nanoparticles: Synthesis, assembly, and optical applications." *The Journal of Physical Chemistry B* 109, no. 29 (2005): 13857–13870.

Nguyen, Van Phuc, Sung Won Kim, Hanna Kim, Hyejin Kim, Kwang Hyuk Seok, Min Jung, Yeh-chan Ahn, and Hyun Wook Kang. "Biocompatible astaxanthin as a novel marine-oriented agent for dual chemo-photothermal therapy." *PloS One* 12, no. 4 (2017): e0174687.

Orecchioni, Marco, Roberto Cabizza, Alberto Bianco, and Lucia Gemma Delogu. "Graphene as cancer theranostic tool: Progress and future challenges." *Theranostics* 5, no. 7 (2015): 710.

Pandey, Priyanka A., Gavin R. Bell, Jonathan P. Rourke, Ana M. Sanchez, Mark D. Elkin, Bryan J. Hickey, and Neil R. Wilson. "Physical vapor deposition of metal nanoparticles on chemically modified graphene: Observations on metal–graphene interactions." *Small* 7, no. 22 (2011): 3202–3210.

Park, Gle, Kyung G. Lee, Seok Jae Lee, Tae Jung Park, Rinbok Wi, and Do Hyun Kim. "Synthesis of graphene-gold nanocomposites via sonochemical reduction." *Journal of Nanoscience and Nanotechnology* 11, no. 7 (2011): 6095–6101.

Pattani, Varun P., Jay Shah, Alexandra Atalis, Anirudh Sharma, and James W. Tunnell. "Role of apoptosis and necrosis in cell death induced by nanoparticle-mediated photothermal therapy." *Journal of Nanoparticle Research* 17 (2015): 1–11.

Pham, Tuan Anh, Byung Choon Choi, Kwon Taek Lim, and Yeon Tae Jeong. "A simple approach for immobilization of gold nanoparticles on graphene oxide sheets by covalent bonding." *Applied Surface Science* 257, no. 8 (2011): 3350–3357.

Pruneanu, Stela, Florina Pogacean, Alexandru R. Biris, Stefania Ardelean, Valentin Canpean, Gabriela Blanita, Enkeleda Dervishi, and Alexandru S. Biris. "Novel graphene-gold nanoparticle modified electrodes for the high sensitivity electrochemical spectroscopy detection and analysis of carbamazepine." *The Journal of Physical Chemistry C* 115, no. 47 (2011): 23387–23394.

Qi, Zeer, Jun Shi, Zheng Zhang, Yuchan Cao, Jingguo Li, and Shaokui Cao. "PEGylated graphene oxide-capped gold nanorods/silica nanoparticles as multifunctional drug delivery platform with enhanced near-infrared responsiveness." *Materials Science and Engineering: C* 104 (2019): 109889.

Qi, Zeer, Jun Shi, Beibei Zhu, Jingguo Li, and Shaokui Cao. "Gold nanorods/graphene oxide nanosheets immobilized by polydopamine for efficient remotely triggered drug delivery." *Journal of Materials Science* 55 (2020): 14530–14543.

Robinson, Joshua T., Scott M. Tabakman, Yongye Liang, Hailiang Wang, Hernan Sanchez Casalongue, Daniel Vinh, and Hongjie Dai. "Ultrasmall reduced graphene oxide with high near-infrared absorbance for photothermal therapy." *Journal of the American Chemical Society* 133, no. 17 (2011): 6825–6831.

Rosenblum, Daniel, Nitin Joshi, Wei Tao, Jeffrey M. Karp, and Dan Peer. "Progress and challenges towards targeted delivery of cancer therapeutics." *Nature Communications* 9, no. 1 (2018): 1410.

Roy, Esha, Prosenjit Mridha, Rinku Baishya, Himangsu Kousik Bora, Rituraj Konwar, and Manash R. Das. "Carbon nanotropes: Potential nanomaterials for drug delivery and biomedical applications." In *Carbon Nanostructures in Biomedical Applications*, pp. 197–227. Cham: Springer International Publishing, 2023.

Saha, Krishnendu, Sarit S. Agasti, Chaekyu Kim, Xiaoning Li, and Vincent M. Rotello. "Gold nanoparticles in chemical and biological sensing." *Chemical Reviews* 112, no. 5 (2012): 2739–2779.

Singh, Priyanka, Santosh Pandit, V. R. S. S. Mokkapati, Abhroop Garg, Vaishnavi Ravikumar, and Ivan Mijakovic. "Gold nanoparticles in diagnostics and therapeutics for human cancer." *International Journal of Molecular Sciences* 19, no. 7 (2018): 1979.

Skrabalak, Sara E., Jingyi Chen, Yugang Sun, Xianmao Lu, Leslie Au, Claire M. Cobley, and Younan Xia. "Gold nanocages: Synthesis, properties, and applications." *Accounts of Chemical Research* 41, no. 12 (2008): 1587–1595.

Spyratou, Ellas, Mersini Makropoulou, Efstathios P. Efstathopoulos, Alexandros G. Georgakilas, and Lembit Sihver. "Recent advances in cancer therapy based on dual mode gold nanoparticles." *Cancers* 9, no. 12 (2017): 173.

Sun, Bingmei, Jinrui Wu, Shaobin Cui, Huanhuan Zhu, Wei An, Qingge Fu, Chengwei Shao, Aihua Yao, Bingdi Chen, and Donglu Shi. "In situ synthesis of graphene oxide/gold nanorods theranostic hybrids for efficient tumor computed tomography imaging and photothermal therapy." *Nano Research* 10 (2017): 37–48.

Tong, Ling, Yan Zhao, Terry B. Huff, Matthew N. Hansen, Alexander Wei, and J.-X. Cheng. "Gold nanorods mediate tumor cell death by compromising membrane integrity." *Advanced Materials* 19, no. 20 (2007): 3136–3141.

Turcheniuk, Kostiantyn, Tetiana Dumych, Rostyslav Bilyy, Volodymyr Turcheniuk, Julie Bouckaert, Volodymyr Vovk, Valentyna Chopyak et al. "Plasmonic photothermal cancer therapy with gold nanorods/reduced graphene oxide core/shell nanocomposites." *RSC Advances* 6, no. 2 (2016): 1600–1610.

Vines, Jeremy B., Jee-Hyun Yoon, Na-Eun Ryu, Dong-Jin Lim, and Hansoo Park. "Gold nanoparticles for photothermal cancer therapy." *Frontiers in Chemistry* 7 (2019): 167.

Vinodgopal, K., B. Neppolian, Ian V. Lightcap, Franz Grieser, Muthupandian Ashokkumar, and Prashant V. Kamat. "Sonolytic design of graphene-Au nanocomposites: Simultaneous and sequential reduction of graphene oxide and Au (III)." *The Journal of Physical Chemistry Letters* 1, no. 13 (2010): 1987–1993.

Wang, Fengyang, Qianqian Sun, Bing Feng, Zhiai Xu, Junying Zhang, Jie Xu, Linlin Lu et al. "Polydopamine-functionalized graphene oxide loaded with gold nanostars and doxorubicin for combined photothermal and chemotherapy of metastatic breast cancer." *Advanced Healthcare Materials* 5, no. 17 (2016): 2227–2236.

Wang, Shouju, Peng Huang, Liming Nie, Ruijun Xing, Dingbin Liu, Zhe Wang, Jing Lin et al. "Single continuous wave laser induced photodynamic/plasmonic photothermal therapy using photosensitizer-functionalized gold nanostars." *Advanced Materials (Deerfield Beach, Fla.)* 25, no. 22 (2013): 3055.

Wang, Xinhuan, Qiusen Han, Ning Yu, Jingying Li, Lin Yang, Rong Yang, and Chen Wang. "Aptamer–conjugated graphene oxide–gold nanocomposites for targeted chemo-photothermal therapy of cancer cells." *Journal of Materials Chemistry B* 3, no. 19 (2015): 4036–4042.

Wang, Zhihua, Xiao Sun, Ting Huang, Jibin Song, and Yudong Wang. "A sandwich nanostructure of gold nanoparticle coated reduced graphene oxide for photoacoustic imaging-guided photothermal therapy in the second NIR window." *Frontiers in Bioengineering and Biotechnology* 8 (2020): 655.

Wu, Yue, Moustafa R. K. Ali, Kuangcai Chen, Ning Fang, and Mostafa A. El-Sayed. "Gold nanoparticles in biological optical imaging." *Nano Today* 24 (2019): 120–140.

Xu, Cheng, Darong Yang, Lin Mei, Qiuhong Li, Haizhen Zhu, and Taihong Wang. "Targeting chemophotothermal therapy of hepatoma by gold nanorods/graphene oxide core/shell nanocomposites." *ACS Applied Materials & Interfaces* 5, no. 24 (2013a): 12911–12920.

Xu, Miao-Qing, Jian-Feng Wu, and Guang-Chao Zhao. "Direct electrochemistry of hemoglobin at a graphene gold nanoparticle composite film for nitric oxide biosensing." *Sensors* 13, no. 6 (2013b): 7492–7504.

Yang, Kai, Shuai Zhang, Guoxin Zhang, Xiaoming Sun, Shuit-Tong Lee, and Zhuang Liu. "Graphene in mice: Ultrahigh in vivo tumor uptake and efficient photothermal therapy." *Nano Letters* 10, no. 9 (2010): 3318–3323.

Yang, Letao, Tae-Hyung Kim, Hyeon-Yeol Cho, Jeffrey Luo, Jong-Min Lee, Sy-Tsong Dean Chueng, Yannan Hou et al. "Hybrid graphene-gold nanoparticle-based nucleic acid conjugates for cancer-specific multimodal imaging and combined therapeutics." *Advanced Functional Materials* 31, no. 5 (2021): 2006918.

Yang, Xiaoying, Xiaoyan Zhang, Zunfeng Liu, Yanfeng Ma, Yi Huang, and Yongsheng Chen. "High-efficiency loading and controlled release of doxorubicin hydrochloride on graphene oxide." *The Journal of Physical Chemistry C* 112, no. 45 (2008): 17554–17558.

Yeh, Yi-Cheun, Brian Creran, and Vincent M. Rotello. "Gold nanoparticles: Preparation, properties, and applications in bionanotechnology." *Nanoscale* 4, no. 6 (2012): 1871–1880.

Zhang, Liming, Jingguang Xia, Qinghuan Zhao, Liwei Liu, and Zhijun Zhang. "Functional graphene oxide as a nanocarrier for controlled loading and targeted delivery of mixed anticancer drugs." *Small* 6, no. 4 (2010): 537–544.

Zhang, Yinan, Dan Xu, Wenqin Li, Jun Yu, and Yu Chen. "Effect of size, shape, and surface modification on cytotoxicity of gold nanoparticles to human HEp-2 and canine MDCK cells." *Journal of Nanomaterials* 2012 (2012): 7–7.

Zhang, Yuan, Jun Qian, Dan Wang, Yalun Wang, and Sailing He. "Multifunctional gold nanorods with ultrahigh stability and tunability for in vivo fluorescence imaging, SERS detection, and photodynamic therapy." *Angewandte Chemie International Edition* 52, no. 4 (2013): 1148–1151.

9 Magnetic Materials for Cancer Hyperthermia and Drug Delivery

Amresh I. Prasad[1] *and Manashjit Gogoi*[2]
[1]Department of Nanotechnology, North-Eastern Hill University, Shillong, India
[2]Department of Biomedical Engineering, North-Eastern Hill University, Shillong, India

9.1 INTRODUCTION

Application of nanoparticles have showed its potential in multidisciplinary branches of science and technologies which includes pharmaceutics, biomedicine, agriculture, environment, physics, chemistry, material science, electronics, information technology, space science and many more [1]. Nanoparticles are known since ancient roman period when they were addressed as small particles, colloids or fine particles. Broadly materials with particle size ranging from 1–100 nm can be defined as nanoparticles [2]. Bulk materials when transformed into nanocrystalline particles depending on the size of the particles the physical properties of the nanomaterials get altered. One significant augmentation in the properties of nanomaterial in comparison with its bulk counterpart is its high effective surface area due to the presence of high number of atoms/molecules on the surface of the particles. This significant high surface area can be harvested for effective drug tagging through various capping agents [3]. The physico-chemical properties of these functionalized nanoparticles make them effective candidate for the various biomedical applications. Nanomaterials can move inside the body without disturbing the normal function due to its small size. Presence of nanomaterial in cells tends to react and these reaction in cells caused changes in cells which includes effect on cell growth and death [4, 5].

Their small size, tuneable shape and enhanced surface properties nanoparticles have showed their potential in medicinal applications such as targeted delivery, imaging, combination therapy, bone and dental repair, and hyperthermia [6]. Nanomaterials have multiple advantages for drug delivery application. The encapsulation of drug in nanomaterials improved biocompatibility, site specific controlled release thus dose required is reduced with prevention of side effects [7, 8].

One of the growing techniques used for elimination of damaged cells and tissue in cancer therapy is use of electromagnetic radiation and heat treatment referred as thermal ablation. Flexibility, low cost, and less invasiveness give thermal ablation therapy advantage over conventional methods. The current heat delivery routes lacks targeting as it faces difficulties in distinguishing between tumors and healthy tissue surroundings [9, 10]. Therefore, a combinational therapy by implying nanomaterial and thermal therapy could be an alternative. The significant attention gain n nanotechnology is due to its potential application in biomedical sector especially use of nanomaterials and nanocomposites for diagnostics and treatment such as thermal therapy. The nanomaterials can be functionalized to bind cancer cell with possibility of selective heating, cell separation and imaging [11–13].

Because of their special magnetic qualities and possible uses in cancer treatment, magnetic materials—particularly, magnetic nanoparticles (MNPs)—have drawn much attention in biomedical research. The properties such as nontoxicity, biocompatibility, injectability, and confined accumulation at the targeted sites are significant in the use of magnetic nanoparticles in clinical and

DOI: 10.1201/9781003799351-9

biomedical applications [14]. Since external magnetic fields may be used to alter these materials, they can be used for drug administration, targeted therapy, and diagnostic imaging. Iron oxide (Fe_3O_4 and γ-Fe_2O_3), cobalt, and their different alloys are important magnetic nanoparticles because of their superparamagnetic characteristics, biocompatibility, and simplicity in functionalization.

In bulk material with time there is no change in direction magnetic moment of the particle as the surrounding thermal energy is less than the particle energy. Whereas when particle size reaches sub-micrometer range the particle energy changes and therefore the magnetic moment direction changes with angle (θ). When the particle size furthered reduced to nano size the magnetic moment direction changes to opposite direction (θ= 180°), this behavior is known as superparamagnetism. Since the room temperature superparamagnetic nanoparticles do not retain any magnetism after magnetic field is removed, these nanoparticles hold biomedical significance [15].

In the latter half of the 20th century, magnetic nanoparticles were first investigated for their potential as contrast agents in magnetic resonance imaging (MRI). The 1950s saw the initial proposal of the theory of magnetic hyperthermia, in which cancer cells are killed by localized heat produced by magnetic nanoparticles. In the decades that followed, developments in nanotechnology broadened their uses, combining chemotherapy and hyperthermia to improve treatment results. Developments in surface modification techniques and synthesis methods have further accelerated their application in targeted drug delivery.

The inherent properties of MNPs opens many new prospects in prominent research and development of diagnostics and therapeutic methodologies [16, 17]. The ability of MNPs response to magnetic field attracted researchers' interest in different theranostic applications. They have become center for nano structure-based nanomedicine science. With use of MNPs it has been possible to magnetically accumulate and release these particles with in the target location [18–22]

MNPs' large surface-to-volume ratio offers a wealth of chemically active sites for biomolecule conjugation. This enables precise engineering and design to allow the MNPs to perform as intended, including therapeutic delivery, target specificity to lesion tissue, long-lasting circulation in the bloodstream, and optical detectability [23, 24]. Because of their magnetic characteristics, MNPs have several uses in medication and gene delivery, diagnostics, and therapies. These applications can be classed as belonging to one or more of the following groups:

(1) Magnetic resonance imaging (MRI) magnetic contrast agents.
(2) The separation by magnetism. To do this, biological or chemical agents that are known to bind to a particular target are used to functionalize magnetic beads, which are then combined in a beaker with a solution that is thought to contain the target. A permanent magnet positioned next to the solution beaker creates a magnetic moment and a field gradient throughout the solution after a predetermined amount of time has passed since the beads and solution came into contact. This separates the targets from the bulk solution that have attached themselves to the magnetized beads.
(3) Immunoassays: MNPs attached to main or secondary antibodies are utilized in immunoassays to quantify and distinguish antigens.
(4) Agents of hyperthermia: a high-frequency alternating magnetic field is applied to selectively heat the MNPs.
(5) Magnetic vectors that, in the case of targeted drug delivery, can be steered toward a specific site using magnetic field gradients.

MNPs are good nanosystems with theranostic applications because they can be used in both therapeutic and diagnostic applications.

This chapter aims to provide an extensive overview of the current state of magnetic materials in cancer hyperthermia and drug delivery. It will cover the synthesis and characterization of magnetic nanoparticles, mechanisms of magnetic hyperthermia, and their application in drug delivery systems. Additionally, it will examine the synergistic potential of combining hyperthermia and drug delivery, address safety and toxicity concerns, and discuss prospects and challenges.

9.1.1 Metallic Magnetic nanoparticles

The outer most distribution of electrons in the electronic orbitals of the metals gives them unique properties and magnetic behavior is one of them. Fe, Ni, Co, Mn are the most discussed and explored transition metals of their class. Among these Fe is mostly used in the compound form, such as oxides and carbonyls, due to its sensitivity toward surface oxidation and high magnetic moment density (220 emu/g) [25]. Fe nanoparticle (65 nm) with cubic body cantered crystalline structure was prepared by Hou and coworkers with PVP functionalized surface. Ni nanoparticles (3.7 nm) was reported with reduction of nickel acetyl acetonate using organic phase at elevated temperature [26, 27].

Iron oxide nanoparticles (IONP) are mainly classified as hematite (α-Fe_2O_3), maghemite (γ-Fe_2O_3), and magnetite (Fe_3O_4) nanoparticles (Figure 9.1). A ferromagnetic nanoparticles with size between 10–20 nm show a unique property known as superparamagnetism [28]. This phenomenon involves nonmagnetic behavior in absence of external magnetic field whereas saturation magnetization due to applied external magnetic field leading to magnetization of nanoparticles. A size dependent property (10–30nm) of single domain magnetic nanoparticles. Among IONP Fe_3O_4 and γ-Fe_2O_3 exhibits room temperature ferrimagnetism thus potential application in magnetic thermal therapy [29]. Four different types of heating mechanism are observed in MNPs. When particle size is greater than 1micron its caused eddy current and hysteresis losses whereas is superparamagnetic particles the heating is due to relaxation losses and in viscous medium it is due to friction losses [30].

9.1.2 Metallic Oxide and Ferrites

One of the most celebrated material with exceptional magnetic properties is Iron Oxide which is exploited to great extent for application in the field of biomedicine due to its cost efficiency, biocompatibility, and chemical stability [31–34]. With extensive research many synthesis route have been reported for the preparation of iron nanoparticles which includes chemical and physical approaches

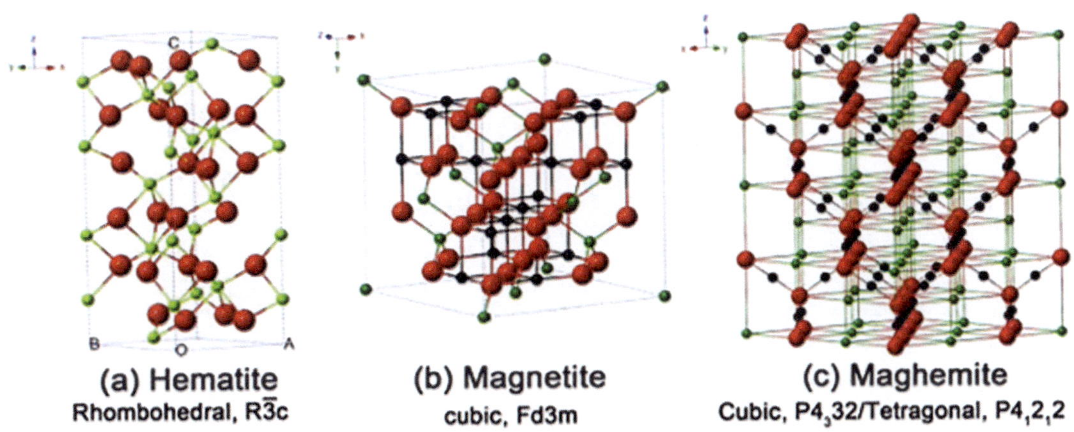

FIGURE 9.1 Crystal structure and crystallographic data of the (a) hematite, (b) magnetite, and (c) maghemite.

Source: The data are sourced from [29].

[26, 35, 36]. Solution-based synthesis is the most used approach. In their approach toward preparation of iron oxide, researchers have focused mainly on surface modification and colloidal stability [31, 37]. In biological systems a biocompatible polymer coated iron oxide shows superior chemical stability with reduced surface oxidation and toxicity. Ferrites are black or dark gray materials. A ferrimagnetic iron oxide is the main constituent of these materials, with various transition metal dopants. MFe_2O_4-type materials with divalent cations (M^{2+}= Zn, Mn, Co, Ni Fe, Pt, Pd etc.) can be synthesized by this technique for improved molecular imaging application [38, 39].

9.1.3 Magnetic Ferrofluids

Ferrofluids are homogenous dispersed solutions of magnetic nanoparticles in a liquid with high colloidal stability. Generally magnetic ferrofluids can be divided into two categories: Ferroluids (> 15 nm) and Magneto rheological fluids (15–40 nm). A colloidal suspension of magnetic nanoparticles (5–10 nm) dispersed in liquid matrix (polar or non-polar) constitutes magneto rheological fluid [40–43]. Furthermore, sometimes attraction between these dispersed nanoparticles is observed which can be prevented treating its surface with surfactants (Figure 9.2). Silica, chitosan, ethylene Glycol, polyvinyl alcohol, Poly acrylic acid are some of the dispersant used for this purpose [44].

9.2 SYNTHESIS METHODS OF MAGNETIC NANOPARTICLES

Tailoring of classical products to cater the specific uses with controlled properties is the latest drifts to material science and engineering. There are many complications in preparation of nanoparticles namely: (i) getting monodispersed nanomaterials with uniform particle size distribution; (ii) Synthesis reproducibility; (iii) obtaining desired crystal phase with high crystallinity; (iv) preferred shape and stability over time. Synthesis by wet chemical method is the most loved route as it is the cheapest way for scale up production. In preparation of monodispersed nanoparticles, a short burst of nucleation followed by controlled growth is important [45]. For monodispersed NPs the most common route is to separate the nucleation and growth steps during synthesis. As we know the NPs have very high surface to volume ratio and to minimize their surface energy the NPs tend to agglomerate. Surface functionalization by surfactant molecule can be employed to prevent agglomeration [46].

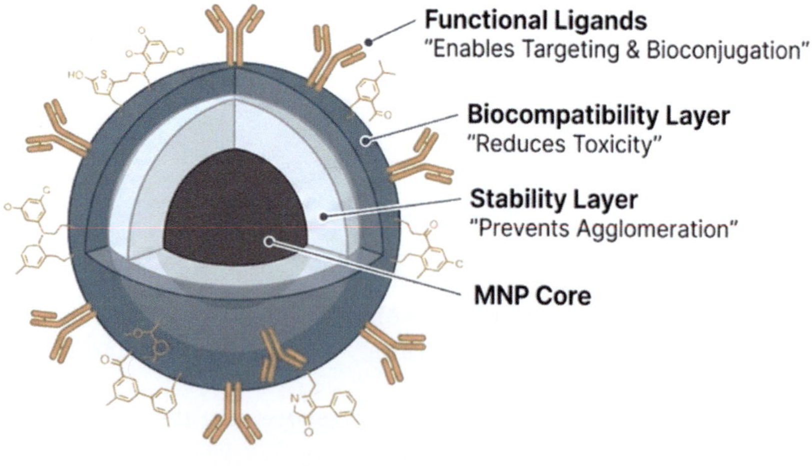

FIGURE 9.2 Surface functionalization of MNPs in ferrofluids.

9.2.1 Co-Precipitation

Co-precipitation is a widely used method for synthesizing iron oxide nanoparticles (Figure 9.3). It is one of the extensively used methods for the preparation of MNPs due to its convenience, use of less harmful materials, and safe procedures.It has significant use in biomedical applications[47, 48]. For the preparation of magnetite nanoparticles from the wet chemical method two main synthesis routes are reported. The first method is partial oxidation of ferrous hydroxide suspension using different oxidizing agents. For example, Fe(II) salt with a mild oxidant such as nitrate ions gives magnetite nanoparticles with spherical morphology and narrow size distribution [49].

Another method is aging of aqueous solution of ferrous and ferric hydroxides in stoichiometric mixture to yield homogeneous spherical magnetite nanoparticles [50]. MNPs are made using an aqueous salt solution and base at ambient or elevated temperature. This technique involves dissolving ferrous (Fe^{2+}) and ferric (Fe^{3+}) salts in an aqueous solution, followed by the addition of a base such as sodium hydroxide (NaOH) or ammonium hydroxide (NH_4OH). The resulting iron oxide nanoparticles are formed through nucleation and growth processes. Parameters such as the concentration of iron salts, the ratio of Fe^{2+} to Fe^{3+}, pH, and temperature are crucial in determining the size and shape of the nanoparticles. For instance, high pH and ionic strength give smaller particles, whereas the use of inert gas medium such as N_2 can be useful in avoiding agglomeration and surface oxidation [37, 51–54]. Temperature is another parameter that governs the particle type. When the temperature is below 80° C, it leads to the formation of magnetite Fe_3O_4, whereas when the temperature is further reduced below 60°C, hematite (Fe_2O_3) is favored. Post-synthesis, surface modification is often required to prevent aggregation and enhance biocompatibility.

A simple reaction is given below:

$$Fe^{2+} + 2Fe^{3+} + 8OH \rightarrow Fe_3O_4 + 4H_2O$$

9.2.2 Thermal Decomposition

The exact control over the size and homogeneity of magnetic nanoparticles is provided by thermal breakdown. Fabrication of different types of metallic magnetic nanoparticles are done via this method most often from organometallic complexes [46]. In presence of hot organic surfactant, the

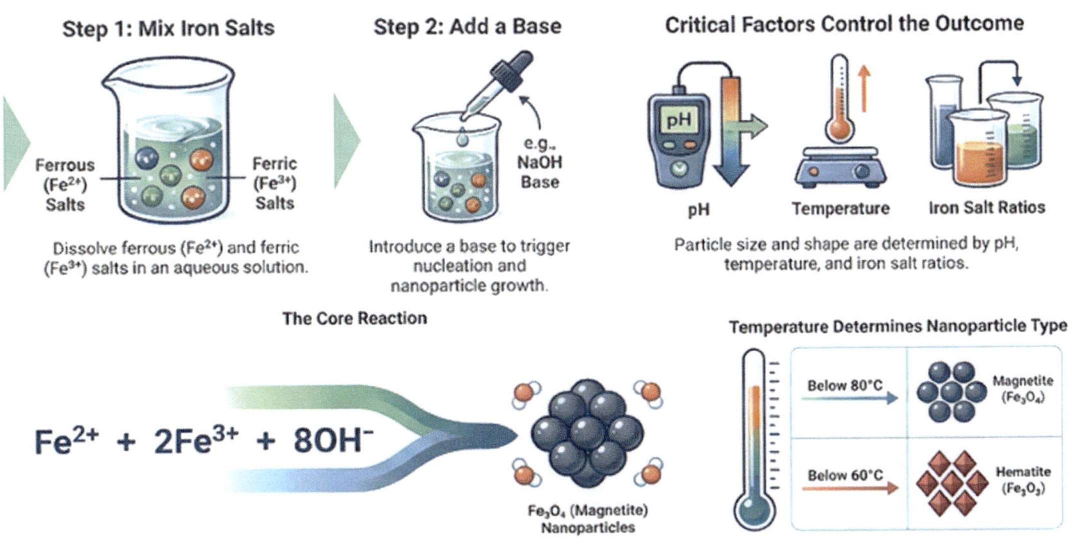

FIGURE 9.3 Synthesis of iron oxide by co-precipitation.

iron precursors decompose to yields highly dispersible, crystalline and size controlled nanoparticles. Using surfactants such as oleic acid, this process involves the high-temperature thermal breakdown of organometallic precursors such as iron pentacarbonyl ($Fe(CO)_5$) or iron oleate as shown in Figure 9.4. The carbonyl group have strong tendency to dissociate under thermal treatment leaving zero valent metal NPs. Monodispersed Fe NPs ranging from 5–19 nm with oleic acid and oleylamine as surfactant are prepared [55]. The composition of the reaction mixture determines the property of the prepared final product. This process yields nanoparticles with excellent magnetic and crystallinity characteristics. However, the procedure calls for high temperatures and chemical solvents, which could present problems with scalability and the environment. Metal NPs synthesized are highly reactive and susceptible to oxidation thus to avoid this significant surface functionalization is required to avoid oxygen penetration.

9.2.3 Hydrothermal Synthesis

Hydrothermal or solvothermal method is a wet chemical method employed in which the aqueous solution crystallizes at high temperature (130°C–250°C) and pressure (0.3–4 MPa). Precursors react at high temperatures and pressures in a sealed autoclave during hydrothermal synthesis (Figure 9.5). Because of this method's great versatility, nanoparticles with different morphologies and compositions can be produced. Narrow-size distributions and well-crystallized nanoparticles can occur in the hydrothermal environment [34, 56, 57]. The properties of the nanoparticles can be precisely tailored by researchers to fulfil certain biomedical applications by varying the solvent type, temperature, and reaction time. A Teflon coated stainless steel autoclave with temperature monitoring is used with solute to obtain crystalline nanoparticles. It is important to note that we cannot attain nanoparticles with particle size less than 10 nm. Rate of reaction is slow and monodispersity is obtained only for short time during the synthesis process.

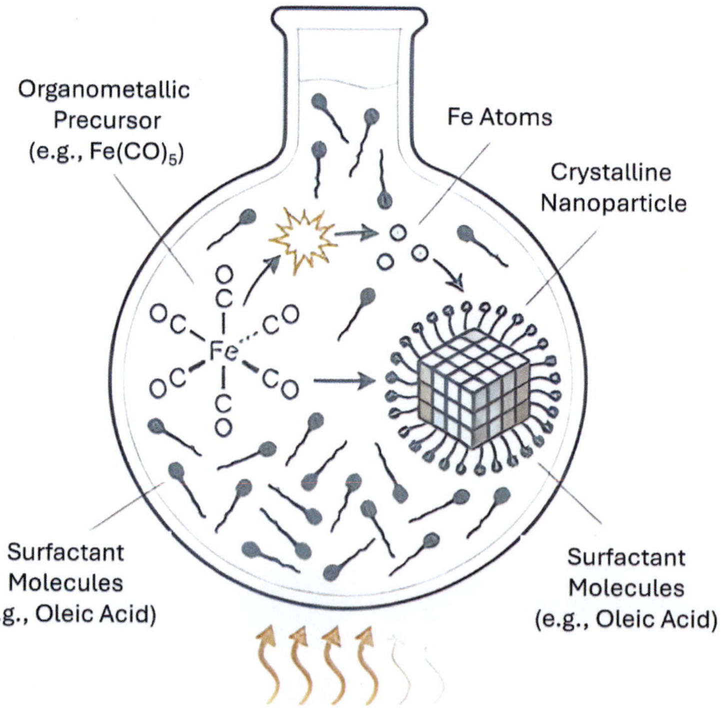

FIGURE 9.4 Synthesis of iron oxide by thermal decomposition method.

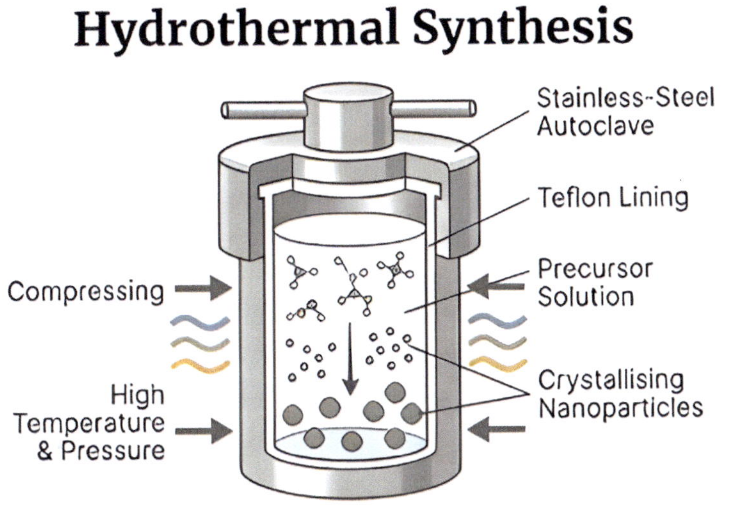

FIGURE 9.5 A schematic illustration of hydrothermal synthesis.

9.2.4 Microemulsion

The process of creating nanoscale droplets of oil-in-water (O/W) or water-in-oil (W/O) emulsions (immiscible liquid) forming thermodynamic stable isotropic dispersion in which the microdomains are stabilized by surfactants thus generating low interfacial tension is known as the microemulsion method (Figure 9.6) [34, 58]. It is also named as reverse micelles method in which surfactants generated monolayers at interface with hydrophilic ends toward water and hydrophobic end facing oil. For the regulated nucleation and development of nanoparticles, these droplets serve as nanoreactors [59, 60]. The types, concentrations, and ratios of water to oil of the surfactants used during synthesis have a significant impact on the properties of the final nanoparticles. This process can produce highly uniform magnetic nanoparticles because it offers exceptional control over particle size and homogeneity. On the other hand, after the completion of reaction the unreacted surfactants can affect the particle properties. Physiochemical properties of Iron core/Iron oxide shell MNPs made using cetyltrimethylammonium bromide (CTAB) and butanol as surfactants are reported [59]. At room temperature a thin film of Fe_3O_4 was formed by controlled oxidation and a silica coating is attained by using 3-aminopropyltrimethoxysilane. A reverse microemulsion method was employed for the synthesis of curcumin loaded MNPs with chitosan functionalized surface for targeted drug delivery carriers in cancer therapy. Similarly, metallic iron particles with gold shell as protection from oxidation is prepared using reverse micelle reaction with CTAB as the surfactant and octane and aqueous reactants as oil and water phase [61].

9.2.5 Sol Gel Method

Another effective method for the preparation of nanostructured MNPs is Sol gel with water as solvent [62]. A colloidal solution namely sol is formed as the precursors undergo hydroxylation or condensation. Removal of solvent by dehydration leads to the formation of gel. The formed colloidal solution can be used in variety of forms, such asfibers, powders, or thin films. Drying of these three-dimensional metal oxide gels gives xerogel with increased crystallinity and decreased porosity (nano powder). Whereas incomplete drying gives aerogels (amorphous and porous) [32, 63, 64]. The reaction parameters are mainly affected by solvents precursors, pH, temperature, solvent type, catalysts, additives and stirring. The resultant material is heat treated to convert it to crystalline state [65].

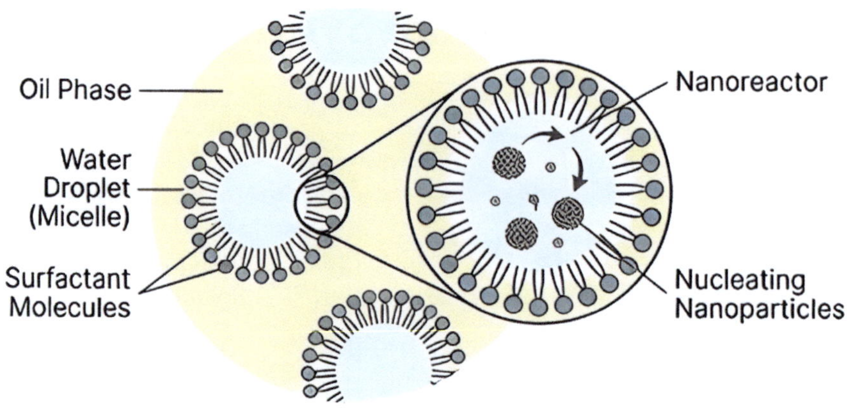

FIGURE 9.6 Various components involved in microemulsion synthesis of nanoparticle.

Metal alkoxides are used in the sol-gel method as the hydroxide group replaces the alkoxide during hydrolysis.

9.2.6 Sonochemical Method

As name suggests in sonochemical method acoustic waves are used to create bubbles in liquid. Acoustic cavitation is created due to the implosive collapse of the bubbles. This implosive collapse causes temporary increase in the temperature and pressure of the reaction mixture as shown in Figure 9.7. The temperature is maintained by continuous water circulation [53, 66, 67]. Selection of type of solvent and precursor decided the particle yield. Usually, low vapor pressure solvent and volatile precursors are used. At room temperature low magnetization amorphous powders are prepared. Following figure shows preparation of strontium ferrite by sonochemical route. This method can also be utilized for preparation of carbon-based materials such as CNT and graphene [68].

9.2.7 Polyol Method

A promising technique for preparation of nanoparticles with uniform particle size with potential application in biomedicine. It's a low temperature preparation technique with precursors containing oxygen such as acetates, peroxides, oxides, and nitrates. The precursors are dissolved in polyol (ethylene glycol, diethylene glycol or dihydroxy ethyl ether) which acts as solvent, reducing agents and also a complexing agent in some cases [50, 69]. In this procedure the dissolved mixture is reflux with diol at temperature range 180°C–200°C (Figure 9.8). A metal diol intermediate is formed which further gets reduced to form metal nanoparticles. Temperature variation can be used to tune particle size during the process. Precipitation kinetics decide the particle shape, size and agglomeration properties. It's an effective method for the preparation of MNPs as various hydroxyl groups on the surface of the nanoparticles prevent surface oxidation. As organic solvent is used the hydrolysis issue due to aqueous solvents can be prevented.

9.2.8 Physical Method

Physical synthesis can primarily be categorized in two approaches: top-down and bottom-up synthesis as shown in Figure 9.9. Top-down synthesis is the mechanical breakdown of bulk materials

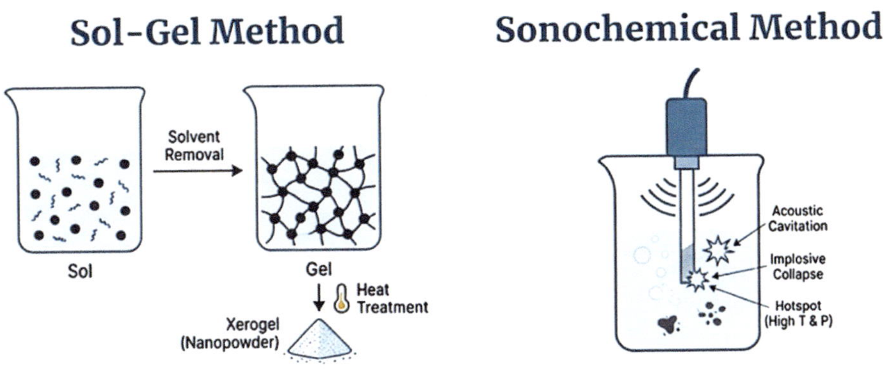

FIGURE 9.7 Sol-gel method and sonochemical method for nanomaterial synthesis.

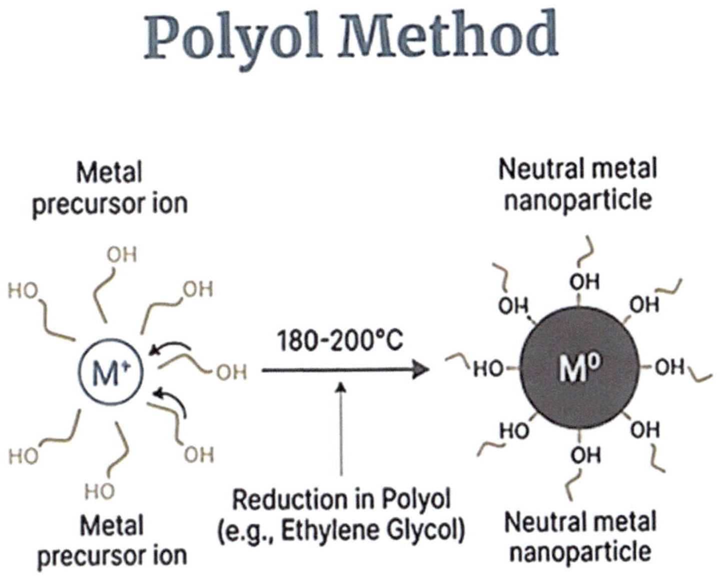

FIGURE 9.8 Sol-gel method and sonochemical method for nanomaterial synthesis.

to nanosized particles, whereas the latter is made by atomic or molecular precursors by condensation or nucleation [70, 71]. The bottom-up approach gives better control and selectivity over the particle size, whereas the top-down approach has many limitations, such as homogeneity, but proves advantageous in production yield. The various physical methods for the synthesis of magnetic nanoparticles include ball milling, laser ablation, wire explosion, inert gas condensation, flame spray pyrolysis, and arc discharge. Ball milling is a simple process where the bulk material is ground into smaller sizes. The working principle is simple—the kinetic energy from the ball to the sample due to the continuous collision leads to the formation of nano- or micro-sized powder particles. Laser ablation is particularly attractive due to the simplicity where high-energy laser is used in a liquid or gaseous environment to vaporize bulk materials, which form nanoparticles on condensation.

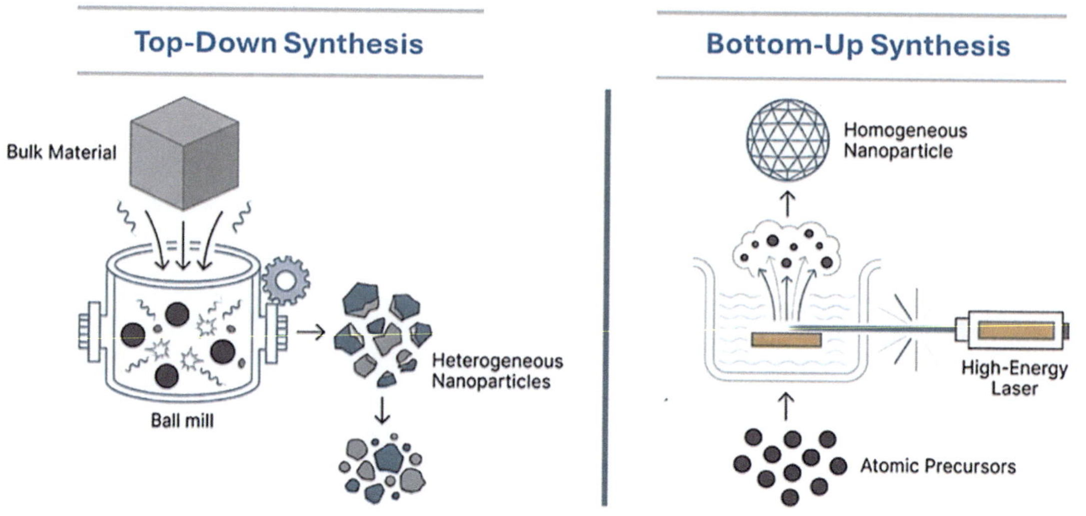

FIGURE 9.9 Top-down and bottom-up approach for the preparation of nanomaterial by physical method.

9.2.9 Biological Method

In bio-mineralization and evolutionary bacteriology magnetostatic bacterial and magnetosomes are studies extensively across many disciplines [72]. The magnetite (Fe_3O_4) or greigite (Fe_3S_4) are surrounded by lipid membranes in magnetotactic bacteria. These magnetosomes have strain dependent shape and size, intrinsic high saturation magnetization, biocompatibility and its perfect dispersion in biological medium holds great significance in bio-nanomedicine [73]. High uniformity in size and shape is found in certain bacterial strains. Reports propose that the magnetosome interaction with the growing nanocrystals facilitates in certain direction thus consequential cuboctahedral, hexagonal, or bullet-shaped magnetosomes [72, 74]. In general a saturated iron ion solution is formed with in the magnetosomes by transporting iron ions into the cell by specific siderophores or even through non-specific mechanism followed by redox reaction [72, 73]. The stoichiometric molar ratio of Fe(III) to Fe(II) is maintained at 2/1 to yield magnetite nanocrystal. The Fe(III) is reduced to Fe(II) for transportation and cellular intake into the magnetosome membrane and finally into hydrous Fe(III) oxide via redox process. One third of hydrous Fe(III) oxide is reduced to Fe(II) to form magnetite. Among all preparation methods, the best suited method for the synthesis of nanoparticle is subject to application in use. Table 9.1 gives the comparative framework for the synthesis methods.

9.3 SURFACE FUNCTIONALIZATION

For magnetic nanoparticles to be more stable, biocompatible, and useful in biomedical applications, their surfaces must be functionalized. Preventing agglomeration, offering steric or electrostatic stability, and introducing functional groups for further bioconjugation are the main goals. These surface functionalized NPs demonstrate superior saturation magnetization, hydrodynamic diameter suitable for theranostic application, better drug binding to the surface [75] and can also serve as catalyst for aromatic compound synthesis such as N-Containing heterocycles [76], photocatalysis [77] and biocatalysis for cancer therapy [78]. NPs with good stability in biological fluids, biodegradability, biocompatibility are essential requirements for biological application. Coating MNPs of biological aqueous solution which are mostly neutral with polymers and surfactants gives NPs anti agglomeration properties with increased biocompatibility [79]. MNPs are coated with different organic and inorganic groups which stabilizes the nanoparticle by covalently binding to these nanoparticles. In situ synthesis, post synthesis grafting, and adsorptions are the various methods by which nanoparticles coating is attained [80]. Surface modification of MNPs gives precise functionalization such as toxicity and pH response. Tuning of core diameter, coating thickness and the targeting ligand can enable nanoprobes to target specific cells and tissues [81, 82].

NPs synthesized in organic phase are found more advantageous in biomedical application due to their monodispersity in size, shape and composition. However, these MNPs show stability due to surfactants, such as oleic acid/oleylamine, and are hydrophobic in nature. The surface of these hydrophobic nanoparticles is often functionalized by surfactant to obtain hydrophilic NPs for biological application (Figure 9.10). An amphiphilic molecule with both hydrophobic and hydrophilic component is used for surfactant addition process through adsorption. The hydrophilic segment is exposed to the solution thus turning into water soluble. Whereas in surfactant exchange the original surfactant is replaced by bifunctional surfactant. One functional group binds tightly with the NPs whereas the other functional group shows polar character [46]. Introduction of amphiphilic

TABLE 9.1
A comparative framework for nanoparticle synthesis.

Method	Size & Shape control	Crystallinity	Scalability/Yield	Key Advantage
Co-precipitation	Moderate	Moderate	High	Simplicity & Cost
Thermal Decomposition	Excellent	High	Moderate	Precision
Hydrothermal	Good	High	Low	Morphology Control
Microemulsion	Exceptional	Variable	Low	Uniformity
Physical Methods	Variable	Variable	High	High Yield
Biological (Magnetosomes)	Exceptional	Excellent	Very Low	Biocompatibility

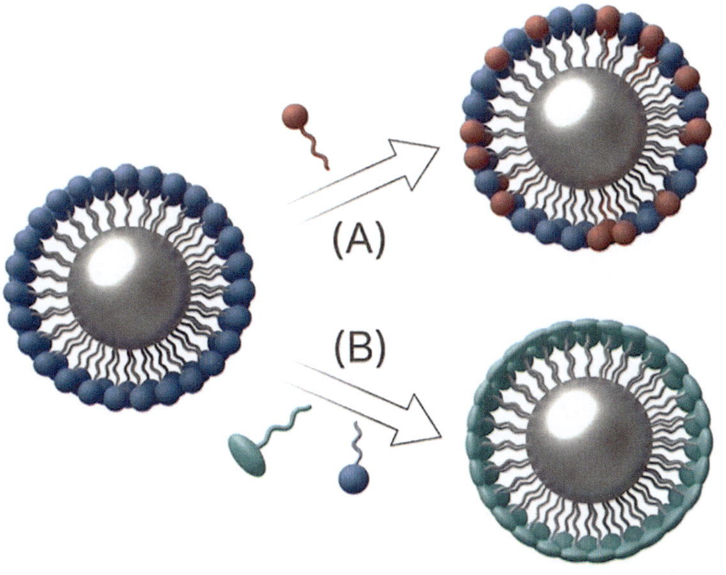

FIGURE 9.10 Schematic illustration of NP surface functionalization via (a) surfactant addition and (b) surfactant exchange.

Source: The data are sourced from [46].

ligands leads to robust double layer around the nanoparticles such as PEG-modified phospholipid coated FeCo NPs. Graphitic shells of FeCo NPs and hydrocarbon chains of phospholipids binds to form hydrophobic double layers whereas the PEG chains provide high water solubility such as polystyrene-poly acrylic acid block copolymer (PS-PAA), tetradecylphosphonate and polyethylene glycol-2-tetradecyl ether [83, 84].

9.3.1 Polymer Coating

Nanoparticles are frequently coated with polymers including dextran, polyvinyl alcohol (PVA), and polyethylene glycol (PEG) which endows particles with important properties. NPs coated with polymers shows better compatibility with organic ingredients, reduced surface oxidation and less susceptibility to leaching. Polymer encapsulation helps in better dispersibility, stability and low toxicity [50]. These polymers offer a hydrophilic shell that decreases non-specific interactions with biological molecules and enhances colloidal stability in biological fluids. PEGylation is frequently used because it can improve the biocompatibility and bloodstream circulation time of nanoparticles. Magnetite nanoparticle encapsulated in polymer are reported by seed precipitation polymerization of methacrylic acid and hydroxyethyl methacrylate [85]. With suitable reaction conditions addition of cross linker and heat results in polydisperse magnetic latex. Inverse emulsion polymerization has reported preparation of superparamagnetic latex [86]. For encapsulation of MNPs and theranostic agents with in the polymeric shell various techniques have been instigated including emulsification, solvent evaporation, spray drying or phase separation technique which determines the size, efficiency and release kinetics of the drug [87].

By harvesting the qualities of liposomes and polymers in nanoparticles creating lipid-polymer hybrid nanoparticles with enhanced encapsulation efficiency stability and good targeting properties improves hydrophilic and lipophilic drug release [88].

9.3.2 Silica Coating

An essential component for superparamagnetic nanocomposite is appropriate tuning of magnetic properties. Another common coating material used for magnetic nanomaterials is silica (SiO_2), which is easy to functionalize and biocompatible and also an effective way to modulate its magnetic properties by heating process [89]. Silica enriched surface has advantage as silanol group present on the surface can react with alcohols and silane coupling agents to give good dispersion in non-aqueous solvents and covalent bonding for specific groups [50]. To attach therapeutic drugs or targeted ligands, silica-coated nanoparticles can be further changed with different functional groups (such as amines or thiols). Additionally, the silica shell acts as a barrier to shield the nanoparticles from one another and improves their stability and dispersibility in aqueous solutions. Hollow spherical γ-Fe_2O_3 coated with silica were prepared using methanol solution with iron ammonium citrate and tetraethoxysilane (TEOS) by aerosol pyrolysis method [90]. A W/O microemulsion process was also used for the preparation of silica-coated iron oxide nanoparticles. The magnetic nanoparticles were prepared by the coprecipitation reaction of ferric and ferrous salt with inorganic base. A thin and uniform coating of silica is attained by base catalyzed hydrolysis and polymerization of TEOS (Figure 9.11).

9.3.3 Ligand Exchange

Ligand exchange is the process of substituting molecules with functional groups for the original surfactants (derived from synthesis). With the use of this technique, bioactive molecules, such as medicines, peptides, or antibodies, can be attached, resulting in more effective treatment and targeted distribution. Thiols, phosphonates, and carboxylates are common ligands utilized in exchange because they can create strong interactions with the surface of nanoparticles.

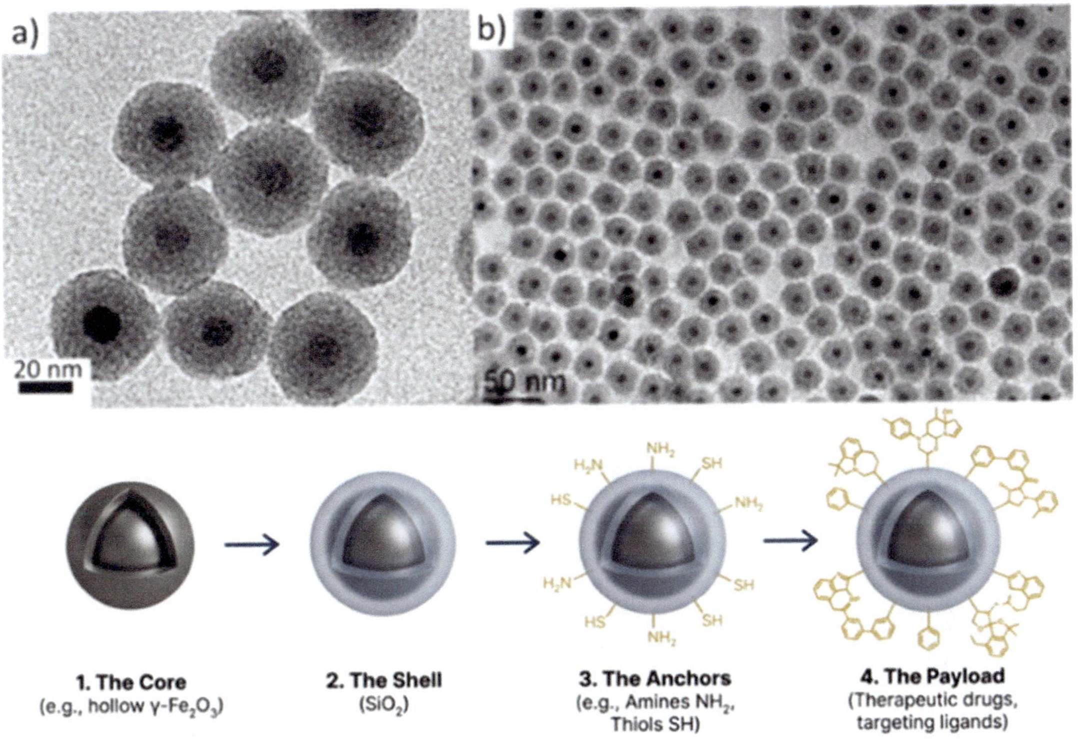

FIGURE 9.11 TEM pictures of silica/iron oxide composites.

Source: The data are sourced from [91].

Because of the strong interaction between the bidentate or multidentate functional groups and MNPs bifunctional ligand exchange should provide better colloidal stability of the MNPs in physiological conditions. Dopamine a bidentate ligand on the surface of IONPs. The ligand coordinates to the surface of IONPs due to improved orbital overlap and reduced steric effect [92]. A mixture of PEG ligands (dopamine-PEG and thiol terminated PEG) for stable FePt NPs in aqueous media, Carboxyl acid terminated dopamine-PEG for Fe/Fe_3O_4 core–shell MNPs and amine-terminated PEG ligand for Fe_3O_4 NPs are few examples [93, 94]. The process was well reported in replacing the hydrophobic ligand with organosilane via dehydration or esterification [46].

9.4 CHARACTERIZATION TECHNIQUES

Proper characterization of magnetic nanoparticles is essential to ensure their suitability for biomedical applications. Various techniques are used to assess their physical, chemical, and magnetic properties.

9.4.1 Transmission Electron Microscopy

Transmission Electron Microscopy (TEM) provides high-resolution images of nanoparticles, allowing detailed analysis of their size, shape, and morphology. It can also reveal the crystallinity of the nanoparticles by providing lattice-resolved images. TEM is crucial for evaluating the uniformity and structural integrity of synthesized nanoparticles.

9.4.2 Dynamic Light Scattering

Dynamic Light Scattering (DLS) measures the hydrodynamic size and size distribution of nanoparticles in suspension. This technique is particularly useful for evaluating the colloidal stability of functionalized nanoparticles in biological fluids. DLS can provide information on particle aggregation and surface modifications.

9.4.3 X-Ray Diffraction (XRD)

XRD is used to determine the crystalline structure and phase purity of nanoparticles. The diffraction patterns obtained can confirm the formation of specific crystal structures and provide information on particle size through Scherrer analysis. XRD is essential for verifying the successful synthesis of the desired magnetic phase.

9.4.4 Vibrating Sample Magnetometry (VSM)

VSM measures the magnetic properties of nanoparticles, including saturation magnetization, coercivity, and remanence. These parameters are crucial for assessing the suitability of nanoparticles for hyperthermia applications. VSM provides insights into the magnetic behavior and efficiency of heat generation under an alternating magnetic field.

9.4.5 Fourier Transform Infrared Spectroscopy (FTIR)

FTIR is employed to identify the chemical bonds, and functional groups present on the surface of nanoparticles. This technique is valuable for confirming successful surface functionalization. FTIR spectra can reveal the presence of specific functional groups, indicating successful attachment of ligands or coatings.

9.5 HYPERTHERMIA AND DRUG DELIVERY

9.5.1 Principles of Hyperthermia

There are many types of thermal treatment being used for cancer therapy which can readily be divided into three types: hyperthermia, thermal ablation (> 45°C) and cryoablation (below −50°C). Hyperthermia which is often called as thermotherapy involves elevating the temperature of cancerous tissues to 41–45°C through electromagnetic energy, which can cause cell death or sensitize cells to other treatments such as chemotherapy and radiation. Temperature above this has cytotoxic effect on cells and is referred as thermal ablation [95]. Magnetic hyperthermia utilizes magnetic nanoparticles to generate localized heat when subjected to an alternating magnetic field. This targeted approach allows for precise control over the temperature increase, minimizing damage to surrounding healthy tissues. The denaturing of cellular and subcellular elements depends on the form, tissue size and temperature distribution. In today's theragnostic hyperthermia is used with other cancer therapies for synergistic effect. Some acidic and poorly oxygenated tumor cells resist radiation [96]. In such cases hyperthermia may induce radiation sensitivity. Similar effects were observed with combination of chemotherapeutic agents and hyperthermia [97, 98].

The acidic environment and inadequate oxygen supply makes the tumor cells more thermosensitive than normal cells [99].The nanoparticle-based magnetic hyperthermia in combination with radio and chemotherapy utilizes the hyper thermosensitivity of cancerous cells. Hyperthermia can effectively be used as sensitizer for radio and chemotherapy which depends on tumor type, drug concentration, temperature and time elapsed between heating and chemotherapy [100, 101].

9.5.2 Heat Generation Mechanisms in Magnetic Nanoparticles

As discussed earlier, the heating mechanism follows four mechanisms, of which relaxation losses are associated with superparamagnetic nanoparticles. The heat generated by magnetic nanoparticles under an alternating magnetic field is primarily due to two mechanisms: Néel relaxation and Brownian relaxation of the particles.

9.5.2.1 Néel Relaxation

Néel relaxation occurs when the magnetic moment within a nanoparticle fluctuates between different directions, leading to energy dissipation as heat. This mechanism is predominant in smaller nanoparticles where the magnetic moment can easily realign. The relaxation time depends on the anisotropy energy barrier and the temperature, influencing the efficiency of heat generation.

9.5.2.2 Brownian Relaxation

Brownian relaxation involves the physical rotation of nanoparticles in the suspension. As the nanoparticles rotate to align with the external magnetic field, frictional forces within the fluid medium generate heat. The generated thermal energy is dissipated to the ambient surroundings through shear stress (Figure 9.12). This mechanism is significant for larger nanoparticles where physical rotation is more feasible. The viscosity of the surrounding medium and the size of the nanoparticles are critical factors affecting Brownian relaxation.

9.5.3 Induction Heating

Nanoparticles dispersed in a solvent are free moving due to Brownian motion. The magnetic nanoparticles face two types of relaxation: Relaxation due to particle rotation (Brownian relaxation) and due to magnetic moment rotation (Néel relaxation). Brownian relaxation is given as:

$$\tau_B = \frac{4\pi\eta r_h^3}{k_B T}$$

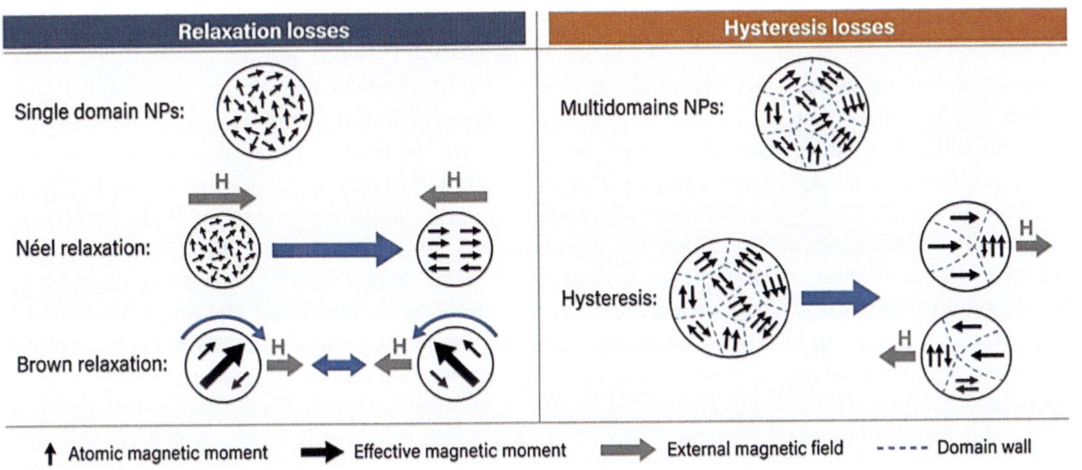

FIGURE 9.12 The Néel relaxation and Brownian mechanism representation of heat generation via MNPs under the atomic magnetic moment.

where η is dynamic viscosity of carrier fluid, r_h is hydrodynamic radius of magnetic nanoparticles. On the other hand, Néel relaxation is represented as:

$$\tau_N = \tau_0 e^{\Delta E/k_B T} = \tau_0 e^{KV/k_B T}$$

where τ_0 is of the order 10^{-9} s and ΔE is anisotropic energy barrier, product of anisotropic energy constant (K) and volume (V), kB is the Boltzmann's constant, and T is the temperature. Thus, dispersed nanoparticles show accelerated particle spin relaxation.

9.5.3.1 Factors Influencing Hyperthermia Efficiency

Several factors affect the efficiency of magnetic hyperthermia:

- Particle Size and Shape: The size and shape of nanoparticles influence their magnetic properties and heat generation capacity. Smaller particles are more effective for Néel relaxation, while larger particles benefit from Brownian relaxation.
- Concentration of Nanoparticles: Higher concentrations can enhance heating but may also cause aggregation, reducing efficiency. Optimal concentrations need to be determined to maximize therapeutic effects without causing adverse side effects.
- Field Strength and Frequency: The strength and frequency of the applied magnetic field must be optimized to maximize heat generation while minimizing damage to healthy tissues. Typically, frequencies in the range of 100–500 kHz are used for medical applications.
- Thermal Conductivity of the Medium: The surrounding medium's thermal conductivity affects heat dissipation and the overall temperature increase in the target area. Efficient heat dissipation ensures uniform heating of the tumor tissue.

Both Néel and Brownian relaxation occur due to exposure of magnetic materials to external alternative magnetic field (AMF) where the field reversal time is shorter than the magnetic relaxation time of the material [102, 103].

9.5.4 Magnetic Nanoparticles for Hyperthermia Treatment

There have been extensive studies reported on innovative MNPs as heat mediators for cancer therapy. The MNPs generate heat by non-intrusive applied alternating magnetic field (AMF) thus causing the cell death by irrevocable physiological changes [104]. Dextran and liposome-coated IONPs have gained substantial clinical recognition among MNPs. Hybrid nano-magnetic systems show higher specific absorption rate (SAR) values due to their increased stability in aqueous mediums. Consequently, they deliver heat directly to the tumor cells without affecting the surrounding cells [105]. Antibody targeting MNPs can cause thermal ablation of tumors under an external alternating magnetic field. Oral squamous cell carcinoma biomarker ($\alpha v\beta 6$) targeting antibodies are incorporated in silica-coated IONPs. They can effectively be targeted to provide favorable therapy for the treatment of oral squamous cell carcinoma [106]. Silica-coated IONPs induce magnetic hyperthermia, and *in vitro* studies indicated they can kill tumor cells (L929 and HeLa cells) effectively under induction heating [107]. Under experimentation, hydroxyapatite-coated iron oxide (IOHAp) nanoparticles killed all MG-63 osteosarcoma cells in 30 min exposure. The internalization of these nanoparticles caused denaturing and oxidation of the cellular system by damaging nucleotides, proteins, and membranes [108]. For an effective clinical application, it is required to have nanomediators for effective heat transfer, thus exhibiting an improved specific absorption rate (SAR). The SAR value highly depends on the material morphology, composition, and magnetic field properties such as frequency (f) and amplitude (H). The aggressive components of the tumor can be regulated by hyperthermia treatment, thus resulting in discontinuation or delay in radiotherapy or surgery in patients [109]. Although magnetic hyperthermia therapy shows encouraging results, the use of magnetic nanoparticles for theranostics is still in its early stage.

9.6 APPLICATIONS OF MAGNETIC NANOPARTICLES IN HYPERTHERMIA

Magnetic nanoparticles have become a new and interesting area of research. The remarkable properties like superparamagnetism, high surface area, and adjustable surface chemistry have fascinated many biomedical researchers. Iron oxide nanoparticles are one of the widely studied magnetic nanoparticles for treating cancer with hyperthermia.

Nanoparticles engineering in combination with alternate magnetic field system, and new methods for targeting tumor makes nanoparticle-induced magnetic hyperthermia a promising treatment. Due to its minimal invasive and multimodal property theranostic there is significant rise in relevance in nanomedicine for cancer treatment.

9.6.1 Preclinical Studies

Preclinical studies involving magnetic hyperthermia have demonstrated their potential to effectively kill cancer cells in vitro and in animal models. These studies focus on optimizing nanoparticle formulations, delivery methods, and treatment parameters to maximize therapeutic efficacy and minimize side effects. For example, studies have shown that magnetic hyperthermia can induce apoptosis and necrosis in cancer cells, enhance the effects of chemotherapy drugs, and inhibit tumor growth in animal models. Bahadur et al. prepared different ferrites—namely, Fe_3O_4, $MnFe_3O_4$, and $CoFe_2O_4$—to evaluate their potential in cancer hyperthermia. $CoFe_2O_4$demonstrated lower SAR and toxicity above 0.2 mg/mL. The lauric acid coating of ferrites proved beneficial in long-term in vivo biocompatibility [110]. Combination therapy of chemo and hyperthermia is gaining importance as an effective cancer modality. Magnetic-liposome-mediated $La_{0.75}Sr_{0.25}MnO_3$ (LSMO) and iron oxide (Fe_3O_4) are developed for self-controlledhyperthermia and chemotherapy. Drug (paclitaxel)-carrying magnetic liposomes were injected into the fibrosarcoma tumor-bearing mice. The result shows a nearly 2.5-fold reduction in tumor growth [111]. Thus, combination therapy has shown remarkable success in cancer treatment. Mesoporous bioactive glass nanoparticles (Fe_3O_4-MBG NPs) show high surface area with entrapped drug release and different pH values (6.4, 7.4 and 8.4). This makes the material safe for tissue regeneration, hyperthermia, and drug delivery [112].

Ningthoujam et al. have developed a hybrid formulation with Fe_3O_4 (YPO_4:Er^{3+}–Yb^{3+}@Fe_3O_4), which has been used for hyperthermia as well as imaging application. The study mainly tests the potential of the hybrid nano-formulation in various applications, such as light conversion, optical heating, hyperthermia, and forensic science [113]. $NaYF_4$:Er^{3+}/Yb^{3+} monodispersed nanoparticles are preparedby the thermolysis method. With Fe_3O_4 the nanoparticles prove beneficial in magnetic and surface plasmon resonance-based hyperthermia [114].

Clinical applications of combined hyperthermia and drug delivery are being explored in various cancer types. These studies aim to establish the safety, effectiveness, and optimal treatment regimens for this multimodal approach. Preliminary clinical trials have shown promising results, indicating that combined therapy can enhance treatment efficacy and reduce side effects. However, further research is needed to translate these findings into routine clinical practice.

9.6.2 Clinical Trials

Several clinical trials have explored the use of magnetic hyperthermia in treating various cancers, including glioblastoma, prostate cancer, and breast cancer. These trials aim to establish the safety, feasibility, and effectiveness of magnetic hyperthermia in human patients. Early-phase clinical trials have shown promising results, with minimal side effects and significant tumor regression. However, large-scale trials are needed to further validate these findings and optimize treatment protocols.

Jordan et al. has worked extensively on magnetic fluid hyperthermia (MFH) to harness the magnetic field induced heat of the nanosized magnetic nanoparticles. The system has proven its efficacy in practical applications in human body for heat treatment in deep regions either by hyperthermia or thermoablation [115]. Depending on temperature applied with respect to time duration this may directly affect the tumor cells or make it more susceptible to radio or chemotherapy [116]. Magnetic fluid hyperthermia is employed to treat prostate cancer. This minimum invasive approach is first clinical application in locally recurrent prostate cancer by injecting nanoparticle suspension transperineally under fluoroscopy guidance [117]. In a report radiosensitizers pimonidazole (PMZ) are encapsulated in temperature sensitive liposomes (TSL) to evaluate the *in vitro* efficacy of TSL-PMZ with hyperthermia and radiotherapy. The results show improved efficacy of radiotherapy in hypoxic condition [118]. In hyperthermia assisted systematic drug delivery system time resolved temperature mapping is crucial. Nanocarrier materials are handy in tumor targeting hyperthermia responsive drug delivery and also as precise nano-thermometer [119].

9.7 MAGNETIC NANOPARTICLES FOR DRUG DELIVERY

Various agents used for drug delivery are called drug carriers. It is vital to see the role of these drug carriers in drug administration for their safety, selectivity and effectiveness to develop systematic drug delivery system (SDDS). Use of nanoparticles for cancer diagnosis and treatment have shown considerable potential due to their high capacity, stability and feasibility of different drug administration routes [120]. MNPs and polymer composites are functionalized and encased with therapeutic drugs which show significance in delivery of targeted drug directly to the disease center under external magnetic field without any additional stress to the body (Figure 9.13). The MNPs due

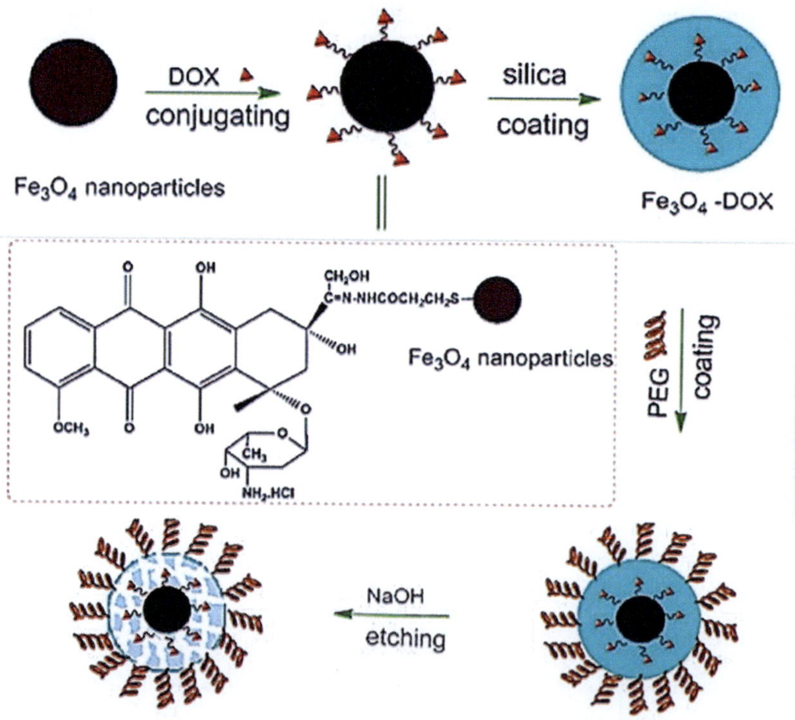

FIGURE 9.13 Synthetic scheme for the development of Doxorubicin loaded magnetic drug delivery system.

Source: The data are sourced from [121].

to their unique biological interactions makes them suitable for MRI contrasting agents. MNPs are effectively been used for diagnosis and treatment namely malignant tumors, cardiovascular and neurological diseases [33]. As a drug carrier, MNPs have effectively been employed for targeted drug delivery through injection (intravenous or intra-arterial).

Immense diversity is observed in drug delivery system which includes both MNPs and targeting drug [122, 123]. The use of magnetic nanoplatforms for delivery of classical anticancer drugs such as cis-platin and doxorubicin is reported. The cytotoxicity of spherical NPs is found to be less in comparison with the cylindrical or oval shaped NPs with increased reactive oxygen species (ROS) concentration [124]. Lung cancer [125], gastric cancer [126], pancreatic cancer [127], hepatocellular carcinoma [128], bone cancer-osteosarcoma [129], blood cancer-leukemia [130], breast cancer [124] are some types of cancer where MNP drug conjugates are used for investigation. Biomaterial research has shown significant progress in recent years to match the theoretical predictions of material science in biomedical applications. Many drug formulations are now commercially available to patients [131].

A magnetic drug formulation with Doxorubicin (DOX) chemically attached to Fe_3O_4 was designed with porous silica shell stabilized with polyethylene glycol (PEG). In $Fe_{3O}^{4\text{-DOX/pSiO}_2}$-PEG silica acts as protective coating and obstruct the DOX thus preventing premature burst release [132]. A pH-dependent polymer Eudragit can be regulated and formulated for targeting any site. The Eudragit coating is often used for colon-targeted drugs [133]. These type of encapsulation of drugs show sustained systematic release thus showing longer drug release profile in comparison with unbounded drug.

9.7.1 Drug Loading Techniques

Various techniques are employed to load drugs onto magnetic nanoparticles:

i. Adsorption: Drugs can be adsorbed onto the surface of nanoparticles through physical or chemical interactions. This method is straightforward but may result in desorption under physiological conditions.
ii. Encapsulation: Nanoparticles can be encapsulated within a polymer or lipid shell that contains the drug. This approach offers controlled release and protection of the drug from degradation.
iii. Covalent Bonding: Drugs can be chemically conjugated to the nanoparticle surface using linker molecules. Covalent bonding ensures stable attachment and controlled release of the drug.

9.7.2 Targeting Mechanisms

MNPs drug targeting involves drug delivery to the tumor site with minimal invasive procedure and thus the effectiveness of the therapy is increased [134, 135]. Cell membrane (~1 μm) permeability is maximum size of NPs allowed whereas in veins the 5 μm is the upper size limit. As the NPs size is typically below the narrowest capillaries there is very less concern over the delivery procedure. There is serious concern over the circulation and clearance of these NPs from body. The positively charged NPs may form nonspecific bonds with negatively charged endothelial layer and on the contrary trapping of high negative NPs by microphages and organs whereas neutral NPs lack steric stability. Therefore, for circulation the NPs needs to have positive or negative surface charge [136, 137].

Targeting mechanisms enhance the delivery of drugs to specific tissues or cells:

- Passive Targeting: Exploits the enhanced permeability and retention (EPR) effect, where nanoparticles accumulate in tumor tissues due to leaky vasculature. This effect is particularly useful for solid tumors with abnormal blood vessels.

- Active Targeting: Involves attaching targeting ligands (e.g., antibodies, peptides) to nanoparticles to specifically bind to receptors overexpressed on cancer cells. This strategy enhances the specificity and efficiency of drug delivery, reducing off-target effects.

9.7.3 Release Kinetics

Controlled release of drugs from nanoparticles is crucial for maintaining therapeutic levels over extended periods. For control release into the circulation usually drug carriers are used. Release kinetics can be tailored by modifying the surface chemistry and composition of the nanoparticles. For instance, pH-sensitive coatings can enable drug release in the acidic environment of tumor tissues, while temperature-sensitive coatings can release drugs in response to hyperthermia. The release profile usually found is either slow due to the diffusion of drugs or trigger release to specific stimuli such as pH, heat, and light [138].

9.8 COMBINED HYPERTHERMIA AND DRUG DELIVERY APPROACHES

The conventional therapy has limitations like toxicity, resistance to drug and tumor penetration. This leads to development of combine strategy by integrating hyperthermia and drug delivery system. This offers enhanced antitumor efficiency with minimum effect on healthy tissues. Hyperthermia causes cytotoxic effect on malignant cells and creates microenvironment which augments co-administered drug. Preclinical literature suggests that the multimodal synergistic approach shows better result.

9.8.1 Synergistic Effects

Combining hyperthermia with drug delivery can have synergistic effects, enhancing the overall therapeutic efficacy. Hyperthermia can increase the permeability of cancer cells, facilitate higher drug uptake and improve treatment outcomes. Additionally, the heat generated by magnetic nanoparticles can accelerate the release of encapsulated drugs, providing a controlled and localized therapeutic effect.

9.8.2 Experimental Models

Experimental models, including in vitro cell cultures and in vivo animal models, are used to study the combined effects of hyperthermia and drug delivery. These models help optimize treatment protocols and understand the underlying mechanisms of synergy. For example, studies using animal models have demonstrated that combined hyperthermia and chemotherapy can significantly inhibit tumor growth and prolong survival compared to either treatment alone.

9.9 SAFETY AND TOXICITY OF MAGNETIC NANOPARTICLES

9.9.1 Biocompatibility

Ensuring the biocompatibility of magnetic nanoparticles is crucial for their safe use in medical applications. Surface coatings and functionalization strategies are employed to reduce cytotoxicity and enhance biocompatibility. For instance, PEGylation can improve the biocompatibility and circulation time of nanoparticles, while minimizing immune recognition and clearance.

9.9.2 Toxicological Studies

Toxicological studies assess the potential adverse effects of magnetic nanoparticles on biological systems. These studies include in vitro cytotoxicity assays, in vivo animal studies, and long-term exposure assessments. MNPs in cancer diagnosis and treatment have shown advantages but their application has observed many restrictions because of their toxicity. Results have shown that while magnetic nanoparticles are generally well-tolerated at therapeutic doses, high concentrations or prolonged exposure can cause toxicity. Factors such as particle size, surface charge, and coating materials significantly influence toxicity profiles. A broad spectrum of magnetic nanoparticles is available. Materials such as cobalt and chromium cannot be employed for biomedical application due to their high toxicity. A nontoxic coating could be helpful in harvesting potentials of such NPs.

9.9.3 Regulatory Aspects

Regulatory guidelines for the clinical use of magnetic nanoparticles are established by agencies such as the FDA and EMA. These guidelines ensure the safety, efficacy, and quality of nanoparticle-based therapies. Key considerations include thorough preclinical testing, rigorous clinical trials, and post-market surveillance to monitor long-term effects and safety.

9.10 PROSPECTS AND CHALLENGES

With recent advances in nanotechnology, magnetic materials have gained prominence in cancer treatment. The precision and minimal invasive treatment offered by magnetic nanoparticles stand out for hyperthermia and magnetically induced drug delivery. Nevertheless, there are significant obstructions that impede its clinical translation. Biocompatibility, toxicity, biodistribution, aggregation, clearance pathway are some of the limiting factors that cause delay in clinical application.

9.10.1 Emerging Trends

Emerging trends in the field include the development of multifunctional nanoparticles, integration with advanced imaging techniques, and personalized medicine approaches. Multifunctional nanoparticles can simultaneously serve as diagnostic agents, therapeutic carriers, and hyperthermia inducers, offering a comprehensive solution for cancer management. Advances in imaging technologies, such as magnetic resonance imaging (MRI) and positron emission tomography (PET), enable real-time monitoring of nanoparticle distribution and therapeutic effects.

9.10.2 Technological Challenges

Technological challenges, such as scalable synthesis, precise control over particle properties, and targeted delivery, must be addressed to advance the clinical application of magnetic nanoparticles. Developing cost-effective and environmentally friendly synthesis methods, improving batch-to-batch consistency, and enhancing targeting efficiency are critical areas of focus. Additionally, overcoming biological barriers, such as the blood-brain barrier, requires innovative approaches to ensure effective delivery to target sites.

9.10.3 Future Directions in Research and Clinical Application

Future research directions include exploring new materials, optimizing treatment protocols, and conducting large-scale clinical trials to establish the efficacy and safety of magnetic nanoparticle-based therapies. Investigating novel materials with superior magnetic properties and biocompatibility, such as rare-earth metal alloys and hybrid nanoparticles, holds promise for enhancing therapeutic outcomes. Furthermore, personalized medicine approaches, where treatments are tailored to individual patients based on genetic and molecular profiles, can maximize the efficacy and minimize the side effects of nanoparticle-based therapies.

9.11 CONCLUSION

This chapter has provided a comprehensive overview of the use of magnetic materials in cancer hyperthermia and drug delivery. Key points include the synthesis and characterization of nanoparticles, mechanisms of hyperthermia, and applications in drug delivery. The integration of hyperthermia and drug delivery offers synergistic therapeutic effects, enhancing treatment efficacy while minimizing side effects. The integration of magnetic hyperthermia and drug delivery holds significant potential for improving cancer treatment outcomes. The ability to target and destroy cancer cells while minimizing side effects represents a major advancement in oncology. The combined approach can enhance the efficacy of existing therapies, reduce drug resistance, and improve patient survival rates.

Continued research and collaboration across disciplines will be essential to fully realize the potential of magnetic nanoparticles in cancer therapy. Advances in nanotechnology, materials science, and biomedical engineering will drive the development of more effective and safer treatments for cancer patients. By addressing the current challenges and leveraging emerging trends, the future of cancer therapy with magnetic nanoparticles looks promising, offering hope for better patient outcomes and improved quality of life.

REFERENCES

[1] K. Chatterjee, S. Sarkar, K. J. Rao, and S. Paria, "Core/shell nanoparticles in biomedical applications," *Advances in Colloid and Interface Science*, vol. 209, pp. 8–39, 2014.

[2] H. Gleiter, "Nanocrystalline materials," in *Advanced Structural and Functional Materials*, W. G. J. Bunk, Ed., Berlin, Heidelberg: Springer, 1991, pp. 1–37.

[3] R. S. Ningthoujam, R. K. Vatsa, A. Kumar, B. N. Pandey, S. Banerjee, and A. K. Tyagi, "Functionalized magnetic nanoparticles: Concepts, synthesis and application in cancer hyperthermia," *Functional Materials: Preparation, Processing and Applications*, vol. 6, pp. 229–260, 2012.

[4] S. F. Medeiros, A. M. Santos, H. Fessi, and A. Elaissari, "Stimuli-responsive magnetic particles for biomedical applications," *International Journal of Pharmaceutics*, vol. 403, no. 1–2, pp. 139–161, 2011.

[5] B. Chen, "Daunorubicin-loaded magnetic nanoparticles of Fe3O4 overcome multidrug resistance and induce apoptosis of K562-n/VCR cells in vivo," *IJN*, p. 201, Sept. 2009

[6] Y. Wang *et al.*, "Multifunctional melanin-like nanoparticles for bone-targeted chemo-photothermal therapy of malignant bone tumors and osteolysis," *Biomaterials*, vol. 183, pp. 10–19, 2018.

[7] M. Baskaran, P. Baskaran, N. Arulsamy, and B. Thyagarajan, "Preparation and evaluation of PLGA-coated capsaicin magnetic nanoparticles," *Pharmaceutical Research*, vol. 34, no. 6, pp. 1255–1263, June 2017.

[8] M. Oroujeni, B. Kaboudin, W. Xia, P. Jönsson, and D. A. Ossipov, "Conjugation of cyclodextrin to magnetic Fe3O4 nanoparticles via polydopamine coating for drug delivery," *Progress in Organic Coatings*, vol. 114, pp. 154–161, 2018.

[9] J. Beik *et al.*, "Nanotechnology in hyperthermia cancer therapy: From fundamental principles to advanced applications," *Journal of Controlled Release*, vol. 235, pp. 205–221, 2016.

[10] E. S. Day, J. G. Morton, and J. L. West, "Nanoparticles for thermal cancer therapy," 2009, Accessed: Oct. 22, 2024.

[11] Z. Ashikbayeva, D. Tosi, D. Balmassov, E. Schena, P. Saccomandi, and V. Inglezakis, "Application of nanoparticles and nanomaterials in thermal ablation therapy of cancer," *Nanomaterials*, vol. 9, no. 9, p. 1195, 2019.

[12] R. L. Manthe, S. P. Foy, N. Krishnamurthy, B. Sharma, and V. Labhasetwar, "Tumor ablation and nanotechnology," *Molecular Pharmaceutics*, vol. 7, no. 6, pp. 1880–1898, Dec. 2010.

[13] R. R. Letfullin, C. B. Iversen, and T. F. George, "Modeling nanophotothermal therapy: Kinetics of thermal ablation of healthy and cancerous cell organelles and gold nanoparticles," *Nanomedicine: Nanotechnology, Biology and Medicine*, vol. 7, no. 2, pp. 137–145, 2011.

[14] A. Ito, M. Shinkai, H. Honda, and T. Kobayashi, "Medical application of functionalized magnetic nanoparticles," *Journal of Bioscience and Bioengineering*, vol. 100, no. 1, pp. 1–11, 2005.

[15] Â. Andrade, R. Ferreira, J. Fabris, and R. Domingues, "Coating nanomagnetic particles for biomedical applications," *Biomedical Engineering-Frontiers and Challenges*, pp. 157–176, 2011.

[16] S. M. Dadfar *et al.*, "Iron oxide nanoparticles: Diagnostic, therapeutic and theranostic applications," *Advanced Drug Delivery Reviews*, vol. 138, pp. 302–325, 2019.
[17] N. T. Thanh, "Clinical applications of magnetic nanoparticles: Design to diagnosis manufacturing to medicine," 2018.
[18] J. R. Sosa-Acosta, C. Iriarte-Mesa, G. A. Ortega, and A. M. Díaz-García, "DNA-Iron oxide nanoparticles conjugates: Functional magnetic nanoplatforms in biomedical applications," in *Surface-Modified Nanobiomaterials for Electrochemical and Biomedicine Applications*, A. R. Puente-Santiago and D. Rodríguez-Padrón, Eds., Topics in Current Chemistry Collections, Cham: Springer International Publishing, 2020, pp. 19–47.
[19] A. A. Tregubov, P. I. Nikitin, and M. P. Nikitin, "Advanced smart nanomaterials with integrated logic-gating and biocomputing: Dawn of theranostic nanorobots," *Chemical Reviews*, vol. 118, no. 20, pp. 10294–10348, Oct. 2018.
[20] M. P. Nikitin, I. V. Zelepukin, V. O. Shipunova, I. L. Sokolov, S. M. Deyev, and P. I. Nikitin, "Enhancement of the blood-circulation time and performance of nanomedicines via the forced clearance of erythrocytes," *Nature Biomedical Engineering*, vol. 4, no. 7, pp. 717–731, 2020.
[21] V. N. Morozov *et al.*, "Generation and delivery of nanoaerosols from biological and biologically active substances," *Journal of Aerosol Science*, vol. 69, pp. 48–61, 2014.
[22] Y.-S. Cho *et al.*, "Cetuximab-conjugated magneto-fluorescent silica nanoparticles for in vivo colon cancer targeting and imaging," *Cancer Letters*, vol. 299, no. 1, pp. 63–71, 2010.
[23] C. Fang and M. Zhang, "Multifunctional magnetic nanoparticles for medical imaging applications," *Journal of Materials Chemistry*, vol. 19, no. 35, pp. 6258–6266, 2009.
[24] J. Estelrich, E. Escribano, J. Queralt, and M. A. Busquets, "Iron oxide nanoparticles for magnetically-guided and magnetically-responsive drug delivery," *International Journal of Molecular Sciences*, vol. 16, no. 4, pp. 8070–8101, 2015.
[25] A. Akbarzadeh, M. Samiei, and S. Davaran, "Magnetic nanoparticles: Preparation, physical properties, and applications in biomedicine," *Nanoscale Research Letters*, vol. 7, no. 1, p. 144, Dec. 2012.
[26] Y. Hou and S. Gao, "Monodisperse nickel nanoparticles prepared from a monosurfactant system and their magnetic properties," *Journal of Materials Chemistry*, vol. 13, no. 7, pp. 1510–1512, 2003.
[27] S. Sun and C. B. Murray, "Synthesis of monodisperse cobalt nanocrystals and their assembly into magnetic superlattices," *Journal of Applied Physics*, vol. 85, no. 8, pp. 4325–4330, 1999.
[28] A. Ali *et al.*, "Synthesis, characterization, applications, and challenges of iron oxide nanoparticles," *NSA*, vol. 9, pp. 49–67, Aug. 2016.
[29] W. Wu, Z. Wu, T. Yu, C. Jiang, and W.-S. Kim, "Recent progress on magnetic iron oxide nanoparticles: Synthesis, surface functional strategies and biomedical applications," *Science and Technology of Advanced Materials*, vol. 16, no. 2, p. 023501, 2015.
[30] A. E. Deatsch and E. E. Evans, "Heating efficiency in magnetic nanoparticle hyperthermia," *Journal of Magnetism and Magnetic Materials*, vol. 354, pp. 163–172, 2014.
[31] M. Mahmoudi, S. Sant, B. Wang, S. Laurent, and T. Sen, "Superparamagnetic iron oxide nanoparticles (SPIONs): Development, surface modification and applications in chemotherapy," *Advanced Drug Delivery Reviews*, vol. 63, no. 1–2, pp. 24–46, 2011.
[32] W. Wu, Q. He, and C. Jiang, "Magnetic iron oxide nanoparticles: Synthesis and surface functionalization strategies," *Nanoscale Researce Letters*, vol. 3, no. 11, p. 397, Nov. 2008.
[33] C. Sun, J. S. Lee, and M. Zhang, "Magnetic nanoparticles in MR imaging and drug delivery," *Advanced Drug Delivery Reviews*, vol. 60, no. 11, pp. 1252–1265, 2008.
[34] A. Lu, E. L. Salabas, and F. Schüth, "Magnetic nanoparticles: Synthesis, protection, functionalization, and application," *Angewandte Chemie International Edition*, vol. 46, no. 8, pp. 1222–1244, Feb. 2007.
[35] L. Yang *et al.*, "Development of receptor targeted magnetic iron oxide nanoparticles for efficient drug delivery and tumor imaging," *Journal of Biomedical Nanotechnology*, vol. 4, no. 4, pp. 439–449, 2008.
[36] Q. Pankhurst, S. Jones, and J. Dobson, "Applications of magnetic nanoparticles in biomedicine: The story so far," *Journal of Physics D: Applied Physics*, vol. 49, no. 50, 2016.
[37] A. K. Gupta and M. Gupta, "Synthesis and surface engineering of iron oxide nanoparticles for biomedical applications," *Biomaterials*, vol. 26, no. 18, pp. 3995–4021, 2005.
[38] O. Veiseh *et al.*, "Specific targeting of brain tumors with an optical/magnetic resonance imaging nanoprobe across the blood-brain barrier," *Cancer Research*, vol. 69, no. 15, pp. 6200–6207, 2009.
[39] T. Hyeon, Y. Chung, J. Park, S. S. Lee, Y.-W. Kim, and B. H. Park, "Synthesis of highly crystalline and monodisperse cobalt ferrite nanocrystals," *The Journalof Physical Chemistry B*, vol. 106, no. 27, pp. 6831–6833, July 2002.

[40] E. Auzans, D. Zins, E. Blums, and R. Massart, "Synthesis and properties of Mn-Zn ferrite ferrofluids" *Journal of Materials Science*, vol. 34, no. 6, pp. 1253–1260, 1999.
[41] S. Odenbach, "Ferrofluids-magnetisable liquids and their application in density separation," *Magnetic and Electrical Separation*, vol. 9, no. 1, pp. 1–25, 1998.
[42] M. T. López-López, A. Gómez-Ramírez, L. Rodríguez-Arco, J. D. G. Durán, L. Iskakova, and A. Zubarev, "Colloids on the Frontier of Ferrofluids. Rheological Properties," *Langmuir*, vol. 28, no. 15, pp. 6232–6245, Apr. 2012.
[43] M. T. López-López, J. D. G. Durán, A. V. Delgado, and F. González-Caballero, "Stability and magnetic characterization of oleate-covered magnetite ferrofluids in different nonpolar carriers," *Journal of Colloid and Interface Science*, vol. 291, no. 1, pp. 144–151, 2005.
[44] M. Kroell, M. Pridoehl, G. Zimmermann, L. Pop, S. Odenbach, and A. Hartwig, "Magnetic and rheological characterization of novel ferrofluids," *Journal of Magnetism and Magnetic Materials*, vol. 289, pp. 21–24, 2005.
[45] T. Hyeon, "Chemical synthesis of magnetic nanoparticles," *Chemical Communications*, no. 8, pp. 927–934, 2003.
[46] N. A. Frey, S. Peng, K. Cheng, and S. Sun, "Magnetic nanoparticles: synthesis, functionalization, and applications in bioimaging and magnetic energy storage," *Chemical Society Reviews*, vol. 38, no. 9, pp. 2532–2542, 2009.
[47] H.-D. Kurland, J. Grabow, G. Staupendahl, W. Andrä, S. Dutz, and M. E. Bellemann, "Magnetic iron oxide nanopowders produced by CO2 laser evaporation," *Journal of Magnetism and Magnetic Materials*, vol. 311, no. 1, pp. 73–77, 2007.
[48] C. Stötzel *et al.*, "Control of the crystal phase composition of $Fe_x O_y$nanopowders prepared by CO_2laser vaporization," *Crystal Growth & Design*, vol. 13, no. 11, pp. 4868–4876, Nov. 2013.
[49] T. Sugimoto and E. Matijević, "Formation of uniform spherical magnetite particles by crystallization from ferrous hydroxide gels," *Journal of Colloid and Interface Science*, vol. 74, no. 1, pp. 227–243, 1980.
[50] P. Tartaj, M. del Puerto Morales, S. Veintemillas-Verdaguer, T. González-Carreño, and C. J. Serna, "The preparation of magnetic nanoparticles for applications in biomedicine," *Journal of Physics D: Applied Physics*, vol. 36, no. 13, p. R182, 2003.
[51] K. Nejati-Koshki *et al.*, "Synthesis and *in vitro* study of cisplatin-loaded $Fe_3 O_4$ nanoparticles modified with PLGA-PEG $_{6000}$ copolymers in treatment of lung cancer," *Journal of Microencapsulation*, vol. 31, no. 8, pp. 815–823, Dec. 2014.
[52] J.-P. Jolivet, M. Henry, and J. Livage, "Metal oxide chemistry and synthesis: From solution to solid state," 2000.
[53] M. Faraji, Y. Yamini, and M. Rezaee, "Magnetic nanoparticles: Synthesis, stabilization, functionalization, characterization, and applications," *JICS*, vol. 7, no. 1, pp. 1–37, Mar. 2010.
[54] D. K. Kim, Y. Zhang, W. Voit, K. V. Rao, and M. Muhammed, "Synthesis and characterization of surfactant-coated superparamagnetic monodispersed iron oxide nanoparticles," *Journal of Magnetism and Magnetic Materials*, vol. 225, no. 1–2, pp. 30–36, 2001.
[55] J. Xie and S. Sun, "Chemical synthesis and surface modification of monodisperse magnetic nanoparticles," in *Nanomaterials: Inorganic and Bioinorganic Perspectives-Encyclopedia in Inorganic Chemistry*, John Wiley & Sons, Ltd, 2008, pp. 482–501.
[56] Y. Wang, C.-X. Yang, and X.-P. Yan, "Hydrothermal and biomineralization synthesis of a dual-modal nanoprobe for targeted near-infrared persistent luminescence and magnetic resonance imaging," *Nanoscale*, vol. 9, no. 26, pp. 9049–9055, 2017.
[57] K. Nejati and R. Zabihi, "Preparation and magnetic properties of nano size nickel ferrite particles using hydrothermal method," *Chemistry Central Journal*, vol. 6, no. 1, p. 23, Dec. 2012.
[58] S. Bedanta, A. Barman, W. Kleemann, O. Petracic, and T. Seki, "Magnetic nanoparticles: A subject for both fundamental research and applications," *Journal of Nanomaterials*, vol. 2013, pp. 1–22, 2013.
[59] K. Kekalo, K. Koo, E. Zeitchick, and I. Baker, "Microemulsion synthesis of iron core/iron oxide shell magnetic nanoparticles and their physicochemical properties," *MRS Proceedings*, vol. 1416, pp. mrsf11-1416-jj05-54, 2012.
[60] R. G. López *et al.*, "Chitosan-coated magnetic nanoparticles prepared in one step by reverse microemulsion precipitation," *International Journal of Molecular Sciences*, vol. 14, no. 10, pp. 19636–19650, 2013.
[61] E. E. Carpenter, "Iron nanoparticles as potential magnetic carriers," *Journal of Magnetism and Magnetic Materials*, vol. 225, no. 1–2, pp. 17–20, 2001.
[62] Q. A. Pankhurst, J. Connolly, S. K. Jones, and J. Dobson, "Applications of magnetic nanoparticles in biomedicine," *Journal of Physics D: Applied Physics*, vol. 36, no. 13, p. R167, 2003.

[63] S. F. Hasany, I. Ahmed, J. Rajan, and A. Rehman, "Systematic review of the preparation techniques of iron oxide magnetic nanoparticles," *Nanoscience Nanotechnology*, vol. 2, no. 6, pp. 148–158, 2012.

[64] S. Sakka, *Handbook of Sol-Gel Science and Technology. 1. Sol-Gel Processing*, vol. 1, Springer Science & Business Media, 2005.

[65] S. Majidi, F. Zeinali Sehrig, S. M. Farkhani, M. Soleymani Golouj eh, and A. Akbarzadeh, "Current methods for synthesis of magnetic nanoparticles," *Artificial Cells, Nanomedicine, and Biotechnology*, vol. 44, no. 2, pp. 722–734, 2016.

[66] E. H. Kim, H. S. Lee, B. K. Kwak, and B.-K. Kim, "Synthesis of ferrofluid with magnetic nanoparticles by sonochemical method for MRI contrast agent," *Journal of Magnetism and Magnetic Materials*, vol. 289, pp. 328–330, 2005.

[67] B. C. Serban *et al.*, "Nanostructured metal oxides semiconductors for oxygen chemiresistive sensing," 2019.

[68] P. A. Kotelnikova *et al.*, "Synthesis of magnetic nanoparticles stabilized by magnetite-binding protein for targeted delivery to cancer cells," *DokladyBiochemistryand Biophysics*, vol. 481, no. 1, pp. 198–200, July 2018.

[69] G. Hemery *et al.*, "Tuning sizes, morphologies, and magnetic properties of monocore versus multicore iron oxide nanoparticles through the controlled addition of water in the polyol synthesis," *Inorganic Chemistry*, vol. 56, no. 14, pp. 8232–8243, July 2017.

[70] A.G. Niculescu, C. Chircov, and A. M. Grumezescu, "Magnetite nanoparticles: Synthesis methods: A comparative review," *Methods*, vol. 199, pp. 16–27, Mar. 2022.

[71] G. Krishna Podagatlapalli, "The fundamentals of synthesis of the nanomaterials, properties, and emphasis on laser ablation in liquids: A brief review," *Discover Nano*, vol. 20, no. 1, p. 98, June 2025.

[72] E. Bäuerlein, "Biomineralization of unicellular organisms: An unusual membrane biochemistry for the production of inorganic nano- and microstructures," *Angewandte Chemie International Edition*, vol. 42, no. 6, pp. 614–641, Feb. 2003.

[73] V. K. Varadan, L. Chen, and J. Xie, *Nanomedicine: Design and Applications of Magnetic Nanomaterials, Nanosensors and Nanosystems*, John Wiley & Sons, 2008.

[74] M. Sarikaya, C. Tamerler, A. K.-Y. Jen, K. Schulten, and F. Baneyx, "Molecular biomimetics: Nanotechnology through biology," *Nature Materials*, vol. 2, no. 9, pp. 577–585, 2003.

[75] Y. Nahar *et al.*, "A facile one-pot synthesis of poly (acrylic acid)-functionalized magnetic iron oxide nanoparticles for suppressing reactive oxygen species generation and adsorption of biocatalyst," *Materials Research Express*, vol. 7, no. 1, p. 016102, 2019.

[76] M. Rajabzadeh, N. Najdi, Z. Zarei, and R. Khalifeh, "CuI immobilized on tricationic ionic liquid anchored on functionalized magnetic hydrotalcite (Fe3O4/HT-TIL-CuI) as a novel, magnetic and efficient nanocatalyst for Ullmann-type C–N coupling reaction," *Journal of Inorganic and Organometallic Polymers and Materials*, vol. 32, no. 7, pp. 2696–2711, 2022.

[77] P. Gupta, R. Tomar, M. Sahni, and S. Chauhan, "Cobalt, nickel and copper doped non-stoichiometric cadmium gallate as a prominent magnetic and photocatalytic material," *Chemical Physics*, vol. 554, p. 111419, 2022.

[78] R. T. P. Da Silva, H. Ribeiro De Barros, D. M. F. Sandrini, and S. I. Córdoba De Torresi, "Stimuli-responsive regulation of biocatalysis through metallic nanoparticle interaction," *Bioconjugate Chemistry*, vol. 33, no. 1, pp. 53–66, Jan. 2022.

[79] N. Kostevšek, "A review on the optimal design of magnetic nanoparticle-based T 2 MRI contrast agents," *Magnetochemistry*, vol. 6, no. 1, p. 11, 2020.

[80] R. Ladj *et al.*, "Polymer encapsulation of inorganic nanoparticles for biomedical applications," *International Journal of Pharmaceutics*, vol. 458, no. 1, pp. 230–241, 2013.

[81] M. Nawaz, Y. Sliman, I. Ercan, M. Lima-Tenório, E. Tenório-Neto, C. Kaewsaneha, A. Elaïssari "Magnetic and pH-responsive magnetic nanocarriers," in *Stimuli Responsive Polymeric Nanocarriers for Drug Delivery Applications*, Elsevier, 2019, pp. 37–85.

[82] A. Shakiba, O. Zenasni, M. D. Marquez, and T. R. Lee, "Advanced drug delivery via self-assembled monolayer-coated nanoparticles," *AIMS Bioengineering*, vol. 4, no. 2, pp. 275–299, 2017.

[83] D. B. Robinson *et al.*, "DNA-functionalized MFe_2O_4 (M = Fe, Co, or Mn) nanoparticles and their hybridization to DNA-functionalized surfaces," *Langmuir*, vol. 21, no. 7, pp. 3096–3103, Mar. 2005.

[84] S.-W. Kim, S. Kim, J. B. Tracy, A. Jasanoff, and M. G. Bawendi, "Phosphine oxide polymer for water-soluble nanoparticles," *Journalof the American Chemical Society*, vol. 127, no. 13, pp. 4556–4557, Apr. 2005.

[85] V. S. Zaitsev, D. S. Filimonov, I. A. Presnyakov, R. J. Gambino, and B. Chu, "Physical and chemical properties of magnetite and magnetite-polymer nanoparticles and their colloidal dispersions," *Journal of Colloid and Interface Science*, vol. 212, no. 1, pp. 49–57, 1999.

[86] K. Wormuth, "Superparamagnetic latex via inverse emulsion polymerization," *Journal of Colloid and Interface Science*, vol. 241, no. 2, pp. 366–377, 2001.

[87] S. Khizar, N. M. Ahmad, N. Zine, N. Jaffrezic-Renault, A. Errachid-el-salhi, and A. Elaissari, "Magnetic nanoparticles: From synthesis to theranostic applications," *ACS Applied Nano Materials*, vol. 4, no. 5, pp. 4284–4306, May 2021.

[88] A. Mukherjee, A. K. Waters, P. Kalyan, A. S. Achrol, S. Kesari, and V. M. Yenugonda, "Lipid–polymer hybrid nanoparticles as a next-generation drug delivery platform: State of the art, emerging technologies, and perspectives," *IJN*, vol. 14, pp. 1937–1952, Mar. 2019.

[89] P. Tartaj and C. J. Serna, "Microemulsion-assisted synthesis of tunable superparamagnetic composites," *Chemistryof Materials*, vol. 14, no. 10, pp. 4396–4402, Oct. 2002.

[90] P. Tartaj, T. González-Carreño, and C. J. Serna, "Single-step nanoengineering of silica coated maghemite hollow spheres with tunable magnetic properties," *Advanced Materials*, vol. 13, no. 21, pp. 1620–1624, Nov. 2001.

[91] S. Mourdikoudis, A. Kostopoulou, and A. P. LaGrow, "Magnetic Nanoparticle Composites: Synergistic Effects and Applications," *Advanced Science*, vol. 8, no. 12, p. 2004951, 2021.

[92] C. Xu *et al.*, "Dopamine as arobust anchor to immobilize functional molecules on the iron oxide shell of magnetic nanoparticles," *Journalof the American Chemical Society*, vol. 126, no. 32, pp. 9938–9939, Aug. 2004.

[93] R. Hong, N. O. Fischer, T. Emrick, and V. M. Rotello, "Surface PEGylation and ligand exchange chemistry of FePt nanoparticles for biological applications," *Chemistryof Materials*, vol. 17, no. 18, pp. 4617–4621, Sept. 2005.

[94] B. Wang, C. Xu, J. Xie, Z. Yang, and S. Sun, "pH controlled release of chromone from chromone-Fe $_3$ O $_4$nanoparticles," *Journalof the American Chemical Society*, vol. 130, no. 44, pp. 14436–14437, Nov. 2008.

[95] E. Cabuy, "Hyperthermia in cancer treatment," *Reliable Cancer Therapies Energy-Based Therapies*, vol. 1, no. 2, pp. 1–48, 2011.

[96] M. W. Dewhirst, Z. Vujaskovic, E. Jones, and D. Thrall, "Re-setting the biologic rationale for thermal therapy," *International Journal of Hyperthermia*, vol. 21, no. 8, pp. 779–790, Dec. 2005.

[97] A. M. Ponce, Z. Vujaskovic, F. Yuan, D. Needham, and M. W. Dewhirst, "Hyperthermia mediated liposomal drug delivery," *International Journal of Hyperthermia*, vol. 22, no. 3, pp. 205–213, Jan. 2006.

[98] R. D. Issels, "Regional hyperthermia in high-risk soft tissue sarcomas," *Current Opinion in Oncology*, vol. 20, no. 4, pp. 438–443, 2008.

[99] A. L. Feldman *et al.*, "Analysis of factors associated with outcome in patients with malignant peritoneal mesothelioma undergoing surgical debulking and intraperitoneal chemotherapy," *JCO*, vol. 21, no. 24, pp. 4560–4567, Dec. 2003.

[100] H. Maeda, J. Wu, T. Sawa, Y. Matsumura, and K. Hori, "Tumor vascular permeability and the EPR effect in macromolecular therapeutics: A review," *Journal of Controlled Release*, vol. 65, no. 1–2, pp. 271–284, 2000.

[101] J. C. Y. Kah *et al.*, "Critical parameters in the pegylation of gold nanoshells for biomedical applications: An *in vitro* macrophage study," *Journal of Drug Targeting*, vol. 17, no. 3, pp. 181–193, Apr. 2009.

[102] M. Suto *et al.*, "Heat dissipation mechanism of magnetite nanoparticles in magnetic fluid hyperthermia," *Journal of Magnetism and Magnetic Materials*, vol. 321, no. 10, pp. 1493–1496, 2009.

[103] A. Hervault and N. T. K. Thanh, "Magnetic nanoparticle-based therapeutic agents for thermo-chemotherapy treatment of cancer," *Nanoscale*, vol. 6, no. 20, pp. 11553–11573, 2014.

[104] P. Das, M. Colombo, and D. Prosperi, "Recent advances in magnetic fluid hyperthermia for cancer therapy," *Colloids and Surfaces B: Biointerfaces*, vol. 174, pp. 42–55, 2019.

[105] J. Jose *et al.*, "Magnetic nanoparticles for hyperthermia in cancer treatment: An emerging tool," *Environmental Scienceand Pollution Research*, vol. 27, no. 16, pp. 19214–19225, June 2020.

[106] C. J. Legge, H. E. Colley, M. A. Lawson, and A. E. Rawlings, "Targeted magnetic nanoparticle hyperthermia for the treatment of oral cancer," *Journalof Oral Pathology &Medicine*, vol. 48, no. 9, pp. 803–809, Oct. 2019.

[107] J. Majeed, L. Pradhan, R. S. Ningthoujam, R. K. Vatsa, D. Bahadur, and A. K. Tyagi, "Enhanced specific absorption rate in silanol functionalized Fe3O4 core–shell nanoparticles: Study of Fe leaching in Fe3O4 and hyperthermia in L929 and HeLa cells," *Colloids and Surfaces B: Biointerfaces*, vol. 122, pp. 396–403, 2014.

[108] S. Mondal *et al.*, "Hydroxyapatite coated iron oxide nanoparticles: A promising nanomaterial for magnetic hyperthermia cancer treatment," *Nanomaterials*, vol. 7, no. 12, p. 426, 2017.

[109] K. Maier-Hauff *et al.*, "Efficacy and safety of intratumoral thermotherapy using magnetic iron-oxide nanoparticles combined with external beam radiotherapy on patients with recurrent glioblastoma multiforme," *Journal of Neurooncology*, vol. 103, no. 2, pp. 317–324, June 2011.

[110] P. Pradhan *et al.*, "Comparative evaluation of heating ability and biocompatibility of different ferrite-based magnetic fluids for hyperthermia application," *Journal BiomedicalMaterials Research*, vol. 81B, no. 1, pp. 12–22, Apr. 2007.

[111] M. Gogoi, M. K. Jaiswal, H. D. Sarma, D. Bahadur, and R. Banerjee, "Biocompatibility and therapeutic evaluation of magnetic liposomes designed for self-controlled cancer hyperthermia and chemotherapy," *Integrative Biology*, vol. 9, no. 6, pp. 555–565, 2017.

[112] M. S. U. Rahman *et al.*, "Magnetic mesoporous bioactive glass for synergetic use in bone regeneration, hyperthermia treatment, and controlled drug delivery," *RSC Advances*, vol. 10, no. 36, pp. 21413–21419, 2020.

[113] A. K. Soni *et al.*, "Smart YPO4:Er–Yb nanophosphor for optical heating, hyperthermia, security ink, cancer endoradiotherapy, and uranyl recovery," *ACS Applied Nano Materials*, Dec. 2020.

[114] A. K. Soni, R. Joshi, B. P. Singh, N. N. Kumar, and R. S. Ningthoujam, "Near-infrared- and magnetic-field-responsive $NaYF_4$:Er^{3+}/Yb^{3+} @SiO_2 @AuNP@Fe_3 O_4nanocomposites for hyperthermia applications induced by fluorescence resonance energy transfer and surface plasmon absorption," *ACS Applied Nano Materials*, vol. 2, no. 11, pp. 7350–7361, Nov. 2019.

[115] U. Gneveckow, A. Jordan, R. Scholz, V. Bruess, N. Waldoefner, J. Ricke, A. Feussner, B. Hildebrandt, B. Rau, P. Wust, "Description and characterization of the novel hyperthermia- and thermoablation-system for clinical magnetic fluid hyperthermia," *Medical Physics*, vol. 31, no. 6, pp. 1444–1451, June 2004.

[116] B. Thiesen and A. Jordan, "Clinical applications of magnetic nanoparticles for hyperthermia," *International Journal of Hyperthermia*, vol. 24, no. 6, pp. 467–474, Jan. 2008.

[117] M. Johannsen, U. Gneveckow, L, Eckelt, A. Feussner, N. Waldöfner, R. Scholz, S. Deger, P. Wust, S. A. Loening, A. Jordan, "Clinical hyperthermia of prostate cancer using magnetic nanoparticles: Presentation of a new interstitial technique," *International Journal of Hyperthermia*, vol. 21, no. 7, pp. 637–647, Nov. 2005.

[118] N. Sadeghi, R. Jan Kok, C. Bo, M. Zandvliet, W. J. C. Geerts, G. Storm, C. T. W. Moonen, T. Lammers, R. Deckers, "Hyperthermia-triggered release of hypoxic cell radiosensitizers from temperature-sensitive liposomes improves radiotherapy efficacy in vitro," *Nanotechnology*, vol. 30, no. 26, p. 264001, Apr. 2019.

[119] R. Deckers, Sara M. Sprinkhuizen, Bart J. Crielaard, Johannes H. Ippel, Rolf Boelens, Chris J. G. Bakker, Gert Storm, Twan Lammers, Lambertus W. Bartels, "Absolute MR thermometry using nanocarriers," *Contrast Media & Molecular Imaging*, vol. 9, no. 4, pp. 283–290, 2014.

[120] A. A. Alavijeh, M. Barati, M. Barati, and H. A. Dehkordi, "The potential of magnetic nanoparticles for diagnosis and treatment of cancer based on body magnetic field and organ-on-the-chip," *Advanced Pharmaceutical Bulletin*, vol. 9, no. 3, p. 360, 2019.

[121] V. V. Mody, A. Cox, S. Shah, A. Singh, W. Bevins, and H. Parihar, "Magnetic nanoparticle drug delivery systems for targeting tumor," *Applied Nanoscience*, vol. 4, no. 4, pp. 385–392, Apr. 2014.

[122] H. Kee, H. Lee, and S. Park, "Optimized Halbach array for focused magnetic drug targeting," *Journal of Magnetism and Magnetic Materials*, vol. 514, p. 167180, 2020.

[123] N. Kiaie, S. H. Emami, S. Rabbani, R. M. Aghdam, and H. A. Tafti, "Targeted and controlled drug delivery to a rat model of heart failure through a magnetic nanocomposite," *Annalsof Biomedical Engineering*, vol. 48, no. 2, pp. 709–721, Feb. 2020.

[124] C. Comanescu, "Magnetic nanoparticles: Current advances in nanomedicine, drug delivery and MRI," *Chemistry*, vol. 4, no. 3, pp. 872–930, 2022.

[125] E. Hatami, P. K. Nagesh, N. Chauhan, M. Jaggi, S. C. Chauhan, and M. M. Yallapu, "In situ nanoparticle self-assembly for combination delivery of therapeutics to non-small cell lung cancer," *ACS Applied Bio Materials*, vol. 5, no. 3, pp. 1104–1119, 2022.

[126] D. Hajializadeh, A. Akhavan Saber, M. Jameh, B. Ahang, A. Moafy, Z. Kohanrooz Bijarpas, R. Saei Masouleh, M. Behzadi Kia, S. Rezaee Mojdehi, A. Salehzadeh, "Potential of apoptosis-inducing by a novel bio-synthesized CoFe2O4@ Ag nanocomposite in gastric cell line at the cellular and molecular level," *Journal of Cluster Science*, vol. 34, no. 1, pp. 359–371, 2023.

[127] J. Zou, S. Chen, Y. Li, L. Zeng, G. Lian, J. Li, S. Chen, K. Huang, Y. Chen, "Nanoparticles modified by triple single chain antibodies for MRI examination and targeted therapy in pancreatic cancer," *Nanoscale*, vol. 12, no. 7, pp. 4473–4490, 2020.

[128] Z. Karahaliloglu, E. Kilicay, and B. Hazer, "PLinaS-g-PEG coated magnetic nanoparticles as a contrast agent for hepatocellular carcinoma diagnosis," *Journal of Biomaterials Science, Polymer Edition*, vol. 31, no. 12, pp. 1580–1603, Aug. 2020.

[129] Y. Fu, G. He, Z. Liu, J. Wang, M. Li, Z. Zhang, Q. Bao, J. Wen, X. Zhu, C. Zhang, W. Zhang, "DNA base pairing-inspired supramolecular nanodrug camouflaged by cancer-cell membrane for osteosarcoma treatment," *Small*, vol. 18, no. 30, p. 2202337, 2022.

[130] P. Zivarpour, J. Hallajzadeh, Z. Asemi, F. Sadoughi, and M. Sharifi, "Chitosan as possible inhibitory agents and delivery systems in leukemia," *Cancer Cell International*, vol. 21, pp. 1–14, 2021.

[131] V. Dalal and S. Biswas, "Nanoscience: Convergence with biomedical and biological applications," in *Functional Bionanomaterials*, D. Thangadurai, J. Sangeetha, and R. Prasad, Eds., Nanotechnology in the Life Sciences, Cham: Springer International Publishing, 2020, pp. 1–25.

[132] F.-H. Chen, L.-M. Zhang, Q.-T. Chen, Y. Zhang, and Z.-J. Zhang, "Synthesis of a novel magnetic drug delivery system composed of doxorubicin-conjugated Fe 3 O 4 nanoparticle cores and a PEG-functionalized porous silica shell," *Chemical Communications*, vol. 46, no. 45, pp. 8633–8635, 2010.

[133] V. Linares, C. J. Yarce, J. D. Echeverri, E. Galeano, and C. H. Salamanca, "Relationship between degree of polymeric ionisation and hydrolytic degradation of Eudragit® E polymers under extreme acid conditions," *Polymers*, vol. 11, no. 6, p. 1010, 2019.

[134] Z. Li *et al.*, "A smart nanoassembly for multistage targeted drug delivery and magnetic resonance imaging," *Advanced Functional Materials*, vol. 24, no. 23, pp. 3612–3620, June 2014.

[135] C. S. Kumar and F. Mohammad, "Magnetic nanomaterials for hyperthermia-based therapy and controlled drug delivery," *Advanced Drug Delivery Reviews*, vol. 63, no. 9, pp. 789–808, 2011.

[136] S.-D. Li and L. Huang, "Pharmacokinetics and biodistribution of nanoparticles," *Molecular Pharmaceutics*, vol. 5, no. 4, pp. 496–504, Aug. 2008.

[137] S. Dong, "Targeted magnetic iron oxide nanoparticles for tumor imaging and therapy," *IJN*, p. 311, Oct. 2008.

[138] S. Singh, S. Singh, J. W. Lillard Jr, and R. Singh, "Drug delivery approaches for breast cancer," *IJN*, vol. 12, pp. 6205–6218, Aug. 2017.

10 Functionalized Nanomaterials for Nanomedicine in Cancer Stem Cell Therapy

Lekhika Pathak,[1,2] *Siddhant Biswas,*[1]
Riya Kanodia,[1] *and Bikul Das*[1,2]
[1]Department of Cancer and Stem Cell Biology, KaviKrishna Laboratory, Indian Institute of Technology Guwahati Research Park, Guwahati, Assam, India
[2]Department of Experimental Therapeutics, Thoreau Laboratory for Global Health, M2D2, University of Massachusetts, Lowell, MA, United States

10.1 INTRODUCTION

Cancer stem cells (CSCs) are a subset of cancer cells with the unique ability to self-renew and differentiate into various types of cancer cells, driving tumor initiation, progression, and metastasis (1). These properties also contribute significantly to the development of drug resistance, a major obstacle in cancer treatment (2, 3). CSCs exhibit multiple drug resistance mechanisms, most notably the over-expression of drug efflux pumps, such as ATP-binding cassette (ABC) transporters, which actively efflux chemotherapeutic agents (4). Additionally, CSCs possess robust DNA repair mechanisms, enabling them to efficiently repair DNA damage induced by chemotherapy and radiotherapy, thus limiting cell death (5). The presence of CSCs within a tumor is strongly associated with poor prognosis and increased tumor aggressiveness across various cancer types, including leukemia, breast, brain, colon, pancreatic, prostate, lung, liver, and skin cancers (6).

Nanomedicine offers a promising approach to overcome CSC-mediated drug resistance. By conjugating ligands specific to CSC surface markers, nanocarriers can selectively target and deliver therapeutic agents to these cells, minimizing damage to healthy stem cells (7). Furthermore, nanocarriers can effectively co-deliver multiple therapeutic agents, including chemotherapeutics, resistance-reversing agents, and differentiation inducers, thereby enhancing their synergistic effects (8, 9). Controlled drug-release strategies, such as stimuli-responsive systems, can further optimize therapeutic efficacy by precisely releasing drugs within the tumor microenvironment (TME) (10). This approach enables the sequential or simultaneous release of drugs in response to specific tumor microenvironmental cues, thereby maximizing therapeutic efficacy while minimizing systemic side effects.

In summary, nanomedicine offers a robust strategy to overcome the therapeutic resistance of CSCs by leveraging precise, multi-agent delivery and controlled release to enhance clinical outcomes.

10.2 MECHANISM OF NANOMEDICINE IN TARGETING CSCS

CSCs are notoriously resistant to conventional therapies such as chemotherapy and radiotherapy and are primary drivers of recurrence and metastasis (6). In this scenario, nanomaterials hold profound significance because their high surface-to-volume ratio; a consequence of their large number of surface atoms-provides unique properties for the efficient targeting of CSCs (11). Building on

DOI: 10.1201/9781003799351-10

these unique physicochemical properties, nanomedicine utilizes diverse platforms such as metallic nanoparticles, liposomes, dendrimers, and quantum dots (QDs) to facilitate control drug release, photothermal/photodynamic therapies, and other advanced modalities in CSC treatment (7, 10).

Recent advancements in nano drug delivery systems (NDDS) have maximized the potential of nanoparticles (NPs) as multifunctional platforms. Their unique attributes including their small size, biocompatibility, and biodegradability enable their diverse application as drug and gene carriers, imaging agents, and photothermal therapeutic (PTT) agents (12). Moreover, active and passive targeting mechanisms enable nanocarriers to provide a great deal of specificity in targeted drug delivery (13). In active targeting, NPs are coupled with peptides, antibodies, and various small molecules that provide the advantages of biocompatibility and reduced cytotoxicity in healthy cells compared to conventional chemotherapy (14, 15). Conversely, passive targeting leads to the preferentially accumulation of NPs within the TME, resulting in higher concentration in the malignant tissues compared to healthy ones due to the enhanced permeability and retention (EPR) effects (16). Tumors have leaky blood vessels and poor lymphatic drainage, allowing NPs to accumulate in the tumor tissue (17). Thus, nanomaterials can be engineered as versatile platform for targeted CSC therapy (Table 10.1). Here, we discuss selected nanotechnology-based therapeutic approaches and their mechanisms site specific delivery. By facilitating site-specific delivery, nanomaterials can engage diverse apoptotic mechanisms to effectively eliminate CSC populations (Figure 10.1).

10.2.1 Carbon Nanomaterials

Carbon-based nanoparticles exhibit strong near-infrared light (NIR) absorption, which enables efficient photothermal conversion. Additionally, the high surface area, simple chemical functionalization, and superior biocompatibility of the carbon-based nanoparticles make them suitable for CSC thermotherapy (18). For CSC-targeted thermotherapy, several kinds of carbon-based nanoparticles have been investigated.

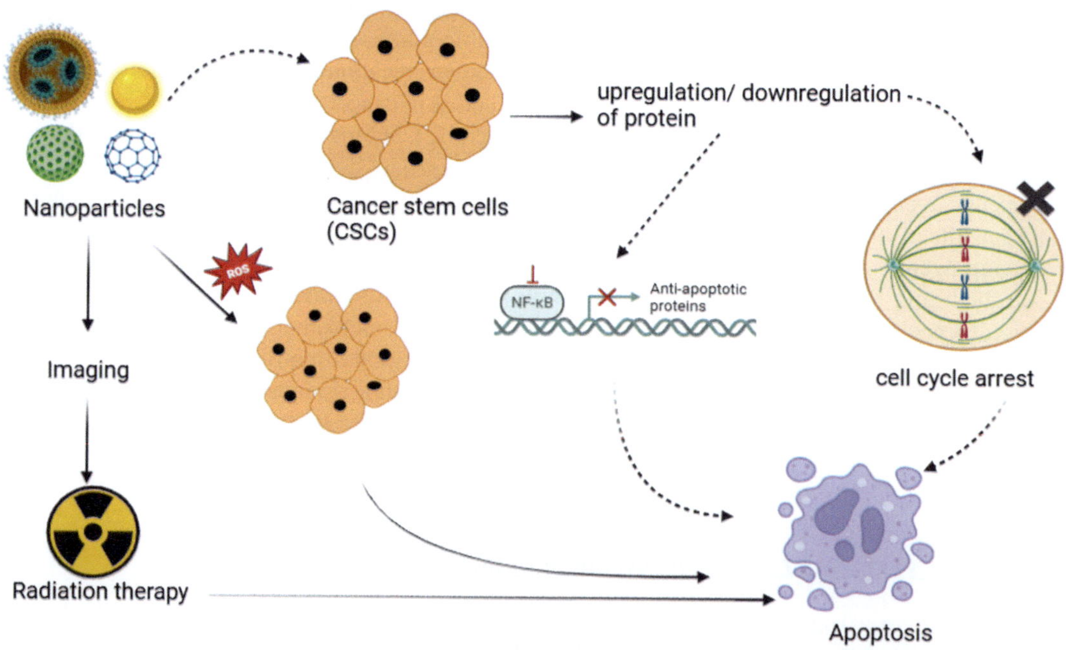

FIGURE 10.1 Schematic representation of the mechanisms for inducing apoptosis by various nanomaterials in CSCs.

(i) **Graphene oxide (GO):** Graphene oxide (GO), a graphene derivative, can be altered easily to act as an outstanding drug and nucleic acid carrier for targeted drug delivery in CSC therapy (19, 20). A study was conducted by Fiorillo *et al.* in 2015 across six independent cancer cell lines; prostate, breast, ovarian, lung, brain and pancreatic cancer. The GO selectively inhibited tumor sphere formation in all these cell lines (19). Another study demonstrated that GO particularly targets CSCs by inducing transdifferentiation of CSCs in glioblastoma (20). These findings suggest that GO may be utilized to eliminate any residual CSCs in order to stop tumor recurrence and distant metastases, thus offering a strategy to accomplish "differentiation-based nano-therapy" (19, 20).

(ii) **Carbon nanotubes (CNTs):** Carbon nanotubes are cylindrical graphene nanostructures, with distinctive characteristics of cell membrane penetrability and high drug-loading ability (21). In 2012, Burke *et al.* showed that breast CSCs (BCSCs) are susceptible to carbon nanotube mediated thermal therapy, which effectively eliminates their long-term proliferate capacity. Thus, the BCSCs, which drive tumor growth and recurrence can be simultaneously eliminated alongside the differentiated bulk tumor cells through nanotube-mediated thermal therapy (22). These CNTs can also induce cell cycle arrest by generating reactive oxygen species (ROS) and disrupting cellular signaling pathways (23). Moreover, Al Faraj *et al.* developed a method using biocompatible multimodal single wall carbon nanotubes (SWCNTs) functionalized with CD44 antibodies, demonstrating enhanced selectivity and efficacy in targeting breast CSCs (24).

(iii) **Nano-diamonds (NDs):** Nano-diamonds, tiny carbon structures shaped like truncated octahedrons, can be customized with various biological and chemical agents, including drugs, targeting molecules, genetic material, and imaging agents (25). Among many nano-material based delivery systems, NDs stand out for their exceptional delivery capabilities and excellent biocompatibility (26). For instance, detonation NDs coated with hyperbranched polyglycerol (dND-PG) and loaded with an anticancer drugs can, upon conjugation with specific targeting ligands, selectively eliminate tumor cells while minimizing off-target cytotoxicity in macrophages (27). Similarly, NDs loaded with the drug Epirubicin through physical adsorption have shown promise in overcoming drug resistance in liver CSCs (11).

10.2.2 Gold Nanoparticles (Au NPs)

Gold nanoparticles, such as spherical gold nanoparticles and gold nanorods, have become popular tools in cancer therapeutic research (28, 29, 30). Their ease of design, structural versatility and excellent biocompatibility (31), render them highly suitable for safe, clinical-grade therapeutic applications. Spherical gold nanoparticles, for example, can be produced in large quantities using a simple method called citrate reduction. More recently, chemists have developed techniques to create gold nanoparticles in various shapes and sizes, including nanorods (32, 33), nanoflowers (34, 35), and nanocages (36, 37). These nanoparticles have unique optical properties that make them ideal for both cancer treatment and imaging. Their ability to absorb, scatter, and interact with light, particularly through a phenomenon called "localized surface plasmon resonance" (LSPR), makes them suitable for photothermal therapy, where they can generate heat to kill cancer cells (38). Additionally, their surfaces can be modified to carry drugs, allowing for targeted drug delivery and improved treatment efficacy.

(i) **Sphere like Au NPs:** Researchers have developed various strategies to use Au NPs for targeting CSCs. Au-NPs are coated on the surface of polystyrene or polypyrrole microspheres to enhance their application in medical diagnosis (39). Au NPs with spherical structure, 20–30 nm in size and with uniform distribution are good for intracellular uptake; thus to target CSCs (40). Additionally, Au NPs can be loaded with chemotherapy drugs to enhance their efficacy and reduce side effects (41). One study demonstrated that Au NPs functionalized with L-aspartate and loaded with chemotherapy drugs could effectively inhibiting the proliferation of hepatocellular carcinoma cells (HCCs) (42). Another study showed that doxorubicin loaded polyethylene glycol coated hollow gold nano-spheres improve the photothermal ablation-chemoembolization therapy of HCC in rats (43). Furthermore, Au NPs conjugated with microRNA-182 could penetrate the blood-brain barrier and target glioblastoma cells, leading to reduced tumor growth and increased survival rates (44). These findings highlight the potential of Au NP-based therapies to target CSCs and improve cancer treatment outcomes. Further research is needed to fully realize the clinical potential of these nanomaterials.

(ii) **Gold nanorods (Au NRs or GNRs):** Gold nanorods (Au NRs) offer significant advantages over spherical gold nanoparticles (Au NPs) in cancer imaging and therapy. Their unique optical properties, strong absorption and scattering of NIR light, make them ideal for these applications (45). NIR light penetrates deeper into tissues and causes less damage to healthy cells, making Au NR-based therapies more effective and less invasive (45, 46). The Au NRs modified with specific aptamers can selectively target and destroy prostate cancer cells and CSCs upon NIR laser irradiation (46). Additionally, Au NR-based photothermal therapy has been shown to effectively eliminate breast CSCs by reducing the number of aldehyde dehydrogenase-positive cells and suppressing the expression of stem cell markers (47).

Au NPs and Au NRs possess several key properties that make them attractive for cancer therapy. They can be easily synthesized in various shapes and sizes, are highly stable and biocompatible, and can be readily modified with targeting molecules and drugs (48). Their unique optical properties facilitate dual-modality imaging and photothermal therapy, making them promising tools for combating cancer.

The nanoparticle-based drug delivery system offers better pharmacokinetic and pharmacodynamic properties (49). More significantly, combinational pharmaceuticals co-loaded in nanomedicines are more effective at killing CSCs than free drugs because they combine the biodistribution and individual pharmacokinetics of combo drugs to produce a set drug ratio (50). However, there are also limitations in addition to the advantages of NDDS based CSC targeted therapeutic strategies.

TABLE 10.1
Types of Nanoparticles and Their Respective Cancer Cell Targets

Nanoparticle	Subtype	Cancer Cell Targets
Carbon nanomaterials	Carbon nanotubes	Breast CSCs, gastric CSCs
	Nanodiamond	Hepatic CSCs
Gold nanoparticles	Sphere Au NPs	Hepatocellular carcinoma, pancreatic and breast stem cells
	Au NRs	Prostate Cancer Stem Cells
Organic nanoparticles	Liposome	Cisplatin-resistant head and neck squamous cell carcinoma, breast cancer stem-cells
	Polymer nanoparticles (PNPs)	Doxorubicin resistant CSCs, CD133+ cells, Caco-2 cells, U87MG and U251 glioma stem cells
DNA nanocarrier	Rod-like DNA origami	Daunorubicin loaded DNA origami drug carrier into resistant leukemia cancer cells
	Aptamer-functionalized DNA origami	Doxorubicin loaded DNA origami into resistant Hela/ADR and MCF-7/ADR cancer cells

10.3 ADVANTAGES AND LIMITATIONS OF NANOMEDICINE CSC THERAPY

Nanomedicine, the application of nanotechnology to medicine, has emerged as a promising approach to target CSC, a subpopulation of cells responsible for tumor initiation, progression, and recurrence. By exploiting the unique properties of nanomaterials, scientists are developing novel therapeutic strategies to overcome the limitations of conventional therapies. One of the key advantages of nanomedicine based CSC therapy is its ability to enhance drug delivery (13, 49). Nanoparticles can encapsulate therapeutic agents, protect them from degradation, and deliver them directly to CSCs, bypassing biological barriers and minimizing systemic toxicity (13). This targeted delivery improves therapeutic efficacy while reducing side effects (51). Additionally, the efficiency of nanomaterials in selective targeting of CSCs can be enhanced by attaching specific ligands or antibodies specific to CSCs (11). This approach not only enhances therapeutic precision but also minimize systemic side effects, thereby improving the overall clinical tolerability for patients. Furthermore, these nanoparticles can be engineered to spatiotemporal control over drug release, thereby optimizing pharmacokinetics and minimizing systemic adverse effects (13, 50).

The significant advantage of nanomedicine is its ability to bypass intrinsic tumor drug resistance mechanisms, a major challenge in clinical oncology (52). A DNA origami-based nanocarrier was constructed for delivery of chemotherapeutic drugs into drug-resistant cancer cells (53, 54). The nanoparticles can also inhibit drug efflux pumps (55), which typically export therapeutic agents from cancer cells, thereby increasing intracellular drug concentration and efficacy. In summary, nanomedicine offers a transformative approach to CSC targeted therapy. By overcoming the limitations of conventional treatments and harnessing the special features of nanomaterials, these strategies provide innovative pathways to effectively eradicate CSC populations and improve clinical outcomes.

Although nanoparticles are mainly made and utilized for medical and therapeutic purposes, the long-term negative effects as well as the limitations of nanoparticles in medicine remain an unknown factor (56). While extensive investigation have been conducted on the toxicology of engineered nanoparticles, public health concerns regarding these materials have increased significantly. The researchers reported that the long term exposure of nanoparticles can be destructive due to their better penetration ability and distinctive toxicity at the nano level (57). While the emergence of nanoparticles-based therapeutics is promising, it is important to acknowledge the existing clinical and technical challenges that remain to be addressed. Standardized regulatory protocols are essential for assessing the potential risks associated with the clinical application of these engineered nanoparticles (58).

While this chapter focuses primarily on the physiochemical properties and functionalization of nanomaterials for CSC-targeted drug delivery, it is important to acknowledge that therapeutic efficacy is also governed by biological targeting strategies. Advanced nanoparticle design often integrates CSC surface biomarkers, such as CD133, CD90, and modulators of key signaling pathways, such as Hedgehog, TGF-ß, to enhance CSC specificity (11).

10.4 CONCLUSION AND FUTURE PERSPECTIVES

The discovery of CSCs has revolutionized our approach to cancer therapy. The drug resistance, recurrence, and self-renewal capabilities of CSCs underscores their complexity within tumors, making their eradication a critical therapeutic priority. While progress has been made in characterizing these cells, distinguishing them from normal stem cells remains a formidable challenge. This specificity is essential for developing targeted therapies that effectively eliminate CSCs while sparing healthy tissues. Further research is required to identify novel CSC specific markers and therapeutic targets.

Therapeutic strategies must be designed to inhibit cancer recurrence and improve patient survival. Conventional treatments often exhibit limitations regarding target specificity, biocompatibility, and physiological stability within the host; consequently, nanoparticle based platforms have emerged as a superior alternative. Nanotechnology offers a promising solution by enabling the precise delivery of therapeutic agents, enhancing drug efficacy, and minimizing systemic toxicity. Furthermore, the TME significantly influences tumor progression and recurrence, nanoparticles are being engineered to interact directly with the TME to modulate these processes (10). Furthermore, critical questions remain regarding the conjugation strategies for active moieties, the preservation of their bioactivity, the stability of the nanoparticle-ligand linkage, long-term metabolic fate and safety profile of these systems in vivo.

A reprogramed CSC phenotype, termed tumor stemness defense (TSD) has been reported to exhibit aggressiveness, therapeutic resistance and the ability to modulate the TME to promote tumor progression (59, 60). Bacteria-induced bystander apoptosis has been demonstrated to effectively target TSD+ CSCs in both *in vitro* and *in vivo* models (59, 60). CSCs often create protective barriers that limit the penetration of therapeutic agents. While bacterial-induced bystander apoptosis is a promising strategy for targeting the TSD phenotype, its clinical success hinges on the precise delivery of bacteria directly into the CSC niche. Nanoparticle-based platforms are essential for overcoming this barrier, as they can be engineered to navigate the tumor architecture and deliver these therapeutic agents specifically to the CSC microenvironment, thereby facilitating a successful, targeted clinical application.

AUTHOR CONTRIBUTIONS

The authors confirm contribution to the chapter as follows: study conception and design: Das B., Pathak L. Draft manuscript preparation: Pathak L, Biswas S, Kanodia R. Figures and table preparation: Biswas S, Kanodia R. Manuscript review and edits: Das B., Pathak L.

ACKNOWLEDGMENTS

The authors express their gratitude to the research team at KaviKrishna Laboratory and the clinical team members at KaviKrishna Telemedicine Care, whose insightful discussions were instrumental in conceptualizing and shaping this chapter.

REFERENCES

1. Batlle E, Clevers H. Cancer stem cells revisited. *Nat Med.* 2017 Oct 6;23(10):1124–1134. https://doi.org/10.1038/nm.4409
2. Shibue T, Weinberg RA. EMT, CSCs, and drug resistance: The mechanistic link and clinical implications. *Nat Rev Clin Oncol.* 2017;14(10):611–629. https://doi.org/10.1038/nrclinonc.2017.44
3. Huang T, Song X, Xu D, et al. Stem cell programs in cancer initiation, progression, and therapy resistance. *Theranostics.* 2020;10(19):8721–8743. Published 2020 Jul 9. https://doi.org/10.7150/thno.41648
4. Moitra K, Lou H, Dean M. Multidrug efflux pumps and cancer stem cells: Insights into multidrug resistance and therapeutic development. *Clin Pharmacol Ther.* 2011 Apr;89(4):491–502. https://doi.org/10.1038/clpt.2011.14
5. Abad E, Graifer D, Lyakhovich A. DNA damage response and resistance of cancer stem cells. *Cancer Lett.* 2020 Apr 1;474:106–117. https://doi.org/10.1016/j.canlet.2020.01.008
6. Chu X, Tian W, Ning J, et al. Cancer stem cells: Advances in knowledge and implications for cancer therapy. *Signal Transduct Target Ther.* 2024 Jul 5;9(1):170. https://doi.org/10.1038/s41392-024-01851-y
7. Luobin L, Wanxin H, Yingxin G, et al. Nanomedicine-induced programmed cell death in cancer therapy: Mechanisms and perspectives. *Cell Death Discov.* 2024 Aug 29;10(1):386. https://doi.org/10.1038/s41420-024-02121-0
8. Dicko A, Mayer LD, Tardi PG. Use of nanoscale delivery systems to maintain synergistic drug ratios in vivo. *Expert Opin Drug Deliv.* 2010 Dec;7(12):1329–1341. https://doi.org/10.1517/17425247.2010.538678
9. Ramsay EC, Dos Santos N, Dragowska WH, Laskin JJ, Bally MB. The formulation of lipid-based nanotechnologies for the delivery of fixed dose anticancer drug combinations. *Curr Drug Deliv.* 2005 Oct;2(4):341–351. https://doi.org/10.2174/156720105774370294
10. Sabit H, Pawlik TM, Radwan F, et al. Precision nanomedicine: Navigating the tumor microenvironment for enhanced cancer immunotherapy and targeted drug delivery. *Mol Cancer.* 2025 Jun 3;24(1):160. https://doi.org/10.1186/s12943-025-02357-z

11. Qin W, Huang G, Chen Z, Zhang Y. Nanomaterials in targeting cancer stem cells for cancer therapy. *Front Pharmacol.* 2017 Jan 18;8:1. https://doi.org/10.3389/fphar.2017.00001
12. Kanaoujiya R, Porwal D, Srivastava S. Applications of nanomaterials for gastrointestinal tumors: A review. *Front Med Technol.* 2022 Sep 1;4:997123. https://doi.org/10.3389/fmedt.2022.997123
13. Yue M, Guo T, Nie DY, Zhu YX, Lin M. Advances of nanotechnology applied to cancer stem cells. *World J Stem Cells.* 2023;15(6):514–529. https://doi.org/10.4252/wjsc.v15.i6.514
14. Thongpon P, Tang M, Cong Z. Peptide-based nanoparticle for tumor therapy. *Biomedicines.* 2025 Jun 9;13(6):1415. https://doi.org/10.3390/biomedicines13061415
15. Zhang L, Zhai BZ, Wu YJ, Wang Y. Recent progress in the development of nanomaterials targeting multiple cancer metabolic pathways: A review of mechanistic approaches for cancer treatment. *Drug Deliv.* 2023 Dec;30(1):1–18. https://doi.org/10.1080/10717544.2022.2144541
16. Bazak R, Houri M, Achy SE, Hussein W, Refaat T. Passive targeting of nanoparticles to cancer: A comprehensive review of the literature. *Mol Clin Oncol.* 2014 Nov;2(6):904–908. https://doi.org/10.3892/mco.2014.356
17. Nakamura Y, Mochida A, Choyke PL, Kobayashi H. Nanodrug delivery: Is the enhanced permeability and retention effect sufficient for curing cancer? *Bioconjug Chem.* 2016 Oct 19;27(10):2225–2238. https://doi.org/10.1021/acs.bioconjchem.6b00437
18. Speranza G. Carbon nanomaterials: Synthesis, functionalization and sensing applications. *Nanomaterials (Basel).* 2021 Apr 9;11(4):967. https://doi.org/10.3390/nano11040967
19. Fiorillo M, Verre AF, Iliut M, et al. Graphene oxide selectively targets cancer stem cells, across multiple tumor types: Implications for non-toxic cancer treatment, via "differentiation-based nano-therapy". *Oncotarget.* 2015 Feb 28;6(6):3553–3562. https://doi.org/10.18632/oncotarget.3348
20. Martelli C, King A, Simon T, Giamas G. Graphene-induced transdifferentiation of cancer stem cells as a therapeutic strategy against glioblastoma. *ACS Biomater Sci Eng.* 2020 Jun 8;6(6):3258–3269. https://doi.org/10.1021/acsbiomaterials.0c00197
21. Shao W, Paul A, Zhao B, et al. Carbon nanotube lipid drug approach for targeted delivery of a chemotherapy drug in a human breast cancer xenograft animal model. *Biomaterials.* 2013;34(38):10109–10119. https://doi.org/10.1016/j.biomaterials.2013.09.007
22. Burke AR, Singh RN, Carroll DL, et al. The resistance of breast cancer stem cells to conventional hyperthermia and their sensitivity to nanoparticle-mediated photothermal therapy. *Biomaterials.* 2012 Apr;33(10):2961–2970. https://doi.org/10.1016/j.biomaterials.2011.12.052
23. Dinicola S, Masiello MG, Proietti S, et al. Multiwalled carbon nanotube buckypaper induces cell cycle arrest and apoptosis in human leukemia cell lines through modulation of AKT and MAPK signaling pathways. *Toxicol In Vitro.* 2015;29(7):1298–1308. https://doi.org/10.1016/j.tiv.2015.05.006
24. Al Faraj A, Shaik AS, Al Sayed B, Halwani R, Al Jammaz I. Specific targeting and noninvasive imaging of breast cancer stem cells using single-walled carbon nanotubes as novel multimodality nanoprobes. *Nanomedicine (Lond).* 2016;11(1):31–46. https://doi.org/10.2217/nnm.15.182
25. Liu KK, Wang CC, Cheng CL, Chao JI. Endocytic carboxylated nanodiamond for the labeling and tracking of cell division and differentiation in cancer and stem cells. *Biomaterials.* 2009;30(26):4249–4259. https://doi.org/10.1016/j.biomaterials.2009.04.056
26. Zhang Y, Cui Z, Kong H, et al. One-shot immunomodulatory nanodiamond agents for cancer immunotherapy. *Adv Mater.* 2016;28(14):2699–2708. https://doi.org/10.1002/adma.201506232
27. Zhao L, Xu YH, Akasaka T, et al. Polyglycerol-coated nanodiamond as a macrophage-evading platform for selective drug delivery in cancer cells. *Biomaterials.* 2014;35(20):5393–5406. https://doi.org/10.1016/j.biomaterials.2014.03.041
28. Wang L, Liu Y, Li W, et al. Selective targeting of gold nanorods at the mitochondria of cancer cells: Implications for cancer therapy. *Nano Lett.* 2011;11(2):772–780.
29. Chen T, Xu S, Zhao T, et al. Gold nanocluster-conjugated amphiphilic block copolymer for tumor-targeted drug delivery. *ACS Appl Mater Interfaces.* 2012;4(11):5766–5774. https://doi.org/10.1021/am301223n
30. Iodice C, Cervadoro A, Palange A, et al. Enhancing photothermal cancer therapy by clustering gold nanoparticles into spherical polymeric nanoconstructs. *Opt Lasers Eng.* 2016;76:74–81. ISSN 0143-8166. https://doi.org/10.1016/j.optlaseng.2015.04.017
31. Ahmad T, Sarwar R, Iqbal A, et al. Recent advances in combinatorial cancer therapy via multifunctionalized gold nanoparticles. *Nanomedicine (Lond).* 2020 May;15(12):1221–1237. https://doi.org/10.2217/nnm-2020-0051
32. Kim D, Choi E, Lee C, et al. Highly sensitive and selective visual detection of Cr(VI) ions based on etching of silver-coated gold nanorods. *Nano Converg.* 2019 Oct 23;6(1):34. https://doi.org/10.1186/s40580-019-0206-1

33. Nikoobakht B, El-Sayed MA. Preparation and growth mechanism of gold nanorods (NRs) using seed-mediated growth method. *Chem Mater*. 2003;15(10):1957–1962. https://doi.org/10.1021/cm020732l
34. Xie J, Zhang Q, Lee JY, Wang DIC. The synthesis of SERS-active gold nanoflower tags for in vivo applications. *ACS Nano*. 2008;2(12):2473–2480. https://doi.org/10.1021/nn800442q
35. Wang Z, Zhang J, Ekman J, et al. DNA-mediated control of metal nanoparticle shape: One-pot synthesis and cellular uptake of highly stable and functional gold nanoflowers. *Nano Lett*. 2010;10(5):1886–1891. https://doi.org/10.1021/nl100675p
36. Skrabalak SE, Chen J, Sun Y, et al. Gold nanocages: Synthesis, properties, and applications. *Acc Chem Res*. 2008;41(12):1587–1595. https://doi.org/10.1021/ar800018v
37. Xia Y, Li W, Cobley CM, et al. Gold nanocages: From synthesis to theranostic applications. *Acc Chem Res*. 2011;44(10):914–924. https://doi.org/10.1021/ar200061q
38. Tian F, Conde J, Bao C, et al. Gold nanostars for efficient in vitro and in vivo real-time SERS detection and drug delivery via plasmonic-tunable Raman/FTIR imaging. *Biomaterials*. 2016;106:87–97. https://doi.org/10.1016/j.biomaterials.2016.08.014
39. Xu T, Li Y, Zhang J, et al., Spherical and polygonal shape of Au nanoparticles coated functionalized polymer microspheres, *Appl Surf Sci*. 2015;345:264–271. https://www.sciencedirect.com/science/article/abs/pii/S0169433215006753
40. Wang J, Liu N, Su Q, et al. Green synthesis of gold nanoparticles and study of their inhibitory effect on bulk cancer cells and cancer stem cells in breast carcinoma. *Nanomaterials (Basel)*. 2022 Sep 24;12(19):3324. https://doi.org/10.3390/nano12193324
41. Huang H, Liu R, Yang J, et al. Gold nanoparticles: Construction for drug delivery and application in cancer immunotherapy. *Pharmaceutics*. 2023 Jul 2;15(7):1868. https://doi.org/10.3390/pharmaceutics15071868
42. Usmani A, Mishra A, Ahmad M. Nanomedicines: A theranostic approach for hepatocellular carcinoma. *Artif Cells Nanomed Biotechnol*. 2018 Jun;46(4):680–690. https://doi.org/10.1080/21691401.2017.1374282
43. Li J, Zhou M, Liu F, et al. Hepatocellular carcinoma: Intra-arterial delivery of doxorubicin-loaded hollow gold nanospheres for photothermal ablation-chemoembolization therapy in rats. *Radiology*. 2016 Nov;281(2):427–435. https://doi.org/10.1148/radiol.2016152510
44. Kouri FM, Hurley LA, Daniel WL, et al. miR-182 integrates apoptosis, growth, and differentiation programs in glioblastoma. *Genes Dev*. 2015 Apr 1;29(7):732–745. https://doi.org/10.1101/gad.257394.114
45. Zhou R, Zhang M, Xi J, et al. Gold nanorods-based photothermal therapy: Interactions between biostructure, nanomaterial, and near-infrared irradiation. *Nanoscale Res Lett*. 2022 Jul 26;17(1):68. https://doi.org/10.1186/s11671-022-03706-3
46. Wang J, Sefah K, Altman MB, et al. Aptamer-conjugated nanorods for targeted photothermal therapy of prostate cancer stem cells. *Chem Asian J*. 2013 Oct;8(10):2417–2422. https://doi.org/10.1002/asia.201300375
47. Xu Y, Wang J, Li X, et al. Selective inhibition of breast cancer stem cells by gold nanorods mediated plasmonic hyperthermia. *Biomaterials*. 2014 May;35(16):4667–4677. https://doi.org/10.1016/j.biomaterials.2014.02.035
48. Kesharwani P, Ma R, Sang L, et al. Gold nanoparticles and gold nanorods in the landscape of cancer therapy. *Mol Cancer*. 2023 Jun 21;22(1):98. https://doi.org/10.1186/s12943-023-01798-8
49. Singh VK, Saini A, Chandra R. The implications and future perspectives of nanomedicine for cancer stem cell targeted therapies. *Front Mol Biosci*. 2017 Jul 21;4:52. https://doi.org/10.3389/fmolb.2017.00052
50. Liu H, Liu M, Zhao Y, Mo R. Nanomedicine strategies to counteract cancer stemness and chemoresistance. *Explor Target Antitumor Ther*. 2023;4:630–656. https://doi.org/10.37349/etat.2023.00157
51. Tiwari H, Rai N, Singh S, et al. Recent advances in nanomaterials-based targeted drug delivery for preclinical cancer diagnosis and therapeutics. *Bioengineering (Basel)*. 2023;10(7):760. Published 2023 Jun 25. https://doi.org/10.3390/bioengineering10070760
52. Zhang C, Zhou X, Zhang H, et al. Recent progress of novel nanotechnology challenging the multidrug resistance of cancer. *Front Pharmacol*. 2022 Feb 14;13:776895. https://doi.org/10.3389/fphar.2022.776895
53. Halley PD, Lucas CR, McWilliams EM, et al. Daunorubicin-loaded DNA origami nanostructures circumvent drug-resistance mechanisms in a Leukemia model. *Small*. 2016 Jan 20;12(3):308–320. https://doi.org/10.1002/smll.201502118. Epub 2015 Nov 19.
54. Pan Q, Nie C, Hu Y, et al. Aptamer-functionalized DNA origami for targeted codelivery of antisense oligonucleotides and doxorubicin to enhance therapy in drug-resistant cancer cells. *ACS Appl Mater Interfaces*. 2020 Jan 8;12(1):400–409. https://doi.org/10.1021/acsami.9b20707. Epub 2019 Dec 18.
55. Ashique S, Garg A, Hussain A, et al. Nanodelivery systems: An efficient and target-specific approach for drug-resistant cancers. *Cancer Med*. 2023 Sep;12(18):18797–18825. https://doi.org/10.1002/cam4.6502
56. Gavas S, Quazi S, Karpiński TM. Nanoparticles for cancer therapy: Current progress and challenges. *Nanoscale Res Lett*. 2021 Dec 5;16(1):173. https://doi.org/10.1186/s11671-021-03628-6

57. Wang C, Lu J, Zhou L, et al. Effects of long-term exposure to Zinc oxide nanoparticles on development, Zinc metabolism and biodistribution of minerals (Zn, Fe, Cu, Mn) in mice. *PLoS One*. 2016 Oct 12;11(10):e0164434. https://doi.org/10.1371/journal.pone.0164434
58. De Jong WH, Geertsma RE, Borchard G. Regulatory safety evaluation of nanomedical products: Key issues to refine. *Drug Deliv Transl Res*. 2022 Sep;12(9):2042–2047. https://doi.org/10.1007/s13346-022-01208-4. Epub 2022 Jul 30.
59. Bhuyan S, Pal B, Pathak L, et al. Targeting hypoxia-induced tumor stemness by activating pathogen-induced stem cell niche defense. *Front Immunol*. 2022 Sep 29;13:933329. https://doi.org/10.3389/fimmu.2022.933329
60. Pathak L, Pal B, Talukdar J, et al. Hypoxia-driven mobilization of altruistic cancer stem cells in platinum-treated head and neck cancer. *Front Immunol*. 2025 Feb 3;15:1336882. https://doi.org/10.3389/fimmu.2024.1336882

Index

Note: Page numbers in *italics* indicate a figure and page numbers in **bold** indicate a table on the corresponding page.

L

M

N

O

P

Q

R

S

T

U

V

W